NEPHROLOGY AND FLUID/ELECTROLYTE PHYSIOLOGY

Neonatology Questions and Controversies

NEPHROLOGY AND FLUID/ELECTROLYTE PHYSIOLOGY

Neonatology Questions and Controversies

Series Editor

Richard A. Polin, MD
Professor of Pediatrics
College of Physicians and Surgeons
Columbia University
Vice Chairman for Clinical and Academic Affairs
Department of Pediatrics
Director, Division of Neonatology
Morgan Stanley Children's Hospital of NewYork-Presbyterian
Columbia University Medical Center
New York, New York

Other Volumes in the Neonatology Questions and Controversies Series

NEPHROLOGY AND FLUID/ELECTROLYTE PHYSIOLOGY

Neonatology Questions and Controversies

William Oh, MD
Professor of Pediatrics
Alpert Medical School of Brown University
Attending Neonatologist
Women and Infants' Hospital
Providence, Rhode Island

Jean-Pierre Guignard, MD
Honorary Professor of Pediatrics
Lausanne University Medical School
Centre Hospitalier Universitaire Vaudois
Lausanne, Switzerland

Stephen Baumgart, MD
Professor of Pediatrics
Children's National Medical Center
Department of Pediatrics
George Washington University School of Medicine
Washington, District of Columbia

Consulting Editor
Richard A. Polin, MD
Professor of Pediatrics
College of Physicians and Surgeons
Columbia University
Vice Chairman for Clinical and Academic Affairs
Department of Pediatrics
Director, Division of Neonatology
Morgan Stanley Children's Hospital of NewYork-Presbyterian
Columbia University Medical Center
New York, New York

SECOND EDITION

ELSEVIER
SAUNDERS

1600 John F. Kennedy Blvd.
Ste 1800
Philadelphia, PA 19103-2899

NEPHROLOGY AND FLUID/ELECTROLYTE PHYSIOLOGY, SECOND EDITION NEONATOLOGY QUESTIONS AND CONTROVERSIES   ISBN: 978-1-4377-2658-9

Notices

Knowledge and best practice in this field are constantly changing. As new research and experience broaden our understanding, changes in research methods, professional practices, or medical treatment may become necessary.

Practitioners and researchers must always rely on their own experience and knowledge in evaluating and using any information, methods, compounds, or experiments described herein. In using such information or methods they should be mindful of their own safety and the safety of others, including parties for whom they have a professional responsibility.

With respect to any drug or pharmaceutical products identified, readers are advised to check the most current information provided (i) on procedures featured or (ii) by the manufacturer of each product to be administered, to verify the recommended dose or formula, the method and duration of administration, and contraindications. It is the responsibility of practitioners, relying on their own experience and knowledge of their patients, to make diagnoses, to determine dosages and the best treatment for each individual patient, and to take all appropriate safety precautions.

To the fullest extent of the law, neither the Publisher nor the authors, contributors, or editors, assume any liability for any injury and/or damage to persons or property as a matter of products liability, negligence or otherwise, or from any use or operation of any methods, products, instructions, or ideas contained in the material herein.

Previous edition copyrighted 2008.

Library of Congress Cataloging-in-Publication Data
Nephrology and fluid/electrolyte physiology neonatology questions and controversies / [edited by] William Oh, Jean-Pierre Guignard, Stephen Baumgart. – 2nd ed.
    p. ; cm. – (Neonatology questions and controversies)
    Includes bibliographical references and index.
    ISBN 978-1-4377-2658-9 (hardcover : alk. paper)
    I. Oh, William. II. Guignard, J.-P (Jean-Pierre) III. Baumgart, Stephen. IV. Series: Neonatology questions and controversies.
    [DNLM: 1. Infant, Newborn, Diseases. 2. Kidney Diseases. 3. Infant, Newborn. 4. Water-Electrolyte Imbalance. WS 320]
    LC classification not assigned
    618.92'01–dc23
                                                                                                      2011051356

Senior Content Strategist: Stefanie Jewell-Thomas
Content Development Specialist: Lisa Barnes
Publishing Services Manager: Jeff Patterson
Senior Project Manager: Anne Konopka
Design Direction: Ellen Zanolle

Printed in The United States of America.

Last digit is the print number: 9   8   7   6   5   4   3   2   1

Contributors

Sharon P. Andreoli, MD
Byron P. and Frances D. Hollett
  Professor of Pediatrics
Department of Pediatrics
James Whitcomb Riley Hospital for
  Children
Indiana University Medical School
Indianapolis, Indiana
  Kidney Injury in the Neonate

Stephen Baumgart, MD
Professor of Pediatrics
Children's National Medical Center
Department of Pediatrics
George Washington University School
  of Medicine
Washington, District of Columbia
  Acute Problems of Prematurity:
  Balancing Fluid Volume and Electrolyte
  Replacements in Very Low Birth Weight
  and Extremely Low Birth Weight
  Neonates

Marie H. Beall, MD
Clinical Professor of Obstetrics and
  Gynecology
David Geffen School of Medicine
University of California, Los Angeles
President
Los Angeles Perinatal Associates
Los Angeles, California
  Water Flux and Amniotic Fluid
  Volume: Understanding Fetal Water
  Flow

Richard D. Bland, MD
Professor of Pediatrics
Stanford University School of Medicine
Stanford, California
  Lung Fluid Balance in Developing
  Lungs and Its Role in Neonatal
  Transition

Farid Boubred, MD
Division of Neonatology
Hopital de la Conception
Assistance Publique-Hôpitaux de
  Marseille, France
Faculte de Medecine
Aix-Marseille Université
Marseille, France
  The Developing Kidney and the Fetal
  Origins of Adult Cardiovascular Disease

Christophe Buffat, PharmD
Assistant Hospitalo-Universitaire
Laboratory of Biochemistry and
  Molecular Biology
Hopital de la Conception
Assistance Publique-Hôpitaux de
  Marseille, France
Aix-Marseille Université
Marseille, France
  The Developing Kidney and the Fetal
  Origins of Adult Cardiovascular Disease

Robert L. Chevalier, MD
David Harrison Distinguished Professor
  of Pediatrics
Department of Pediatrics
The University of Virginia
Charlottesville, Virginia
  Obstructive Uropathy: Assessment of
  Renal Function in the Fetus

Andrew T. Costarino, MD
Professor of Anesthesiology and
  Pediatrics
Department of Anesthesiology
Thomas Jefferson University School of
  Medicine
Philadelphia, Pennsylvania
Chairman
Department of Anesthesiology &
  Critical Care Medicine
Alfred I. duPont Hospital for Children
Wilmington, Delaware
  Edema

Andrea Dotta, MD
Division of Newborn Medicine
Bambino Gesù Children's Hospital and
  Research Institute
Rome, Italy
  *Renal Modulation: Arginine Vasopressin
  and Atrial Natriuretic Peptide*

Francesco Emma, MD
Division Head
Division of Nephrology and Dialysis
Bambino Gesù Children's Hospital and
  Research Institute
Rome, Italy
  *Renal Modulation: Arginine Vasopressin
  and Atrial Natriuretic Peptide*

Daniel I. Feig, MD, PhD
Professor of Pediatrics
Director
Division of Pediatric Nephrology
University of Alabama, Birmingham
Birmingham, Alabama
  *Renal Urate Metabolism in the Fetus
  and Newborn*

Joseph T. Flynn, MD, MS
Director
Pediatric Hypertension Program
Seattle Children's Hospital
Professor
Department of Pediatrics
University of Washington School of
  Medicine
Seattle, Washington
  *Neonatal Hypertension: Diagnosis and
  Management*

Jean-Bernard Gouyon, MD
Neonatology
Centre Etudes Perinatales de l'Ocean
  Indien CHR de la Reunion
GHSR Reunion Island, France
  Glomerular Filtration Rate in Neonates

Jean-Pierre Guignard, MD
Honorary Professor of Pediatrics
Lausanne University Medical School
Centre Hospitalier Universitaire
  Vaudois
Lausanne, Switzerland
  *Glomerular Filtration Rate in
  Neonates, Use of Diuretics in the
  Newborn*

Lucky Jain, MD, MBA
Richard W. Blumberg Professor &
  Executive Vice Chairman
Department of Pediatrics
Emory University School of Medicine
Atlanta, Georgia
  *Lung Fluid Balance in Developing
  Lungs and Its Role in Neonatal
  Transition*

Pedro A. Jose, MD, PhD
Director
Center for Molecular Physiology
  Research
Children's National Medical Center
Professor
Pediatrics and Medicine
George Washington University School
  of Medicine & Public Health
Washington, District of Columbia
  *Renal Modulation: The Renin-
  Angiotensisn-Aldosterone System*

Sarah D. Keene, MD
Assistant Professor of Pediatrics
Division of Neonatal/Perinatal Medicine
Emory University
Atlanta, Georgia
  *Lung Fluid Balance in Developing
  Lungs and Its Role in Neonatal
  Transition*

Yosef Levenbrown, DO
Fellow in Pediatric Critical Care
Thomas Jefferson University School of
  Medicine
Department of Anesthesiology and
  Critical Care Medicine
Alfred I. duPont Hospital for Children
Wilmington, Delaware
  Edema

John M. Lorenz, MD
Professor of Clinical Pediatrics
Division of Neonatology
Columbia University
New York, New York
  Potassium Metabolism

Ran Namgung, MD, PhD
Professor of Pediatrics
Department of Pediatrics
Yonsei University College of Medicine
Seoul, Korea
  *Perinatal Calcium and Phosphorus
  Metabolism*

Aruna Natarajan, MD, DCh, PhD
Associate Professor of Pediatrics,
   Pharmacology and Physiology
Attending Pediatric Intensivist
Georgetown University Hospital and
   School of Medicine
Washington, District of Columbia
   *Renal Modulation: The Renin-
   Angiotensin-Aldosterone System*

William Oh, MD
Professor of Pediatrics
Alpert Medical School of Brown
   University
Attending Neonatologist
Women and Infants' Hospital
Providence, Rhode Island
   *Body Water Changes in the Fetus and
   Newborn: Normal Transition After
   Birth and the Effects of Intrauterine
   Growth Aberration*

Michael G. Ross, MD, MPH
Professor of Obstetrics and Gynecology
   and Public Health
David Geffen School of Medicine
University of California Los Angeles
   School of Public Health
Los Angeles, California
   *Water Flux and Amniotic Fluid Volume:
   Understanding Fetal Water Flow*

Istvan Seri, MD, PhD
Professor of Pediatrics
Department of Pediatrics
Division of Neonatal Medicine
Keck School of Medicine
University of Southern California
Center for Fetal and Neonatal Medicine
Children's Hospital Los Angeles
Los Angeles, California
University of Southern California
   Medical Center
Los Angeles, California
   *Acid Base Homeostasis in the Fetus and
   Newborn*

Umberto Simeoni, MD
Professor of Pediatrics
Division of Neonatology
Hôpital de La Conception
Assistance Publique-
   Hôpitaux de Marseille, France
Faculté de Médecine & INSERM
   UMR608
Aix-Marseille Université
Marseille, France
   *The Developing Kidney and the Fetal
   Origins of Adult Cardiovascular Disease*

Endre Sulyok, MD, PhD, DSc
Professor of Pediatrics
Faculty of Health Sciences
University of Pécs
Pécs, Hungary
   *Renal Aspects of Sodium Metabolism in
   the Fetus and Neonate*

Reginald C. Tsang, MBBS
Professor Emeritus of Pediatrics
Division of Neonatology
Cincinnati Children's Hospital Medical
   Center
Cincinnati, Ohio
   *Perinatal Calcium and Phosphorus
   Metabolism*

Daniel Vaiman, PhD
Institut Cochin
INSERM 1016
Genetics and Development Department
   Universite Paris Descartes
Paris, France
   *The Developing Kidney and the Fetal
   Origins of Adult Cardiovascular
   Disease*

Jeroen P.H.M. van den Wijngaard, PhD
Biomedical Engineering and Physics
Academic Medical Center
University of Amsterdam
Department of Medical Physics
Academic Medical Center
University of Amsterdam
Amsterdam, the Netherlands
   *Water Flux and Amniotic Fluid Volume:
   Understanding Fetal Water Flow*

Martin van Gemert, PhD
Professor of Clinical Applications of
  Laser Physics
Director
The Laser Center
Academic Medical Center
University of Amersterdam
Amsterdam, the Netherlands
  Water Flux and Amniotic Fluid Volume:
  Understanding Fetal Water Flow

Marc Zaffanello, MD
Professor, Pediatrician
Department of Life and Reproduction
  Sciences
University of Verona
Verona, Italy
  Renal Modulation: Arginine Vasopressin
  and Atrial Natriuretic Peptide

Israel Zelikovic, MD
Director
Division of Pediatric Nephrology
Rambam Medical Center
Director and Associate Professor
Laboratory of Developmental
  Nephrology
Department of Physiology and
  Biophysics
Rappaport Faculty of Medicine and
  Research Institute
Technion-Israel Institute of Technology
Haifa, Israel
  Hereditary Tubulopathies

Series Foreword

Richard A. Polin, MD

> *"Medicine is a science of uncertainty and an art of probability."*
>
> —William Osler

Controversy is part of every day practice in the NICU. Good practitioners strive to incorporate the best evidence into clinical care. However, for much of what we do, the evidence is either inconclusive or does not exist. In those circumstances, we have come to rely on the teachings of experienced practitioners who have taught us the importance of clinical expertise. This series, "Neonatology Questions and Controversies," provides clinical guidance by summarizing the best evidence and tempering those recommendations with the art of experience.

To quote David Sackett, one of the founders of evidence-based medicine:

> *Good doctors use both individual clinical expertise and the best available external evidence* and neither alone is enough. *Without clinical expertise, practice risks become tyrannized by evidence, for even excellent external evidence may be inapplicable to or inappropriate for an individual patient. Without current best evidence, practice risks become rapidly out of date to the detriment of patients.*

This series focuses on the challenges faced by care providers who work in the NICU. When should we incorporate a new technology or therapy into every day practice, and will it have positive impact on morbidity or mortality? For example, is the new generation of ventilators better than older technologies such as CPAP, or do they merely offer more choices with uncertain value? Similarly, the use of probiotics to prevent necrotizing enterocolitis is supported by sound scientific principles (and some clinical studies). However, at what point should we incorporate them into every day practice given that the available preparations are not well characterized or proven safe? A more difficult and common question is when to use a new technology with uncertain value in a critically ill infant. As many clinicians have suggested, sometimes the best approach is to do nothing and "stand there."

The "Questions and Controversies" series was developed to highlight the clinical problems of most concern to practitioners. The editors of each volume (Drs. Bancalari, Oh, Guignard, Baumgart, Kleinman, Seri, Ohls, Maheshwari, Neu, and Perlman) have done an extraordinary job in selecting topics of clinical importance to every day practice. When appropriate, less controversial topics have been eliminated and replaced by others thought to be of greater clinical importance. In total, there are 56 new chapters in the series. During the preparation of the "Hemodynamics and Cardiology" volume, Dr. Charles Kleinman died. Despite an illness that would have caused many to retire, Charlie worked until near the time of his death. He came to work each day, teaching students and young practitioners and offering his wisdom and expertise to families of infants with congenital heart disease. We are dedicating the second edition of the series to his memory. As with the first edition, I am indebted to the exceptional group of editors who chose the content and edited each of the volumes. I also wish to thank Lisa Barnes (content development specialist at Elsevier) and Judy Fletcher (publishing director at Elsevier), who provided incredible assistance in bringing this project to fruition.

Foreword

Interest in the care of the premature baby developed more than 100 years ago. Nevertheless, newborn babies had to wait until the 1940s for investigators to focus on their immature kidneys. Jean Oliver, Edith Louise Potter, George Fetterman and Robert Vernier were among the first to study and describe the structures of the immature kidney. Most of the basic knowledge on the function of the neonatal kidney was also developed between the early 1940s and the early 1970s. While Homer Smith at New York University College of Medicine was in the process of establishing the basic concepts of mature renal physiology, two investigators explored the function of the immature kidney and founded the scientific basis of modern perinatal nephrology: Henry Barnett at Albert Einstein College of Medicine in New York and Reginald McCance at the University of Cambridge in the UK. Quantification of glomerular filtration rate was established, first in infants, then in term neonates and later on in tiny premature neonates. The ability of the immature kidney to modify the glomerular ultrafiltrate, to dilute or concentrate the urine, to get rid of an acid load, to produce and respond to various hormones, and to maintain constant the neonate's body fluid volume and composition, was subsequently investigated. When it became clear that dysfunction and dysgenesis of the kidney could have long lasting consequences, fetal developmental studies were conducted with the aim of understanding the pathogenesis of renal diseases and dysfunctions from the early days of gestation.

Studies on the key role played by the placenta in maintaining the homeostasis of the fetus, as well as research on the formation and function of the fetal and the postnatal kidney have grown exponentially in the last decades. A bewildering amount of results, sometimes contradictory, has been produced, clarifying many yet unsolved problems, but also raising new questions. The interpretation of published clinical or experimental data, as well as the establishment of practical guidelines most often based on poorly or ill-controlled clinical trials generated controversies that sometimes disconcerted the physician in charge of still-unborn or newly-born infants.

The purpose of this new series entitled *Neonatology Questions and Controversies* is to discuss precisely the scientific basis of perinatal medicine. It also aims to present a rational, critical analysis of current concepts in different fields related to fetuses and newborn infants. To cover the various topics presented in this *Nephrology and Fluid/Electrolyte Physiology* volume, such as placental and perinatal physiology, pathophysiology and pathology, the editors gathered a distinguished group of contributors who are all leading experts in their respective fields. It is our conviction that physicians and students will benefit from this authoritative source of critical knowledge to improve the fate of fetuses and neonates under their care.

We thank all our contributors for their dedication and generous cooperation.

Jean-Pierre Guignard, MD

Preface

A preface is to give the editors the opportunity to review the events since the publication of the previous edition; update, add, or delete the various chapters; and thank the authors for their efforts and expertise in their contribution.

Since the publication of the first edition of this monograph 3 years ago, the survival rates of newborn infants in this country and abroad has been maintained at a healthy pace. The quality of life of most survivors is good. These achievements are the results of many evidence-based management strategies developed and implemented by dedicated care providers of this population. An important component of these strategies is the fluid and electrolyte therapy and management of various renal disorders of the high-risk infants. We believe that our first edition has filled the role of providing new knowledge and treatment modalities to the care providers. The book's popularity among our readership is evident by the high volume of sales and the publication of a Spanish version for our Latin American colleagues in South America and elsewhere (*Ediciones Journal*, Buenos Aires, 2011).

In addition to updating all of the chapters in the first edition with the addition of numerous references, the editors have added six new chapters to this edition. We mourned the passing of a talented and esteemed author, Dr. Karl Bauer. One of us (Dr. Oh), who was Dr. Bauer's mentor, took the responsibility of writing a chapter that expands the contents of Dr. Bauer's original chapter to include the body fluid changes during the transitional period. We also believe that urate, calcium, and phosphorus metabolisms are important parts of fluid and electrolyte management in the perinatal period. We were very fortunate to have successfully recruited Drs. Ron Namrung and Reginald C. Tsang, two authorities in this field, to write the chapter on perinatal calcium and phosphorus metabolism and Dr. Daniel Feig, an expert in perinatal urate metabolism, to write a chapter on this important subject. In addition, we added a chapter on neonatal hypertension written by Dr. Joseph Flynn, who is well known in this field. Recognizing that there are two areas in neonatal nephrology and fluid and electrolyte therapy that deserve inclusion in this publication—hereditary tubulopathies and the use of diuretics in newborns—we have asked Dr. Israel Zelikovic and one of us (Dr. Guignard) to fill those gaps.

We would like to express our deepest gratitude to all of the authors for their hard work in updating and writing new chapters in this book. We believe that with the update and the six new chapters, this book will continue to serve our dedicated physicians, nurses, and other allied health care providers as a reference in providing fluid and electrolyte therapy and management of renal diseases in this most vulnerable population. We anticipate that optimal management of these conditions, along with other management strategies, will continue to contribute to good outcomes among high-risk infants.

William Oh, MD

Jean-Pierre Guignard, MD

Stephen Baumgart, MD

Contents

SECTION C

The Kidney: Normal Development and Hormonal Control

SECTION D

Special Problems

NEPHROLOGY AND FLUID/ELECTROLYTE PHYSIOLOGY

Neonatology Questions and Controversies

Placenta and Fetal Water Flux

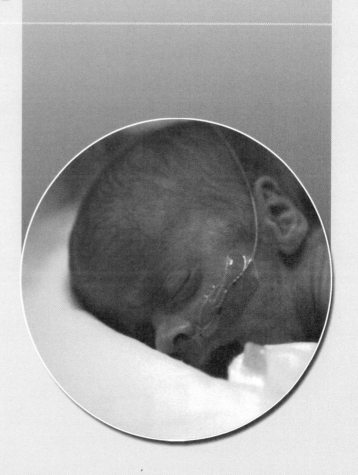

CHAPTER 1

Water Flux and Amniotic Fluid Volume: Understanding Fetal Water Flow

Marie H. Beall, MD, Jeroen P.H.M. van den Wijngaard, PhD,
Martin van Gemert, PhD, Michael G. Ross, MD, MPH

- Clinical Scenarios
- Fetal Water
- Mechanisms of Water Flow
- Aquaporins
- Conclusion

In a term human gestation, the amount of water in the fetal compartments, including the fetus, placenta, and amniotic fluid (AF), may exceed 5 L; in pathologic states, the amount may be much more because of excessive AF or fetal hydrops. Water largely flows from the maternal circulation to the fetus via the placenta, and the rate of fetal water acquisition depends on placental water permeability characteristics. In the gestational compartment, water is circulated between the fetus and AF. In the latter part of pregnancy, an important facet of this circulation is water flux from the AF to the fetal circulation across the amnion. Normal AF water dynamics are critical because insufficient (oligohydramnios) or excessive (polyhydramnios) amounts of AF are associated with impaired fetal outcome even in the absence of structural fetal abnormalities. This chapter reviews data regarding the placental transfer of water and examines the circulation of water within the gestation, specifically the water flux across the amnion, as factors influencing AF volume. Finally, some controversies regarding the mechanics of these events are discussed.

Clinical Scenarios

Water flux in the placenta and chorioamnion is a matter of more than theoretical interest. Clinical experience in humans suggests that altered placental water flow occurs and can cause deleterious fetal effects in association with excessive or reduced AF volume.

Maternal Dehydration

Maternal dehydration has been associated with reduced fetal compartment water and oligohydramnios. As an example, the following case has been reported: A 14-year-old girl was admitted at 33 weeks' gestation with cramping and vaginal spotting. A sonogram indicated oligohydramnios and an AF index (AFI) of 2.6 cm (reference range, 5–25 cm) with normal fetal kidneys and bladder. On hospital day 2, the AFI was 0 cm. Recorded maternal fluid balance was 8 L in and 13.6 L out. Serum sodium was 153 mEq/L. Diabetes insipidus was diagnosed and treated with intranasal desmopressin acetate. The oligohydramnios resolved rapidly, and the patient delivered a healthy 2700-g male infant at 38 weeks' gestation.[1]

Reduced Maternal Plasma Oncotic Pressure

Maternal malnutrition may predispose patients to increased fetal water transfer and polyhydramnios. We recently encountered a patient who illustrated this condition: A 35-year-old gravida 4, para 3 presented at 32 to 33 weeks of gestation complaining of premature labor. On admission, the maternal hematocrit was 18.9% and hemoglobin was 5.6 g/dL with a mean corpuscular volume of 57.9 fL. Blood chemistries were normal except that the patient's serum albumin was 1.9 g/dL (reference range, 3.3–4.9 g/dL). A diagnosis of maternal malnutrition was made. On ultrasound examination, the AFI was 24.5 cm, and the fetal bladder was noted to be significantly enlarged consistent with increased urine output. Premature labor was thought to be attributable to uterine overdistension. Subsequently, the patient delivered a 1784-g male infant with Apgar scores of 3 at 1 minute and 7 at 5 minutes. The infant was transferred to the neonatal intensive care unit for significant respiratory distress.

As described below, although the forces driving normal maternal-to-fetal water flux are uncertain, changes in the osmotic–oncotic difference between the maternal and fetal sera can affect the volume of water flowing from the mother to the fetus. In the first case, presumably because of an environment of increased maternal osmolality, less water crossed the placenta to the fetus. Similarly, maternal dehydration caused by water restriction (in a sheep model)[2] or caused by hot weather (in humans)[3] have been associated with reduced AF volumes. Conversely, reduced maternal oncotic pressure likely contributed to increased maternal-to-fetal water transfer in the second patient. Fetal homeostatic mechanisms then led to increased fetal urine output and increased AF volume. Similarly, studies with DDAVP (desmopressin) in both humans[4] and sheep[5] have demonstrated that a pharmacologic reduction in maternal serum osmolality can lead to an increase in AF. As these examples illustrate, fetal water flow is a carefully balanced system that can be perturbed with clinically significant effect. The material presented below will detail the mechanisms regulating fetal–maternal–AF fluid homeostasis.

Fetal Water

Placental Water Flux

Net water flux across the placenta is relatively small. In sheep, a water flow to the fetus of 0.5 mL/min[6] is sufficient for fetal needs at term. By contrast, tracer studies suggest that the total water exchanged (i.e., diffusionary flow) between the ovine fetus and the mother is much larger, up to 70 mL/min.[7] Most of this flow is bidirectional, resulting in no net accumulation of water. Although the mechanisms regulating the maternal–fetal flux of water are speculative, the permeability of the placenta to water changes with gestation,[8] suggesting that placental water permeability may be a factor in regulating the water available to the fetus.

Although fetal water may derive from sources other than transplacental flux, these other sources appear to be of minor importance. Water could, theoretically, pass from the maternal circulation to the AF across the fetal membranes (i.e., transmembrane flow), although this effect is thought to be small,[9] partly because the AF is hypotonic compared with maternal serum. The driving force resulting from osmotic and oncotic gradients between hypotonic, low-protein AF and isotonic maternal serum is far greater than that induced by maternal vascular versus AF hydrostatic pressure. Any direct water flux between maternal serum and AF should therefore be from the fetus to the mother. In addition, a small amount of water is produced as a byproduct of fetal metabolic processes. Because these alternative routes contribute only a minor proportion of the fetal water, it is apparent that the fetus is dependent on placental flux for the bulk of water requirements.

Fetal Water Compartments

In gestation, water is partitioned between the fetus, placenta and membranes, and AF. Although term human fetuses may vary considerably in size, an average fetus contains 3000 mL of water, of which about 350 mL is in the vascular compartment. In addition, the placenta contains another 500 mL of water. More precisely, the volume of fetal and placental water is proportionate to the fetal weight. AF volume is less correlated with fetal weight. The AF is a fetal water depot,[10] and in normal human gestations at term, the AF volume may vary from 500 mL to more than 1200 mL.[11] In pathologic states, the AF volume may vary more widely. Below we present what is known regarding the formation of AF, the circulation of AF water, and the mechanisms controlling this circulation.

Amniotic Fluid Volume and Composition

During the first trimester, AF is isotonic with maternal plasma[12] but contains minimal protein. It is thought that the fluid arises either from a transudate of fetal plasma through nonkeratinized fetal skin or maternal plasma across the uterine decidua or placental surface.[13] With advancing gestation, AF osmolality and sodium concentration decrease, a result of the mixture of dilute fetal urine and isotonic fetal lung liquid production. In comparison with the first half of pregnancy, AF osmolality decreases by 20 to 30 mOsm/kg H_2O with advancing gestation to levels approximately 85% to 90% of maternal serum osmolality[14] in humans, although there is no osmolality decrease in the AF near term in rats.[15] AF urea, creatinine, and uric acid increase during the second half of pregnancy, resulting in AF concentrations of the urinary byproducts two to three times higher than those of fetal plasma.[14]

Concordant with the changes in AF content, AF volume changes dramatically during human pregnancy (Fig. 1-1). The average AF volume increases progressively from 20 mL at 10 weeks to 630 mL at 22 weeks and to 770 mL at 28 weeks' gestation.[16] Between 29 and 37 weeks' gestation, there is little change in volume. Beyond 39 weeks, AF volume decreases sharply, averaging 515 mL at 41 weeks. When the pregnancy becomes postdate, there is a 33% decline in AF volume per week[17-19] consistent with the increased incidence of oligohydramnios in postterm gestations.

Fetal Water Circulation

Amniotic fluid is produced and resorbed in a dynamic process with large volumes of water circulated between the AF and fetal compartments (Fig. 1-2). During the latter half of gestation, the primary sources of AF include fetal urine excretion and fluid secreted by the fetal lung. The primary pathways for water exit from the AF include removal by fetal swallowing and intramembranous (IM) absorption into fetal blood. Although some data on these processes in the human fetus are available, the bulk of the information about fetal AF circulation derives from animal models, especially sheep.

Urine Production

In humans, fetal urine production changes with increasing gestation. The amount of urine produced by the human fetus has been estimated by the use of ultrasound

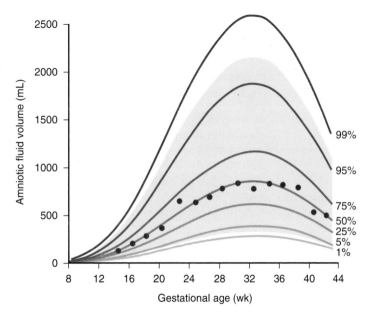

Figure 1-1 Normal range of amniotic fluid volume in human gestation. (From Brace RA, Wolf EJ. Normal amniotic fluid volume changes throughout pregnancy. *Am J Obstet Gynecol.* 1989;161(2):382-388, used with permission.)

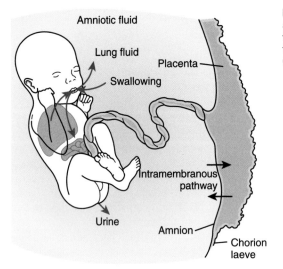

Figure 1-2 Water circulation between the fetus and amniotic fluid (AF). The major sources of AF water are fetal urine and lung liquid; the routes of absorption are through fetal swallowing and intramembranous flow (see text).

assessment of fetal bladder volume,[20] although the accuracy of these measurements has been called into question. Exact human fetal urine production rates across gestation are not established but appear to be in the range of 25% of body weight per day or nearly 1000 mL/day near term.[20,21]

In near-term ovine fetuses, 500 to 1200 mL/day of urine is distributed to the AF and allantoic cavities.[22,23] During the last third of gestation, the fetal glomerular filtration rate (GFR) increases in parallel to fetal weight, with a similar but variable increase in reabsorption of sodium, chloride, and free water.[24] Fetal urine output can be modulated, as numerous endocrine factors, including arginine vasopressin, atrial natriuretic factor, aldosterone, and prostaglandins, have been demonstrated to alter fetal renal blood flow, GFR, or urine flow rates.[25,26] Importantly, physiologic increases in fetal plasma arginine vasopressin significantly increase fetal urine osmolality and reduce urine flow rates.[27,28]

Lung Fluid Production

It appears that all mammalian fetuses normally secrete fluid from their lungs. The absolute rate of fluid production by human fetal lungs has not been estimated; the fluid production rate has been extensively studied in the ovine fetus only. During the last third of gestation, the fetal lamb secretes an average of 100 mL/day per kg fetal weight. Under physiological conditions, half of the fluid exiting the lungs enters the AF, and half is swallowed.[29] Therefore, an average of approximately 165 mL/day of lung liquid enters the AF near term. Fetal lung fluid production is affected by physiologic and endocrine factors, but nearly all stimuli have been demonstrated to reduce fetal lung liquid production, with no evidence of stimulated production and nominal changes in fluid composition. Increased arginine vasopressin,[30] catecholamines,[31] and cortisol,[32] even acute intravascular volume expansion,[33] decrease lung fluid production. Given this lack of evidence of bidirectional regulation, it appears that, unlike the kidneys, the fetal lungs may not play an important role in the maintenance of AF volume homeostasis. Current opinion is that fetal lung fluid secretion is likely most important in providing pulmonary expansion, which promotes airway and alveolar development.

Fetal Swallowing

Studies of near-term pregnancies suggest that the human fetus swallows an average of 210 to 760 mL/day[34] of AF, which is considerably less than the volume of urine produced each day. However, fetal swallowing may be reduced beginning a few days before delivery,[35] so the rate of human fetal swallowing is probably underestimated.

Little other data on human fetal swallowed volumes is available. In fetal sheep, there is a steady increase in the volume of fluid swallowed over the last third of gestation. In contrast to a relatively constant daily urine production/kg body weight, the daily volume swallowed increases from approximately 130 mL/kg per day at 0.75 term to more than 400 mL/kg per day near term.[36] A series of studies have measured ovine fetal swallowing activity with esophageal electromyograms and swallowed volume using a flow probe placed around the fetal esophagus.[37] These studies demonstrate that fetal swallowing increases in response to dipsogenic (e.g., central or systemic) hypertonicity[38] or central angiotensin II[39] or orexigenic (central neuropeptide Y[40]) stimulation and decreases with acute arterial hypotension[41] or hypoxia.[29,42] Thus, near-term fetal swallowed volume is subject to periodic increases as mechanisms for "thirst" and "appetite" develop functionality, although decreases in swallowed volume appear to be more reflective of deteriorating fetal condition.

Intramembranous Flow

The amount of fluid swallowed by the fetus does not equal the amount of fluid produced by both the kidneys and the lungs in either human or ovine gestation. As the volume of AF does not greatly increase during the last half of pregnancy, another route of fluid absorption is needed. This route is the IM pathway.

The IM pathway refers to the route of absorption between the fetal circulation and the amniotic cavity directly across the amnion. Although the contribution of the IM pathway to the overall regulation and maintenance of AF volume and composition has yet to be completely understood, results from in vivo and in vitro studies of ovine membrane permeability suggest that the permeability of the fetal chorioamnion is important for determining AF composition and volume.[43-45] This IM flow, recirculating AF water to the fetal compartment, is thought to be driven by the significant osmotic gradient between the hypotonic AF and isotonic fetal plasma.[46] In addition, electrolytes (e.g., Na^+) may diffuse down a concentration gradient from fetal plasma into the AF, and intraamniotic peptides (e.g., arginine vasopressin[47,48]) and other electrolytes (e.g., Cl^-) may be recirculated to the fetal plasma.

Although it has never been directly measured in humans, indirect evidence supports the presence of IM flow. Studies of intraamniotic ^{51}Cr injection demonstrated the appearance of the tracer in the circulation of fetuses with impaired swallowing.[49] Additionally, alterations in IM flow may contribute to AF clinical abnormalities because membrane ultrastructure changes are noted with polyhydramnios or oligohydramnios.[50]

Experimental estimates of the net IM flow averages 200 to 250 mL/day in fetal sheep and likely balances the flow of urine and lung liquid with fetal swallowing under homeostatic conditions. Filtration coefficients have been calculated,[51] although IM flow rates under control conditions have not been directly measured. Mathematical models of human AF dynamics also suggest significant IM water and electrolyte fluxes,[52,53] but transmembranous flow (AF to maternal) is extremely small compared with IM flow.[54,55]

This detailed understanding of fetal fluid production and resorption provides little explanation as to how AF volume homeostasis is maintained throughout gestation and does not account for gestational alterations in AF volume or postterm or acute-onset oligohydramnios. As an example, the acute reduction in fetal swallowing in response to hypotension or hypoxia seen in the ovine model would not produce the reduced AF volume noted in stressed human fetuses. For this reason, recent research has addressed the regulation of water flow in the placenta and fetal membranes. We will discuss the possible mechanisms for the regulation of fetal water flow, beginning with a review of the general principles of membrane water flow.

Mechanisms of Water Flow

Biologic membranes exist, in part, to regulate water flux. Flow may occur through cells (i.e., transcellular) or between cells (i.e., paracellular), and the type of flow affects the composition of the fluid crossing the membrane. In addition, transcellular flow may occur across the lipid bilayer or through membrane channels or pores (i.e., aquaporins [AQPs]); the latter route is more efficient because the water permeability of the lipid membrane is low. Because the AQPs allow the passage of water only (and sometimes other small nonpolar molecules), transcellular flow is predominantly free water. Paracellular flow occurs through relatively wide spaces between cells and consists of both water and solutes in the proportions present in the extracellular space; large molecules may be excluded. Although water molecules can randomly cross the membrane by diffusion without net water flow, net flow occurs only in response to concentration (osmotic) or pressure (hydrostatic) differences.

Osmotic and hydrostatic forces are created when there is a difference in osmotic or hydrostatic pressure on either side of the membrane. Osmotic differences arise when there is a difference in solute concentration across the membrane. For this difference to be maintained, the membrane permeability of the solute must be low (i.e., a high reflection coefficient). Commonly, osmotic differences are maintained by charged ions such as sodium or large molecules such as proteins (also called oncotic pressure). These solutes do not cross the cell membrane readily. Osmotic differences can be created locally by the active transport of sodium across the membrane with water following because of the osmotic force created by the sodium imbalance. It should be noted that although the transport of sodium is active, water flux is always a passive, non–energy-dependent process. Hydrostatic differences occur when the pressure of fluid is greater on one side of the membrane. The most obvious example is the difference between the inside of a blood vessel and the interstitial space. Hydrostatic differences may also be created locally by controlling the relative direction of two flows. Even with equal initial pressures, a hydrostatic difference will exist if venous outflow is matched with arterial inflow (countercurrent flow). The actual movement of water in response to these gradients may be more complex as a result of additional physical properties, including unstirred layer effects and solvent drag.

Net membrane water flux is a function of the membrane properties and the osmotic and hydrostatic forces. Formally, this is expressed as the Starling equation:

$$Jv = LpS(\Delta P - \sigma RT(c_1 - c_2))$$

where Jv is the volume flux; LpS is a description of membrane properties (hydraulic conductance times the surface area for diffusion); ΔP is the hydrostatic pressure difference; and $-\sigma RT(c_1 - c_2)$ is the osmotic pressure difference, with T being the temperature in degrees Kelvin, R the gas constant in Nm/Kmol, σ the reflection coefficient (a measure of the permeability of the membrane to the solute), and c_1 and c_2 the solute concentrations on the two sides of the membrane. Experimental studies most often report the membrane water permeability (a characteristic of the individual membrane). Permeability is proportionate to flux (amount of flow per second per cm^2 of membrane) divided by the concentration difference on different sides of the membrane (amount per cubic cm). Membrane water permeabilities are reported as the permeability associated with flux of water in a given direction and under a given type of force or as the diffusional permeability. Because one membrane may have different osmotic versus hydrostatic versus diffusional permeabilities,[56] an understanding of the forces driving membrane water flow is critical for understanding flow regulatory mechanisms. This area remains controversial, but the anatomy of placenta and membranes suggests possible mechanisms for promoting water flux in one direction.

Mechanism of Placental Water Flow
Placental Anatomy[57,58]

The placenta is a complex organ, and the anatomic variation in the placentas of various species is substantial. Rodents have often been used for the study of placental water flux because primates and rodents share a hemochorial placental structure. In hemochorial placentas, the maternal blood is contained in sinuses in direct contact with one or more layers of fetal epithelium. In humans, this epithelium is the syncytiotrophoblast, a layer of contiguous cells with few or no intercellular spaces. Beneath the syncytium, there are layers of connective tissue and fetal blood vessel endothelium. (In early pregnancy, human placentas have a layer of cytotrophoblast underlying the syncytium; however, by the third trimester, this layer is not continuous and is therefore not a limiting factor for placental permeability.) The human placenta is therefore monochorial. Guinea pig placentas are also monochorial; the fetal vessels are covered with connective tissue that is in turn covered with a single layer of syncytium.[59] In mice, the layer immediately opposed to the maternal blood is a cytotrophoblast layer, covering two layers of syncytium. Because of the presence of three layers in much of the placenta, the mouse placenta is labeled trichorial. Similar to the case in humans, the mouse cytotrophoblast does not appear to be continuous, suggesting that the cytotrophoblast layer does not limit membrane permeability. The rat placenta is similar to that of the mouse.

The syncytium is therefore a common structure in all of these placental forms and a likely site of regulation of membrane permeability. In support of this hypothesis, membrane vesicles derived from human syncytial brush border were used to evaluate the permeability of the placenta. At 37° C, the osmotic permeability of apical vesicles was $1.9 \pm 0.06 \times 10^{-3}$ cm/s; the permeability of basal membrane (fetal side) vesicles was higher at $3.1 \pm 0.20 \times 10^{-3}$ cm/s.[60] The difference between the basal and apical sides of the syncytiotrophoblasts was taken to indicate that the apical (maternal) side of the trophoblast was the rate-limiting structure for water flow through the placenta. In all placentas, the fetal blood is contained in vessels, suggesting that fetal capillary endothelium may also serve as a barrier to flow between maternal and fetal circulations. Experimental evidence suggests, however, that the capillary endothelium is a less significant barrier to small polar molecules than the syncytium.[58]

Although sheep have been extensively used in studies of fetal physiology and placental permeability, their placentas differ from those of humans in important respects. The sheep placenta is classified as epitheliochorial, meaning that the maternal and fetal circulations are contained within blood vessels with maternal and fetal epithelial layers interposed between them. In general, compared with the hemochorial placenta, the epithelialchorial placenta would be expected to demonstrate decreased water permeability based on the increase in membrane layers. In addition, the forces driving water permeability may differ between the two placental types because the presence of maternal vessels in the sheep placenta increases the likelihood that a hydrostatic pressure difference could be maintained favoring water flux from maternal to fetal circulations.

In all of the rodent placentas, fetal and maternal blood circulate in opposite directions (countercurrent flow), potentially increasing the opportunity for exchange between circulations based on local differences. The direction of maternal blood circulation in human placentas is from the inside to the outside of the placental lobule and therefore at cross-current to the fetal blood flow[61] (Fig. 1-3). Unlike in mice and rats, investigation has not revealed countercurrent blood flow in ovine placentas.[62]

The preceeding is not intended to imply that there are not important differences between human and rodent placentas. The human placenta is organized into cotyledons, each with a central fetal vessel. Fetal–maternal exchange in the mouse and rat placenta occurs in the placental labyrinth. In addition, rats and mice have an "inverted yolk sac placenta," a structure with no analogy in the primate placenta. Readers are referred to Faber and Thornberg[57] and Benirschke[63] for additional details.

Controversies in Placental Flow

In the placenta, the flux of water may be driven by either hydrostatic or osmotic forces. Hydrostatic forces can be developed in the placenta by alterations in the flow in maternal and fetal circulations. Osmotic forces may be generated locally by active

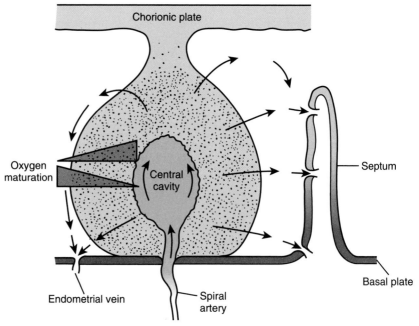

A

Figure 1-3 Maternal blood flow in the human placenta. Blood flow proceeds from the spiral artery to the center of the placental lobule. Blood then crosses the lobule laterally, exiting through the endometrial vein. This creates a gradient in oxygen content from the inside to the outside of the lobule because of the changing oxygen content of the maternal blood. (From Hempstock J, Bao YP, Bar-Issac M, et al. Intralobular differences in antioxidant enzyme expression and activity reflect the pattern of maternal arterial bloodflow within the human placenta. *Placenta*. 2003;24(5):517-523, used with permission.)

transport of solutes such as sodium or by depletion of solute from the local peri-membrane environment (caused by the so-called "unstirred layer" effect). The relative direction of maternal and fetal blood flows can be concurrent, countercurrent, crosscurrent, or in part combinations of these flows,[64] and differences in the direction of blood flow may be important in establishing either osmotic or hydrostatic gradients within the placenta. It has not been possible to directly study putative local pressure or osmotic differences at the level of the syncytium; therefore, theories regarding the driving forces for placental water flux are inferences from available data.

Water may be transferred from mother to fetus driven osmotically by the active transport of solutes such as sodium.[65] In rats, inert solutes such as mannitol and inulin are transferred to the maternal circulation from the fetus more readily than from the mother to fetus,[66] and conversely, sodium is actively transported to the fetus in excess of fetal needs. This was taken to indicate that water was being driven to the fetal side by a local osmotic effect created by the sodium flux. Water with dissolved solutes then differentially crossed from fetus to mother, probably by a paracellular route. Perfusion of the guinea pig placenta with dextran-containing solution demonstrates that the flow of water can also be influenced by colloid osmotic pressure.[67] In sheep, intact gestations have yielded estimates of osmotic placental water flow of 0.062 mL/kg min per mOsm/kg H_2O.[68] The importance of osmotically driven water flow in sheep is uncertain because the same authors found that the maternal plasma was consistently hyperosmolar to the fetal plasma. Theoretical considerations have been used, however, to argue that known electrolyte active transport and a modest hydrostatic pressure gradient could maintain maternal-to-fetal water flow against this osmotic gradient.[69]

Others have argued that the motive force for water flux in the placenta is hydrostatic. In perfused placentas of guinea pigs, reversal of the direction of the fetal flow reduced the rate of water transfer,[70] and increasing the fetal-side perfusion pressure increased the fetal-to-maternal water flow in both the perfused guinea pig placentas[71] and in an intact sheep model.[72] Both findings suggest that water transfer is flow dependent.

As a whole, the available data suggest that either osmotic or hydrostatic forces can promote placental water flux. The actual motive force in normal pregnancy is uncertain and may vary with the species, the pregnancy stage, or both. Whatever the driving force, at least some part of placental water flux involves the flow of solute-free water transcellularly, suggesting the involvement of membrane water channels in the process.

Mechanism of Intramembranous Flow

Membrane Anatomy

In sheep, an extensive network of microscopic blood vessels is located between the outer surface of the amnion and the chorion,[73] providing an extensive surface area available for IM flow. In primates, including humans, IM fluxes likely occur across the fetal surface of the placenta because the amnion and chorion are not vascularized per se. The close proximity of fetal blood vessels to the placental surface provides accessibility to the fetal circulation, explaining the absorption of AF technetium[46] and arginine vasopressin[48] into the fetal serum in subhuman fetal primates after esophageal ligation. In vitro experiments with isolated layers of human amnion and chorion have also demonstrated that the membranes act as selective barriers of exchange.[74]

Studies in the ovine model suggest that the IM pathway can be regulated to restore homeostasis. Because fetal swallowing is a major route of AF fluid resorption, esophageal ligation would be expected to increase AF volume significantly. Although AF volume increased significantly 3 days after ovine fetal esophageal occlusion,[75] longer periods (9 days) of esophageal ligation reduced AF volume in preterm sheep.[76] Similarly, esophageal ligation of fetal sheep over a period of 1 month did not increase AF volume.[77] In the absence of swallowing, normalized AF volume suggests an increase in IM flow. In addition, IM flow markedly increased after the infusion of exogenous fluid to the AF cavity.[78] Collectively, these studies suggest that AF resorption pathways and likely IM flow are under dynamic feedback regulation. That is, AF volume expansion increases IM resorption, ultimately resulting in a normalization of AF volume. Importantly, factors downregulating IM flow are less studied, and there is no functional evidence of reduced IM resorption as an adaptive response to oligohydramnios, although AQP water channel expression in the amnion may be decreased (see below). Studies have revealed that prolactin reduced the upregulation of IM flow because of osmotic challenge in the sheep model[79] and reduced diffusional permeability to water in human amnion[80] and guinea pig[81] amnion, suggesting that downregulation of IM flow is possible.

Controversies Regarding Intramembranous Flow

The specific mechanism and regulation of IM flow is key to AF homeostasis. A number of theories have been put forward to account for the observed results. Esophageal ligation of fetal sheep resulted in the upregulation of fetal chorioamnion vascular endothelial growth factor (VEGF) gene expression.[82] It was proposed that VEGF-induced neovascularization potentiates AF water resorption. These authors also speculated that fetal urine or lung fluid (or both) may contain factors that upregulate VEGF. Their further studies demonstrated an increased water flow despite a constant membrane diffusional permeability (to technetium) in animals in which the fetal urine output had been increased by an intravenous volume load and a concurrent flow of water and solutes against a concentration gradient by the IM route.[83,84] Finally, artificial regulation of the osmolality and oncotic pressure of the AF revealed that the major force promoting IM flow in sheep was osmotic; however, there was an additional flow of about 24 mL/h, which was not osmotic dependent. Because protein was also transferred to the fetal circulation, this flow was believed to be similar to fluid flow in the lymph system.[85]

These findings, in aggregate, have been interpreted to require active bulk fluid flow across the amnion; Brace et al[84] have proposed that this fluid transport occurs via membrane vesicles (bulk vesicular flow), as evidenced by the high prevalence of amnion intracellular vesicles seen in electron microscopy.[86] This theory is poorly accepted because vesicle water flow has not been demonstrated in any other tissue and is highly energy dependent. Most others believe that IM flow occurs through conventional para- and transcellular channels, driven by osmotic and hydrostatic forces. Mathematical modeling indicates that relatively small IM sodium fluxes could be associated with significant changes in AF volume, suggesting that sodium flux may be a regulator of IM flow,[53] although the observation that IM flow was independent of AF composition suggests that other forces (e.g., hydrostatic forces) may also drive IM flow.[87]

Importantly, upregulation of VEGF or sodium transfer alone cannot explain AF composition changes after fetal esophageal ligation because AF electrolyte composition indicates that water flow increases disproportionately to solute flow.[76] The passage of free water across a biological membrane without solutes is a characteristic of transcellular flow, a process mediated by water channels in the cell membrane. Although water flow through these channels is passive, the expression and location of the channels can be modulated to regulate water flux. We will review the characteristics of AQP water channels and then comment on the evidence that AQPs may be involved in regulating gestational water flow.

Aquaporins

Aquaporins are cell membrane proteins approximately 30 kD in size (26–34 kD). Similarities in amino acid sequence suggest that the three-dimensional structure of all AQPs is similar. AQP proteins organize in the cell membrane as tetramers; however, each monomer forms a hydrophilic pore in its center and functions independently as a water channel[88] (Fig. 1-4). Although all AQPs function as water channels, some AQPs also allow the passage of glycerol, urea, and other small

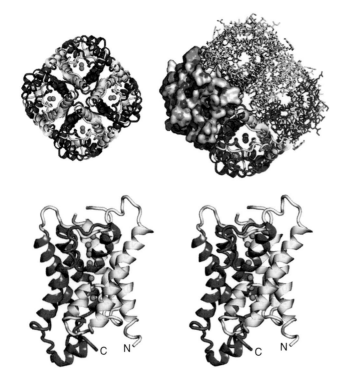

Figure 1-4   Structure of aquaporin (bovine AQP0). *Upper left* shows the structure from the extracellular side of the membrane. *Upper right* shows each monomer in a different format. *Lower figure* shows a side view of an AQP monomer, extracellular side upper. The two figures are to be viewed in crossed-eye stereo. C and N, ends of the protein. (From Harries WE, Akhavan D, Miercke LJ, Khademi S, Stroud RM. The channel architecture of aquaporin 0 at a 2.2-A resolution. *Proc Natl Acad Sci U S A.* 2004 Sep 28;101(39):14045-50, used with permission.)

nonpolar molecules. These have also been called aquaglyceroporins. Multiple AQPs have been identified ($\leq$13, depending on the mammalian species). Some are widely expressed throughout the body; others appear to be more tissue specific.

AQP function depends on cellular location. In the kidneys, several AQPs are expressed in specific areas of the collecting duct: whereas AQP3 and AQP4 are both present in the basolateral membrane of the collecting duct principal cells, AQP2 is present in the apical portion of the membrane of these same cells.[89] The presence of these different AQPs on opposite membrane sides of the same cell is important for the regulation of water transfer across the cell because altered AQP properties or AQP expression may differentially regulate water entry from the collecting duct lumen and water exit to the interstitial fluid compartment. Absence of the various renal AQPs leads to renal concentrating defects, particularly, the absence of AQP2 in humans is responsible for nephrogenic diabetes insipidus.

Aquaporin function is also dependent on the cellular milieu. This regulation may occur through the insertion or removal of AQP into the membrane from the intracellular compartment. For example, in the renal tubule, AQP2 is transferred from cytoplasm vesicles to the apical cell membrane in response to arginine vasopressin[90] or forskolin.[91] AQP8 is similarly transferred from hepatocyte vesicles to the cell membrane in response to dibutyryl cyclic AMP (cAMP) and glucagon.[92] In longer time frames, the expression of various AQPs may be induced by external conditions. For example, AQP3 expression in cultured keratinocytes is increased when the cell culture medium is made hypertonic.[93] In summary, AQPs are important in the regulation of water flow across biological membranes, and their expression and activity can be regulated according to the hydration status of the organism.

Aquaporins in Placentas and Membranes

Four AQPs (i.e., AQP1, 3, 8, and 9) have been widely reported in the placenta and fetal membranes of a variety of species, and alterations in the expression of these AQPs have been related to changes in AF volume. Reports also describe the finding of AQP4[94] and AQP5[95] in human placenta or membranes, but no information is available relating these AQPs to AF volume changes, and they will not be further considered here. AQP1 mRNA and protein have been demonstrated in ovine,[96] mouse,[97] and human[98] placentas associated with the placental vessels. Ovine placental AQP1 expression levels are highest early in pregnancy, with a decline thereafter, although there is an increase in expression near term.[99] AQP1 protein expression has been demonstrated in the fetal chorioamnion at term in human gestations[100] associated with amnion epithelium and cytotrophoblast of the chorion.[97] AQP3 message and protein has been demonstrated in the placentas and fetal chorioamnion of humans[100,101] and mice[97] and in sheep placentas,[96,99] and mRNA has been found in rat placentas.[102] In humans, AQP3 protein is expressed on the apical membranes of the syncytiotrophoblast[101] on amnion epithelium and cytotrophoblast of the chorion.[103] AQP3 has also been demonstrated on the trophoblasts of mice.[97] AQP8 mRNA has been detected in mouse,[104] sheep,[99] and human placentas and in human fetal chorioamnion.[105] AQP9 protein and mRNA have been demonstrated in human placentas.[101]

Evidence suggests that AQPs may be involved in the regulation of placental water flow. In mice, AF volume is positively correlated with placental AQP3 mRNA expression.[97] In humans with abnormalities of AF volume, message for AQP3 and AQP9 is decreased in placentas in polyhydramnios,[106,107] and message for AQP3 is increased in placentas in oligohydramnios.[108] This has been interpreted as a compensatory change tending to increase maternal-to-fetal water flow. Data on placental AQP1[108,109] and AQP8[107,110] in human pathology have been inconsistent, making these AQPs less likely to be key regulators of placental water flow.

Aquaporin and Intramembranous Water Flow

AQP 1, 3, 8, and 9 have all been demonstrated in human amniochorion, and AQP 1, 3, and 9 have been found to be associated with amnion epithelium and cytotrophoblast of the chorion. IM flow may therefore also be through AQPs. There is evidence that AQP1 is necessary for normal AF homeostasis. Mice lacking the AQP1 gene have significantly increased AF volume,[111] and in normal mice, AF volume was negatively correlated with AQP1 expression.[97] In conditions with pathologic AF volume, AQP1, 3, 8, and 9 expression are increased in human amnion derived from patients with increased AF volumes,[57,106,107,110-113] and AQP1 and AQP3 are decreased in the amnion of patients with oligohydramnios.[108,109] These changes were postulated to be a response to, rather than a cause of, the AF volume abnormalities. Alterations in AQP expression may also be a cause of AF volume abnormalities; AQP1 protein increased in sheep fetal chorioallantoic membranes in response to fetal hypoxia, suggesting increased IM flow as a mechanism for the oligohydramnios associated with fetal compromise.[114] Finally, AQP expression in the chorioamnion is subject to hormonal regulation. In work done in our laboratory, AQP3, AQP8, and AQP9 expression is upregulated in cultured human amnion cells after incubation with cAMP or forskolin, a cAMP-elevating agent.[115,116] These data together support the hypothesis that AQPs, specifically AQP1, are important mediators of water flow out of the gestational sac across the amnion.

In summary, we propose the following model for human fetal water flow. Water crosses from the maternal to fetal circulation in the placenta, perhaps under the influence of local osmotic differences created by the active transport of sodium. Transplacental water flow, at least in the maternal-to-fetal direction, is through AQP water channels. Membrane permeability in the placenta is therefore subject to regulation by up- or downregulating the number of AQP channels in the membrane. There is no evidence of acute changes in placental water permeability, but changes in permeability have been described over time; these could be attributable to changes in the expression of AQPs with advancing gestation. AQP3 is expressed on the apical membrane of the syncytiotrophoblasts; the membrane barrier thought to be rate limiting for placental water flux, and its expression increases with gestation. AQP3 is therefore a candidate for the regulation of placental water flow.

In the gestational compartment, water circulates between the fetus and the AF. The available evidence suggests that the IM component of this flow is mediated by AQPs, specifically by AQP1. IM flow can be altered over gestation and in response to acute events (e.g., increased AF volume). These alterations in IM flow are likely affected by alterations in the membrane expression of AQP1. Normally, AQP1 expression in the amnion decreases with gestation associated with increasing AF volume, but expression can be increased by various humeral factors, polyhydramnios, or fetal acidosis.

Conclusion

The circulation of water between mother and fetus and within the fetal compartment is complex, and the mechanisms regulating water flow remain poorly understood. Water flow across the placenta must increase with increasing fetal water needs and must be relatively insensitive to transient changes in maternal status. Water circulation within the gestation must sustain fetal growth and plasma volume while also allowing for appropriate amounts of AF for fetal growth and development.

Experimental data suggest that placental water flow is affected by both hydrostatic and osmotic forces and that both transcellular and paracellular water flow occurs. IM water flow is more likely to be osmotically driven, although there are other contributing forces as well. The observation that water crosses the membrane in excess of solutes suggests a role for AQP water channels in placental and IM water flow. Experimental data have confirmed the expression of AQPs in the placenta and fetal membranes, as well as modulation of this expression by a variety of factors. AQP3 is an exciting prospect for the regulation of placental water flow given its cellular location and association with AF volume. AQP1 has been implicated in the mechanism of IM flow using a variety of experimental models. The availability of agents known to regulate the expression of AQPs suggests the possibility of treatments for AF volume abnormalities based on the stimulation or suppression of the appropriate water channel.

References

1. Hanson RS, Powrie RO, Larson L. Diabetes insipidus in pregnancy: a treatable cause of oligohydramnios. *Obstet Gynecol.* 1997;89(5 Pt 2):816-817.
2. Schreyer P, Sherman DJ, Ervin MG, et al. Maternal dehydration: impact on ovine amniotic fluid volume and composition. *J Dev Physiol.* 1990;13(5):283-287.
3. Sciscione AC, Costigan KA, Johnson TR. Increase in ambient temperature may explain decrease in amniotic fluid index. *Am J Perinatol.* 1997;14(5):249-251.
4. Ross MG, Cedars L, Nijland MJ, Ogundipe A. Treatment of oligohydramnios with maternal 1-deamino-[8-D-arginine] vasopressin-induced plasma hypoosmolality. *Am J Obstet Gynecol.* 1996;174(5):1608-1613.
5. Ross MG, Nijland MJ, Kullama LK. 1-Deamino-[8-D-arginine] vasopressin-induced maternal plasma hypoosmolality increases ovine amniotic fluid volume. *Am J Obstet Gynecol.* 1996; 174(4):1118-1125.
6. Lumbers ER, Smith FG, Stevens AD. Measurement of net transplacental transfer of fluid to the fetal sheep. *J Physiol.* 1985;364:289-299.
7. Faichney GJ, Fawcett AA, Boston RC. Water exchange between the pregnant ewe, the foetus and its amniotic and allantoic fluids. *J Comp Physiol [B].* 2004;174(6):503-510.
8. Jansson T, Powell TL, Illsley NP. Gestational development of water and non-electrolyte permeability of human syncytiotrophoblast plasma membranes. *Placenta.* 1999;20(2-3):155-160.
9. Brace RA. Progress toward understanding the regulation of amniotic fluid volume: water and solute fluxes in and through the fetal membranes. *Placenta.* 1995;16(1):1-18.
10. Moore TR. Amniotic fluid dynamics reflect fetal and maternal health and disease. *Obstet Gynecol.* 2010;116(3):759-765.
11. Goodwin JW, Godden JO, Chance GW. *Perinatal Medicine: The Basic Science Underlying Clinical Practice.* Baltimore, MD: The Williams and Wilkins; 1976.
12. Campbell J, Wathen N, Macintosh M, et al. Biochemical composition of amniotic fluid and extra-embryonic coelomic fluid in the first trimester of pregnancy. *Br J Obstet Gynaecol.* 1992;99(7):563-565.
13. Faber JJ, Gault CF, Green TJ, et al. Chloride and the generation of amniotic fluid in the early embryo. *J Exp Zool.* 1973;183(3):343-352.
14. Gillibrand PN. Changes in the electrolytes, urea and osmolality of the amniotic fluid with advancing pregnancy. *J Obstet Gynaecol Br Commonw.* 1969;76(10):898-905.
15. Desai M, Ladella S, Ross MG. Reversal of pregnancy-mediated plasma hypotonicity in the near-term rat. *J Matern Fetal Neonatal Med.* 2003;13(3):197-202.
16. Brace RA, Wolf EJ. Normal amniotic fluid volume changes throughout pregnancy. *Am J Obstet Gynecol.* 1989;161(2):382-388.
17. Gadd RL. The volume of the liquor amnii in normal and abnormal pregnancies. *J Obstet Gynaecol Br Commonw.* 1966;73(1):11-22.
18. Beischer NA, Brown JB, Townsend L. Studies in prolonged pregnancy. 3. Amniocentesis in prolonged pregnancy. *Am J Obstet Gynecol.* 1969;103(4):496-503.
19. Queenan JT, Von Gal HV, Kubarych SF. Amniography for clinical evaluation of erythroblastosis fetalis. *Am J Obstet Gynecol.* 1968;102(2):264-274.
20. Rabinowitz R, Peters MT, Vyas S, et al. Measurement of fetal urine production in normal pregnancy by real-time ultrasonography. *Am J Obstet Gynecol.* 1989;161(5):1264-1266.
21. Fagerquist M, Fagerquist U, Oden A, Blomberg SG. Fetal urine production and accuracy when estimating fetal urinary bladder volume. *Ultrasound Obstet Gynecol.* 2001;17(2):132-139.
22. Ross MG, Ervin MG, Rappaport VJ, et al. Ovine fetal urine contribution to amniotic and allantoic compartments. *Biol Neonate.* 1988;53(2):98-104.
23. Wlodek ME, Challis JR, Patrick J. Urethral and urachal urine output to the amniotic and allantoic sacs in fetal sheep. *J Dev Physiol.* 1988;10(4):309-319.
24. Robillard JE, Matson JR, Sessions C, Smith Jr FG. Developmental aspects of renal tubular reabsorption of water in the lamb fetus. *Pediatr Res.* 1979;13(10):1172-1176.
25. Robillard JE, Weitzman RE. Developmental aspects of the fetal renal response to exogenous arginine vasopressin. *Am J Physiol.* 1980;238(5):F407-F414.
26. Lingwood B, Hardy KJ, Coghlan JP, Wintour EM. Effect of aldosterone on urine composition in the chronically cannulated ovine foetus. *J Endocrinol.* 1978;76(3):553-554.
27. Lingwood B, Hardy KJ, Horacek I, et al. The effects of antidiuretic hormone on urine flow and composition in the chronically-cannulated ovine fetus. *Q J Exp Physiol Cogn Med Sci.* 1978; 63(4):315-330.
28. Ervin MG, Ross MG, Leake RD, Fisher DA. V1- and V2-receptor contributions to ovine fetal renal and cardiovascular responses to vasopressin. *Am J Physiol.* 1992;262(4 Pt 2):R636-R643.
29. Brace RA, Wlodek ME, Cock ML, Harding R. Swallowing of lung liquid and amniotic fluid by the ovine fetus under normoxic and hypoxic conditions. *Am J Obstet Gynecol.* 1994;171(3):764-770.
30. Ross MG, Ervin G, Leake RD, et al. Fetal lung liquid regulation by neuropeptides. *Am J Obstet Gynecol.* 1984;150(4):421-425.
31. Lawson EE, Brown ER, Torday JS, et al. The effect of epinephrine on tracheal fluid flow and surfactant efflux in fetal sheep. *Am Rev Respir Dis.* 1978;118(6):1023-1026.
32. Dodic M, Wintour EM. Effects of prolonged (48 h) infusion of cortisol on blood pressure, renal function and fetal fluids in the immature ovine foetus. *Clin Exp Pharmacol Physiol.* 1994;21(12):971-980.

33. Sherman DJ, Ross MG, Ervin MG, et al. Ovine fetal lung fluid response to intravenous saline solution infusion: fetal atrial natriuretic factor effect. *Am J Obstet Gynecol.* 1988;159(6):1347-1352.
34. Pritchard JA. Fetal swallowing and amniotic fluid volume. *Obstet Gynecol.* 1966;28(5):606-610.
35. Bradley RM, Mistretta CM. Swallowing in fetal sheep. *Science.* 1973;179(77):1016-1017.
36. Nijland MJ, Day L, Ross MG. Ovine fetal swallowing: expression of preterm neurobehavioral rhythms. *J Matern Fetal Med.* 2001;10(4):251-257.
37. Sherman DJ, Ross MG, Day L, Ervin MG. Fetal swallowing: correlation of electromyography and esophageal fluid flow. *Am J Physiol.* 1990;258(6 Pt 2):R1386-R1394.
38. Xu Z, Nijland MJ, Ross MG. Plasma osmolality dipsogenic thresholds and c-fos expression in the near-term ovine fetus. *Pediatr Res.* 2001;49(5):678-685.
39. El-Haddad MA, Ismail Y, Gayle D, Ross MG. Central angiotensin II AT1 receptors mediate fetal swallowing and pressor responses in the near term ovine fetus. *Am J Physiol Regul Integr Comp Physiol.* 2004;288(4):R1014-R1020.
40. El-Haddad MA, Ismail Y, Guerra C, et al. Neuropeptide Y administered into cerebral ventricles stimulates sucrose ingestion in the near-term ovine fetus. *Am J Obstet Gynecol.* 2003;189(4): 949-952.
41. El-Haddad MA, Ismail Y, Guerra C, et al. Effect of oral sucrose on ingestive behavior in the near-term ovine fetus. *Am J Obstet Gynecol.* 2002;187(4):898-901.
42. Sherman DJ, Ross MG, Day L, et al. Swallowing: response to graded maternal hypoxemia. *J Appl Physiol.* 1991;71(5):1856-1861.
43. Lingwood BE, Wintour EM. Amniotic fluid volume and in vivo permeability of ovine fetal membranes. *Obstet Gynecol.* 1984;64(3):368-372.
44. Gilbert WM, Newman PS, Eby-Wilkens E, Brace RA. Technetium Tc 99m rapidly crosses the ovine placenta and intramembranous pathway. *Am J Obstet Gynecol.* 1996;175(6):1557-1562.
45. Lingwood BE, Wintour EM. Permeability of ovine amnion and amniochorion to urea and water. *Obstet Gynecol.* 1983;61(2):227-232.
46. Gilbert WM, Brace RA. The missing link in amniotic fluid volume regulation: intramembranous absorption. *Obstet Gynecol.* 1989;74(5):748-754.
47. Ervin MG, Ross MG, Leake RD, Fisher DA. Fetal recirculation of amniotic fluid arginine vasopressin. *Am J Physiol.* 1986;250(3 Pt 1):E253-E258.
48. Gilbert WM, Cheung CY, Brace RA. Rapid intramembranous absorption into the fetal circulation of arginine vasopressin injected intraamniotically. *Am J Obstet Gynecol.* 1991;164(4):1013-1018.
49. Queenan JT, Allen Jr FH, Fuchs F, et al. Studies on the method of intrauterine transfusion. I. Question of erythrocyte absorption from amniotic fluid. *Am J Obstet Gynecol.* 1965;92:1009-1013.
50. Hebertson RM, Hammond ME, Bryson MJ. Amniotic epithelial ultrastructure in normal, polyhydramnic, and oligohydramnic pregnancies. *Obstet Gynecol.* 1986;68(1):74-79.
51. Gilbert WM, Brace RA. Novel determination of filtration coefficient of ovine placenta and intramembranous pathway. *Am J Physiol.* 1990;259(6 Pt 2):R1281-R1288.
52. Mann SE, Nijland MJ, Ross MG. Mathematic modeling of human amniotic fluid dynamics. *Am J Obstet Gynecol.* 1996;175(4 Pt 1):937-944.
53. Curran MA, Nijland MJ, Mann SE, Ross MG. Human amniotic fluid mathematical model: determination and effect of intramembranous sodium flux. *Am J Obstet Gynecol.* 1998;178(3):484-490.
54. Anderson DF, Faber JJ, Parks CM. Extraplacental transfer of water in the sheep. *J Physiol.* 1988;406:75-84.
55. Anderson DF, Borst NJ, Boyd RD, Faber JJ. Filtration of water from mother to conceptus via paths independent of fetal placental circulation in sheep. *J Physiol.* 1990;431:1-10.
56. Capurro C, Escobar E, Ibarra C, et al. Water permeability in different epithelial barriers. *Biol Cell.* 1989;66(1-2):145-148.
57. Faber JJ, Thornberg KL. *Placental Physiology: Structure and Function of Fetomaternal Exchange.* New York., NY: Raven; 1983.
58. Stulc J. Placental transfer of inorganic ions and water. *Physiol Rev.* 1997; 77(3):805-836.
59. Georgiades P, Ferguson-Smith AC, Burton GJ. Comparative developmental anatomy of the murine and human definitive placentae. *Placenta.* 2002;23(1):3-19.
60. Jansson T, Illsley NP. Osmotic water permeabilities of human placental microvillous and basal membranes. *J Membr Biol.* 1993;132(2):147-155.
61. Hempstock J, Bao YP, Bar-Issac M, et al. Intralobular differences in antioxidant enzyme expression and activity reflect the pattern of maternal arterial bloodflow within the human placenta. *Placenta.* 2003;24(5):517-523.
62. Makowski EL, Meschia G, Droegemueller W, Battaglia FC. Distribution of uterine blood flow in the pregnant sheep. *Am J Obstet Gynecol.* 1968;101(3):409-412.
63. Benirschke K. Comparative Placentation. Available at http://medicine ucsd.edu/cpa/homefs.html.
64. Schroder HJ. Basics of placental structures and transfer functions. In: Brace RA, Ross MG, Robillard JE, eds. *Reproductive and Perinatal Medicine Vol. XI, Fetal & Neonatal Body Fluids.* Ithaca, NY: Perinatology Press; 1989:187-226.
65. Stulc J, Stulcova B, Sibley CP. Evidence for active maternal-fetal transport of Na+ across the placenta of the anaesthetized rat. *J Physiol.* 1993;470:637-649.
66. Stulc J, Stulcova B. Asymmetrical transfer of inert hydrophilic solutes across rat placenta. *Am J Physiol.* 1993;265(3 Pt 2):R670-R675.
67. Schroder H, Nelson P, Power G. Fluid shift across the placenta: I. The effect of dextran T 40 in the isolated guinea-pig placenta. *Placenta.* 1982;3(4):327-338.

68. Ervin MG, Amico JA, Leake RD, et al. Arginine vasotocin-like immunoreactivity in plasma of pregnant women and newborns. *West Soc Ped Res Clin Res*. 1985;33:115A.

69. Conrad Jr EE, Faber JJ. Water and electrolyte acquisition across the placenta of the sheep. *Am J Physiol*. 1977;233(4):H475-H487.

70. Schroder H, Leichtweiss HP. Perfusion rates and the transfer of water across isolated guinea pig placenta. *Am J Physiol*. 1977;232(6):H666-H670.

71. Leichtweiss HP, Schroder H. The effect of elevated outflow pressure on flow resistance and the transfer of THO, albumin and glucose in the isolated guinea pig placenta. *Pflugers Arch*. 1977;371(3):251-256.

72. Brace RA, Moore TR. Transplacental, amniotic, urinary, and fetal fluid dynamics during very-large-volume fetal intravenous infusions. *Am J Obstet Gynecol*. 1991;164(3):907-916.

73. Brace RA, Gilbert WM, Thornburg KL. Vascularization of the ovine amnion and chorion: a morphometric characterization of the surface area of the intramembranous pathway. *Am J Obstet Gynecol*. 1992;167(6):1747-1755.

74. Battaglia FC, Hellegers AE, Meschia G, Barron DH. In vitro investigations of the human chorion as a membrane system. *Nature*. 1962;196:1061-1063.

75. Fujino Y, Agnew CL, Schreyer P. Amniotic fluid volume response to esophageal occlusion in fetal sheep. *Am J Obstet Gynecol*. 1991;165(6 Pt 1):1620-1626.

76. Matsumoto LC, Cheung CY, Brace RA. Effect of esophageal ligation on amniotic fluid volume and urinary flow rate in fetal sheep. *Am J Obstet Gynecol*. 2000;182(3):699-705.

77. Wintour EM, Barnes A, Brown EH, et al. Regulation of amniotic fluid volume and composition in the ovine fetus. *Obstet Gynecol*. 1978;52(6):689-693.

78. Faber JJ, Anderson DF. Regulatory response of intramembranous absorption of amniotic fluid to infusion of exogenous fluid in sheep. *Am J Physiol*. 1999;277(1 Pt 2):R236-R242.

79. Ross MG, Ervin MG, Leake RD. Bulk flow of amniotic fluid water in response to maternal osmotic challenge. *Am J Obstet Gynecol*. 1983;147(6):697-701.

80. Leontic EA, Tyson JE. Prolactin and fetal osmoregulation: water transport across isolated human amnion. *Am J Physiol*. 1977;232(3):R124-R127.

81. Holt WF, Perks AM. The effect of prolactin on water movement through the isolated amniotic membrane of the guinea pig. *Gen Comp Endocrinol*. 1975;26(2):153-164.

82. Matsumoto LC, Bogic L, Brace RA, Cheung CY. Fetal esophageal ligation induces expression of vascular endothelial growth factor messenger ribonucleic acid in fetal membranes. *Am J Obstet Gynecol*. 2001;184(2):175-184.

83. Daneshmand SS, Cheung CY, Brace RA. Regulation of amniotic fluid volume by intramembranous absorption in sheep: role of passive permeability and vascular endothelial growth factor. *Am J Obstet Gynecol*. 2003;188(3):786-793.

84. Brace RA, Vermin ML, Huijssoon E. Regulation of amniotic fluid volume: intramembranous solute and volume fluxes in late gestation fetal sheep. *Am J Obstet Gynecol*. 2004;191(3):837-846.

85. Faber JJ, Anderson DF. Absorption of amniotic fluid by amniochorion in sheep. *Am J Physiol Heart Circ Physiol*. 2002;282(3):H850-H854.

86. Wynn RM, French GL. Comparative ultrastructure of the mammalian amnion. *Obstet Gynecol*. 1968;31(6):759-774.

87. Anderson D, Yang Q, Hohimer A, et al. Intramembranous absorption rate is unaffected by changes in amniotic fluid composition. *Am J Physiol Renal Physiol*. 2005;288(5):F964-F968.

88. Knepper MA, Wade JB, Terris J, et al. Renal aquaporins. *Kidney Int*. 1996;49(6):1712-1717.

89. Nielsen S, Frokiaer J, Marples D, et al. Aquaporins in the kidney: from molecules to medicine. *Physiol Rev*. 2002;82(1):205-244.

90. Klussmann E, Maric K, Rosenthal W. The mechanisms of aquaporin control in the renal collecting duct. *Rev Physiol Biochem Pharmacol*. 2000;141:33-95.

91. Tajika Y, Matsuzaki T, Suzuki T, et al. Aquaporin-2 is retrieved to the apical storage compartment via early endosomes and phosphatidylinositol 3-kinase-dependent pathway. *Endocrinol*. 2004;145(9):4375-4383.

92. Gradilone SA, Garcia F, Huebert RC, et al. Glucagon induces the plasma membrane insertion of functional aquaporin-8 water channels in isolated rat hepatocytes. *Hepatology*. 2003;37(6):1435-1441.

93. Sugiyama Y, Ota Y, Hara M, Inoue S. Osmotic stress up-regulates aquaporin-3 gene expression in cultured human keratinocytes. *Biochim Biophys Acta*. 2001;1522(2):82-88.

94. De FM, Cobellis L, Torella M, et al. Down-regulation of aquaporin 4 in human placenta throughout pregnancy. *In Vivo*. 2007;21(5):813-817.

95. Liu H, Zheng Z, Wintour EM. Aquaporins and fetal fluid balance. *Placenta*. 2008;29(10):840-847.

96. Johnston H, Koukoulas I, Jeyaseelan K, et al. Ontogeny of aquaporins 1 and 3 in ovine placenta and fetal membranes. *Placenta*. 2000;21(1):88-99.

97. Beall MH, Wang S, Yang B, et al. Placental and membrane aquaporin water channels: correlation with amniotic fluid volume and composition. *Placenta*. 2007;28(5-6):421-428.

98. Liu HS, Song XF, Hao RZ. [Expression of aquaporin 1 in human placenta and fetal membranes]. *Nan Fang Yi Ke Da Xue Xue Bao*. 2008;28(3):333-336.

99. Liu H, Koukoulas I, Ross MC, et al. Quantitative comparison of placental expression of three aquaporin genes. *Placenta*. 2004;25(6):475-478.

100. Mann SE, Ricke EA, Yang BA, et al. Expression and localization of aquaporin 1 and 3 in human fetal membranes. *Am J Obstet Gynecol.* 2002;187(4):902-907.
101. Damiano A, Zotta E, Goldstein J, et al. Water channel proteins AQP3 and AQP9 are present in syncytiotrophoblast of human term placenta. *Placenta.* 2001;22(8-9):776-781.
102. Umenishi F, Verkman AS, Gropper MA. Quantitative analysis of aquaporin mRNA expression in rat tissues by RNase protection assay. *DNA Cell Biol.* 1996;15(6):475-480.
103. Wang S, Amidi F, Beall M, et al. Aquaporin 3 expression in human fetal membranes and its up-regulation by cyclic adenosine monophosphate in amnion epithelial cell culture. *J Soc Gynecol Investig.* 2006;13(3):181-185.
104. Ma T, Yang B, Verkman AS. Cloning of a novel water and urea-permeable aquaporin from mouse expressed strongly in colon, placenta, liver, and heart. *Biochem Biophys Res Commun.* 1997;240(2): 324-328.
105. Wang S, Kallichanda N, Song W, et al. Expression of aquaporin-8 in human placenta and chorio-amniotic membranes: evidence of molecular mechanism for intramembranous amniotic fluid resorption. *Am J Obstet Gynecol.* 2001;185(5):1226-1231.
106. Zhu XQ, Jiang SS, Zou SW, et al. [Expression of aquaporin 3 and aquaporin 9 in placenta and fetal membrane with idiopathic polyhydramnios.] *Zhonghua Fu Chan Ke Za Zhi.* 2009;44(12): 920-923.
107. Zhu X, Jiang S, Hu Y, et al. The expression of aquaporin 8 and aquaporin 9 in fetal membranes and placenta in term pregnancies complicated by idiopathic polyhydramnios. *Early Hum Dev.* 2010;86(10):657-663.
108. Zhu XQ, Jiang SS, Zhu XJ, et al. Expression of aquaporin 1 and aquaporin 3 in fetal membranes and placenta in human term pregnancies with oligohydramnios. *Placenta.* 2009;30(8):670-676.
109. Hao RZ, Liu HS, Xiong ZF. [Expression of aquaporin-1 in human oligohydramnios placenta and fetal membranes.] *Nan Fang Yi Ke Da Xue Xue Bao.* 2009;29(6):1130-1132.
110. Huang J, Qi HB. [Expression of aquaporin 8 in human fetal membrane and placenta of idiopathic polyhydramnios.] *Zhonghua Fu Chan Ke Za Zhi.* 2009;44(1):19-22.
111. Mann SE, Ricke EA, Torres EA, Taylor RN. A novel model of polyhydramnios: amniotic fluid volume is increased in aquaporin 1 knockout mice. *Am J Obstet Gynecol.* 2005;192(6):2041-2044.
112. Mann S, Dvorak N, Taylor R. Changes in aquaporin 1 expression affect amniotic fluid volume. *Am J Obstet Gyn.* 2004;191, S132.
113. Mann SE, Dvorak N, Gilbert H, Taylor RN. Steady-state levels of aquaporin 1 mRNA expression are increased in idiopathic polyhydramnios. *Am J Obstet Gynecol.* 2006;194(3):884-887.
114. Bos HB, Nygard KL, Gratton RJ, Richardson BS. Expression of aquaporin 1 (AQP1) in chorioallantoic membranes of near term ovine fetuses with induced hypoxia. *J Soc Gynecol Invest.* 2005;12(2 suppl):333A.
115. Wang S, Chen J, Au KT, Ross MG. Expression of aquaporin 8 and its up-regulation by cyclic adenosine monophosphate in human WISH cells. *Am J Obstet Gynecol.* 2003;188(4):997-1001.
116. Wang S, Amidi F, Beall MH, Ross MG. Differential regulation of aquaporin water channels in human amnion cell culture. *J Soc Gynecol Invest.* 2005;12(2 suppl):344A.

CHAPTER 2

Body Water Changes in the Fetus and Newborn: Normal Transition After Birth and the Effects of Intrauterine Growth Aberration*

William Oh, MD

- Body Fluid Compartments
- Body Water in Fetal Growth Aberration
- Transitional Changes of Body Water After Birth
- Clinical Implications of Transitional Body Water Changes in Preterm Very Low Birth Weight Infants

Body Fluid Compartments

Water is the most abundant element of body composition. It is divided into two compartments: Intracellular water (ICW) and extracellular water (ECW); the latter is further divided into interstitial fluid and plasma volume (Fig. 2-1). Several methods are available for the measurements of body water in human infants. The general principle has been the use of an indicator that is infused to the subject, allowing for equilibration, and then obtaining a plasma sample to calculate the volume of interest using the principle of dilution with the following formula: $V = I \div Pl\ I$, in which V is volume of the compartment being measured, I is the amount of indicator infused, and Pl I is plasma concentration of infused indicator. Various indicators measure different body water compartments depending on their location of distribution. Table 2-1 shows the water compartments that can be measured with various indicators used.

In early gestation (24 weeks), the total body water (TBW) is very high (≈86% of body weight), and most of it (60%) is in the ECW compartment. With increasing gestational age and with growth, the TBW content decreases. The decline is primarily attributable to an increase in solids components of the body composition with growth as evidenced by an increase in the ICW compartment and a decline of the ECW compartment. At term, the TBW is down to 78% of body weight with 44% being in the ECW compartment, 34% in the ICW compartment and the rest (22%) being solid body mass. At 1 year of age, the TBW is approximately 70% of body weight; most of it is in the ICW (42%), and the rest is in the ECW. Solids account for approximately 30% of body weight.[1,2] These changes also mean that a preterm infant born at 28 weeks' gestation will have a high TBW and ECW.

It should be noted that the changes in body composition discussed above do not distinguish the variation as a result of intrauterine growth aberration. The latter can be in the form of macrosomia (large for gestational age [LGA]) or intrauterine growth restriction (IUGR; also known as small for gestational age [SGA]). Their body fluid characteristics are described below.

---

*This chapter is dedicated to the late Karl Bauer, MD, a friend and fond colleague. The author has adapted many of the contents of his chapter in the first edition of this publication.

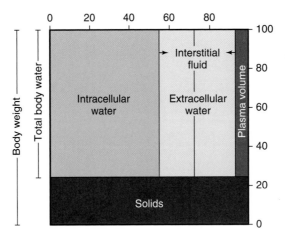

Figure 2-1   Body water distribution in a term newborn infant.

Body Water in Fetal Growth Aberration

Large for Gestational Age

This is a heterogeneous group of infants that consists of those with accelerated fetal growth as a result of poorly controlled maternal diabetes mellitus, maternal constitutional obesity without diabetes, and genetic predisposition to enhanced fetal growth.

The data on body water in LGA infants are sparse. The only information published in the literature is that of Clapp et al,[3] who used D_2O dilution technique to measure TBW and found that in seven infants of diabetic mothers (not all LGA), the value is lower than those of infants with nondiabetic mothers (73% vs. 80% body weight). It should be noted that not all of the infants of diabetic mothers were LGA; they had birth weights ranging from 1430 to 3495 g.

In the absence of good data on directly measured body water content, one may try to make an estimation of this parameter by indirect assessment of the data on body composition in these subjects.

Using dual energy x-ray absorptiometry (DEXA), Hammami et al[4] measured the body composition of 47 LGA term infants and compared the results with a group of gestational age-matched appropriate for gestational age (AGA) infants. They found that the LGA infants had a higher absolute amount of body fat, lean body mass, and mineral contents. When expressed as a percent of body weight, the LGA had higher total body fat and mineral contents but less lean body mass. They also found that the increase in total body fat was highest among LGA infants whose mothers had impaired glucose tolerance during pregnancy.

Table 2-1   INDICATORS USED FOR BODY WATER IN HUMANS*

Body Water Compartment	Indicator
Total body water	Antipyrine stable isotope of water (D_2O or $H_2^{18}O$)
Extracellular water	Bromide, sucrose, inulin
Plasma volume	Evans blue

*The other body composition can be calculated by using the following formula:
Solids = Body weight − Total body water
Intracellular water = Total body water − Extracellular water
Interstitial water = Extracellular water − Plasma volume

Intrauterine Growth Restriction or Small for Gestational Age

In contrast to LGA infants, there is abundant information regarding the body water composition of infants with IUGR.

As in LGA infants, infants with IUGR comprise a heterogeneous group resulting from maternal factors, placental pathology, or fetal causes. Maternal factors include such conditions as maternal undernutrition; maternal disease (e.g., preeclampsia, toxemia of pregnancy); or maternal exposure to adverse environmental factors such as smoking, alcohol, or substance abuse. Placental pathology includes such conditions as placental vascular disease (e.g., preeclampsia resulting in placental vascular insufficiency and placental anomalies). Fetal causes include genetic abnormalities and fetal infection. The clinical diagnosis of a SGA infant, which is also used in most body composition studies, does not differentiate between the different etiologies for impaired growth and is a categorical rather than a continuous description of growth impairment. All of these limitations complicate the interpretation of body composition measurements.

Body Water and Solids in Intrauterine Growth Restriction or Small for Gestational Age Infants

During normal intrauterine growth, TBW content decreases from 94% of body weight in the first trimester of pregnancy to 78% at term caused by the accumulation of body solids during growth.[1,2] In the first two thirds of gestation, body solids increase because of the accretion of protein and minerals, and there is little fat deposition. We know from postmortem chemical analyses that at 27 weeks' gestation, 86% of body weight is water, 12% is fat-free dry solids, and only 2% is fat.[5] In vivo measurements in AGA preterm infants with a birth weight below 1500 g showed a TBW content of 83%,[6] and no fat was detectable by dual photon absorptiometry using [153]Gd magnetic resonance tomography (MRT) in preterm infants.[7] During the last trimester of gestation, the proportion of body solids increases from 14% to 24% of body weight because of the deposition of body fat, which is 2% of body weight at 27 weeks' gestation and 10% to 15% of body weight at birth.[5]

Normal intrauterine growth critically depends on the delivery of sufficient nutrients to the fetus via the placenta. When nutrient delivery was reduced by uterine artery ligation during experimental IUGR in rats, TBW was increased, reflecting the reduced deposition of body fat and protein.[8] In human neonates born after IUGR, the TBW content of the body was also increased compared with normal intrauterine growth. In SGA preterm neonates, the mean TBW content was 62 mL/kg higher than in AGA preterm neonates,[9] and in SGA term neonates, the mean TBW content was increased by 76 mL/kg[10] or by 102 mL/kg,[11] respectively. No reduction in TBW was found in only one study of a small group of SGA neonates with a wide range of gestational ages[12] (Table 2-2).

The relative increase in TBW in SGA neonates is caused by the reduction in body solids, not by an accumulation of excess water caused by a disturbed fluid homeostasis. In preterm SGA neonates, the higher body water content reflects the reduced deposition of protein and minerals because during the first two thirds of gestation, the fetal body consists of water and fat-free dry solids, but there is little deposition of fat. A reduction in fetal lean mass during IUGR has been demonstrated by ultrasound measurements of the cross-sectional lean body area of the fetal thigh.[13] A reduced protein and mineral deposition early in gestation is likely to disrupt organ development. In fact, preterm SGA neonates have a higher mortality rate and more chronic lung disease than gestational age-matched preterm AGA neonates,[14] and SGA preterm neonates are still smaller and lighter at 3 years of age than AGA preterm neonates.[15] A recent study by Zeitlin et al[16] confirmed this association.

Different from preterm SGA neonates, the increase in body water content in term SGA neonates reflects primarily the reduced deposition of fat. The accumulation of fat is the primary cause of the physiologic reduction in TBW during normal growth throughout the third trimester of gestation. Aside from body water measurements, several lines of evidence indicate that adipose tissue is indeed reduced in SGA term neonates. Reduced abdominal wall fat thickness measured by

Table 2-2 TOTAL BODY WATER (TBW) AND EXTRACELLULAR VOLUME (ECV) IN APPROPRIATE FOR GESTATIONAL AGE (AGA) AND SMALL FOR GESTATIONAL AGE (SGA) HUMAN NEONATES

Reference	Subjects	Patients (n)		TBW (mL/kg)	Significance	Method
Cassady and Milstead[11] (1971)	Term (37–43 wk)	AGA SGA	12 23	688 ± 16 790 ± 13	P < .001	Indicator dilution (antipyrine)
Hartnoll et al[9] (2000)	Preterm (25–30 wk)	AGA SGA	35 7	906 (833–954) 844 (637–958)	P = .019	Indicator dilution ($H_2^{18}O$)
Cheek et al[10] (1984)	Term (≥37 wk)	AGA SGA	7 6	749 825	Not reported	Indicator dilution (D_2O)
vd Wagen et al[12] (1986)	GA (34–40 wk)	AGA SGA	11 10	780 ± 38 776 ± 13	NS	Indicator dilution (D_2O)
Author	Subjects	Patients (n)		ECV (mL/kg)	Significance	Method
Cassady[44] (1970)	Term (≥37 wk)	AGA SGA	13 20	376 ± 20 419 ± 45	P = .025	Indicator dilution (bromide)
Cheek et al[10] (1984)	Term (≥37 wk)	AGA SGA	7 6	361 ± 16 395 ± 35	Not reported	Indicator dilution (bromide)
vd Wagen et al[12] (1986)	GA (34–40 wk)	AGA SGA	11 10	355 ± 55 344 ± 35	NS	Indicator dilution (sucrose)

GA, gestational age; NS, not significant.

ultrasonography in a late gestation fetus was found during IUGR.[17] The percentage of adipose tissue estimated from dual photon absorptiometry using [153]Gd MRT was 2% in SGA term neonates compared with 13% in AGA term neonates,[7] and thinner skin folds in SGA term neonates indicated a thinner subcutaneous fat layer.[18] A study by Lapillonne et al[19] using DEXA analysis also found a reduced fat content in SGA near-term and term infants, although the difference did not reach statistical significance because of the small sample size.

No conclusions about the effect of altered body composition of SGA neonates on the risk for neonatal complications or long-term outcome can be drawn from body fluid compartment measurements because studies including body composition measurements are usually small, and no clinical outcomes are reported. Yet from anthropometric studies that include large numbers of neonates, the prognostic utility of body composition estimated from anthropometry can be analyzed. Body weight below a certain cutoff point is the parameter most often used to diagnose impaired fetal growth. In future studies of fetal growth restriction, weight deficit should be quantified and expressed on a continuous scale (e.g., as a standard deviation score) instead of using a fixed cut-off value. The more severe the weight reduction, the higher the risk of neonatal morbidity and mortality for SGA neonates regardless of the cause of the growth deficit[20] and the higher the risk of low intellectual performance in adulthood.[21]

Another issue that complicates the interpretation of body water changes and IUGR is the categorization of these infants as having symmetric or asymmetric IUGR. Whereas the former is often defined by clinicians as having growth restriction affecting all three morphometric parameters (weight, length, and head circumference), the latter defines the group that has growth restriction affecting the weight but not the length or head circumference. It is unclear if symmetric versus asymmetric growth restriction is a relevant predictor of childhood growth in addition to weight deficit. Whereas term neonates with asymmetric IUGR were more likely to demonstrate catch-up growth than preterm neonates with symmetric IUGR, preterm SGA neonates had restriction of childhood growth regardless of having symmetric or asymmetric IUGR at birth.[15] Reduced adipose tissue thickness is a more sensitive predictor for neonatal complications in SGA neonates than weight because symptomatic SGA neonates with hypoglycemia or polycythemia (or both) had a thinner subcutaneous fat layer than asymptomatic SGA neonates, but there was no difference in body weight or length between the two groups.[22]

In summary, fetal growth aberration significantly affects body composition. Accelerated fetal growth results in increase in body solids and fat with a relative decrease in body water. IUGR, on the other hand, results in reduction in body fat with a relative increase in body water. Note that the body water changes in both situations are relative without an absolute increase in actual contents.

Transitional Changes of Body Water after Birth

Although the mechanism is unknown, there is a universal contraction of ECW in infants soon after birth associated with a weight loss of 7% to 15% of body weight by the end of the first week. The magnitude of contraction is inversely proportional to maturity. Term infants have an average of 5% to 7% weight loss during the first week (reflecting contraction of ECW),[23] but very low birth weight (VLBW)[24] and extremely low birth weight (ELBW)[25] infants may lose 10% to 15% of body weight, respectively, during that same time frame (Fig. 2-2). This study confirmed the earlier studies[26,27] showing that the magnitude of reduction of ECW is directly proportional to its content. It should be noted that these studies represented cross-sectional data and did not distinguish the type of infants with reference to growth aberration.

It is apparent that the removal of the ECW is through the renal route. The evidence for this is not direct but implied based on the concurrence of reduction in ECW, weight loss, natriuretic diuresis, and negative sodium balance.[28,29] There is also evidence that diuresis during the first week of life is associated with an improvement in respiratory distress.[30]

There are virtually no data available in regards to the postnatal body fluid transition in LGA infants. However, there is a significant body of literature in regards to IUGR. Postnatal weight loss in seven SGA preterm neonates (birth weight <5th percentile) with a mean gestational age of 35 weeks was only 5% and was accompanied by a proportionate reduction in body water and body solids.[31] This study included no information about fluid intake or diuresis and no AGA control group.

In another study comparing five SGA preterm neonates (mean gestational age, 35 weeks) with 14 weight-matched AGA neonates (mean gestational age, 31 weeks), the SGA neonates had a maximal postnatal weight loss of only 2% compared with a maximal postnatal weight loss of 8% in the AGA control infants. On days 4 to 6 of life, the SGA neonates had already regained birth weight, and there was no detectable change in TBW or body solids; at the same postnatal age, body weight and TBW in the AGA neonates were significantly lower than at birth.[32] There were no differences in day-to-day fluid and energy intake during the first week of life in the SGA and AGA groups; however, the AGA infants had a higher urine output during this time. A possible reason for the attenuated postnatal increase in urine output in SGA preterm neonates was their altered hemodynamic adaptation. SGA preterm neonates did not show the postnatal increase in cardiac output observed in the AGA neonates.

Wadhawan et al[33] recently analyzed a large database from the National Institute of Child Health & Human Development Neonatal Research Network to compare the postnatal weight loss of SGA ($n = 1248$) versus AGA infants ($n = 8213$) and association with the risk of death or bronchopulmonary dysplasia (BPD). They found that the SGA infants had less prevalence of postnatal weight loss than the AGA infants (81.2% vs. 93.7%, respectively; $P < .001$). The association between postnatal weight loss and death or BPD was also similar between SGA and AGA groups. They suggest that clinicians who consider the association between early postnatal weight loss and risk of death or BPD should do so independent of gestation or birth weight status.[33] The postnatal weight loss data also confirmed the previous observations.[31,32]

More recently, Varma et al[34] analyzed a group of AGA ELBW infants ($n = 102$) and concluded that the maximal postnatal weight loss was more related to maturity than to clinical determinants. The association between postnatal weight loss and clinical morbidity clearly needs further study.

Clinical implications of Transitional Body Water Changes in Preterm Very Low Birth Weight Infants

Fluid therapy in the immediate neonatal period in preterm and low birth weight neonates has the following objectives: It (1) allows for the physiologic postnatal contraction of the extracellular volume to occur, (2) aims at a postnatal weight loss of about 10% of body weight, (3) aims at a negative fluid and sodium balance on days 1 to 3 of life, and (4) minimizes transepidermal water loss.[35] These objectives can be achieved with restricted water intakes and sequentially monitoring water and electrolyte balance by using the daily intake, output, weight changes, and serum

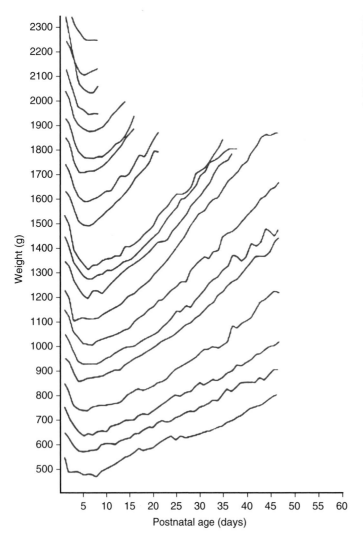

Figure 2-2 Body weight change in low birth weight infants. Weight changes of infants at 100-g intervals are shown. (From Shaffer SG, Quimiro CL, Anderson JV, Hall RT. Postnatal weight changes in low birth weight infants. *Pediatrics.* 1987;79:702-705, with permission.)

Table 2-3 BODY WEIGHT CHANGES, INTAKE, OUTPUT, ESTIMATED INSENSIBLE WATER LOSS (ILW), AND CALCULATED INTAKE THE NEXT 24 HOURS IN A 1.0-KG INFANT AT BIRTH

Age	Weight (g)	Intake (mL/kg)	Urine (mL/kg)	Serum (Na mEq/L)	Estimated IWL	Fluid Next 24 h	Sodium (mEq/kg)
Birth	1,000	—	—	—	50	70[†]	0
24 h	970	70	20	140	80*	100[†]	1
48 h	950	100	48	140	72	120[§]	1
72 h	930	120	68	140	72	140	2
7 d	980[¶]	140	60	140	50	140[•]	2

*Estimated insensible water loss = Intake − Urine output − Weight changes = 70 − 20 + 30 = 80.
[†]10% glucose.
[‡]Amino acid added.
[§]Fat emulsion added.
[¶]A gain of 20 g from the previous 24 hours.
[•]IWL + Urine + Stool + Weight gain = 50 + 60 + 10 + 20 = 140.

electrolyte concentrations (particularly sodium) data in adjusting the appropriate amount of intake to achieve theses goals. Failure to do so will result in either dehydration if inadequate amount of fluid is given or increased risk of patent ductus arteriosus (PDA), necrotizing enterocolitis (NEC) and perhaps chronic lung disease if excess fluid is given.[35-39] There is also suggestive evidence that sodium restriction during the first week of life to produce a negative sodium balance can achieve the same goals as fluid restriction.[40,41] The physiologic rationale behind the latter is that if sodium intake exceeds the requirement, the sodium retention will result in water excess producing the same result as in excess water intake with positive water balance.

Maintaining a negative water and sodium balance during the first week is the key to successful fluid and electrolyte management of VLBW infants and even more so for ELBW infants because the latter are at much higher risk for the morbidities already described. The following case presentation illustrates how a clinician can balance the fluid and electrolyte status of an ELBW infant by paying close attention to daily body weight changes in the process of prescribing the daily fluid and electrolyte.

Let's take the case of a 1.0 kg AGA infant admitted to the neonatal intensive care unit with respiratory distress who was being cared for in a hybrid humidified incubator (Giraffe OmniBed, GE Healthcare). The latter is a new high-technology incubator that has been shown to be very effective in maintaining body temperature and fluid balance in VLBW infants.[42] The initial fluid order consisted of 70 mL/kg of 10% glucose without electrolytes. The volume is based on the estimated insensible water loss for this infant of 50 mL/kg and an additional 20 mL/kg for estimated water required to excrete approximately 5 mOsm/kg of endogenous solute load. Table 2-3 illustrates the potential scenario in body weight changes, intake, output data, and estimated insensible water loss as well as the rationale for the prescribed fluid, electrolyte, and nutrition intake for this infant. The scenario clearly shows that systematic data collection, interpretation, and forward calculation of intakes needed ensure negative fluid and sodium balance in this infant during the first 72 hours. Note that the ECW contraction generally ceases at day 4 to 6 of life; thus, the weight should be unchanged. By day 6 of life, the body weight should begin to increase at 20 to 30 g/kg, which reflects anabolic or the beginning of growth phase. A useful way of ensuring the appropriate fluid balance is achieved is to plot the weight changes on a daily basis using a standard growth chart as the one shown in Figure 2-3.

There is essentially no clinical trial about fluid therapy for LGA as well as SGA neonates. From the body water measurements we know that despite their "wrinkled" appearance, SGA neonates are not dehydrated at birth. Rather, severely growth restricted neonates have an expanded extracellular volume. The only study providing data on fluid therapy in the immediate neonatal period report an attenuated

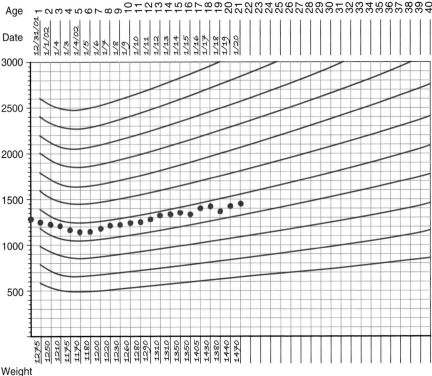

Figure 2-3 Weight changes during the first 3 weeks of life of a very low birth weight infant.

postnatal weight loss in SGA preterm infants receiving the same amount of fluid intake as weight-matched AGA preterm infants.[43] This study suggests that SGA preterm neonates do not need extra fluid intake in the immediate neonatal period but rather a cautious approach to fluid prescription. It is probably fair to state that the description of fluid therapy above is appropriate for VLBW infants of various growth categories. However, future clinical trials to confirm this statement are desirable.

References

1. Friis-Hansen B. Changes in body water compartments during growth. *Acta Paediatr.* 1957;46(suppl 110):1-68.
2. Friis-Hansen B. Body water compartments in children: changes during growth and related changes in body composition. *Pediatrics.* 1961;28:169-181.
3. Clapp WM, Butterfield LJ, O'Brien D. Body water compartment in premature infants with special reference to the effects of the respiratory distress syndrome and of maternal diabetes and toxemia. *Pediatrics.* 1962;29:883-889.
4. Hammami M, Walters JC, Hockman EM, et al. Disproportionate alterations in body composition of large for gestational age neonates. *J Pediatr.* 2001;138:817-821.
5. Ziegler EE, O'Donnell AM, Nelson SE, Fomon SJ. Body composition of the reference fetus. *Growth.* 1976;40:329-341.
6. Bauer K, Bovermann G, Roithmaier A, et al. Body composition, nutrition, and fluid balance during the first two weeks of life in preterm neonates weighing less than 1500 grams. *J Pediatr.* 1991;118; 615-620.
7. Petersen S, Gotfredsen A, Knudsen FU, Lean body mass in small for gestational age and appropriate for gestational age infants. *J Pediatr.* 1988;113:886-889.
8. Hohenauer L, Oh W. Body composition in experimental intrauterine growth retardation in the rat. *J Nutr.* 1969;99:358-361.
9. Hartnoll G, Betremieux P, Modi N. Body water content of extremely preterm infants at birth. *Arch Dis Child Fetal Neonatal Ed.* 2000;83:F56-F59.
10. Cheek DB, Wishart J, MacLennan A, Haslam R. Cell hydration in the normally grown, the premature, and the low weight for gestational age infant. *Early Hum Dev.* 1984;10:75-84.
11. Cassady G, Milstead RR. Antipyrine space studies and cell water estimates in infants of low birth weight. *Pediatr Res.* 1971;5:673-682.

12. vd Wagen A, Okken A, Zweens J, Zijlstra WG. Body composition at birth of growth-retarded newborn infants demonstrating catch-up growth in the first year of life. *Biol Neonate.* 1986;49:121-125.
13. Padoan A, Rigano S, Ferrazzi E, et al. Differences in fat and lean mass proportions in normal and growth restricted fetuses. *Am J Obstet Gynecol.* 2004;191:1459-1464.
14. Lal MK, Manktelow BN, Draper ES, Field DJ. Chronic lung disease of prematurity and intrauterine growth retardation: a population-based study. *Pediatrics.* 2003;111:483-487.
15. Strauss RS, Dietz WH. Growth and development of term children born with low birth weight: effects of genetic and environmental factors. *J Pediatr.* 1998;133:67-72.
16. Zeitlin J, El Ayoubi M, Jarreau PH, et al. Impact of fetal growth restriction on mortality and morbidity in a very preterm birth cohort. *J Pediatr.* 2010;157(5):733-739.
17. Gardeil F, Greene R, Stuart B, Turner MJ. Subcutaneous fat in the fetal abdomen as a predictor of growth restriction. *Obstet Gynecol.* 1999;94:209-212.
18. Brans YW, Sumners JE, Dweck HS, Cassady G. A noninvasive approach to body composition in the neonate: dynamic skinfold measurement. *Pediatr Res.* 1974;8:215-222.
19. Lapillonne A, Braillon P, Claris O, et al. Body composition in appropriate and in small for gestational age infants. *Acta Paediatr.* 1997;86:196-200.
20. Kramer MS, Olivier M, McLaen FH, et al. Impact of intrauterine growth retardation and body proportionality on fetal and neonatal outcome. *Pediatrics.* 1990;85:707-713.
21. Bergvall N, Iliadou A, Johannsson S, et al. Risks for low intellectual performance related to being born small for gestational age are modified by gestational age. *Pediatrics.* 2006;117:e460-e467.
22. Drossou V, Diamanti E, Noutsia H, et al. Accuracy of anthropometric measurements in predicting symptomatic SGA and LGA neonates. *Acta Paediatr.* 1995;84:1-5.
23. Cheek DB, Wishart J, MacLennan A, Haslam R. Cell hydration in the normally grown, the premature, and the low weight for gestational age infant. *Early Hum Dev.* 1984;10:75-84.
24. Shaffer SG, Quimiro CL, Anderson JV, Hall RT. Postnatal weight changes in low birth weight infants. *Pediatrics.* 1987;79:702-705.
25. Pauls J, Bauer K, Versmold H. Postnatal body weight curves for infants below 1000g birth weight receiving early enteral and parenteral nutrition. *Eur J Pediatr.* 1998;157:416-421.
26. Dancis J, O'Connell JR, Holt LE. A grid for recording the weight of preterm infants. *J Pediatr.* 1948;33:570-572.
27. Brosius KK, Ritter DA, Kenny JD. Postnatal growth curve of the infant with extremely low birth weight who was fed enterally. *Pediatrics.* 1984;74:778-782.
28. Ross BS, Cowett RM, Oh W. Renal functions of low birth weight infants during the first two months of life. *Pediatr Res.* 1977;11:1162-1164.
29. Siegel SR, Oh W. Renal function as a marker of human fetal maturation. *Acta Paediatr Scand.* 1976;65: 481-485.
30. Bidiwala KS, Lorenz JM, Kleinman LI. Renal function correlates of diuresis in preterm infant. *Pediatrics.* 1988,82:50-58.
31. vd Wagen A, Okken A, Zweens J, Zijlstra WG. Composition of postnatal weight loss and subsequent weight gain in small for dates newborn infants. *Acta Paediatr Scand.* 1985;74:57-61.
32. Leipälä JA, Boldt T, Turpeinen U, et al. Cardiac hypertrophy and altered hemodynamic adaptation in growth-restricted preterm infants. *Pediatr Res.* 2003;53:989-993.
33. Wadhawan R, Perritt R, Laptook AR, et al. Association between early postnatal weight loss and death or broncho-pulmonary dysplasia in small and appropriate for gestational age extremely low birth weight infants. *J Perinatology.* 2007;27:359-364.
34. Varma, RP, Shibli S, Fang H, et al. Clinical determinants and utility of early postnatal maximum weight loss in fluid management of extremely low birth weight infants. *Early Human Dev.* 2009,85: 59-64.
35. Modi N. Management of fluid balance in the very immature neonate. *Arch Dis Child Fetal Neonatal Ed.* 2004;89:F108-F111.
36. Bell EF, Warburton D, Stonestreet BS, Oh W. High volume fluid intake predisposes premature infants to necrotizing enterocolitis. *Lancet.* 1979;2:90.
37. Bell EF, Warburton D, Stonestreet BS, Oh W. Effect of fluid administration of the development of symptomatic patent ductus arteriosus and congestive heart failure in premature infants. *N Engl J Med.* 1980;302:598-604.
38. Bell EF, Acarregui MJ. Restricted versus liberal water intake for preventing morbidity and mortality in preterm infants. *Cochrane Database Syst Rev.* 2001;3:CD000503.
39. Bell EF, Acarregui MJ. Restricted versus liberal water intake for preventing morbidity and mortality in preterm infants. *Cochrane Database Syst Rev.* 2000;2:CD000503.
40. Hartnoll G, Betremieux P, Modi N. Randomized controlled trial of postnatal sodium supplementation on oxygen dependency and body weight in 25–30 week gestational age infants. *Arch Dis Child.* 2000;85:F29-F32.
41. Hartnoll G, Betremieux P, Modi N. Randomized controlled trial of postnatal sodium supplementation on body composition in 25–30 week gestational age infants. *Arch Dis Child.* 2000;82(1):F24-F28.
42. Kim, SM, Lee, EY Chen J, et al. Improved care and growth outcomes by using hybrid humidified incubators in very preterm infants. *Pediatrics.* 2010;125(1):e137-e145.
43. Bauer K, Cowett RM, Howard GM, et al. Effect of intrauterine growth retardation on postnatal weight change in preterm infants. *J Pediatr.* 1993;123:301-306.
44. Cassady G. Body composition in intrauterine growth retardation. *Pediatr Clin North Am.* 1970;17:79-99.

Electrolyte Balance during Normal Fetal and Neonatal Development

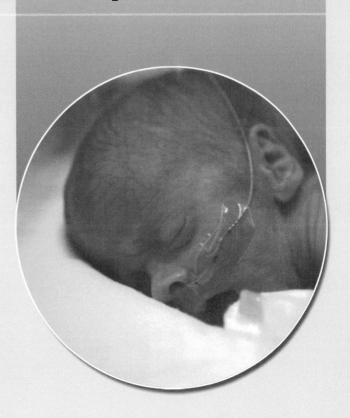

CHAPTER 3

Renal Aspects of Sodium Metabolism in the Fetus and Neonate

Endre Sulyok, MD, PhD, DSc

3

- Body Water Compartments
- Body Water Compartments and Initial Weight Loss
- Physical Water Compartments
- Sodium Homeostasis
- Disturbances in Plasma Sodium Concentrations
- Sodium Homeostasis and Acid–Base Balance

Sodium and volume homeostasis in fetuses and neonates has been the subject of intensive research for decades. Several aspects of the developmental changes in renal sodium handling have been revealed. It is now apparent that in addition to the intrinsic limitations of tubular transport of sodium by the immature kidney, extra-renal factors play an important role in maintaining sodium balance. In this chapter, an attempt has been made to summarize our current knowledge of the sodium homeostasis in fetuses and neonates and to present a revised concept of perinatal redistribution of body fluids. In the light of recent clinical, experimental, and molecular biological research, our understanding of the developmental changes in salt and water metabolism is greatly improved, and consequently, a more targeted approach can be applied to the clinical management of healthy and sick neonates.

Body Water Compartments

Body water is distributed in well-defined compartments that undergo marked developmental changes. Whereas total body water (TBW) and extracellular water (ECW) gradually decrease, intracellular water (ICW) increases as the gestation advances. The decrease of ECW is mainly confined to the interstitial water (ISW); the plasma water remains relatively unaffected.[1]

Individual estimates of body water compartments over this period vary greatly and are related to several factors, including intrauterine growth rate, gender, pregnancy pathology, mode of delivery, maternal fluid management during labor, neonatal renal function, and postnatal fluid intake.

The perinatal redistribution of body fluid compartments is associated with changes in ionic composition of tissue water. Accordingly, at the early stage of development, the body has high sodium and low potassium contents that progress to the opposite with increasing maturation.

As shown by Ziegler et al,[2] the sodium and chloride content per 100 g fat-free weight, the principal electrolytes of ECW, decrease, but protein, phosphorous, magnesium and potassium content, the major constituents of the ICW, increase. More specifically, body sodium decreased progressively from 9.9 mEq at 24 weeks' gestation to 8.7 mEq at term as opposed to the steady increase of body potassium from 4.0 mEq to 4.6 mEq during the same period of gestation.[2]

When individual tissues of various species were analyzed separately, there were variations in the rate of chemical development, possibly reflecting differences in their functional maturation. Interestingly, the developmental pattern of brain electrolytes in fetal sheep and guinea pigs followed paraboloid relationships with gestational age; brain sodium and chloride content reached its peak value in the second part of gestation, which was mirrored by the minimum value of brain potassium.[3] This phenomenon may represent corresponding alterations in the volume of ECW or in the transport activity of the Na^+/K^+ exchanger. It is also of interest that when distinct brain areas representing various stages of phylogenetic development were investigated, brain water content and sodium concentration were found to vary from high for the youngest cortex to low for the oldest medulla, with the respective values for other brain areas falling between these extremes.[4]

Cell Volume Regulation

The volume and composition of body fluid compartments are strictly controlled. ECW is under neuroendocrine control, and the final regulation is accomplished by the kidney through retaining or excreting solutes and fluids. By contrast, ICW volume is regulated by osmotically-driven passive water flux across the cell membrane.

In this regard, it is to be noted that cells of the brain and transporting epithelia respond to perturbations of ECW osmolality, not only with inducing the appropriate water flow in or out of cells, but also with gaining or losing cellular organic and anorganic osmolytes to limit osmotic water flux and to preserve cell volume. This volume regulatory response (VRR) develops in the brain of ovine fetuses in a region- and age-related fashion. Namely, in fetuses with 60% of gestation, this VRR is impaired when compared with more mature animals, and it starts operating in the younger cortex then in the phylogenetically older medulla.[5] It is to be stressed that the elevated tissue sodium levels, and more importantly, the elevated sodium to potassium ratio in the developing brain indicates that the process of "chemical maturation" has not been completed,[6] and the immature brain is not capable of controlling its volume by ionic movements but rather by the accumulation or extrusion of the predominant organic osmolyte (i.e., taurine).[7]

In addition to the well-defined VRR by the cellular osmolytes, the cell membrane itself is also involved in the adaptation of cells to osmotic challenges. Brain-specific water channel membrane protein, aquaporin 4 (AQP4), is widely distributed in cells at the blood–brain and brain–cerebrospinal fluid interfaces, where it facilitates water movement.

AQP4 protein is expressed abundantly in a highly polarized distribution in ependymal cells and astroglial membranes facing capillaries and forming the glia limitans.[8]

A growing body of evidence suggests that complete lack, reduced expression, mislocalization, deficient membrane anchoring, and dysfunction of brain AQP4 limit transmembrane water flux and provide first-line defense mechanisms to maintain cerebral water balance and to protect brain volume.[9]

In support of this notion, Manley et al[10] demonstrated that AQP4 deficiency protected the brain and reduced edema formation in mice exposed to acute water intoxication and focal ischemic stroke. Compared with their wild-type counterparts, the AQP4 knockout mice had less brain water content, better neurologic outcome, and improved survival. Almost simultaneously, our group, using a different experimental model, came essentially to the same conclusion. Namely, we found that in response to severe systemic hyponatremia, a rapid increase occurred in the immunoreactivity of astroglial AQP4 protein without significant changes in AQP4 mRNA levels or subcellular distribution of AQP4 protein. According to our interpretation, the hypoosmotic stress-related posttranscriptional AQP4 protein changes may potentially be accounted for by enhanced phosphorylation and subsequent altered conformation and immunogenicity of the channel protein.[11] Phosphorylated AQP4 has been shown to have reduced water conductivity.[12] Furthermore, the dystrophin-associated protein (DAP) complex that connects extracellular matrix components to the cytoskeleton is closely related to AQP4. Neuronal dystrophin isoform and the related proteins are co-localized with brain AQP4 in the astrocyte endfeet, and AQP4 is markedly reduced in dystrophin or α-syntrophin deficient states. Dystrophin-null mice subjected to water intoxication had delayed ICW accumulation and prolonged survival.[13] These observations indicate that whereas functioning AQP4 favors development of brain edema, AQP4 deficiency protects against edemagenesis when animals are challenged by pathological conditions known to cause brain water accumulation.

Recent studies on the ontogeny of the expression of brain AQP4 protein and mRNA in four mammalian species, including humans, have revealed their very low levels at the early stage of gestation and their gradual increase as the gestation progressed to term.[14,15] AQP4 protein expression levels in rat cerebellum during different stages of postnatal development have proved to be hardly detectable in the first week, increasing from 2% of adult levels on day 7 to 25% and 63% on days 14 and 28, respectively.[16] These observations provide suggestive evidence that the low expression of AQP4 may limit transmembranous water flux and may contribute to maintaining water balance in the maturing brain, which has no fully developed osmolyte-related VRR.

Fetal Sodium Metabolism

The dynamic interactions between maternal and fetal circulation and amniotic fluid (AF) throughout gestation ensure fetal homeostasis and supply nutrients, solutes, and water for growth. The placenta and fetal membranes play an essential role in regulating transport processes because they behave like a low-permeability barrier or contain specific transcellular transport mechanisms. In general, minerals that are contained in the plasma at low concentrations and are mainly intracellular or sequestered in bones (K^+, Mg, Ca, phosphate) are transported to the fetus actively, but the transfer of major extracellular ions (Na^+, Cl^-) has great interspecies variations and may occur through active or passive transport.[17]

To accomplish normal fetal growth, the accretion rate of sodium and potassium has been estimated to be 1.8 mmol/kg/day, and the volume of transplacental water flux is approximately 20 mL/kg/day in near-term human fetuses.[18]

Fetal plasma sodium concentrations are stable in relation to gestational age of 18 to 40 weeks and are not significantly different from maternal plasma sodium concentrations or are slightly lower, which allows passive sodium flow to the fetus.[19] It has been well documented, however, that the placental syncytiotrophoblast is equipped with transport systems needed for transcellular sodium transfer. Sodium flux from mother to fetus is 10 to 100 times higher than the rate of sodium accretion by the fetus, indicating that most of the sodium transferred to the fetus returns to the mother by paracellular diffusion, so the transplacental sodium flux is bidirectional and nearly symmetrical.[20]

Amniotic Fluid Dynamics

Although there are fairly wide variations, the volume and composition of AF undergo characteristic changes during gestation.[21] Its volume increases from 40 mL at 11 weeks' gestation to approximately 700 mL at 25 weeks' gestation and then increases further to reach its maximum of about 920 mL at 35 weeks' gestation. Later in gestation, it begins to decrease to about 720 mL at term followed by a more marked reduction in postterm pregnancies. During the first trimester of gestation, osmolality and electrolyte composition of the AF correspond to fetal plasma. When the fetus begins to void hypotonic urine at approximately 11 weeks of gestation, AF osmolality decreases progressively with advancing gestational age to reach the value of 250 to 260 mOsm/L near term. Sodium concentration in fetal urine decreases accordingly and contributes to the generation of hypotonic AF. The low AF osmolality provides an osmotic driving force for the outward water flow across the intra- and transmembranous pathways. The volume and composition of AF during late gestation are therefore determined by fetal urine and lung fluid secretion as the two primary sources of AF, and fetal swallowing and intramembranous absorption as the two primary routes of amniotic water clearance (Fig. 3-1). Quantitative estimates for the dynamic state of AF sodium are presented in Table 3-1.

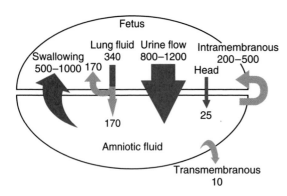

Figure 3-1 Schematic presentation of water flows into and out of the amniotic space in late gestation. Arrow size is proportional to flow rate. (From Gilbert WM, Brace RA. Amniotic fluid volume and normal flows to and from the amniotic cavity. *Semin Perinatol.* 1993;17:150-157, with permission.)

B

Mechanisms of Placental Sodium Transfer

Convincing evidence has been provided to indicate that in rats and pigs, the maternal–fetal sodium flux is accomplished by active transcellular transport, which is saturable, highly dependent on temperature, and can be inhibited by ouabain added to the fetal side.[22] The presence of Na^+, K^+-ATPase in the trophoblast plasma membrane has been demonstrated.[23] Moreover, in rat placentas, the activity and expression of the α-subunit of Na^+, K^+-ATPase increase is parallel with the maternal–fetal sodium flux during the last trimester of pregnancy.[24] These observations are in line with the conclusion that the sodium-pump enzyme serves as the major common pathway of sodium extrusion from the syncytiotrophoblast at the fetal side of the membrane. Attempts to explore the sites of sodium entry at the brush-border plasma membrane (maternal side facing) have identified several mechanisms. The Na^+/H^+ exchanger (NHE) family of transport proteins has been shown to be present in the placental microvillous plasma membrane. These transport proteins mediate the electroneutral exchange of extracellular Na^+ for intracellular H^+ and play a role in regulating intracellular pH, transepithelial Na transport and cell volume homeostasis.

Three isoforms of the NHE protein family (NHE1, NHE2, and NHE3) have been detected in the microvillous membrane of syncytiotrophoblast. NHE1 proved to be the predominant isoform responsible for the amiloride-sensitive maternofetal sodium transfer.[25] NHE activity increases over gestation, and the amiloride-sensitive Na^+ uptake by the microvillous membrane is markedly elevated in term placentas compared with first trimester placentas.[26] A similar gestational pattern was seen for the expression of NHE1 and NHE2 mRNA. NHE1 protein expression did not change over gestation, but NHE2 and NHE3 protein showed a marked increase in their

Table 3-1 SODIUM AND VOLUME METABOLISM IN HUMAN AMNIOTIC FLUID

	Amniotic Fluid		Urine		Lung		Flow Calculations	
Gestational age (wk)	Volume (mL)	Na (mEq/L)	Volume (mL)	Na (mEq/L)	Volume (mL)	Na (mEq/L)	IM_D (mL)	S_D (mL)
11	40	135	11	122	0	140	1	10
15	151	135	49	110	2	140	9	37
20	393	135	122	89	10	140	42	83
25	665	135	239	71	27	140	112	147
30	872	134	427	57	58	140	241	239
35	924	131	728	50	114	140	438	403
40	726	126	1211	50	169	140	701	686

IM_D, dynamic intramembranous flow; S_D, dynamic swallowed volume.
From Curran MA, Nijland MJM, Mann SE, Ross MG. Human amniotic fluid mathematical model: determination and effect of intramembranous sodium flux. *Am J Obstet Gynecol.* 1998;178:484-490.

expression between the second trimester and term.[27] Interestingly, when placental NHE1 activity and expression were compared between normally grown and growth-retarded preterm and full-term infants, both the expression and activity of NHE1 were lower in the growth-retarded group delivered preterm. It has been suggested that the limited Na^+/H^+ exchange may contribute to the development of fetal acidosis frequently seen in these infants without apparent birth asphyxia.[28] Studies to reveal the control mechanisms of Na^+ transport by NHE in brush-border membrane vesicles isolated from human placental villous tissue have shown that whereas ethylisopropylamiloride, the specific inhibitor of the transporter, decreased Na uptake by 98%, benzamil, the Na channel blocker, had no effect. Similarly, the activity of NHE remained unaffected by cyclic AMP (cAMP), phorbol ester, insulin, angiotensin II, or parathyroid hormone (PTH), all known to regulate Na^+/H^+ exchange by the isoform present in the renal brush-border membrane.[29] Aldosterone and cortisol have a rapid non-genomic stimulatory effect on the activity of NHE in human placental syncytiotrophoblast at term. This effect, however, could only be observed in placentas from female babies, possibly because of the low expression of gluco- and mineralocorticoid receptors (MRs) and 11-β-hydroxysteroid dehydrogenase-2 (11-βHSD2) mRNA in placentas from male babies.[30] These observations suggest that estrogen may also have an important role in regulating the expression and function of NHE in placental membranes.

In addition to the Na^+/H^+ antiporter, other transport mechanisms have been assumed to be involved in the passive entry of Na^+ into the trophoblast from the maternal side. Furosemide-sensitive Na^+, K^+, $2Cl^-$ co-transporter and hydrochlorothiazide-sensitive Na-Cl co-transporter appear to be absent from placental brush-border membrane vesicles,[22] although bumetanide-sensitive Na^+, K^+, $2Cl^-$ co-transporter has been shown to be expressed in BeWo cells, a human trophoblastic cell line.[31] The involvement of epithelial sodium channel (ENaC) in placental sodium transport has not been confirmed; however, there has been suggestive evidence for the presence and gestational increase of ENaC-α-subunit in the allantoic membrane and trophoblast of porcine placentas.[32] Moreover, functional α-ENaC has been detected in the apical membrane of normal human syncytiotrophoblast, but neither mRNA nor protein expression of α-ENaC could be identified in preeclamptic placentas, suggesting the role for placental sodium transport in the pathophysiology of preeclampsia.[33] The substrate-specific (phosphate, amino acids) co-transporter mediated Na uptake by the microvillous membrane of the syncytiotrophoblast has been widely accepted.[29]

The placenta has been claimed to act as a nutrient sensor because placental transport functions are altered according to the maternal nutrient supply. Indeed, whereas intrauterine growth restriction is associated with the reduction of a number of placental transporters, accelerated fetal growth is characterized by increased activity in these transporters. Evidence has been provided that these placental transport alterations are the result of specific regulation rather than representing a consequence of altered fetal growth.[34]

Fetal Homeostatic Reactions

Fetal sheep infused intravascularly with normal saline had a modest increase in AF volume and a substantial increase in urine flow rate. These increases roughly equaled the intramembranous absorption that occurred in parallel with an increase in vascular endothelial growth factor (VEGF) gene expression in the amnion, chorion, and placenta. Based on these findings, it has been suggested that the increased intramembranous absorption induced by volume-loading diuresis may be mediated by VEGF via stimulating active transport processes.[35]

Persistent fetal diuresis can also be induced by maternal administration of DDAVP (desmopressin) combined with oral water load. Water retention results in maternal hyponatremia followed by a slow decline in fetal plasma sodium and increased fetal urine flow. Fetal diuresis has been assumed to be attributable to fetal hyponatremia rather than to the reduction in maternal-to-fetal osmotic gradient. This notion appears to be supported by the close inverse relationship of fetal urine flow rate to fetal plasma sodium concentration and by the persistent diuresis despite placental osmotic equilibrium.[36]

Furthermore, to maintain sodium homeostasis in the fetus of sodium-depleted, severely hyponatremic pregnant rats, net sodium transfer to the growing fetus increases markedly against a significant sodium concentration gradient between maternal and fetal plasma.[37] By contrast, long-term hypertonic NaCl infusion into late-gestation fetal sheep caused a significant increase in fetal plasma sodium, chloride, and osmolality, but their values in the maternal plasma remained unaltered. Most of the infused sodium and chloride was excreted by fetuses in large volumes of hypotonic urine. There was a transient increase in AF volume with unchanged osmolality and sodium concentration. Interestingly, because the infused NaCl was retained neither in the fetus nor in the AF, it has been suggested that NaCl was lost from the fetal into the maternal compartment despite osmotic and concentration gradients favoring the opposite direction of transfer.[38]

Fetal sheep undergoing continuous drainage of fetal fluids in late gestation attempt to maintain their salt and water balance by a compensatory reduction in renal sodium excretion. The decrease in fetal renal sodium excretion, however, accounted for only about 11% of total sodium conservation; the rest of the compensation was achieved by the mother.[39]

All of these observations can be regarded as strong evidence that the fetal sodium and volume homeostasis is effectively regulated and when challenged by depletion or loading fetomaternal control mechanisms comes into operation to restore volume and salt balance to normal. The control of fetal homeostatic mechanisms operating to limit or enhance salt and fluid flux across the kidney or fetal membrane barriers has not been clearly defined. However, there have been reports that in addition to the traditional volume regulatory hormones, prolactin plays an important role. Namely, fetal prolactin has been shown to be released in response to increasing cord serum sodium concentration and osmolality. Fetal prolactin in turn has a significant positive correlation with AF sodium concentration and osmolality but an inverse relationship with AF volume, suggesting the suppression of hypotonic fetal urine excretion.[40] The additional roles of maternal and AF prolactin, derived from maternal decidua in fetal-AF salt and water balance, have also been proposed.[41] In good agreement with these findings, we have demonstrated significantly elevated plasma prolactin levels in full-term newborn infants presenting with idiopathic edema[42] and an increase in plasma prolactin in sodium-depleted low birth weight (LBW) premature infants and its restoration to normal levels when supplemental sodium was given.[43]

Body Water Compartments and Initial Weight Loss

Soon after birth, redistribution of body fluid compartments occurs, which is a subject of controversy. Most authors agree that early postnatal weight loss corresponds to the isotonic contraction of ECW and the disposal of excess sodium and water through the kidney.[44] It is greater and lasts longer in infants with less advanced maturation.[45] The weight loss and the contraction of ECW is a physiologic adaptation to extrauterine life rather than dehydration or starvation, in as much as body solids increase and nitrogen balance is positive during the period of weight loss. Longitudinal studies to assess changes in body composition of preterm neonates with and without respiratory distress syndrome (RDS) during the immediate postnatal period support this notion. Providing adequate nutritional support, postnatal weight loss and loss of TBW is accompanied by a steady increase in the accretion of body solids. The rate of increase, however, proved to be greater in healthy preterm infants than in those with RDS.[46] Contrasting reports have been published by others showing some evidence for tissue catabolism and for failure to gain solids.[47-49]

In addition to renal excretion, a fluid "shift" from ECW to ICW has also been described, but this is more likely a result of ECW loss than growth in cell mass.[50]

In LBW premature infants, the initial weight loss of 15% or more is confined to the extravascular ECW. Plasma volume remains unchanged, and there are no clinical signs of dehydration or hypovolemic circulatory failure. Plasma protein levels that would reflect a shift in oncotic pressure differences favoring water loss from interstitium into the vascular space do not change.[51]

It has recently been shown that the interstitium has its own regulation; its volume and sodium content are controlled by local, tissue-specific molecular mechanisms. In animals on high-salt diets, tissue sodium is bound to glycosaminoglycans (GAGs) and stored in the skin interstitium in excess of water. The water-free sodium fraction generates local hypertonicity, which initiates regulatory cascade, including macrophage-driven and tonicity-responsive enhancer binding protein (TonEBP), and VEGF-C–mediated hyperplasia of lymphocapillary network. The expanded subcutaneous lymphatic system collects tissue fluid from the interstitial extracellular space and drains sodium and water back to the circulation.[52] This mechanism may also be implicated in the selective reduction of the interstitium that occurs in early postnatal life because all elements of the system are present in the neonatal tissues. The GAG content of the immature skin is particularly elevated, which can bind and store sodium and can increase local tonicity. A compromised function of this local regulatory pathway may result in retention of interstitial fluid and persistent expansion of ECF compartment with related morbidities.

Renal salt wasting and hyponatremia during early postnatal weight loss in LBW prematures is not compatible with isotonic contraction of ECW; rather, it indicates that these infants are not capable of maintaining the volume of their ECW within the physiologic limits.

Cheek[53] has developed the concept that there was a significant decrease in cell water content rather than in ECW during the first days of life. MacLaurin,[54] using thiocyanate as a marker for ECW, identified ICW as the source of neonatal water loss. In this study, ICW fell in parallel with TBW, ECW rose slightly, and plasma volume remained constant. He argued that ECW is more effectively maintained than ICW during adaptation to early extrauterine life. In good agreement with these observations, Coulter and Avery[55] demonstrated a paradoxical reduction in hydration of fat-free body mass (mL water/100 g fat-free body mass) in neonatal rabbit pups, which correlated with increasing weight gain during the first 72 hours of life. The extent of relative reduction in tissue water varied considerably among individual tissues; the greatest losses were observed in the skin (24%) and skeletal muscle (5%–8%). Whereas lean body mass and skin and skeletal muscle water related inversely to weight gain and fluid intake, the liver and brain related directly. Based on these findings, the authors concluded that there is an ICW reservoir located mainly in the skin and muscle from which water is released in a regulated manner according to the actual need. Thus, when sufficient fluid intake is provided, the superfluous ICW is rapidly released and excreted. However, when fluid intake is restricted, the release is considerably slower and contributes to maintaining circulating plasma volume.[55]

The mechanisms triggering and controlling the process of initial weight loss have not been clearly established. Recently, it has been proposed that the postnatal decrease in pulmonary vascular resistance and the subsequent increase of left atrial return result in the release of atrial natriuretic peptide (ANP), which induces sodium chloride and water diuresis.[56,57] However, plasma ANP does not correlate with either urinary flow rate or urinary sodium excretion.[58]

Physical Water Compartments

To reconcile the apparently conflicting views on the source of neonatal water loss, a concept has been recently put forward implying that not only the compartmentalization but also the mobility of tissue water is of importance in neonatal body fluid redistribution. Accordingly, motionally distinct water fractions have been established—the free bulky water and the relatively constrained, slow-motion bound water. From this latter fraction, water can be liberated in a regulated manner according to the actual need of volume regulation irrespective of its location in the cellular or extracellular phase.[59]

The Principle of Physical Water Compartments

The term *physical water compartments* designates the physical state of tissue water and implies interactions between dipole water molecules and tissue biopolymers, including proteins and GAGs. The interaction of the polar solid surface of intra- or extracellular macromolecules with water results in the formation of the dynamic structure of polarized water multilayer. The degree of water polarization depends on the number of exposed active, polar groups of the water-polarizing macromolecules. The first oriented layer of water molecules on the surfaces can induce a second layer to orient, the second will likewise influence the third, and so on. As a result, a picture of hydrophilic surfaces bounded by a coat of structured water emerges. The range of interactions generating the polarized water multilayer has been variously suggested extending from nanometers to several micrometers. With respect to the electrical polarization and spatial orientation of tissue water, intra- and extracellular macromolecules therefore create microcompartments with different size and stability. The extent of water polarization is assumed to be proportional to the limitation of tissue water mobility.[60,61]

Determination of Motionally Distinct Water Fractions

Proton nuclear magnetic resonance (H^1-NMR) measurements have been applied to assess quantitative changes in tissue water mobility because they provide an estimate of the physical state of tissue water, including volume fraction, proton residence time, and intrinsic magnetic relaxation rate within the compartments. The theoretical basis for this estimate is that the magnetic relaxation rates for ordered (bound) water protons are faster than those for non-ordered (free) water protons. For quantitative assessment of tissue water fractions with different mobility, multicomponent analysis of the T_2 relaxation decay curves has been applied.[62]

Physical Water Compartments during the Early Postnatal Period

In a series of recent studies, we attempted to quantitate the free and bound water fractions in the skin, skeletal muscle, brain, and liver of two groups of newborn rabbits during the first 3 to 4 days of life. Rabbit pups of one group were nursed conventionally by their mothers, suckling ad libitum, and the other group included pups separated from their mothers and completely withheld from fluid intake.[59]

Biexponential analysis of the T_2 relaxation curves revealed that the bound water fractions amounted to 42% to 47% in the skin, 50% to 57% in the muscle, and 34% to 40% in the liver, respectively, of the total tissue water. This pattern of distribution did not change either with age or fluid intake. By contrast, the percent contribution of bound water fraction in the brain fell progressively from 61% at birth to 3% to 4% at the age of 72 to 96 hours. In response to complete fluid deprival, the reduction of bound water fraction was accelerated to attain a value of as low as 4% already on the first day of life.

Using triexponential analysis, we found that most of the skin (48%–64%) and muscle water (54%–64%) is loosely bound followed by the free (skin, 26%–45%; muscle, 25%–32%) and tightly bound water fractions (skin: 6%–14%; muscle, 10%–16%). Postnatal age and fluid intake had no apparent influence on this pattern of partition. In the brain, loosely bound water (48%–94%) also predominated over the free (3%–49%) and tightly bound water fraction (3%–29%). Starving pups responded to fluid deprivation with a three- to sixfold decrease in the tightly bound water and with a simultaneous fourfold increase in the free water fractions.

The postnatal increase of the free water fraction can be regarded as supportive evidence for restructuring brain water to maintain brain volume.

The different water mobility in individual newborn rabbit tissues and its response pattern to complete withdrawal of fluid intake appear to be the result of the differences in water content, water-free chemical composition, qualitative or quantitative alterations in macromolecular compounds, and metabolic activity of the tissues investigated.

Role of Hyaluronan in the Perinatal Lung and Brain Water Metabolism

Hyaluronan (HA), with its polyanionic nature and gel-like properties, has been claimed to be the major macromolecular compound controlling water mobility and water balance in the lung.[63] During the fetal and neonatal periods, HA concentration in the lung tissue is elevated and inversely proportional to the maturity of the neonate. Its role as a determinant of tissue water content during pulmonary adaptation has been established.[64]

Recently, parameters of lung water metabolism and lung HA concentrations have been studied simultaneously in the late fetal and early postnatal periods. It has been demonstrated that whereas that the T_2-derived free water fraction increased, the bound water fraction decreased progressively with advancing maturation. HA correlated positively with total lung water but not with the bound water fraction. The elimination of lung fluid, therefore, is associated with an increase in free water at the expense of bound water fraction.

The underlying mechanisms of the release of water molecules from macromolecular bindings remain to be established as HA does not appear to be directly involved in this process.[65]

Parameters of brain water metabolism and brain HA concentration undergo similar developmental changes. With increasing maturation, the motionally constrained bound water is restructured to freely moving water fraction, and it proves to be independent of total brain water and tissue HA content.[66]

On the basis of these observations, one can conclude that in addition to the well-defined channel-mediated water transport and a reduction in ECW, the redistribution of the bound to free water fraction is an important but still unappreciated mechanism of the physiologic dehydration of immature lung and brain.

Role of Hyaluronan in Neonatal Renal Concentration

The possible involvement of renal papillary HA in renal water handling has also been proposed. A large amount of HA is accumulated in the inner medulla and papilla that limits water flow by influencing interstitial hydrostatic pressure.[67]

Inducing water diuresis by increased body hydration results in elevated HA content in renal papilla, but opposite changes are seen after water deprivation. As a result, renal papillary HA positively correlates with urine flow rate, and there is an inverse relationship of papillary HA to urine osmolality. These findings support the notion that increased papillary interstitial HA can antagonize renal tubular water reabsorption.[68]

In the light of these observations, it is relevant to postulate that the impaired concentration performance of the immature kidney can be accounted for, not only by the decreased corticopapillary osmotic gradient and diminished renal tubular responsiveness to arginine vasopressin (AVP), but also by the markedly elevated HA content-related limited water flow in the neonatal renal papilla. This additional mechanism may be of great importance in neonatal adaptation when excess water needs to be excreted.[69]

Sodium Homeostasis

Sodium chloride balance is normally maintained by renal sodium conservation and excretion over a broad range of intakes. Newborn infants are limited in conserving sodium when challenged by sodium restriction and in excreting sodium when challenged by a sodium load.

Renal Sodium Excretion under Basal Conditions

In the first week of life, urinary sodium excretion and fractional sodium excretion, in particular, are high and are inversely proportional to the maturity of the neonate[70-74] (Fig. 3-2). Premature infants of less than 35 weeks' gestation have an obligatory sodium loss with subsequent negative sodium balance, which is believed to be a physiologic measure for adjustments to extrauterine existence. It is assumed

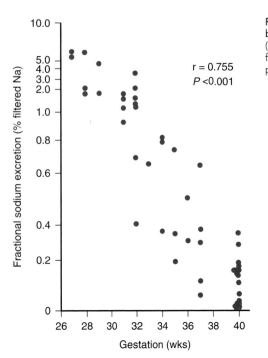

Figure 3-2 Scattergram showing the inverse correlation between fractional sodium excretion and gestational age. (From Siegel BR, Oh W. Renal function as a marker of human fetal maturation. *Acta Paediatr Scand.* 1976;65:481-485, with permission.)

r = 0.755

P <0.001

to result from isotonic contraction of expanded ECW present at birth and the disposal of excess extracellular sodium through the kidney. This concept has been supported by the observation that the practice of giving a high fluid and sodium intake to replace water and sodium loss was associated with an increased incidence of patent ductus arteriosus (PDA), cardiac failure, bronchopulmonary dysplasia (BPD), necrotizing enterocolitis (NEC), and intracranial hemorrhage (ICH), all conditions known to relate to fluid overload and protracted expansion of ECW.

Tang et al[46] have shown that loss of body water after birth occurs to the same extent in healthy preterm infants and in babies with RDS and is unrelated to the volume of fluid administered.

Bell and Acarregui[75] reviewed the results of randomized trials on water restriction and BPD and concluded that although there is a trend for lower incidence of BPD in preterm infants who received restricted fluid intake during the first days of life, the difference is not statistically significant. Based on the result of this meta-analysis, the most prudent prescription for water intake to premature infants seems to be careful restriction of water intake so that physiologic needs are met without allowing significant dehydration.

Recently, Oh et al[76] demonstrated that higher fluid intake and less weight loss during the first 10 days of life were associated with an increased risk of BPD.

Sodium, along with chloride concentration in plasma, often falls to low levels, and urinary sodium excretion remains high relative to plasma sodium. It has become apparent, therefore, that the redistribution of body fluid compartments alone does not account for the high rate of urinary sodium excretion, but rather may be caused by renal immaturity.[77-79]

This contention is supported by the gestational age-related changes in sodium balance and in the activity of the renin–angiotensin–aldosterone system (RAAS) in 1-week-old newborn infants with gestational ages of 31 to 41 weeks. It has been demonstrated that in response to renal salt wasting and to the subsequent negative sodium balance, premature infants augmented their plasma renin activity above values found for full-term infants. Plasma renin activity correlated positively with urinary sodium excretion, but negatively with sodium balance. Plasma aldosterone concentration did not change with gestational age; urinary aldosterone excretion, however, increased steadily as the gestation advanced. The clear dissociation between

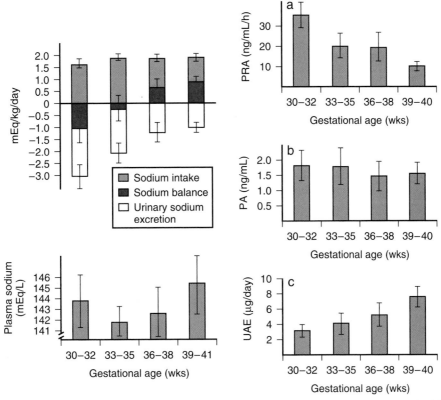

Figure 3-3 Sodium balance and the activity of the renin-angiotensin-aldosterone system in 1-week-old newborn infants with gestational ages of 30 to 41 weeks. PA, plasma aldosterone concentration; PRA, plasma renin activity; UAE, urinary aldosterone excretion. (From Sulyok E, Németh M, Tényi J, et al. Relationship between maturity, electrolyte balance and the function of the renin-angiotension-aldosterone system in newborn infants. *Biol Neonate*. 1979;35:60-65, with permission.)

plasma renin activity and aldosterone status strongly suggests that the adrenal glands of premature infants do not respond adequately to stimulation in the first week of life. Urinary aldosterone excretion was found to relate inversely to renal sodium excretion, but directly to sodium balance (Fig. 3-3). These findings indicate that the improvement of renal sodium conservation and establishment of positive sodium balance with increasing maturation is causally related to aldosterone secretion and/ or renal tubular aldosterone reactivity.[80]

Clinical and experimental studies attempting to define the nephron segments responsible for urinary sodium loss indicate that the higher fractional sodium excretion in premature infants is caused by deficient proximal and distal tubular reabsorption of sodium. With advancing gestational and postnatal ages, significant improvement occurs in renal sodium conservation.[81,82]

Aldosterone-mediated distal reabsorption improves more rapidly to keep up with the sodium load presented to this nephron site.[83,84] According to the concept of glomerulotubular imbalance, there is a morphologic and functional preponderance of glomeruli to proximal tubules in immature nephrons. Consequently, it is argued that a greater fraction of glomerular filtrate escapes proximal tubular reabsorption.[85,86]

Indeed, in the neonatal kidney, the volume of proximal tubules (the membrane area available for reabsorption), the net oncotic pressure favoring reabsorption and the capacity of transporters involved in active sodium reabsorption are reduced.[87-89]

It is of note, however, that the distal nephron also exhibits immature sodium transport characteristics consisting of high passive permeability, low baseline active transport, and mineralocorticoid unresponsiveness with low density and activity of aplical Na^+ channels.[90,91]

Molecular Basis of Proximal Tubular Sodium Reabsorption

The sodium transporting capacity of the proximal tubule undergoes maturational changes. Most of the luminal sodium uptake is mediated by the NHE via electroneutral exchange of extracellular Na^+ for intracellular H^+. The NHEs are a widely distributed family of transport proteins containing six members (NHE 1–6). They have 10–12-transmembrane spanning domains with an intracellular C-terminal region. Their amino acid sequences show 45% to 65% homology. The six isoforms vary in terms of cellular location to the apical or basolateral membrane, amiloride sensitivity, and mode of regulation.[92]

NHE3, which predominantly mediates sodium-dependent apical proton secretion in the proximal tubules, is stimulated by the low intracellular sodium generated and maintained by basolateral Na^+, K^+-ATPase. Membrane vesicles isolated from animals at different stages of maturation and in vitro microperfusion studies using neonatal juxtamedullary proximal convoluted tubules have shown a lower rate of bicarbonate transport, decreased Na^+, K^+-ATPase, and NHE activity in immature compared with mature animals.[88,89,93]

The postnatal maturation of NHE and the subsequent improvement of bicarbonate transport may be accelerated by adrenocortical steroid stimulation of either NHE and Na^+, K^+-ATPase or direct, receptor-mediated angiotensin II stimulation of NHE. More recently, parallel maturation of apical NHE activity, NHE3 mRNA expression, and NHE3 protein levels has been demonstrated, which can be accelerated with glucocorticoids in newborn rabbits but not with angiotensin II in fetal sheep.[94,95] Furthermore, thyroid hormones and the surge in circulating catecholamine levels and increased sympathetic nerve activity at birth have also been claimed to enhance NHE activity.[96,97]

Because glucocorticoids upregulate α-adrenergic receptor mRNA expression in proximal tubules, glucocorticoids may also potentiate the effect of catecholamines to increase NHE activity.[98] On the other hand, dopamine inhibits NHE-mediated sodium uptake by proximal tubule segments and tonic inhibition of fetal proximal tubular NHE activity by dopamine has been documented.[99]

It is of note that the progressive increase in renal Na^+-H^+ exchange with advancing gestational and postnatal age was described long before the discovery of the NHE system.[100]

Another way for sodium entry into the proximal tubular cells is the sodium-dependent phosphate co-transport system (Na-Pi). The transport is electrogenic and involves the co-transport of three sodium ions and one phosphate anion. Three distinct isoforms of mammalian Na-Pi (1–3) have been identified. All are expressed in the proximal tubule cells, but Na-Pi2 is exclusively located in the brush-border membrane and has a predominant role in proximal tubular Pi reabsorption. It has been documented that the transport rates of Na-Pi were substantially higher in brush-border membrane vesicles obtained from newborns than those from adults. The high transport capacity of the Na-Pi co-transport system in the newborn kidney, however, is associated with low adaptability to changes in dietary Pi intake. Interestingly, the expression of the Na-Pi mRNA levels in newborns was similar or lower than those in adult rats, suggesting that the increased protein levels and activity of the co-transporter early in life may be accounted for by posttranscriptional regulation. PTH has been shown to inhibit, but growth hormone and insulin-like growth factor increase the Na-Pi-mediated sodium and phosphate uptake.[101]

Sodium uptake by the proximal tubule cells can also be achieved by Na–amino acid and Na-glucose co-transporters located in the brush-border membrane. Sodium-coupled amino acid and glucose transport are developmentally regulated having low activity during the fetal and neonatal period followed by a steady increase as the maturation progresses. The limited co-transport of Na with amino acids and glucose is responsible for the low threshold of amino acid and glucose reabsorption and contributes to the generalized aminoaciduria and glucosuria frequently seen in early life. On the other hand, it appears to constrain quantitatively important Na influx into the brush-border membrane vesicles, thereby diminishing proximal tubular sodium reabsorption.[102]

Molecular Basis of Distal Tubular Sodium Reabsorption

There have been several reports to reveal developmental regulation of sodium transport in the cortical collecting duct (CCD), a nephron segment that plays an important role in determining sodium excretion in the final urine. Vehaskari,[90] using isolated perfused rabbit CCD at three different postnatal ages, has found that the maturation of sodium transport occurs in two stages: first the high passive sodium permeability decreases to mature levels during the first 2 weeks of life followed by the second stage, an increase in active transport capacity and simultaneous development of mineralocorticoid responsiveness. Vehaskari[90] assumed that the immaturity of active sodium transport may be attributed to intracellular mechanisms that limit transcellular sodium flux. These may include (1) incomplete polarization of the principal cells, (2) decreased basolateral Na^+, K^+-ATPase activity, (3) decreased apical Na permeability caused by a decreased number of Na channels, and (4) decreased conductance of the existing channels.

The amiloride-sensitive ENaC is made of three homologous subunits, named α, β, and γ ENaC. The α-ENaC subunit expressed alone is for channel function and can drive sodium absorption. The β and γ subunits have been demonstrated to stabilize the channel and to allow proper insertion into the membrane. The expression of the three subunits together induces a multiple increase in the amiloride-sensitive sodium flux compared with the α-ENaC alone.[103] The expression profile of α-ENaC mRNA is very similar to that of α_1 Na^+, K^+-ATPase mRNA, a constituent of the sodium pump involved in active transepithelial sodium transport. During gestation, there is a gradual rise in the renal expression of both α-ENaC and α_1 Na^+, K^+-ATPase mRNA, which reaches a plateau after birth. Furthermore, α-ENaC mRNA correlates directly with α_1 Na^+, K^+-ATPase mRNA, suggesting that the renal expression of these transporters is regulated by common factors during the perinatal period.[104]

Further studies to explore the cellular mechanisms of the limitation of active sodium transport in the distal nephron have shown that in microdissected rat nephron segments all three ENaC mRNA subunits were exclusively detected from the distal convoluted tubule to the outer medullary collecting duct. The levels of their expression, however, proved to be very low during the late fetal period, but they increased rapidly to reach adult level within 24 to 72 hours after birth. The authors have suggested that the low ENaC subunit gene expression is a potentially limiting factor in Na transport in the very immature kidney only; impaired translation or impaired targeted trafficking of the channel protein may also be implicated.[105]

As channel proteins are redistributed to the apical membrane, they undergo hormone-dependent processing, which includes proteolytic cleavage and further glycosylation of the channel subunits.[106] These biochemical pathways may be compromised in the perinatal period and may limit the accumulation of mature channel protein at the apical surface.

To get some more insight into the underlying mechanisms of the low net sodium absorption by the developing CCD, intensive research has been performed on the apical membrane ion conductance and channel expression during the late fetal and early postnatal period. It has been clearly demonstrated that the low rate of sodium absorption in the early neonatal period can be attributed to the paucity of conducting apical ENaCs in principal cells of the CCD and to the lower open probability of these channels in the first week than later after the second week of life.[107]

A markedly increased abundance of the transcripts of all three ENaC subunits has been observed in the last 3 to 4 days of fetal life in rats. After birth, only modest changes could be detected with increasing α and decreasing β and γ subunits. Interestingly, as the kidney matures, the expression of the ENaC subunits is redistributed from the inner medullary collecting duct to the CCD.[108]

The perinatal upregulation of ENaC activity appears to be related to the perinatal surge of adrenocortical steroid hormones because the trend and time course of the two events run parallel. In contrast to this notion, the developmental expression of the three subunits of ENaC did not differ between corticotropin-releasing hormone knockout mice and wild-type animals, indicating that the endogenous corticosteroids have no influence on the perinatal expression of ENaC. Interestingly, exogenous, synthetic glucocorticoids (dexamethasone) significantly enhanced prenatal expression of α subunit but did not affect the expression of β and γ subunits of renal ENaC.[109]

The different response is assumed to be the result of metabolization of the endogenous glucocorticoids by the kidney. In fact, abundant 11 β-HSD2 mRNA expression has been noted in fetal mouse kidney, so it is relevant to suggest that this enzyme inactivates endogenous glucocorticoids and by co-localizing with MRs is involved in protecting steroid receptors and in controlling glucocorticoid action in developing renal tissues.[110]

In a comprehensive study, Martinerie et al[111] made an attempt to characterize the developmental pattern of the expression of MR isoforms, 11 β-HSD2 and α-ENaC, the key players of the mineralocorticoid signaling pathway in murine and human kidneys. During renal development, a biphasic temporal expression of MR was demonstrated with a transient peak between 15 and 24 weeks of gestation followed by low MR expression in late gestational and neonatal kidney and a progressive increase thereafter. This cyclic MR expression was tightly correlated with the evolution of 11-β-HSD2 and α-ENaC, implying that the low renal MR expression at around birth may be involved in renal tubular unresponsiveness to aldosterone and compromised sodium handling by the immature kidney.[111]

In addition to the ENaC expression, the ontogenetic expression patterns of other sodium transport proteins have also been examined to define the sodium entry pathways during nephrogenesis. Using high-resolution histochemical techniques and in situ hybridization, these transport proteins have been found to begin to be expressed in early nascent tubular segments. Along with the structural differentiation and segmental specialization of this distal nephron, cells committed to active sodium transport exhibit transporters, including bumetanide-sensitive Na^+, K^+, $2Cl^-$ co-transporter, Na-Cl co-transporter, and Na/Ca exchanger.[112] The physiologic significance of the transcription of these transport proteins early during development, before the excretory function of the kidney is established, needs to be defined.

Other Factors Influencing Renal Sodium Handling

In addition to renal immaturity, any increase in glomerular filtration rate (GFR), urine output, and fractional sodium excretion contributes to renal salt wasting. Lorenz et al[113] identified three distinct phases of fluid and electrolyte homeostasis in LBW premature infants with or without RDS during the first days of life. The low urine output of the first day (prediuretic phase) is followed by spontaneous diuresis and natriuresis during the second and third days independent of fluid intake (diuretic phase). The onset, duration, and extent of diuresis appear to be variable. The high rate of urine flow and sodium excretions is assumed to be the result of abrupt increases of GFR and fractional sodium excretion subsequent to the reabsorption of residual fetal lung fluid and expansion of extracellular space. During the postdiuretic phase, GFR remains unchanged, and urine flow and sodium excretion decrease to values intermediate between those observed in the prediuretic and diuretic phases and begin to vary appropriately in response to changes in fluid intake.[113,114]

Premature infants receiving a high intravenous (IV) fluid load have a high renal sodium loss and an exaggerated sodium deficit. To maintain sodium balance and normal plasma sodium level with IV infusions, sodium and fluid intake should be restricted or extra sodium should be given.

Bueva and Guignard[115] also concluded that by providing restricted fluid intake with low sodium (1–2 mEq/kg/day), premature infants with birth weights of 1000 to 1500 g have fractional sodium excretion not higher than 2.2% and are able to maintain sodium balance. In this group of preterm neonates, plasma sodium concentration, however, fell to a level of 132 mEq/L at postnatal age of 15 to 16 days. In their view, the high rate of sodium excretion is iatrogenic in nature and may be caused by the liberal fluid intake. The concept, therefore, that salt wasting in preterm neonates is the result of renal immaturity and NaCl supplement should be given to prevent or correct sodium depletion is wrong. In their study, fluid intake was 80 mL/kg on the first day and then increased by 20 mL/kg/day to reach 150 mL/kg/day by the end of the first week.

More recently, Delgado et al[116] conducted a longitudinal prospective study of very LBW (VLBW) premature infants with gestational ages of 23 to 31 weeks to measure parameters of sodium balance weekly for 5 weeks. Fluid intake did not exceed 150 mL/kg/day in any gestational and postnatal age group, and sodium intake was also kept at a relatively low level of less than 4 mEq/kg/day. An inverse relationship was found between fractional sodium excretion and gestational age, and fractional sodium excretion fell progressively in each age group with increasing postnatal age (Fig. 3-4). A state of positive sodium balance was not consistently detected until after approximately 32 weeks of gestational age. Unfortunately, the postnatal course of plasma sodium was not presented, but the unique value of this report is the measurement of α-ENaC mRNA expression in human kidney homogenates obtained from fetuses of 20 to 36 weeks' gestation. Most importantly, they could demonstrate for the first time the developmental regulation of the expression of α-ENaC, the channel protein that mediates the final excretion of sodium during gestation in humans. They identified a significant increase of approximately 25% in α-ENaC mRNA abundance between 20 and 36 weeks of gestational age.

This study is of primary importance to underscore that inefficient sodium handling is an intrinsic feature of the immature kidney, albeit variations in sodium and fluid intake may modify the rate of urinary sodium excretion and subsequently the sodium balance.

Because the current clinical practice of fluid management of LBW premature infants is quite variable, it is imperative to establish clinical and laboratory parameters that dictate sodium and water intake to meet the optimal needs of infants at various gestational and postnatal ages.

Several approaches have been applied to assess liberal or restricted fluid therapy including determination of urine flow rate; osmolality and sodium excretion; body weight changes with or without plasma sodium levels; and measurements of ECW, TBW, and body solids. Occasionally, hormone parameters controlling salt and water balance have also been determined. Another approach is to relate fluid therapy to the incidence, severity, and mortality of neonatal pathologies known to be associated with fluid overload. Using different approaches, different conclusions could be drawn. However, by integrating the available data, a unified concept may emerge that could be considered for planning neonatal fluid therapy.

However, the renal responses to variations in sodium and water intake are often unpredictable; therefore, individualized fluid and electrolyte therapy is needed (Table 3-2).

Renal Sodium Excretion in Response to Salt Loading

The renal response of the newborn to salt loading is blunted compared with that of the adult. Low GFR is a limiting factor, although the difference in sodium excretory response between newborns and adults still exists when correction is made for GFR. Studies using free water clearance and the technique of distal nephron blockade have identified the distal nephron as the site where fractional sodium reabsorption increases as development proceeds.[117,118]

The augmented distal tubular sodium transport is assumed to be mediated by the high concentration of plasma aldosterone. This assumption is supported by the diminished response of the renin-angiotensin-aldosterone (RAAS) to suppression by volume expansion with isotonic saline infusion.[119] However, in newborn dogs, most of the increase in sodium load to the distal nephron, which occurs during NaCl expansion, is reabsorbed in the thick ascending limb of the loop of Henle, and it is independent of aldosterone stimulation.[120]

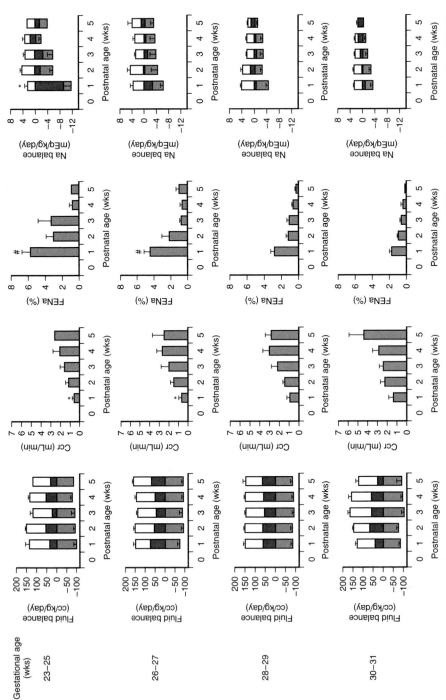

Figure 3-4 Gestational and postnatal age-related changes in fluid balance, creatinine clearance (CCr), fractional sodium excretion (FENa), and sodium balance in premature infants of 23 to 31 weeks' gestation during the first 5 weeks of life. (From Delgado MM, Rohatgi R, Khan S, et al. Sodium and potassium clearances by the maturing kidney: clinical-molecular correlates. *Pediatr Nephrol.* 2003;18:759-767, with permission.)

Table 3-2 DAILY TOTAL FLUID INTAKE IN PREMATURE INFANTS WITH BIRTH WEIGHT LESS THAN 1500 G DURING THE FIRST 10 DAYS OF LIFE (ML/KG)*

			Neonatal Research Network			
			BPD-Free Survivors		Death or BPD	
Age (days)	Iowa	Lausanne	Intake (mL/kg/day)	Weight Loss (%)	Intake (mL/kg/day)	Weight Loss (%)
1	65–75	80	No data		No data	
2	75–80	100	118	0.4	136	0.1
3	90–95	120	134	3.8	158	2.8
4		140	147	7.3	170	6.7
5		150	154	9.7	171	8.1
6		150	157	8.7	169	7.4
7	120–130	150	156	8.1	165	6.3
8	130	150	153	6.4	163	4.7
9	130	150	152	4.7	159	3.3
10	≈135	150	150	3.1	158	1.8

*Initial weight loss of no more than 12% to 15% of birth weight was allowed. In the Neonatal Research Network, the study subjects had mean birth weight and gestational age of 736 g and 25.4 weeks in the bronchopulmonary dysplasia (BPD) group and 815 g and 26.7 weeks in the BPD-free survivors group.
Adapted from Bell EF, Acarregui MJ. Restricted versus liberal water intake for preventing morbidity and mortality in preterm infants. *Cochrane Database Syst Rev.* 2001;(1):CD000503; Bueva A, Guignard J-P. Renal function in preterm neonates. *Pediatr Res.* 1994;36:572-577; and Oh W, Poindexter BB, Perritt R, et al. Association between fluid intake and weight loss during the first ten days of life and risk of bronchopulmonary dysplasia in extremely low birth weight infants. *J Pediatr.* 2005;147:786-790.

When a dose of 0.12 g/kg NaCl is administered orally to premature and term neonates during the first week of life, a significantly higher natriuretic response occurs in premature infants of 29 to 35 weeks' gestation than in term infants. When the natriuretic response to salt challenge is followed in a premature infant until its expected term, the response diminishes to a value characteristic for term neonates. However, the renal capacity to excrete a sodium load is still much lower in premature infants than in children 8 to 14 years of age.[72,121]

The postnatal development of the natriuretic response to salt challenge is accelerated by dietary manipulation. Chronic sodium loading augmented a natriuretic response to acute volume expansion in pre-weaned rats, but the renal response is incomplete and independent of GFR and plasma ANP levels.[122]

Infants receiving a high-salt diet before being given a salt load have a greater capacity to excrete sodium than those on a low-salt diet. In some studies, sodium is more rapidly excreted when given as $NaHCO_3$ than as NaCl. Others have found no difference in the rate of excretion of sodium as bicarbonate versus sodium as chloride in response to loading doses in the dog. However, the mechanism of natriuresis is probably different. With sodium chloride loading, sodium delivered to the distal nephron is reabsorbed with chloride in the thick ascending limb of Henle loop, but with sodium bicarbonate loading, sodium is reabsorbed in the late distal and cortical collecting tubules in exchange for potassium and H^+.[123]

It is of interest that bicarbonate excretion appears to be largely independent of sodium excretion during the period of spontaneous diuresis. Bicarbonate is effectively retained, and the major anion accompanying excreted sodium is chloride, not bicarbonate.[124]

Intestinal Sodium Transport

Sodium absorption from the gastrointestinal tract is efficient. Fecal sodium excretion is usually less than 10% of the intake in VLBW premature infants and does not vary significantly with age over the period of 2 to 7 postnatal weeks.[78]

Al-Dahhan et al,[125] investigating the development of intestinal sodium handling, report that stool sodium loss correlates inversely with postconceptional age and parallels urinary sodium excretion, although at much lower absolute values. By contrast, experimental evidence suggests that amiloride-sensitive, electrogenic sodium absorption in the distal colon is more efficient in newborn than in adult rabbits, and it is assumed to be accounted for by the high circulating aldosterone levels in neonates.[126]

Studies on the ontogeny of colonic sodium transport in early childhood have shown the highest sodium absorption rate in preterm infants with gestational ages of 30 to 33 weeks. This decreases in parallel with the decrease of plasma aldosterone as gestational and postnatal ages advance. It has been postulated, therefore, that the maturation of colonic sodium absorption precedes that of the renal tubular sodium reabsorption, and it functions as a major self-conserving mechanism that counterbalances urinary sodium loss.[127]

Disturbances in Plasma Sodium Concentrations

Early-Onset Hyponatremia

Hyponatremia (plasma sodium <130 mEq/L) occurring in the first week of life is designated as an early type of hyponatremia. It is attributed to water retention, but sodium depletion may also contribute. It occurs in association with excessive free water infusion into the mother with perinatal pathology causing non-osmotic release of antidiuretic hormone[128] and with salt-restricted parenteral fluid regimen.[129]

Placental permeability to sodium in human fetuses increases as gestation progresses so that free water is more readily retained early than late in gestation.[130]

Infants born to mothers on a diet deficient in sodium are also at risk for early hyponatremia.[131]

Late-Onset Hyponatremia

This is usually the result of a combination of inadequate sodium intake, renal salt wasting, and free water retention. Accordingly, its incidence, severity, and duration are influenced by the maturity of the neonate and the feeding protocol applied. In the early study by Roy et al,[79] when fluid intake was liberal (150–200 mL/kg/day) and only 1.6 m/Eq/kg/day sodium was given, late hyponatremia occurred in 30% to 40% of VLBW infants (Fig. 3-5). When the daily sodium intake was increased to 3 mEq/kg/day, late hyponatremia was reduced to less than 10% and was practically eliminated when sodium intake was further increased.[78,79]

Shaffer and Meade[132] observed lower plasma sodium concentration in infants receiving 1 mEq/kg/day than in those receiving 3 mEq/kg/day sodium over 30 days; however, the pattern of sodium balance remained similar.

Lorenz et al[133] maintained plasma sodium in the normal range when they administered a low-sodium intake (≈1 m/Eq/kg/day) and restricted fluid (60–80 mL/kg/day), resulting in a weight loss of 13% to 15%. This approach tested the hypothesis that hyponatremia is accounted for mainly by the high-volume formula intake, natriuresis, and associated water retention. These authors conclude that given the lack of adverse effects of their low sodium and free water regimen and the absence of hyponatremia, this regimen was appropriate for VLBW infants. They concluded that no sodium supplement is needed.

Costarino et al[129] compared a salt-restricted parenteral fluid regimen with a sodium-supplemented maintenance regimen (3–4 mEq/kg/day) for the treatment of extremely LBW (ELBW) infants during the first 5 days of life. Whereas maintenance sodium intake resulted in a nearly zero sodium balance, sodium-restricted infants continued to excrete urinary sodium at a high rate, which promoted more negative balance. No differences were noted between the two groups in urine output, GFR, urinary sodium excretion, and osmolar clearance. However, serum sodium concentrations were significantly higher in maintenance infants than in restriction infants despite the increased fluid intake in the former. Clinical outcome was not affected by sodium intake except for the lower incidence of BPD in the sodium-restricted

Figure 3-5 Postnatal course of plasma Na⁺, K⁺, and Cl⁻ concentrations in very low birth weight infants. Admission (Adm.) specimen is the baseline specimen at a mean age of 18 days. (From Day GM, Radde IC, Balfe JW, Chance GW. Electrolyte abnormalities in very low birth weight infants. *Pediatr Res.* 1976;10:522-526, with permission.)

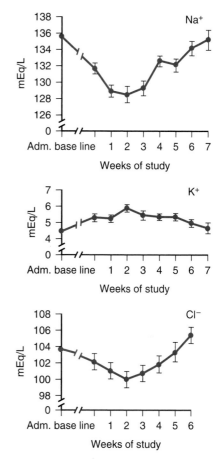

group. The authors conclude that sodium intake should be restricted and the least amount of IV fluid should be provided to maintain serum sodium concentration in the normal range. However, their study was limited to the first week of life, and the authors did not obtain reliable information toward defining sodium requirements during the second and third weeks, a period of rapid growth, when late hyponatremia develops. In fact, longitudinal studies reveal that preterm infants on a low-sodium diet, who have renal salt wasting, sustain a protracted sodium loss. In this setting, limiting water intake does not address the sodium deficit; it aggravates volume depletion.

The study by Wilkins[134] argues against sodium restriction; LBW infants excreted excessive amounts of sodium and severe sodium depletion developed during the first 2 weeks regardless of plasma sodium concentration. However, after some initial increase, plasma sodium decreased progressively and often culminated in profound and prolonged hyponatremia.

Interestingly, Shaffer et al[135] noted late hyponatremia in association with reduced ECW in six of 18 infants who were born at 32 weeks' gestational age. This finding indicates that endocrine reactions often do not normalize sodium and water balance but lead to sodium chloride losses. Consequently, sodium chloride supplements are needed.

In a randomized controlled trial, Hartnoll et al[136,137] compared the effects of early (on the second day after birth) and delayed (when weight loss of 6% of birth weight was achieved) sodium supplementation of 4 mmol/kg/day on body composition and sodium balance in infants of 25 to 30 weeks' gestational age. In the delayed group, there was a significant reduction in TBW and ECW by the end of the first week, but body solids accrued more rapidly in the early group. By day 14, significant differences in body composition were no longer seen. Sodium balance was negative in both groups after the first day, and fractional sodium excretion did not differ. It was concluded that early supplementation can delay the physiological water loss, which may cause an increased risk of continuing oxygen requirement not mediated by alterations in pulmonary artery pressure, but rather by retaining interstitial lung fluid, lowering lung compliance, and exacerbating respiratory compromise.

Bell and Acarregui[138] also reported a significant association of restricted fluid intake with increased postnatal weight loss, reduced risk of PDA and NEC, and a clear tendency to reduce the risk of BPD, ICH, and death.

Early introduction (0–24 hr. vs. 36–48 hr.) of total parenteral nutrition (TPN) and moderate sodium combined with restricted fluid intake had no apparent influence on serum sodium and potassium levels but caused a reduced diuresis and lower postnatal weight loss in association with better weight gain at days 14 and 21 after birth. With respect to the similar clinical outcomes, maintained fluid balance and improved energy status and growth in the early intervention group early initiation of TPN with restricted fluid intake is recommended.[139]

Our own supplementation policy proposes to give extra sodium at a dose of 3 to 5 mmol/kg/day and 1.5 to 2.5 mmol/kg/day for 8 to 21 days and 22 to 35 days, respectively. Delayed sodium supplementation does not interfere with cardiopulmonary adaptation but ensures positive sodium balance and maintains normal plasma sodium concentrations. Moreover, supplemental sodium prevents the excessive activation of RAAS, and plasma renin activity, plasma aldosterone concentration, and urinary aldosterone excretion remain within the limits characteristic for healthy full-term neonates[140] (Fig. 3-6).

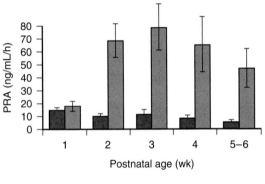

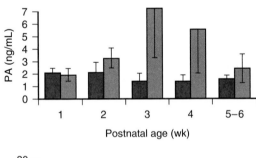

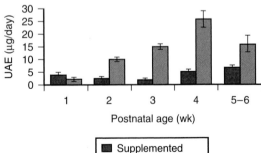

Figure 3-6 Postnatal development of plasma renin activity (PRA), plasma aldosterone concentration (PA), and urinary aldosterone excretion (UAE) in premature infants with and without NaCl supplementation during the first 6 weeks of life. (From Sulyok E, Németh M, Tényi I, et al. Relationship between the postnatal development of the renin-angiotensin-aldosterone system and electrolyte and acid-base status of the NaCl-supplemented premature infants. In: Spitzer A, ed. *The Kidney during Development*. Morphology and Function. New York: Masson Publishing, 1982, pp. 272-281, with permission.)

■ Supplemented
■ Non-supplemented

Reduction of flow-dependent urinary sodium excretion[141] and maintaining positive sodium balance by providing restricted fluid intake may carry the risks that the sodium requirements for growth are not met. Moreover, under the conditions of low sodium and fluid intake, a positive sodium balance can be achieved by excessive activation of RAAS only, which indicates some extent of volume depletion, marginal somatic stability, and still undefined long-term consequences.

Early Hypernatremia

In early hypernatremia, plasma sodium exceeds 150 mEq/L. Repeated administration of hypertonic sodium bicarbonate solution to "correct" acidosis in critically ill LBW neonates who have compromised renal function is the most common cause of neonatal hypernatremia. This hypernatremia can be reduced or avoided by decreasing the concentration of the sodium bicarbonate given and the amount infused. VLBW infants are also at risk for developing hypernatremia from extremely high insensible water loss. This is augmented when radiant warmers and phototherapy are used[142] and by the limited ability of the immature kidney to concentrate urine and reabsorb free water.[143]

Attempts should be made to reduce insensible water loss, carefully monitor water balance, and adjust water intake appropriately to prevent hypernatremia. Hypernatremia occasionally occurs after the first week of life in premature infants who are receiving NaCl supplementation and inadequate free water.

Clinical Consequences of Inadequate Sodium Intake

Premature infants fed breast milk or those fed low-sodium formula who develop renal salt wasting often become sodium depleted and hyponatremic. Premature infants with late hyponatremia generally are asymptomatic. However, some develop apnea and neurologic symptoms such as irritability and convulsion.

Sodium chloride makes a major contribution to plasma osmolality. As a result, the decrease in plasma sodium is accompanied by a parallel decline in plasma osmolality. A decrease in cell solute content, which occurs in chronic hyponatremia, lowers the increase in cell volume that initially occurs with hyponatremia. The concentrations of intracellular organic osmolytes decrease; these include taurine, myoinositol, phosphocreatine, glutamate, glutamine, and glycerophosphorylcholine. Central AVP and ANP have also been shown to participate in brain volume regulation. When the brain is exposed to severe hyponatremia, AVP accelerates and ANP reduces cellular water accumulation.[144] AVP action is V_1-receptor mediated, and it has been claimed to stimulate water flux via AQP4, the brain-specific water channels, directly.[145]

It has also been proposed that the V_1-receptor is coupled with the sodium channel and AVP primarily enhances cellular sodium uptake, which is followed by the passive, osmotically driven channel-mediated water transport. This possibility is supported by the observations that specific blockers of the sodium channel (benzamil, amiloride analogues) prevent cellular swelling and an increase in brain water content.[146] These findings may have relevance to hyponatremic premature infants because during the period of early or late hyponatremia, preterm infants may encounter increased AVP secretion.[147]

During correction of hyponatremia, the reaccumulation of organic osmolytes is delayed after the return of plasma sodium to normal. Rapid correction of hyponatremia may be associated with neurologic lesions, typically designated as central pontine myelinolysis, although sustained deprivation of organic solute alone may also have adverse effects.[148]

Central pontine myelinolysis is a rare condition characterized by a symmetrically sited central pontine lesion with a loss of myelin and an absence of inflammation. Its pathogenesis is not clearly defined, but there have been reports implicating apoptosis-mediated death of oligodentrocytes as a significant contributor to the demyelination. Proapoptotic markers have been detected in glial cell cytoplasm, and there is evidence of activated caspaces to initiate proteolytic cascade.[149]

Others have assumed the role of blood–brain barrier disruption, activation of the complement cascade, complement-induced oligodentrocyte lysis and immunologic destruction of white matter in the process of demyelinolysis.[150] This immune-mediated mechanism is supported by the prevention of blood–brain barrier disruption and of the severe neurologic impairment when dexamethasone treatment was applied.[151]

Sodium deficiency during gestation in rats is associated with impaired brain growth and alterations in brain cholesterol, protein, and RNA content.[152] Accordingly, there are data indicating that neonatal sodium deficiency may have unfavorable influences on later development of cognitive and mental functions,[153] and severe hyponatremia (duration and rate of correction) may be a risk factor for sensorineural hearing loss, cerebral palsy, ICH, and increased mortality in neonates who experienced perinatal asphyxia.[154] Furthermore, LBW newborn infants encountering neonatal hyponatremia had increased sodium intake as adolescents.[155]

Sodium depletion has been associated with retarded growth in height and weight in animals and humans, and 3 mM/kg/day sodium chloride supplementation in VLBW premature infants has been shown to improve growth, protein synthesis, and bone mineralization.[156] Young rats with diet-induced sodium deficiency have reduced RNA concentrations and exhibit decreased rates of protein synthesis in skeletal muscle.[157]

It has been suggested that ECF volume contraction and hyponatremia reduce growth factor-stimulated Na^+-H^+ exchange activity, decrease muscle intracellular pH, and impair DNA synthesis and cell growth.[158] Premature infants with late hyponatremia have been shown to have reduced concentrating performance because of their blunted renal response to AVP. The limited renal tubular sodium reabsorption and the hyponatremic state may hinder the establishment of intrarenal osmotic gradient and impair renal response to AVP, thus preventing excessive water retention and further worsening of hyponatremia.[159]

Since Barker[160] put forward the hypothesis of fetal origin of some adult diseases, many studies have been published to confirm the association of LBW and hypertension in adult life. Despite the great progress that has been made in our understanding of the effect of fetal programming on subsequent organ function and adult disease, the underlying mechanisms still remain to be clearly established. Several lines of evidence have been provided, however, that a reduction in nephron number, enlargement of glomerular volume, and alterations in renal sodium handling and adrenocortical hormones are likely to have an impact on blood pressure.[161]

It is also to be considered that in LBW premature infants the responses of salt-retaining hormones to renal salt wasting and sodium depletion, particularly the excessively activated RAAS, may have far-reaching consequences on the later course of blood pressure control. Indeed, it may trigger inflammatory response and oxygen-derived free radical production and may compromise endothelial function as reflected by the elevation of asymmetric dimethylarginine, a marker and mediator of endothelial dysfunction.[162] It appears likely that not the systemic or brain renin–angiotensin system (RAS) but rather the intrarenal RAS with upregulated angiotensin II type I receptor is involved in this process. In support of this notion, angiotensin-converting enzyme inhibitor has been demonstrated to have a long-lasting suppressive effect on the development of hypertension.[163]

Clinical Consequences of Excessive Sodium Intake

Excessive use of hypertonic sodium bicarbonate for the correction of severe metabolic acidosis associated with perinatal asphyxia and RDS causes hypernatremia. Inadvertent sodium load may also contribute; it was found to amount to 5.8 mEq/kg/day on day 1 followed by a steady decline to a level of 1.8 mEq/kg/day on day 5 in premature infants with birth weights less than 1000 g.[164] Hypernatremia increases the risk of neonatal ICH in term and preterm infants. Increased sodium intake on each of the first 3 days after birth is associated with grade II to IV intraventricular hemorrhage in VLBW infants even after adjustments for gestational age, severity of illness, respiratory factors, and gender.[165] The rapid osmotic shift of fluid from ICW leads to cell dehydration, brain shrinkage, and tearing of the cerebral capillaries.[166]

In immature animals, cerebral cell volume regulation is well developed to maintain brain size in the face of hypernatremic stress. The elevated brain water content is associated with an increased concentration of osmoprotective molecules. During development, there is a parallel decline in brain water, total electrolyte, and organic osmolyte contents. The percentage contribution of inorganic solutes to osmoprotection is greater than that of organic solutes in immature animals than in adult animals, and among the individual organic osmolytes, taurine is the most prominent cerebral osmolyte. In support of this notion, taurine levels are elevated in the immature brain, and cerebral taurine best correlates with brain water content in normonatremic developing animals.[7]

High fluid and sodium chloride administration, which offsets the physiologic contraction of ECF volume in the first week of life, has severe consequences that include inducing PDA, cardiac failure, BPD, ICH, and NEC. A second problem is that LBW infants who are fed formula with extra sodium chloride to promote growth retain salt and water, as evidenced by AVP-mediated reduction in free water clearance[167] and development of delayed-onset peripheral edema, signs of increased intracranial pressure, and congestive heart failure.[168]

In full-term newborn infants, variations in sodium intake had immediate and long-term effects on blood pressure. Infants kept on low sodium during the first 6 months of life encountered lower blood pressure at the end of the trial and 15 years later.[169] By contrast, high sodium intake in late gestation or in infancy generates oxygen free radicals and low-grade inflammation that may cause endothelial dysfunction and hypertension later in life.

In view of the widespread untoward clinical consequences of inadequate or excessive sodium intake, sodium supplementation in LBW neonates should be tailored to their individual needs, determined by close monitoring of sodium and water balance and some relevant endocrine parameters. The optimal timing, dosage, and route of sodium supplementation remain to be established.

Sodium Homeostasis and Acid–Base Balance

Studies from our laboratory provided evidence that acid–base regulation and renal sodium handling are closely related in the neonatal period.[170]

The limited capacity of the immature kidney to excrete H^+ is associated with an obligatory sodium loss. The maturation of renal acidifying processes with increasing gestational and postnatal age results in a progressive increase in renal Na^+-H^+ exchange and in a steady decline in sodium excretion.

Furthermore, metabolic acidosis has been shown to enhance renal sodium excretion, and the acidosis-induced urinary sodium loss has been found to follow a developmental pattern; the lower the birth weight and the younger the age of the neonate, the less pronounced was the sodium excretory response.

Renal salt wasting, in turn, has been shown to contribute to the development of late metabolic acidosis.

All of these observations are in line with the low activity of renal NHE3 in early life and its steady increase with advancing maturation.

References

1. Friis-Hansen B. Body water compartments in children. Changes during growth and related changes in body composition. *Pediatrics.* 1961;28:169-181.
2. Ziegler EE, O'Donnell AM, Nelson SE, Fomon SJ. Body composition of the reference fetus. *Growth.* 1976;40:329-341.
3. Bradbury MWB, Crowder J, Desai S, et al. Electrolytes and water in the brain and cerebrospinal fluid of the foetal sheep and guinea-pig. *J Physiol.* 1972;227:591-610.
4. Aprison MH, Lukenbill A, Segar WE. Sodium, potassium, chloride and water content of six discrete parts of the mammalian brain. *J Neurochem.* 1960;5:150-155.
5. Stonestreet BS, Oen-Hsiao JM, Petersson KH, et al. Regulation of brain water during acute hyperosmolality in ovine fetuses, lambs, and adults. *J Appl Physiol.* 2003;94:1491-1500.
6. Widdowson EM, Dickerson JWT. The effect of growth and function on the chemical composition of soft tissues. *Biochem J.* 1960;77:30-43.

7. Trachtman H, Yancey PH, Gullans SR. Cerebral cell volume regulation during hypernatremia in developing rats. *Brain Res*. 1995;693:155-162.

8. Nielsen S, Nagelhus EA, Amiry-Moghaddam M, et al. Specialized membrane domains for water transport in glial cells: high-resolution immunogold cytochemistry of aquaporin-4 in rat brain. *J Neurosci*. 1997;17:171-180.

9. Sulyok E, Vajda Z, Dóczi T, Nielsen S. Aquaporins and the central nervous system. *Acta Neurochirurgica*. 2004;146:955-960.

10. Manley GT, Fujimura M, Ma T, et al. Aquaporin-4 deletion in mice reduces brain edema after acute water intoxication and ischemic stroke. *Nat Med*. 2000;6:159-163.

11. Vajda ZS, Promeneur D, Dóczi T, et al. Increased aquaporin-4 immunoreactivity in rat brain in response to systemic hyponatraemia. *Biochem Biophys Res Commun*. 2000;270:495-503.

12. Han Z, Wax MB, Patil RV. Regulation of aquaporin-4 water channels by phorbol ester-dependent protein phosphorylation. *J Biol Chem*. 1998;273:6001-6004.

13. Vajda ZS, Pedersen M, Füchtbauer E-M, et al. Delayed onset of brain edema and mislocalization of aquaporin-4 in dyshophin-null transgenic mice. *Proc Natl Acad Sci U S A*. 2002;99:13131-13136.

14. Johansson PA, Dziegielewska KM, Ek CJ. Aqaporin-1 in the choroid plexuses of developing mammalian brain. *Cell Tissue Res*. 2005;322:353-364.

15. Gömöri É, Pál J, Ábrahám H, et al. Fetal development of membrane water channel proteins aquaporin-1 and aquaporin-4 in the human brain. *Int J Dev Neurosci*. 2006;24:295-305.

16. Wen H, Nagelhus EA, Amiry-Moghaddam M, et al. Ontogeny of water transport in rat brain: postnatal expression of the aquaporin-4 water channel. *Eur J Neurosci*. 1999;11:935-945.

17. Štulc J. Placental transfer of inorganic ions and water. *Physiol Rev*. 1997;77:805-836.

18. Wilbur WJ, Power GG, Longo LL. Water exchange in the placenta: a mathematical model. *Am J Physiol*. 1978;235:R181-R199.

19. Gozzo ML, Noia G, Bargaresi G, et al. Reference intervals for 18 clinical chemistry analytes in fetal plasma samples between 18 and 40 weeks of pregnancy. *Clin Chem*. 1998;44:683-685.

20. Flexner LD, Cowie DB, Hellman MD, et al. The permeability of the human placenta to sodium in normal and abnormal pregnancies and the supply of sodium to the human fetus as determined with radioactive sodium. *Am J Obstet Gynecol*. 1948;55:469-480.

21. Curran MA, Nijland MJM, Mann SE, Ross MG. Human amniotic fluid mathematical model: determination and effect of intramembranous sodium flux. *Am J Obstet Gynecol*. 1998;178:484-490.

22. Štulc J, Štulcová B, Sibley CP. Evidence for active maternal-fetal transport of Na$^+$ across the placenta of the anaesthetized rat. *J Physiol (London)*. 1993;470:637-649.

23. Boyd CAR, Chipperfield AR, Steele LW. Separation of the microvillous (maternal) form the basal (fetal) plasma membranes of human term placenta: methods and physiological significance of marker enzyme distribution. *J Develop Physiol*. 1979;1:361-377.

24. Brownbill P, Atkinson DE, Glazier JD, et al. Changes in unidirectional maternofetal ^{22}Na clearance (K$_{mf}$) and Na$^+$-K$^+$-ATPase α-subunit expression by the placenta of the anesthetized rat during the last third of gestation (Abstract). *J Physiol (London)*. 1993;476:368P.

25. Speake PF, Mynett KJ, Glazier JD, et al. Activity and expression of Na$^+$/H$^+$ exchanger isoforms in the syncytiotrophoblast of the human placenta. *Pflügers Archives*. 2005;450:123-130.

26. Mahendran D, Byrne S, Donnai P, et al. Na$^+$ transport, H$^+$ concentration gradient dissipation and system A amino acid transporter activity in purified microvillons plasma membrane isolated from first trimester human placenta: comparison to the term microvillous membrane. *Am J Obstet Gynecol*. 1994;171:1534-1540.

27. Hughes JL, Doughty IM, Glazier JD, et al. Activity and expression of the Na$^+$/H$^+$ exchanger in the microvillous plasma membrane of the syncytiotrophoblast in relation to gestation and small for gestational age birth. *Pediatr Res*. 2000;48:652-659.

28. Johansson M, Glazier JD, Jansson T, et al. Na$^+$/H$^+$ exchange is reduced in the microvillous membranes isolated form preterm IUGR pregnancies. *Placenta*. 2001;22:A66.

29. Brunette MG, Leclerc M, Claveau D. Na$^+$ transport by human placental brush border membranes: are there several mechanisms? *J Cell Physiol*. 1996;167:72-80.

30. Speake PF, Glazier JD, Greenwood SL, Sibley CP. Aldosterone and cortisol acutely stimulate Na$^+$/H$^+$ exchanger activity in the syncytiotrophoblast of the human placenta: effect of fetal sex. *Placenta*. 2010;31:289-294.

31. Zhao H, Hundal HS. Identification and biochemical localization of Na$^+$, K$^+$, 2Cl$^-$ cotransporter in the human placental cell line BeWo. *Biochem Biophys Res Commun*. 2000;274:43-48.

32. Page KR, Ashworth CJ, McArdle HJ, et al. Sodium transport across the chorioallantoic membrane of porcine placenta involves the epithelial sodium channel (ENaC). *J Physiol*. 2003;547:849-857.

33. DelMonaco S, Assef Y, Damiano A, et al. Characterization of epithelial sodium channel in human pre-eclampsia syncytiotrophoblast. *Medicina*. 2006;66:31-35.

34. Jansson T, Powell TL. IFPA 2005 Award in Placentology Lecture. Human Placental Transport in altered fetal growth: does the placenta function as a nutrient sensor? A review. *Placenta*. 2006;(Suppl A):S91-S97.

35. Daneshmand SS, Cheung CY, Brace RA. Regulation of amniotic fluid volume by intramembranous absorption in sheep: role of passive permeability and vascular endothelial growth factor. *Am J Obstet Gynecol*. 2003;188:786-793.

36. Roberts TJ, Nijland MJM, Williams L, Ross MG. Fetal diuretic response to maternal hyponatremia: contribution of placental sodium gradient. *J Appl Physiol*. 1999;87:1440-1447.

37. Kirksey A, Pike RI, Callahan AJ. Some effects of high and low sodium intakes during pregnancy in the rat II. Electrolyte concentrations of maternal plasma, muscle, bone and brain and of placenta, amniotic fluid, fetal plasma and total fetus in normal pregnancy. *J Nutr*. 1962;77: 43-51.

38. Powell TL, Brace RA. Fetal fluid responses to long-term 5 M NaCl infusion: where does all the salt go? *American J Physiol*. 1991;261:R412-R419.

39. Gibson KJ, Lumbers ER. Effects of continuous drainage of fetal fluids on salt and water balance in fetal sheep. *J Physiol*. 1996;494:443-450.

40. Pullano JG, Cohen-Addad N, Apuzzio JJ, et al. Water and salt conservation in the human fetus and newborn. I. Evidence for a role of fetal prolactin. *J Clin Endocrinol Metab*. 1989;69: 1180-1186.

41. Riddick DH, Maslar IA. The transport of prolactin by human fetal membranes. *J Clin Endocrinol Metab*. 1991;52:220-224.

42. Ertl T, Sulyok E, Bódis J, Csaba IF. Plasma prolactin levels in full-term newborn infants with idiopathic edema: Response to furosemide. *Biol Neonate*. 1986;49:15-20.

43. Ertl T, Sulyok E, Varga L, Csaba IF. Postnatal development of plasma prolactin level in premature infants with and without NaCl supplementation. *Biol Neonate*. 1983;44:219-223.

44. Arant BS. Fluid therapy in the neonate: concept in transition. *J Pediatr*. 1982;101:387-389.

45. Shaffer SG, Quimiro CL, Andreson JV, Hall RT. Postnatal weight changes in low birth weight infants. *Pediatrics*. 1987;79:702-705.

46. Tang W, Ridout D, Modi N. Influence of respiratory distress syndrome on body composition after preterm birth. *Arch Dis Child*. 1997;77:F28-F31.

47. Bauer K, Bovermann G, Roithmaier A, et al. Body composition, nutrition and fluid balance during the first two weeks of life in preterm neonates weighing less than 1500 grams. *J Pediatr*. 1991;118: 615-620.

48. Van der Wagen A, Okken J, Zweens J, Zijlstra WG. Composition of postnatal weight loss and subsequent weight gain in small for dates newborn infants. *Acta Paediatr Scand*. 1985;74: 57-61.

49. Heimler R, Doumas BT, Jendrzejczak BM, et al. Relationship between nutrition, weight change, and fluid compartments in preterm infants during the first week of life. *J Pediatr*. 1993;122: 110-114.

50. Cheek DB, Wishart J, MacLennan A, Haslam R. Cell hydration in the normally grown, the premature and the low weight for gestational age infants. *Early Hum Dev*. 1984;10:75-84.

51. Thomas JL, Reichelderfer TE. Premature infants: analysis of serum during the first seven weeks. *Clin Chem*. 1968;14:272-280.

52. Machnik A, Neuhofer W, Jantsch J, et al. Macrophages regulate salt-dependent volume and blood pressure by a vascular endothelial growth factor-C-dependent buffering mechanism. *Nat Med*. 2009;15:545-552.

53. Cheek DB. Extracellular volume: its structure and measurement and the influence of age and disease. *J Pediatr*. 1961;58:103-125.

54. MacLaurin JC. Changes in body water distribution during the first two weeks of life. *Arch Dis Child*. 1966;41:286-291.

55. Coulter DM, Avery ME. Paradoxical reduction in tissue hydration with weight gain in neonatal rabbit pups. *Pediatr Res*. 1980;14:1122-1126.

56. Tulassay T, Seri I, Rascher W. Atrial natriuretic peptide and extracellular volume contraction after birth. *Acta Paediatr Scand*. 1987;76:444-446.

57. Bierd TM, Kattwinkel L, Chevalier RL, et al. Interrelationship of atrial natriuretic peptide, atrial volume, and renal function in premature infants. *J Pediatr*. 1990;116:753-759.

58. Shaffer SG, Geer PG, Goetz KL. Elevated atrial natriuretic factor in neonates with respiratory distress syndrome. *J Pediatr*. 1986;109:1028-1033.

59. Sulyok E. Physical water compartments: a revised concept of perinatal body water physiology. *Physiol Res*. 2005;55:133-138.

60. Ling GN. *A Revolution in the Physiology of the Living Cell*. Malabar, FL: Krieger Publishing Co; 1992.

61. Israelachvili J, Wennerström H. Role of hydration and water structure in biological and colloidal interactions. *Nature*. 1996;379:217-225.

62. Mulkern RV, Bleier AR, Adzamil IK, et al. Two-site exchange revisited: a new method for extracting exchange parameters in biological systems. *Biophys J*. 1989;55:221-232.

63. Hällgren R, Samuelsson T, Laurent TC, Moding J. Accumulation of hyaluronan (hyaluronic acid) in the lung in adult respiratory distress syndrome. *Am Rev Respir Dis*. 1989;139:682-687.

64. Allen SJ, Sedin EG, Jonzon A, et al. Lung hyaluronan during development: a quantitative and morphological study. *Am J Physiol*. 1991;260:H1449-H1454.

65. Sedin EG, Bogner P, Berényi E, et al. Lung water and proton magnetic resonance relaxation in preterm and term rabbit pups: their relation to tissue hyaluronan. *Pediatr Res*. 2000;48: 554-559.

66. Sulyok E, Nyúl Z, Bogner P, et al. Brain water in fetal and newborn rabbits as assessed by H'-NMR relaxometry: its relation to tissue hyaluronan. *Biol Neonate*. 2001;79:62-72.

67. Hällgren R, Gerdin B, Tufveson G. Hyaluronic acid accumulation and redistribution in rejecting rat kidney graft: relationship to the transplantation edema. *J Exp Med*. 1990;171:2063-2076.
68. Hansell P, Göransson V, Odling C, et al. Hyaluronan content in the kidney in different states of body hydration. *Kidney Int*. 2000;58:2061-2068.
69. Sulyok E, Nyul Z. Hyaluronan-related limited concentration by the immature kidney. *Med Hypotheses*. 2005;65:1058-1061.
70. Ross B, Cowett RM, ad Oh W. Renal functions of low birth weight infants during the first two months of life. *Pediatr Res*. 1977;11:1162-1164.
71. Sulyok E, Heim T, Soltész Gy, Jászai V. The influence of maturity on renal control acidosis in newborn infants. *Biol Neonate*. 1972;21:418-435.
72. Aperia A, Broberger O, Thodenius K, Zetterström R. Developmental study of the renal response to an oral salt load in preterm infants. *Acta Paediatr Scand*. 1974;63:517-524.
73. Arant BS. Developmental pattern of renal functional maturation compared in the human neonate. *J Pediatr*. 1978;92:705-712.
74. Siegel SR, Oh W. Renal function as a marker of human fetal maturation. *Acta Paediatr Scand*. 1976;65:481-485.
75. Bell EF, Acarregui MJ. Restricted versus liberal water intake for preventing morbidity and mortality in preterm infants. *Cochrane Database Syst Rev*. 2001;(1):CD000503.
76. Oh W, Poindexter BB, Perritt R, et al. Association between fluid intake and weight loss during the first ten days of life and risk of bronchopulmonary dysplasia in extremely low birth weight infants. *J Pediatr*. 2005;147:786-790.
77. Sulyok E. The relationship between electrolyte and acid-base balance in the premature infant during early postnatal life. *Biol Neonate*. 1971;17:227-237.
78. Day GM, Radde IC, Bafle JW, Chance GW. Electrolyte abnormalities in very low birthweight infants. *Pediatr Res*. 1976;10:522-526.
79. Roy RN, Chance CW, Radde IC, et al. Late hyponatremia in very low birth weight infants (1.3 kilograms). *Pediatr Res*. 1976;10:526-531.
80. Sulyok E, Németh M, Tényi J, et al. Relationship between maturity, electrolyte balance and the function of the renin-angiotensin-aldosterone system in newborn infants. *Biol Neonate*. 1979;35:60-65.
81. Sulyok E, Varga F, Gyory E, et al. On the mechanism of renal sodium handling in newborn infants. *Biol Neonate*. 1980;37:75-79.
82. Rodriguez-Soriano J, Vallo A, Oliveros R, Castillo G. Renal handling of sodium in premature and full-term neonates: a study using clearance method during water diuresis. *Pediatr Res*. 1983;17:1013-1016.
83. Sulyok E, Varga F, Gyory E, et al. Postnatal development of renal sodium handling in premature infants. *J Pediatr*. 1979;95:787-792.
84. Leslie GI, Arnold JD, Gyory AZ. Postnatal changes in proximal and distal tubular sodium reabsorption in healthy very low-birth-weight infants. *Biol Neonate*. 1991;60:108-113.
85. Haycock GB, Aperia A. Salt and the newborn kidney. *Pediatr Nephrol*. 1991;5:65-70.
86. Edelmann CM, Spitzer A. The maturing kidney. A modern view of well-balanced infants with imbalanced nephrons. *J Pediatr*. 1969;75:509-519.
87. Schwartz GJ, Evan AP. Development of solute transport in rabbit proximal tubule. III. Na^+, K^+-ATPase activity. *Am J Physiol*. 1984;246:F845-F852.
88. Baum M. Neonatal rabbit juxtamedullary proximal convoluted tubule acidification. *J Clin Invest*. 1990;85:499-506.
89. Beck JC, Lipkowitz MS, Abramson RG. Ontogeny of Na/H antiporter activity in rabbit renal brush border membrane vesicles. *J Clin Invest*. 1991;87:7067-7076.
90. Vehaskari VM. Ontogeny of cortical collecting duct sodium transport. *Am J Physiol*. 1994;267:F49-F54.
91. Satlin LM, Palmer LG. Apical Na^+ conductance in maturing rabbit principal cell. *Am J Physiol*. 1994;266:F57-F65.
92. Counillon L, Pouysségur J. The expanding family of eukaryotic Na^+/H^+ exchangers. *J Biol Chem*. 2000;275:1-4.
93. Guillery EN, Karniski LP, Mathews MS, Robillard JE. Maturation of proximal tubule Na^+/H^+ antiporter activity in sheep during transition from fetus to newborn. *Am J Physiol*. 1994;267:F537-F545.
94. Baum M, Quigley R. Glucocorticoids stimulate rabbit proximal convoluted tubule acidification. *J Clin Invest*. 1993;91:110-114.
95. Guillery EN, Karniski LP, Mathews MS, et al. Role of glucocorticoids in the maturation of renal cortical Na^+/H^+ exchanger activity during fetal life in sheep. *Am J Physiol*. 1995;268:F710-F717.
96. Kinsella JL, Sacktor B. Thyroid hormones increase Na^+-H^+ exchange activity in renal brush border membranes. *Proc Natl Acad Sci U S A*. 1985;82:3606-3610.
97. Mazursky JE, Segar JL, Smith BA, et al. Rapid increase in renal sympathetic nerve activity (RSNA) during the transition form fetal to newborn life (Abstract). *Clin Res*. 1993;41:A329.
98. Guillery EN, Porter CC, Jose PA, et al. Developmental regulation of the $\alpha_{1\beta}$ - adrenoceptor in the sheep kidney. *Pediatr Res*. 1993;34:124-128.
99. Gesek FA, Schoolwerth AC. Hormonal interactions with the proximal Na^+-H^+ exchanger. *Am J Physiol*. 1990;258:F514-F521.

100. Kerpel-Fronius E, Heim T, Sulyok E. The development of the renal acidifying processes and their relation to acidosis in low-birth-weight infants. *Biol Neonate*. 1970;15:156-168.
101. Spitzer A, Barac-Nieto M. Ontogeny of renal phosphate transport and the process of growth. *Pediatr Nephrol*. 2001;16:763-771.
102. Holtbäck U, Aperia A. Molecular determinants of sodium and water balance during early human development. *Semin Neonatol*. 2003;8:291-299.
103. Canessa CM, Schild L, Buell G, et al. Amiloride-sensitive epithelial Na$^+$ channel is made of three homologous subunits. *Nature*. 1994;367:463-467.
104. Dagenais A, Kothary R, Berthiaume Y. The α subunit of the epithelial sodium channel in the mouse: developmental regulation of its expression. *Pediatr Res*. 1997;42:327-334.
105. Vehaskari VM, Hempe JM, Manning J, et al. Developmental regulation of ENaC subunit mRNA levels in rat kidney. *Am J Physiol*. 1998;247:C1661-C1666.
106. Ergonul Z, Frinot G, Palmer L. Regulation of maturation and processing of ENaC subunits in rat kidney. *Am J Physiol*. 2006;291:F683-F693.
107. Satlin LM, Palmer LG. Apical Na$^+$ conductance in maturing rabbit principal cell. *Am J Physiol*. 1996;270:F391-F397.
108. Watanabe S, Matsushita K, McCray PB, Stokes JB. Developmental expression of the epithelial Na$^+$ channel in kidney and uroepithelia. *Am J Physiol*. 1999;276:F304-F314.
109. Nakamura K, Stokes JB, McCray PB. Endogenous and exogenous glucocorticoid regulation of ENaC mRNA expression in developing kidney and lung. *Am J Physiol*. 2002;283:C762-C772.
110. Brown RW, Diaz R, Robson AC, et al. The ontogeny of 11 β-hydroxysteroid dehydrogenase type 2 and mineralocorticoid receptor gene expression reveal intricate control of glucocorticoid action in development. *Endocrinology*. 1996;137:794-797.
111. Martinerie L, Viengchareun S, Delezoide A-L, et al. Low renal mineralocorticoid receptor expression at birth contributes to partial aldosterone resistance in neonates. *Endocrinology*. 2009;150:4414-4424.
112. Schmitt R, Ellison DH, Farman N, et al. Developmental expression of sodium entry pathways in rat nephron. *Am J Physiol*. 1999;276:F367-F381.
113. Bidiwala KS, Lorenz JM, Kleinman LI. Renal function correlates of postnatal diuresis in preterm infants. *Pediatrics*. 1988;82:50-58.
114. Lorenz JM, Kleinman LI, Ahmed G, Makarian K. Phases of fluid and electrolyte homeostasis in the extremely low birth weight infants. *Pediatrics*. 1995;95:484-489.
115. Bueva A, Guignard J-P. Renal function in preterm neonates. *Pediatr Res*. 1994;36:572-577.
116. Delgado MM, Rohatgi R, Khan S, et al. Sodium and potassium clearances by the maturing kidney: clinical-molecular correlates. *Pediatr Nephrol*. 2003;18:759-767.
117. Aperia A, Elinder G. Distal tubular sodium reabsorption in the developing rat kidney. *Am J Physiol*. 1981;240:F487-F491.
118. Kleinman LI. Renal sodium reabsorption during saline loading and distal blockade in newborn dog. *Am J Physiol*. 1975;228:1407-1408.
119. Drukker A, Goldsmith DI, Spitzer A, et al. The renin-angiotensin system in newborn dog: developmental pattern of response to acute saline loading. *Pediatr Res*. 1980;14:304-307.
120. Kleinman LI, Banks RO. Segmental nephron sodium and potassium reabsorption in newborn and adult dogs during saline expansion. *Proc Soci Exp Biol Med*. 1983;173:231-237.
121. Aperia A, Broberger O, Thodenius K, Zetterström R. Renal response to an oral salt load in newborn full-term infants. *Acta Paediatr Scand*. 1972;61:670-676.
122. Muchant DG, Tornhill BA, Belmonte DC, et al. Chronic sodium loading augments natriuretic response to acute volume expansion in the preweaned rat. *Am J Physiol*. 1995;269:R15-R22.
123. Lorenz JM, Kleinman LI, Disney TA. Lack of anion effect on volume expansion natriuresis in the developing canine kidney. *J Develop Physiol*. 1986;8:395-410.
124. Ramiro-Tolentino SB, Markarian K, Kleinman LI. Renal bicarbonate excretion in extremely low birth weight infants. *Pediatrics*. 1996;98:256-261.
125. Al-Dahhan J, Haycock GB, Chantler C, Stimmler L. Sodium homeostasis in term and preterm neonates II. Gastrointestinal aspects. *Arch Dis Child*. 1983;58:343-345.
126. O'Loughlin EV, Hunt DM, Kreutzmann D. Postnatal development of colonic electrolyte transport in rabbits. *Am J Physiol*. 1990;258:G447-G453.
127. Jenkins HR, Fenton TR, McIntosh N, et al. Development of colonic sodium transport in early childhood and its regulation by aldosterone. *Gut*. 1990;31:194-197.
128. Rees L, Brook CGD, Shaw JCL, Forsling MR. Hyponatraemia in the first week of life in preterm infants. Part 1. Arginine vasopressin secretion. *Arch Dis Child*. 1984;59:414-422.
129. Costarino AT, Gruskay JA, Corcoran L, et al. Sodium restriction versus daily maintenance replacement in very low birth weight premature neonates: a randomized, blind therapeutic trial. *J Pediatr*. 1992;120:99-106.
130. Sibley CP, Boyd DH. Mechanisms of transfer across the human placenta. In Polin PA, Fox WW, *Fetal and Neonatal Physiology*. Philadelphia: WB Saunders, 1998; pp. 77-89.
131. Lelong-Tissier M-C, Retbi J-M, et al. Hyponatremie maternofoetale carentielle par regime desodé au cours d'une grosesse multiple. *Archives Francaises de Pédiatric*. 1977;34:64-70.
132. Shaffer SG, Meade VM. Sodium balance and extracellular volume regulation in very low birth weight infants. *J Pediatr*. 1989;115:285-290.
133. Lorenz JM, Kleinman LI, Kotagal UR, Reller MD. Water balance in very low-birth-weight infants: relationship to water and sodium intake and effect on outcome. *J Pediatr*. 1982;101:423-432.

134. Wilkins BH. Renal function in sick very low birth weight infants: 3. Sodium, potassium and water excretion. *Arch Dis Child*. 1992;67:1154-1161.
135. Shaffer SG, Bradt SK, Meade VM, Hall RT. Extracellular fluid volume changes in very low-birth-weight infants during first 2 postnatal months. *J Pediatr*. 1987;111:124-128.
136. Hartnoll G, Bétrémieux P, Modi N. Randomised controlled trial of postnatal sodium supplementation on body composition in 25 to 30 week gestational age infants. *Arch Dis Child*. 2000;82: 24-28.
137. Hartnoll G, Bétrémieux P, Modi N. Randomised controlled trial of postnatal sodium supplementation in infants of 25-30 weeks gestational age: effects on cardiopulmonary adaptation. *Arch Dis Child*. 2001;85:29-32.
138. Bell EF, Acarregui MJ. Restricted versus liberal water intake for preventing morbidity and mortality in preterm infants. *Cochrane Database Syst Rev*. 2008;1:CD000503.
139. Elstgeest LE, Martens SE, Lopriore E, et al. Does parenteral nutrition influence electrolyte and fluid balance in the preterm infants in the first days after birth? *PLOS ONE*. www.plosone.org. 2010;5: 1-6.
140. Sulyok E, Németh M, Tényi I, et al. Relationship between the postnatal development of the renin-angiotensin-aldosterone system and electrolyte and acid-base status of the NaCl-supplemented premature infants. In: Spitzer A, ed. *The Kidney during Development. Morphology and Function (pp. 272–281)*. New York: Masson Publishing USA, Inc.; 1982.
141. Satlin LM, Sheng S, Woda CB, Kleyman TR. Epithelial Na$^+$ channels are regulated by flow. *Am J Physiol Renal Physiol*. 2001;280:F1010-F1018.
142. Bell EF, Heidrich GA, Cashore WJ, Oh W. Combined effect of radiant warmer and phototherapy on insensible water loss in low-birth-weight infants. *J Pediatr*. 1979;94:810-813.
143. Rees L, Shaw JCL, Brook CDG, Forsling ML. Hyponatraemia in the first week of life in preterm infants. Part II. Sodium and water balance. *Arch Dis Child*. 1984;59:423-429.
144. Vajda ZS, Pedersen M, Dóczi T, et al. Effects of centrally administered arginine vasopressin and atrial natriuretic peptide on the development of brain edema in hyponatremic rat. *Neurosurgery*. 2001;49:697-705.
145. Gunnarson E, Zelenina M, Aperia A. Regulation of brain aquaporins. *Neuroscience*. 2004;129: 947-955.
146. Sulyok E, Pál J, Vajda S, Steier R, Dóczi T. Benzamil prevents brain water accumulation in hyponatremic rats. *Acta Neurochirurgica*. 2009;151:1121-1125.
147. Sulyok E, Kovács L, Lichardus B, et al. Late hyponatremia in premature infants: role of aldosterone and arginine vasopressin. *J Pediatr*. 1985;106:990-994.
148. Lien Y-HH, Shapiro JI, Chan L. Study of brain electrolytes and organic osmolytes during correction of chronic hyponatremia. Implications for the pathogenesis of central pontine myelinolysis. *Acta Neuropathol*. 1991;103:590-598.
149. DeLuca GC, Nagy ZS, Esiri MM, Davey P. Evidence for a role for apoptosis in central pontine myelinolysis. *Acta Neuropathol*. 2002;103:590-598.
150. Baker EA, Tian Y, Adler S, Verbalis JG. Blood-brain barrier disruption and complement activation in the brain following rapid correction of chronic hyponatremia. *Exp Neurol*. 2000;165: 221-230.
151. Sigamura Y, Murase T, Takefuji S, et al. Protective effect of dexamethasone on osmotic-induced demyelination in rats. *Exp Neurol*. 2005;192:178-183.
152. Bursey RG, Watson ML. The effect of sodium restriction during gestation on offspring brain development in rats. *Am J Clin Nutr*. 1983;37:43-51.
153. Aviv A, Kobayashi T, Higashino H, et al. Chronic sodium deficit in the immature rats: its effect on adaptation to sodium excess. *Am J Physiol*. 1982;242:E241-E247.
154. Moritz ML, Ayus JC. New aspects in the pathogenesis, prevention and treatment of hyponatremic encephalopathy in children. *Pediatr Nephrol*. 2010;25:1225-1238.
155. Shirazki A, Weintraub Z, Reich D, et al. Lowest neonatal serum sodium predicts sodium intake in low birthweight children. *Am J Physiol*. 2007;292:R1683-R1689.
156. Mbiti MJ, Aysi AK, Orinda DA. Sodium supplementation in very low birth weight infants fed on their mothers milk: II Effects on protein and bone metabolism. *East Afr Med J*. 1992;69: 627-630.
157. Wassner SJ. Altered growth and protein turnover in rats fed sodium deficient diet. *Pediatr Res*. 1989;26:608-613.
158. Ray PE, Lyon RC, Ruley EJ, Holliday MA. Sodium or chloride deficiency lowers muscle intracellular pH in growing rats. *Pediatr Nephrol*. 1996;10:33-37.
159. Kovács L, Sulyok E, Lichardus B, et al. Renal response to arginine vasopressin in premature infants with late hyponatraemia. *Arch Dis Child*. 1986;61:1030-1032.
160. Barker DJP. The developmental origins of adult disease. *J Am Coll Nutr*. 2004;23:588-595.
161. Luyckx VA, Brenner BM. Low-birth-weight, nephron number, and kidney disease. *Kidney Int*. 68 Supplement, 2005;97:S68-S72.
162. Vida G, Sulyok E, Lakatos O, Ertl T, et al. Plasma levels of asymmetric dimethylarginine in premature neonates: its possible involvement in developmental programming of chronic diseases. *Acta Paediatr*. 2009;98:437-441.
163. Manning J, Vehaskari VM. Postnatal modulation of prenatally programmed hypertension by dietary Na and ACE inhibition. *Am J Physiol*. 2005;288:R80-R84.
164. Bartley JH, Nagy S, Frank M, Bhatia J. Inadvertent sodium load in the first 5 days of life in extremely low birth weight infants. *J Perinatol*. 2004;24:593.

165. Barnette AR, Myers BJ, Berg CS, Inder TE. Sodium intake and intraventricular hemorrhage in preterm infants. *Ann Neurol*. 2010;67:817-823.
166. Simmons MA, Adock EW, Bard H. Hypernatremia and intracranial hemorrhage in neonates. *N Engl J Med*. 1974;291:6-10.
167. Sulyok E, Rascher W, Baranyai Zs, et al. The influence of NaCl supplementation on vasopressin secretion and renal water excretion in premature infants. *Biol Neonate*. 1993;64:201-208.
168. Hornich H, Amiel-Tison C. Retention hydrosaline chez les enfants de faible poids de naissnace. *Archives Francaises de Pédiatrie*. 1977;34:206-218.
169. Geleijnse JM, Hofman A, Witteman JCM, et al. Long-term effects of neonatal sodium restriction on blood pressure. *Hypertension*. 1997;29:913-917.
170. Sulyok E, Varga F. Renal aspects of neonatal sodium homeostasis. *Acta Paediatrica Hungarica*. 1983;24:23-35.

3

CHAPTER 4

Potassium Metabolism

John M. Lorenz, MD

- Normal Metabolism
- Developmental Physiology
- Clinical Relevance

Normal Metabolism

Total body potassium (K) in an adult male is about 50 mmol/kg of body weight and is influenced by age; sex; and, very importantly, muscle mass. Approximately 98% of the total body K is found in the intracellular fluid (ICF) space at a concentration of 100 to 150 mmol/L, depending on the cell type. This high intracellular [K$^+$] is essential for many basic cellular processes. In plasma water, the concentration of K is only 3.5 to 5 mmol/L. (In interstitial fluid water, with which ICF K is in equilibrium, [K$^+$] is 7% to 8% higher because of the Gibbs-Donnan equilibrium.) This steep [K$^+$] gradient from the ICF to extracellular fluid (ECF) compartment is maintained by active transport of K into the cell in exchange for sodium, which is mediated by sodium–potassium–triphosphatase (Na$^+$, K$^+$-ATPase) in the cell membrane. Most of the total body K is contained in muscle. This gradient is the major determinate of the resting membrane potential across the cell membrane, affecting muscle excitability and contractility.

Figure 4-1 shows the distribution and regulation of total body K in normal adults.

K homeostasis requires appropriate internal distribution of K and maintenance of an appropriate external K balance. *Regulation of the internal K balance* refers to the regulation of the critical concentration K gradient across cell membranes. Quantitatively, skeletal muscle is the most important cell type in this process because the great majority of total body and intracellular K is contained within muscle cells. *Regulation of the external K balance* refers to the regulation of total body K content. Although maintenance of total body K balance depends on excretion of K, predominantly by the kidney, this is a relatively slow process. In adults, daily K intake (50–100 mmol/day) exceeds the total K content of the ECF and only approximately 50% of oral K load is excreted in the following 4 to 6 hours. Of the retained K, 80% to 90% is rapidly transported from the ECF to the ICF space. Thus, life-threatening hyperkalemia would result were it not for the temporary, but rapid, extracellular to intracellular translocation of the transient excess of K.

Regulation of Internal K Balance[1]

The regulation of K distribution across cell membranes is critical for cellular function. Whereas uptake of K into cells is active in exchange for Na driven by Na$^+$, K$^+$-ATPase, the efflux of K from the cell is passive and depends on the type, density, and open probability of K-specific channels in various cell types. Figure 4-2 illustrates the factors affecting internal K balance.

An acute increase in plasma [K$^+$] decreases the concentration gradient against which the Na$^+$, K$^+$-ATPase pump must operate and thereby favors cellular uptake of

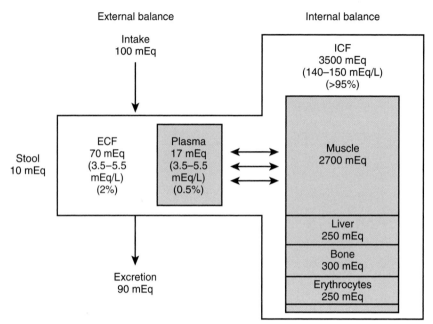

Figure 4-1 Total-body potassium distribution and regulation in a 70-kg adult under normal conditions. ECF, extracellular fluid; ICF, intracellular fluid. (From Williams ME, Epstein FH. Internal exchanges of potassium. In Seldin DW, Giebisch G (eds). The regulation of potassium balance. New York, Raven Press, 1989, pp. 3-29, with permission.)

K. A chronic increase in K intake sufficient to increase plasma [K^+] increases insulin-stimulated cellular K uptake by increasing Na^+, K^+-ATPase abundance in muscle cells. An acute decrease in plasma [K^+] decreases cellular K uptake by increasing the concentration gradient. A chronic decrease in K intake sufficient to decrease plasma [K+] decreases insulin stimulated cellular K uptake by decreasing Na^+, K^+-ATPase abundance in muscle cells.

Insulin stimulates the cellular uptake of K by hepatocytes and muscle cells, independent of its affect on glucose transport, by inducing an increase in Na^+, K^+-ATPase activity. β-Adrenergic stimulation promotes K uptake by hepatocytes, skeletal, and cardiac muscle via β-2 receptors. Conversely, β-adrenergic blockade impairs

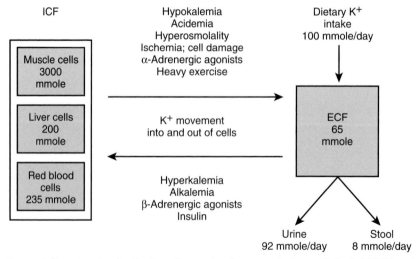

Figure 4-2 Factors influencing the distribution of potassium between the intracellular fluid (ICF) and extracellular fluid (ECF) compartments. (Modified from Schafer J. Renal regulation of potassium, calcium and magnesium. In Johnson LR (ed). Essential medical physiology. Amsterdam/Boston: Elsevier Academic Press, 3rd ed, 2003, pp. 437-446, with permission.)

cellular uptake of K. Insulin and the β-adrenergic system are important components of the extrarenal defense against hyperkalemia and act in both physiological and pathological concentrations. α-Adrenergic receptor stimulation promotes efflux of K from hepatocytes. The role of aldosterone in modulating internal K balance is uncertain.

Acute administration or the production of acid with an associated anion to which the cell membrane is relatively impermeable (i.e., exogenous hydrochloric acid, ammonium chloride, or endogenous acidosis of uremia) promotes K efflux from cells.[2] In this situation, K and sodium (Na) exit the cell in exchange for the excess ECF protons, which are buffered intracellularly, to maintain electroneutrality across the cell membrane. However, with organic acidemia (e.g., lactic acidemia), the associated anion diffuses into the cell more freely and thus is not associated with K efflux. During respiratory acidosis, the increment in plasma [K+] for any given change in pH is greater than with organic acidemia, but less than with mineral acidemia. An increase in the diffusion of bicarbonate (HCO_3) into cells as the result of an increase in plasma [HCO_3^-], independent of ECF pH, may be associated with the concomitant uptake of K. Respiratory alkalosis does not promote much shift of K across cell membranes.

The shift of water out of cells with severe ECF hyperosmolarity increases the intracellular [K^+], promoting K efflux from cells. Impairment of Na^+, K^+-ATPase activity by hypoxia (or loss of Na^+, K^+-ATPase activity with cell death) results in the movement of K out of the cell down its concentration gradient.

Regulation of External K Balance

Total body K content is a reflection of the balance between K intake and output. K intake depends on the quantity and type of intake. Under normal conditions, the average adult takes in about 50 to 100 mmol/day of K, about the same amount as Na. K output occurs through three primary routes: urine, gastrointestinal tract, and skin.

Renal Potassium Excretion[3]

The kidney is the major excretory organ for K and is primarily responsible for the regulation of external K balance. K is freely filtered across the glomerulus. As shown

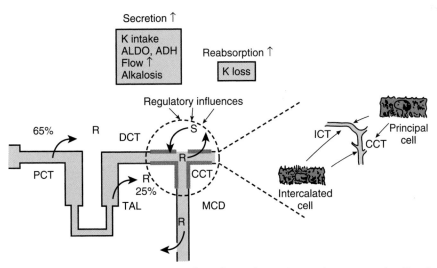

Figure 4-3 Summary of potassium (K) transport along the nephron. *Arrows* demonstrate the direction of net K transport. The percentages of the filtered K load remaining at specific nephron sites are shown. The collecting duct system is indicated by the *hatched portion* of the nephron. ADH, antidiuretic hormone; ALDO, aldosterone; CCT, cortical collecting tubule; DCT, distal convoluted tubule; ICT, initial connecting tubule; MCD, medullary collecting duct; PCT, proximal convoluted tubule; R, reabsorption; S, secretion; TAL, thick ascending limb of the loop of Henle. (From Giebisch G, Wang W. Potassium transport from clearance to channels to pumps. Kidney Int 1996;49:1624, with permission.)

in Figure 4-3, 60% to 70% of the filtered K is reabsorbed in the proximal tubule. Reabsorption in this tubular segment is the result of solvent drag (dependent on active Na transport and a high permeability of the paracellular pathway to K) and by the positive transepithelial voltage in the second half of this segment (Fig. 4-4). Net K reabsorption continues in the loop of Henle. In the thick ascending limb of the loop of Henle, K is reabsorbed across the apical cell membrane by means of a Na-K-2Cl cotransporter. This co-transporter is driven by the electrochemical gradient generated by Na$^+$, K$^+$-ATPase in the basolateral membrane, which favors Na entry across the luminal membrane (Fig. 4-4). Reabsorption in this nephron segment results in the delivery of only 10% of the filtered K to the distal renal tubule (Fig. 4-3). Thus, the balance of regulated, active K secretion and regulated, active K reabsorption in the distal tubule, specifically in the late distal tubule and cortical collecting tubule (CCT), determines the magnitude of renal K excretion.[4] Principal cells are responsible for K secretion, and intercalated cells are responsible for K reabsorption in the late distal tubule and CCT. Note that transport across the apical membrane is different in each nephron segment or cell type, but basolateral membrane transport is similar.[4]

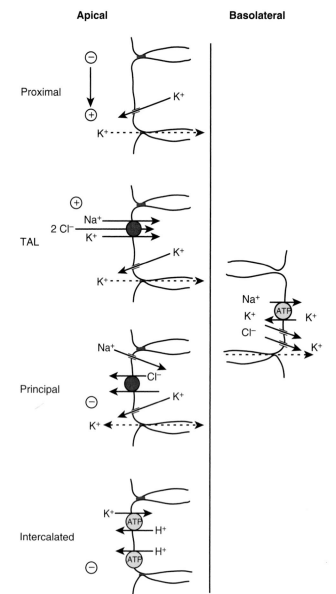

Apical   **Basolateral**

Proximal

TAL

Principal

Intercalated

Figure 4-4 Cell models of potassium (K) transport along the nephron. Transport across the apical membrane is different in each nephron segment or cell type, but basolateral membrane transport is similar. ATP, adenosine triphosphate; TAL, thick ascending limb of the loop of Henle. (From Giebisch G, Wang W. Potassium transport from clearance to channels to pumps. Kidney Int 1996;49:1624, with permission.)

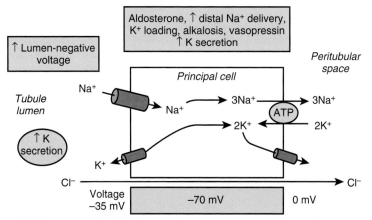

Figure 4-5 Cell model of a principal cell with overview of factors known to regulate potassium (K) secretion. (From Giebisch GH. A trail of research on potassium. Kidney Int 2002;62:1498, with permission.)

K secretion by principal cells is effected by the active exchange of K for Na across the basolateral membrane, driven by Na^+, K^+-$ATPase^5$ (Fig. 4-5). A lumen-negative voltage is generated across the late distal tubule and CCT by the apical entry of Na into the principal cell down its concentration gradient via epithelial sodium channels (ENaCs), driven by the extrusion of Na from the principal cell across the basolateral membrane by Na^+, K^+-ATPase. Intracellular K passively diffuses down a favorable electrochemical gradient via K channels in the apical membrane. Under baseline conditions, K transverses the apical membrane of the principal cell via an ATPase sensitive, small conductance (SK) channel with a high open probability. Maxi-K channels are high conductance K channels in the apical membrane, but are present at low density and low opening probability under baseline conditions. Whereas SK channels are responsible for baseline K secretion, flow-dependent K secretion (see below) is thought to be mediated by maxi-K channels. The magnitude of transport of K across the principal cell then is determined by the electrochemical gradient across the late distal tubule and CCT and the permeability of the apical membrane of the principal cell to Na and K. The latter is a function of the number and open probability of ion specific apical membrane channels. K secretion is strongly stimulated by an increase in the tubular fluid flow rate in the late distal tubule and CCT. This is the result of both a more favorable electrochemical gradient and increased permeability of the luminal membrane to K. The higher the tubular flow rate, the slower the rise in [K^+] along the late distal tubule and CCT as secreted K is more rapidly diluted in the greater volume of tubular fluid transversing the late distal tubule and CCT. Any associated increase in Na delivery to the late distal tubule and CCT also increases the concentration gradient driving Na across the apical membrane. High tubular flow rates also increase the permeability of the principal cell membrane to K by activating maxi-K channels.[6] Therefore, K secretion in the late distal tubule and CCT is regulated by factors that affect the electrochemical gradient or apical membrane permeability to Na or K. Because urinary K excretion is largely the result of K secretion in the late distal tubule and CCT under most conditions, these factors then determine urinary K excretion.

An acute increase in plasma [K^+] as the result of high K intake produces a more favorable electrochemical gradient for K secretion in the late distal tubule and CCT, increases the density of SK channels in the apical membrane, and stimulates aldosterone secretion. Aldosterone stimulates K secretion in the late distal tubule and CCT by increasing the density of ENaCs (by recruitment of intracellular channels and de novo synthesis) and increasing Na^+, K^+-ATPase activity in the basolateral membrane of principal cells (by recruitment of intracellular pumps and de novo synthesis). Na^+, K^+-ATPase activity is coupled to SK density in the apical membrane—increased pump activity increases SK density, and decreased pump activity decreases SK density. A chronic increase in K intake results in increased capacity of the principal cell for K secretion, a process referred to as *K adaptation*. It results from an increase in the density of SK and maxi-K channels and increased activity of ENaCs in the apical membrane and increased Na^+, K^+-ATPase activity in the basolateral membrane under baseline conditions. These changes are independent of aldosterone but depend on increased plasma $[K^+]$.

A decrease in plasma $[K^+]$ as a result of decreased K intake or increased K excretion decreases K secretion in the distal tubule and CCT by decreasing Na^+, K^+-ATPase activity in the basolateral membrane of principal cells, redistributing SK channels from the apical membrane into the cell, reducing distal tubular flow rate, and inhibiting aldosterone secretion. These changes decrease sodium reabsorption via ENaCs, which in turn decrease the driving force for K secretion. In addition, hypokalemia promotes potassium reabsorption by intercalated cells in the late distal tubule and CCT (see below). A chronic decrease in K intake results in decrease SK channel abundance, and H^+,K^+-ATPase abundance consistent with K conservation.

Acute metabolic acidosis reduces K secretion by decreasing $[K^+]$ in the principal cell, which reduces the electrochemical gradient for K secretion, and by decreasing tubular fluid pH, which inhibits apical SK activity. The effect of chronic metabolic acidosis is complex; it depends on associated changes in filtered chloride (Cl) and HCO_3, distal tubular flow rate, and aldosterone. Acute respiratory and metabolic alkalosis stimulate K secretion in the late distal tubule and CCT by increasing the electrochemical gradient for K secretion and increasing tubular fluid pH. The latter increases the permeability of the apical membrane of the principal cell to K by increasing the duration that SK channels remain open. A K-Cl co-transporter in the apical membrane may also be involved in the increase in K secretion in response to metabolic alkalosis. While mediating only a modest amount of K secretion at physiological tubular fluid $[Cl^-]$, this co-transporter is activated when the tubular fluid $[HCO_3^-]$ or pH rises.[7] Metabolic alkalosis also stimulates the basolateral uptake of K.

Vasopressin has both apical and peritubular sites of action on the principal cell that stimulate K secretion. It may stimulate SK channels and K-Cl co-transporters in the apical membrane. It is unlikely that vasopressin is involved in the physiologic regulation of urinary K excretion. However, it may sustain K excretion in the face of reductions in distal tubular flow rate (e.g., during extracellular volume contraction).

Intercalated cells in the late distal tubule and CCT primarily function in H^+/HCO_3^- transport. However, under conditions of chronic K depletion, intercalated cells reabsorb K by the active exchange of a single K^+ for a proton catalyzed by hydrogen, potassium-triphosphatase (H^+,K^+-ATPase) in the apical membrane[4] (Fig. 4-4). K depletion increases the activity of H^+,K^+-ATPase in the apical membrane; decreases apical membrane K permeability (channel not shown in Fig. 4-4), reducing the back leak of K into the lumen down its electrochemical gradient; and increases basolateral membrane K permeability. Both metabolic acidosis and Na depletion also increase K^+-H^+ exchange across the apical membrane of the intercalated cell.

Intestinal Potassium Excretion

Under normal conditions, loss of K through the gastrointestinal tract is only 5% to 10% of dietary intake. The bulk of dietary K intake is reabsorbed in the small intestine. Analogous to the kidney, gastrointestinal K output is primarily a balance of regulated, active K secretion and regulated, active K reabsorption in the colon. Active K secretion in the colon is driven by basolateral uptake of K via Na^+, K^+-ATPase. Movement of K across the apical membrane, down its electrochemical concentration gradient, occurs via a Na-K-2Cl co-transporter. K reabsorption is active, mediated by a colonic apical H^+,K^+-ATPase. Aldosterone, glucocorticoids, epinephrine, and prostaglandins increase stool K content. Indomethacin and K depletion reduce it.

Intestinal K excretion assumes a significant role in maintaining external K balance in severe renal insufficiency as the result of increase in colonic basolateral membrane Na^+, K^+-ATPase, when as much as 30% to 80% of K intake may be excreted in the feces. Chronic K deprivation sufficient to decrease plasma [K⁺] increases colonic apical [K⁺], which increases colonic K reabsorption.

Sweat Gland Potassium Excretion

Human excretory sweat [K⁺] is 5 to 10 mmol/L, so K losses from the skin in sweat are negligible under baseline conditions. This route of K excretion is not subject to feedback control.

Plasma [K⁺]

Extracellular fluid [K⁺] is a function of both internal and external K balance. Because the ICF K pool is 50-fold that of the ECF, changes in internal K balance can result in acute, dramatic, life-threatening changes in ECF [K⁺]. On the other hand, changes in ECF [K⁺] as the result of changes in external K balance usually occur more slowly and are buffered by homeostatic changes in internal K balance. As a result, plasma [K⁺] concentration is a late indicator of changes in external K balance.

Feedback and Feedforward Control of Plasma [K⁺][8]

Changes in plasma [K⁺] trigger appropriate changes in internal and external K balance mechanisms as described above via classic feedback control as illustrated in the top of Figure 4-6. This feedback control is robust, but can be slow to respond to perturbations in external K balance. Evidence is emerging of *feedforward* control of internal and external K balance in response to changes in dietary K intake (i.e., appropriate changes in internal and external K balance in response to these dietary changes) *in the absence of or before associated changes in plasma [K⁺]*, as illustrated in the bottom of Figure 4-6.

After a meal, pancreatic insulin secretion is stimulated by absorption of glucose and amino acids, which in turn stimulates the cellular uptake of K by hepatocytes and muscle cells independent of plasma [K⁺]. Glucagon secretion in response to a protein (and thereby K) -rich meal increases the glomerular filtration rate (GFR), which increases distal tubular flow rate and increases the transtubular K gradient (the ratio of urine to plasma [K⁺] ÷ the ratio of urine to plasma osmolality). Both of these effects stimulate K secretion in the late distal tubule and CCT. In addition, as yet unidentified K sensors (probably in the splanchnic bed) rapidly stimulate renal potassium secretion and insulin-stimulated extracellular K uptake in response to a K-containing meal in the absence of or before any associated increase in plasma [K⁺].

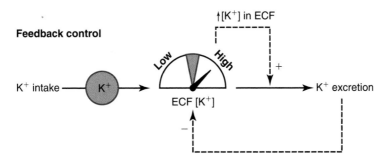

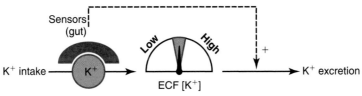

Figure 4-6   Schematic illustration of the control of extracellular fluid (ECF) [K⁺] via feed*back* (*top*) versus feedfor*ward* control (*bottom*). (From Youn JH, McDonough AA. Recent advances in understanding integrative control of potassium homeostasis. Annu Rev Physiol 2009;71:384, with permission.)

Modest decreases in dietary K intake do not result in even transient changes in plasma [K$^+$]. Reduced intake is able to be sensed in the absence of even minor changes in plasma [K$^+$] and, via unidentified signaling pathways, reduces both insulin stimulated cellular K uptake and renal K excretion by redistributing SK channels from the apical membrane into the cell.

Feedforward control is more rapid and more precise than, but not as robust as, feedback control. The combination of both provides rapid, precise, and robust control of plasma [K$^+$].

Developmental Physiology

Unlike adults, in whom K homeostasis requires that the external K balance be zero, the external K balance must be positive for the growth of fetuses and neonates. Changes in fetal and neonatal total body K content during development are shown in Figure 4-7. This is a reflection, at least in part, of an increase in muscle mass and ICF [K$^+$] in muscle during development.[9] K metabolism in fetuses and neonates reflects this K requirement.

Fetus

K is actively transported across the placenta from the mother to the fetus. The plasma [K$^+$] in canine fetuses nearly always exceeds maternal plasma [K$^+$] under basal conditions.[10] Human fetal plasma [K$^+$] is also higher than that of the mother at term, but not significantly so at 16 to 22 weeks.[11] Thus, maternal–placental–fetal K metabolism is appropriately geared toward supplying the fetus with the K necessary for growth. The estimated maximum K accretion rate in utero is 0.8 mmol/kg/day.

The fetus is also buffered against maternal K deficiency. Despite a 35% decrease in plasma [K$^+$] and 28% decrease in intercellular [K$^+$] of skeletal muscle in pregnant female dogs fed a K-deficient diet throughout gestation, there was no difference in

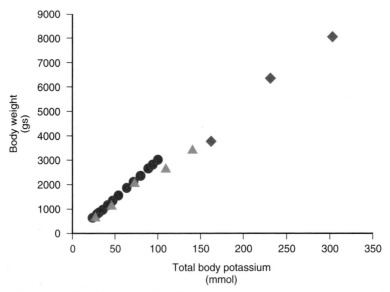

Figure 4-7 Total-body potassium (K) versus body weight. ●, derived from neutron activation analysis of cadavers (live births of nutritionally adequate mothers surviving 1–10 days). (Data from Ellis KJ. Body composition of the neonate. In RM Cowett (ed). Principles of neonatal-perinatal metabolism. New York, Springer-Verlag 1998, pp. 1077-1095.) ▲, chemical analysis of cadavers. (Data from Widdowson EM, Dickerson JWT. Chemical composition of the body. In Comar CL, Bonner F (eds). Mineral metabolism, vol 2, part A. New York, Academic Press, 1964, pp. 2-247.) ◆, sequential total body K by whole-body 40K counting in 76 breast- or formula-fed, normally growing, term infants at 0.5, 3, and 6 months of age. (Data from Butte NF, Hopkinson JM, Wong WW, Smith EO, Ellis KJ. Body composition during the first two years of life: an updated reference. Pediatr Res 47:578-585, 2000.)

fetal plasma [K⁺], fetal total body K, fetal dry weight, or litter size at near term compared with control subjects.[10] Despite a 50% decrease in plasma [K⁺] and 30% decrease in intercellular [K⁺] of skeletal muscle of rat dams fed a K-deficient diet from days 2 to 5 to day 21 of gestation, there was no change in fetal plasma [K⁺] and only a 10% decrease in fetal total body K at 22 days of gestation.[12] Similar results were found when acute K deficiency was induced in rat dams at 14 or 16 days of gestation by peritoneal dialysis with isotonic $NaHCO_3$.[13] On the other hand, fetuses do not seem to be buffered against excess maternal K. Serum [K⁺] of pups of rat dams infused with KCl to maintain serum [K⁺] greater than 10 mmol/L for 2 hours also exceeded 10 mmol/L.[12]

Neonate

Internal Potassium Metabolism

There are no data regarding whether there are quantitative differences between newborns and adults in the effect of factors controlling the distribution of K between the ICF and ECF spaces. However, studies in newborns confirm that β-catecholamine[14] and insulin administration stimulate the movement of K from the ECF to ICF space.[15,16]

Renal Potassium Metabolism

Thirteen to 15 days old rat pups have been shown to have the capacity to secrete potassium under basal conditions.[17] Even low birth weight (and presumably preterm) infants are capable of urinary K excretion at a rate in excess of the rate of K filtration across the glomerulus during K or $NaHCO_3$ loading (or loading of both) in the first month of life, indicating net tubular K secretion.[18] In newborn dogs, urinary K excretion is largely the result of amiloride-sensitive K secretion under basal conditions and during K loading.[19] Amiloride is known to selectively block sodium conductance across the luminal membrane in the distal tubule via inhibition of ENaCs. This then suggests that urinary K excretion under basal and K loaded conditions is largely the result of K secretion in the distal nephron (as is the case in adults) and that the cellular mechanisms of K secretion in this segment are similar to those in adults.

However, the rate of K excretion per unit body or kidney weight during exogenous K loading is lower in immature than mature animals.[19] In newborn infants, K secretion (as indicated indirectly by the calculated transtubular K concentration gradient in the distal nephron) was lower in preterm infants (mean gestational age, 29.3 ± 2.7 weeks) in the first 2 weeks of life than in term infants under basal conditions but similar to that in 1- to 2-week-old term infants during 3 to 5 weeks of life.[20] There was also a significant positive correlation between K secretion and postmenstrual age in the preterm infants. However, the relevance of these results to the developmental changes in K secretory capacity is unclear because no information is provided about the rate of K administration. In general, the limited K secretory capacity of the immature distal nephron is clinically relevant only under conditions of K excess.

Data in newborn dogs suggest that K secretion in response to K loading is not limited by basolateral Na⁺, K⁺-ATPase activity.[21,22] In vivo studies in suckling rats indicate that [Na⁺] in distal tubular fluid is greater than 35 mmol/L (as in adult rats) and therefore should not restrict K secretion.[23] Plasma aldosterone concentration is higher in preterm and term infants than in adults,[24,25] and the density of aldosterone binding sites, receptor affinity, and degree of nuclear binding of hormone receptors are similar in immature and mature rats.[24] However, clearance studies in fetuses and neonates and immature and mature rats demonstrate a relative insensitivity of the immature kidney to aldosterone,[24-26] presumably because of a postreceptor phenomenon. Studies in developing rabbits suggest that K secretion in the CCT in this species is limited by a paucity of SK channels.[27] In a study of single-nephrectomy specimens from 20 to 36 week's gestation infants, steady-state expression of mRNA encoding the SK channel did not change during this period and was only

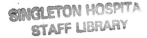

approximately one-third of that in nephrectomy specimens from 7-month-old subjects.[28] This could be expected to result in a decreased K secretory capacity of the immature distal tubule. Woda et al[6] have also shown the lack of response to increased tubular flow rate in developing rabbits as a result of the delayed expression of maxi-K channels. However, the kaliuresis associated with postnatal diuresis and natriuresis in preterm infants[29] and the development of hypokalemic hypochloremic metabolic alkalosis in association with loop diuretic therapy in newborns (see below) suggest that this finding may not be relevant to human infants.

On the other hand, K reabsorption increased in parallel to the increase in the filtered K load with increasing gestational age in a study of infants at 23 to 31 weeks of gestation on days 4 to 5 of life, so that urinary K excretion remained low and unchanged over this period of gestation.[30]

Intestinal K Metabolism

Although the neonatal intestine is certainly capable of reabsorbing dietary K, the relative capacity of the neonatal colon for net K secretion is unknown. However, when K load stimulated levels of colonic Na^+, K^+-ATPase activity in premature, term, and 4-day-old Sprague-Dawley rats were measured, enzyme activity increased in response to K loading in all three groups, demonstrating that preterm and term rats are capable of colonic adaptation to chronic K loading.[31]

Na^+, K^+-ATPase activity, H^+,K^+-ATPase activity, and K transport were measured in the colons of near-term rat pups immediately after delivery without feeding, 10-day-old rat pups maintained with their dams, and adult (50-day-old) Sprague-Dawley rats fed a regular diet.[32] H^+,K^+-ATPase activity was absent in the near-term colon, but activity was twice the adult level in the infant colon. Although colonic Na^+, K^+-ATPase activity increased progressively with maturation, the ratio of H^+,K^+-ATPase to Na^+, K^+-ATPase activity was threefold higher in the rat pups than in the adult rat colon. As a result, K uptake in the colon was almost threefold higher. Thus, after birth, the infant rat colon adapts postnatally, probably in response to feeding, by increasing colonic reabsorption in excess of the adult to promote the greater K reabsorption required for growth.

Feedback and Feedforward Control of Plasma [K^+]

The data discussed above confirm the existence of feedback control of plasma [K^+] in the newborn, although at least in the case of the renal response to a K load, less robust than in adults. There are no data regarding feedforward control in the newborn. However, although the dietary intake of breast- and formula-fed infants is relatively high (~2–3 mmol/100 kcal or 2–3 mmol/kg/day) compared with adults (~1.5 mmol/kg/day), the feedforward control of plasma [K^+] might be expected to be less important than in adults because of the regularity and frequency of feeding in the newborn period. However, it might be expected to be more important during fasting.

Clinical Relevance

Perturbations in internal or external K balance on usual K intakes (1–3 mmol/kg/day) are unusual in neonates except under a few circumstances.

Hyperkalemia

Spurious Hyperkalemia

Hyperkalemia in the neonatal intensive care unit is most commonly spurious secondary to red blood cell hemolysis in the whole-blood sample.

Nonoliguric Hyperkalemia

Plasma [K^+] increases in the first 24 to 72 hours after birth in very premature infants even in the absence of exogenous K intake or renal failure.[29,33,34] This increase results from the transcellular movement of K from the ICF space to the ECF space.[34] This shift occurs at a time when the renal K excretion is restricted by the low GFR and relatively low fractional excretion of Na, which limits sodium and water delivery to the distal nephron.[29] The reason for and appropriateness of this shift are not understood. However, it is known to result in hyperkalemia in 25% to 50% of infants weighing less than 1000 g at birth or born at less than 28 weeks' gestation.[29,35-40] The magnitude of this shift correlates roughly with the degree of prematurity, but it does not seem to occur (or at least is not clinically significant) after 30 to 32 weeks' gestation.[34] The most effective strategy for managing nonoliguric hyperkalemia when renal secretory capacity is so restricted is to stimulate the movement of K back from the ECF to ICF space with albuterol inhalation[14] or insulin[15,16] therapy.

Even without albuterol or insulin therapy, plasma [K$^+$] falls with the onset of physiologic diuresis and natriuresis, as the associated increase in delivery of water and Na to the distal nephron results in marked kaliuresis. In fact, many infants with nonoliguric hyperkalemia become hypokalemic after the onset of diuresis and natriuresis if K administration is not initiated as plasma [K$^+$] declines.[29]

Renal Failure

As in adults, an acute severe reduction in GFR severely reduces water and Na delivery to the distal nephron and thus restricts K secretion.

Hypokalemia
Loop and Thiazide Diuretics

Hypokalemia commonly results from loop and diuretic therapy[41] (Fig. 4-8). This is primarily the result of the stimulation of distal K secretion by the increased delivery

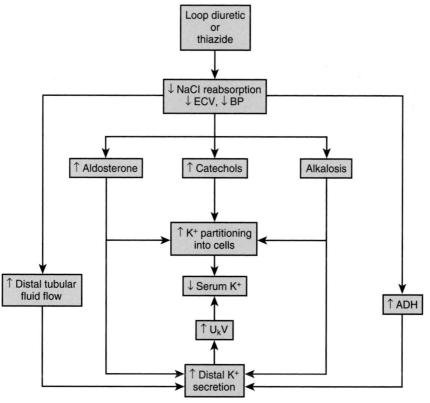

Figure 4-8 Effects of loop and thiazide diuretics on internal potassium (K) balance and K transport in the distal nephron. ADH, antidiuretic hormone; BP, blood pressure; ECV, extracellular volume. (From Wilcox CS. Diuretics and potassium. In Seldin DW, Giebisch G (eds). Regulation of potassium balance. New York, Raven Press, 1989, pp. 325-345, with permission.)

of water and Na delivery. However, increases in aldosterone, catecholamines, vaso-pressin, and alkalosis (caused by contraction of the ECF) also result in enhanced cellular uptake of K from the ECF space.

Alkalosis

The predominant cause of hypokalemia with metabolic or respiratory alkalosis is negative external K balance. An increase in plasma $[HCO_3^-]$ also produces a rapid decrease in plasma $[K^+]$, which is caused by enhanced cellular uptake of K from the ECF space.

References

1. Rosa RM, Eckstein FH. Extrarenal potassium metabolism. In: Seldin DW, Giebisch G, eds. *The kidney: physiology and pathophysiology.* New York: Raven Press; 2000:1515-1574.
2. Andrógue HF, Madias NE. Changes in plasma potassium concentration during acid and base disturbances. *Am J Med.* 1981;71:454.
3. Berliner RW. Renal mechanisms for K excretion. *Harvey Lect.* 1961;55:141–171.
4. Giebisch G, Wang W. Potassium transport from clearance to channels to pumps. *Kidney Int.* 1996;49:1624.
5. Giebisch GH. A trail of research on potassium. *Kidney Int.* 2002;62:1498.
6. Woda CB, Bragin A, Kleyman TR, et al. Flow-dependent K^+ secretion in the cortical collecting duct is mediated by a maxi-K channel. *AJP.* 2001;49:F793.
7. Amorim JBO, Bailey MA, Musa-Aziz R, et al. Role of luminal anion and pH in distal potassium secretion. *Am J Physiol.* 2003;284:F381.
8. Youn JH, McDonough AA. Recent advances in understanding integrative control of potassium homeostasis. *Annu Rev Physiol.* 2009;71:381-401
9. Dickerson JWT, Widdowson EM. Chemical changes in skeletal muscle during development. *Biochem J.* 1960;74:247.
10. Servano CV, Talbert LM, Welt LG. Potassium deficiency in the pregnant dog. *J Clin Invest.* 1964;43:27.
11. Bengtsson B, Gennser G, Nilsson E. Sodium, potassium, and water content of human fetal, neonatal, and maternal plasma and red blood cells. *Acta Paediatr Scand.* 1970;59:192.
12. Dancis J, Springer D. Fetal homeostasis in maternal malnutrition: potassium and sodium deficiency in rats. *Pediatr Res.* 1970;4:345.
13. Stewart EL, Welt LG. Protection of the fetus in experimental potassium depletion. *Am J Physiol.* 1961;200:824.
14. Singh DS, Sadiq HF, Noguchi A, et al. Efficacy of albuterol inhalation in treatment of hyperkalemia in premature infants. *J Pediatr.* 2002;141:16.
15. Malone TA. Glucose and insulin versus cation-exchange resin for the treatment of hyperkalemia in very low birth weight infants. *J Pediatr.* 1991;118:121.
16. Hu PS, Su BH, Peng CT, et al. Glucose and insulin infusion versus kayexalate for early treatment of non-oliguric hyperkalemia in very-low-birth-weight infants. *Acta Paediatr Taiwan.* 1999;40:314.
17. Lelievre-Pegorier M, Merlet-Benichou C, Roinel N, et al. Developmental pattern of water and electrolyte transport in rat superficial nephrons. *Am J Physiol.* 1983;245:F15.
18. Tudvad F, McNamara MA, Barnett HL. Renal response of premature infants to administration of bicarbonate and potassium. *Pediatrics.* 1954;13:4.
19. Lorenz JM, Kleinman LI, Disney TA. Renal response of the newborn dog to potassium loading. *Am J Physiol.* 1986;251:F513.
20. Nako Y, Ohki Y, Harigaya A, et al. Transtubular potassium concentration gradient in preterm neonates. *Pediatr Nephrol.* 1999;13:880.
21. Lorenz JM, Manuli MA, Browne LE. Chronic potassium supplementation of newborn dogs increases cortical Na, K-ATPase but not urinary potassium excretion. *J Dev Physiol.* 1990;13:181.
22. Lorenz JM, Manuli MA, Browne LE. The role of cortical Na,K-ATPase in distal nephron potassium secretion by the immature canine kidney. *Pediatr Res.* 1991;30:457.
23. Aperia A, Elinder G. Distal tubular sodium reabsorption in the developing rat kidney. *Am J Physiol.* 1981;240:F487.
24. Sulyok E, Nemeth M, Tenyi I, et al. Relationship between maturity, electrolyte balance, and the function of the renin-angiotensin-aldosterone system in newborn infants. *Bio Neonate.* 1979;35:60.
25. Stephenson G, Hammet M, Hadaway G, et al. Ontogeny of renal mineralocorticoid receptors and urinary electrolyte responses in rats. *Am J Physiol.* 1984;247:F665.
26. Van Acker KJ, Sharpe SL, Deprettere AJ, et al. Renin-angiotensin-aldosterone system in the healthy infant and child. *Kidney Int.* 1979;16:196.
27. Benchimol C, Zavilowitz B, Satlin LM. Developmental expression of ROMK mRNA in rabbit cortical collecting duct. *Pediatr Res.* 2002;47:46.
28. Satlin LM. Developmental regulation of expression of renal potassium secretory channels. *Curr Opin Nephrol Hyperten.* 2004;13:445.
29. Lorenz JM, Kleinman LI, Markarian K. Potassium metabolism in extremely low birth weight infants in the first week of life. *J Pediatr.* 1997;131:81.
30. Delgado MM, Rohati R, Khan S, et al. Sodium and potassium clearances by the maturing kidney: clinical-metabolic correlates. *Pediatr Nephrol.* 2003;18:759.

31. Aizman RI, Celsi G, Grahnquist L, et al. Ontogeny of K$^+$ transport in the distal rat colon. *Am J Physiol.* 1996;271:G268.
32. Verma RP, Horvath K, Blochin B, et al. Maturational response of colonic and renal Na+, K(+)-ATPase activity to K+ load and betamethasone in preterm rats. *J Lab & Clini Med.* 1994;12:676.
33. Usher R. The respiratory distress syndrome of prematurity. I. Changes in potassium in the serum and the electrocardiogram and effects of therapy. *Pediatrics.* 1959;24:562.
34. Sato K, Kondo T, Iwao H, et al. Internal potassium shift in premature infants: cause of nonoliguric hyperkalemia. *J Pediatr.* 1995;126:109.
35. Gruskay J, Costarino AT, Polin RA, et al. Nonoliguric hyperkalemia in the premature infant weighing less than 1000 grams. *J Pediatr.* 1988;113:381.
36. Fukada Y, Kojima T, Ono A, et al. Factors causing hyperkalemia in premature infants. *Am J Perinatology.* 1989;6:76.
37. Sato K, Kondo T, Iwao H, et al. Sodium and potassium in red blood cells of premature infants during the first few days: risk of hyperkalemia. *Acta Paediatr Scand.* 1991;80:899.
38. Shaffer SG, Kilbride HW, Hayes LK, et al. Hyperkalemia in very low birth weight infants. *J Pediatr.* 1992;121:275–279.
39. Stefano JL, Norman ME, Morales MC, et al. Decreased erythrocyte Na+ K+-ATPase activity associated with cellular potassium loss in extremely low birth weight infants with nonoliguric hyperkalemia. *J Pediatr.* 1993;122:276–284.
40. Stefano JL, Norman ME: Nitrogen balance in extremely low birth weight infants with nonoliguric hyperkalemia. *J Pediatr.* 1993;123:632.
41. Wilcox CS. Diuretics and potassium. In: Seldin DW, Giebisch G, eds. *The regulation of potassium balance (pp. 325–345).* New York: Raven Press; 1989.

4

CHAPTER 5

Renal Urate Metabolism in the Fetus and Newborn

Daniel I. Feig, MD, PhD

Uric acid is the primary endpoint of purine disposal pathways in humans and primates. Most other animals have the hepatic enzyme urate oxidase that further metabolizes uric acid to a more water-soluble molecule, allantoin (Fig. 5-1).[1] Loss of this enzyme during hominid evolution to three different silencing mutations some 24, 16, and 13 million years ago[2,3] results in the accumulation of uric acid in the bloodstream and risk for urate-mediated pathology. Urate generation rate varies significantly depending on the turnover of purines, which can be effected by diet, cell damage, and cell turnover.[4] The kidneys are responsible for most (70%–80%) of urate clearance.[5] Thus, perturbations of glomerular filtration or tubular reabsorption or active excretion can cause significant changes in serum uric acid concentrations. The combination of a lack of urate oxidase and efficient tubular reabsorption leads to the higher serum levels of uric acid in humans.[6] In neonates and infants, because of rapid changes in glomerular filtration rate (GFR), serum uric acid concentrations can vary significantly.[7]

Uric Acid in Human Disease

Uric acid was first noted to be associated with human disease in the mid-1800s. First associated with inflammatory gout, uric acid was also implicated in hypertension and cardiovascular and renal disease as early as 1879.[8] In the 1970s to 1990s, a number of epidemiologic studies demonstrated an association between serum uric acid and cardiovascular disease.[9-18] Although most suggested an independent risk contribution, some demonstrated by multiple logistic regression that uric acid was not independent of other more conventional risk factors, such as renal function, obesity, hypertension, and hypercholesterolemia.[19] Belief in a direct pathogenic role for uric acid waned during the 1990s as, despite epidemiologic evidence, no plausible physiologic mechanism could be established.

Between 1999 and 2004, several investigators used rodent models of mild hyperuricemia to investigate the pathophysiology of uric acid disorders. Because genetic knockouts of rodent urate oxidase tended to lead to renal failure and death by several weeks of age, the models of mild to moderate hyperuricemia based on the pharmacologic inhibition of urate oxidase[20-22] were used. Such experiments revealed that a rise in serum uric acid led to an increase in both systolic and diastolic blood pressure within 1 to 2 weeks.[20] Initial blood pressure response was mediated by activation of the renin–angiotensin system and downregulation of circulating nitric oxide[20,23-25] and could be promptly reversed by reduction of serum uric acid or renin–angiotensin system blockade. Sustained hyperuricemia leads to a different pathophysiology. If rats that have had hyperuricemic hypertension for a couple of

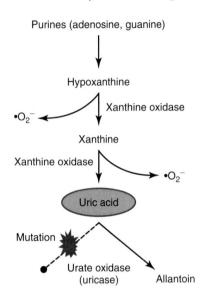

Purines (adenosine, guanine)

Hypoxanthine

Xanthine oxidase

$\cdot O_2^-$

Xanthine

Xanthine oxidase

$\cdot O_2^-$

Uric acid

Mutation

Urate oxidase
(uricase)

Allantoin

Primates   *Non-primates*

Figure 5-1 Metabolism of uric acid. Uric acid is the endproduct of purine disposal metabolism. Xanthine oxidase catalyzes the oxidation of both xanthine and hypoxanthine to uric acid. A byproduct of these reactions is superoxide radical. Nonprimates have the enzyme urate oxidase that metabolizes uric acid to allantoin. Humans and higher primates have lost the activity of urate oxidase through a series of mutations.

months are allowed to normalize their uric acid by withdrawal of the urate oxidase inhibitor, the blood pressure will return to normal as long as the rats remain on a low-sodium diet. If fed a high-sodium diet, the formally hyperuricemic rats have a sodium sensitive hypertension that is irreversible even with no further exposure to hyperuricemia.[21] This results from uric acid–mediated geometric changes in the renal afferent arterioles that then cause a shift in the pressure–natriuresis curve.[26] That is to say that a high systemic blood pressure is required to excrete dietary sodium load.

A large number of epidemiologic studies have linked serum uric acid and risk of arterial hypertension[27]; however, the most direct evidence for a mechanistic link comes from studies in adolescents. It was found that serum uric acid was above 5.5 mg/dL in 89% of adolescents with untreated new-onset primary hypertension, but was elevated in fewer than 30% of subjects with secondary hypertension and nearly absent in healthy control participants. The relationship of uric acid to systolic blood pressure was linear with each 1 mg/dL increase in serum uric acid being associated with an 8 mm Hg increase in systolic blood pressure.[28] In a randomized, double-blind, placebo-controlled, cross-over trial of uric acid reduction, adolescents with newly diagnosed hypertension and hyperuricemia were randomized to placebo followed by allopurinol (a xanthine oxidase inhibitor) or allopurinol followed by placebo for 4 weeks, each separated by a 2-week washout period.[29] In subjects whose uric acid was decreased below 5.0 mg/dL, 86% became normotensive.

Uric acid has also been associated with several other conditions. For well over a century, uric acid crystal deposition has been known to contribute causatively to the development of gout.[30] Hyperuricemia also independently predicts a reduction in renal function in the general population.[31-33] Clinically, an elevated uric acid both induces and accelerates established renal disease by mediating renal vasoconstriction, endothelial dysfunction, and renin activation and inducing microvascular lesions that impair autoregulation and cause glomerular hypertension.[34-37] Even in the context of normal renal function, elevated serum uric acid is associated with greater risk of renal functional decline.[32,38] Recent clinical studies suggest that lowering uric acid may slow renal disease progression in subjects with hyperuricemia and chronic kidney disease.[39] Hyperuricemia also predicts hyperinsulinemia,[40] diabetes,[15,41-44] and weight gain.[14] High-fructose intake accelerates renal disease with identical features as hyperuricemia[45]; fructose also activates endothelial, renal tubular, and hepatic cells, and some of the effects are mediated by uric acid.[46-48] Finally, uric acid may induce inflammation. Serum uric acid levels correlate with C-reactive protein (CRP) levels and with microalbuminuria in humans[49,50] and in experimental models, uric acid stimulates CRP synthesis in human vascular cells,[51] and uric acid reduction causes CRP levels to decrease.[39,52]

Uric Acid in Diseases of Fetuses and Newborns

The spectrum of uric acid associated-disease in newborns is different from that of older children and adults. Developmentally, the earliest onset of hyperuricemia is seen in preeclampsia. Although many of the symptoms can be explained by excessive placental production of sFLT1 (fms-like tyrosine kinase), a soluble vascular endothelial growth factor (VEGF) antagonist, leading to partial blockade of VEGF and severe endothelial dysfunction,[53] uric acid is consistently elevated in preeclampsia. It is not clear whether uric acid is causative or merely associated with the condition, but higher maternal levels of uric acid during early pregnancy are predictive of the disease.[54] Uric acid can readily cross the placenta so that maternal hyperuricemia is transmitted to the developing fetus. Urate supersaturation of urine in newborns can result in the presence of an orange-pink paste seen in diapers that have precipitated many visits to emergency departments and pediatrician's offices, but generally disturbs parents much more than infants and can truly be considered a normal variant.[55,56] At higher urinary concentrations, uric acid can cause perinatal kidney stones[57] or severe melamine–urate stones in infants exposed to melamine-contaminated formulas.[58] Premature infants with hyperuricemia are at greater risk for the development of retinopathy of prematurity.[59] As in older children, higher uric acid levels are seen in neonates with hypertension, with a mean value of 3.8 mg/dL compared with 3.4 mg/dL[60] in nonhypertensive children.[3]

Elevated uric acid concentrations are not necessarily always disadvantageous. Uric acid is a potentially potent antioxidant and could play a protective role against reactive oxygen species. Allantoin is the primary, stable oxidation product of uric acid, so some groups have assayed allantoin to uric acid ratios to assess the severity of oxidant exposure and found much higher allantoin levels in infants with severe chronic lung disease.[61]

Generation of Uric Acid

In fetuses and neonates, the generation of uric acid is entirely attributable to the metabolism of endogenous purines. Although high-purine foods, including beef, lamb, shellfish, and beer, can be important contributors to gout flares in adults, breast milk and infant formula are very low in purines.[62] Cell turnover and the concomitant release of purines from nucleic acids can provide a purine load that raises serum uric acid.[63] This is important in tumor lysis syndrome and possibly during severe tissue injury, but the urate-generation rate in newborns is likely more closely linked to the relative efficiency of hepatic xanthine oxidase and metabolic purine recovery via 5-phosphoribosyl-1-pyrophosphate (PRPP). The metabolism of sugars may also play a role in urate homeostasis. Figure 5-2 illustrates the overlapping metabolism of fructose and glucose.[64] The initial step of glucose metabolism is the 6 phosphorylation by glucokinase (also called hexokinase). The source of both the energy for the reaction and the phosphate is adenosine triphosphate (ATP). Glucokinase is inhibited by adenosine diphosphate (ADP), which prevents acute intracellular ATP depletion and accumulation of low-energy moieties as substrate for purine disposal pathways. In contrast, fructokinase, the enzyme that initiates the metabolism of fructose, is not inhibited by ADP, so cellular loading with fructose can lead to increased urate generation.[65] The dominant sugar in breast milk and some infant formulas is lactose, a disaccharide of glucose and galactose. Some synthetic infant formulas use sucrose, a disaccharide of glucose and fructose, or high-fructose corn syrup, 45% sucrose and 55% fructose, so they could theoretically contribute to increased urate production; however, this possibility has not been tested in clinical trials.

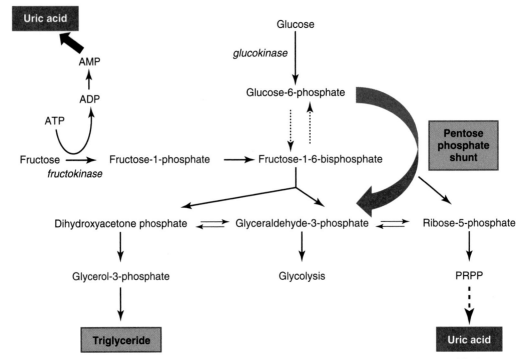

Figure 5-2 Interrelationship between sugar and purine metabolism. The diagram depicts a simplified version of glucose and fructose metabolism. Glucokinase is inhibited by adenosine diphosphate (ADP) whereas fructokinase is not. This results in the production of excess ADP and adenosine monophosphate (AMP) as a result of fructose consumption, which can then be metabolized to uric acid as a result of purine disposal. On the *right side* of the figure, ribose-5-phosphate is the initiation step of purine salvage, so alterations in that pathway can also lead to changes in uric acid concentration.

Glomerular Filtration Rate

Because uric acid is freely filtered by the glomerulus, the serum uric acid concentrations in neonates partly depend on the GFR. Neonates, particularly preterm neonates, have reduced GFR relative to older or later gestation children. Table 5-1 shows the serum creatinine and GFR of pre- and full term infants.[7,66,67] In children of less than 28 weeks' gestation, the GFR is quite low but increases with age, reaching mature levels within the first months of life.[68] Serum creatinine falls in parallel.

Table 5-1 MEAN SERUM CREATININE, GLOMERULAR FILTRATION RATE, AND URIC ACID VALUES AT VARIOUS GESTATIONAL AND POSTNATAL AGES

Age	Serum Creatinine (mg/dL)	Glomerular Filtration Rate (mL/min/1.73m²)	Serum Uric Acid (mg/dL)	Fractional Excretion of Uric Acid (%)
≤28 weeks' gestation	0.66–1.31	13.4 ± 7.9	ND	ND
29–32 weeks' gestation	0.59–1.18	21.9 ± 16	3.6 ± 0.6	70 ± 22
33–36 weeks' gestation	0.40–1.05	32.4 ± 12	3.0 ± 0.7	48 ± 17
37–42 weeks' gestation	0.34–0.85	41 ± 15	2.6 ± 0.5	39 ± 14
2–8 weeks	0.20–0.60	66 ± 25	1.8 ± 0.5	16.5 ± 12.1
2 months–1 year	0.10–0.30	96 ± 22	2.2 ± 0.8	15.2 ± 10.1

ND, not determined.
Data from Rudd et al,[7] Ichida,[65] Schwartz et al,[66] Tsukahara et al,[67] Vieux et al,[68] Basu et al,[69] and Stapleton.[70]

Similarly, serum uric acid falls with advancing age, suggesting that some of the control of urate clearance is purely filtration.[69] The fractional excretion of uric acid and the urine urate-to-creatinine ratios are extremely high in preterm neonates but are much lower in full-term and older infants.[69,70] This may be in part compensatory for the higher serum uric acid levels, but may also represent a degree of immaturity of the tubular reabsorption mechanisms. Because branching nephrogenesis is at least partially abrogated by preterm delivery, some permanent loss in nephron mass and renal reserve is expected and may have deleterious late effects on urate clearance in formally premature infants.[71]

Proximal Tubular Urate Transport

Uric acid is freely filtered through the glomerulus; however, more than 90% is reabsorbed in the proximal tubule. Because of its hydrophobicity and negative charge, it is unlikely that there is significant paracellular transport, leaving the transcellular transport as the dominant mechanism (Fig. 5-3).

The most active transporter on the luminal membrane is the urate anion transporter 1 (URAT-1), which is a high-throughput anion exchanger located at the luminal membrane of the proximal tubule. URAT-1 primarily exchanges luminal uric acid for monocarboxylates, including lactate, nicotinate, and pyrazinecarboxylic acid. URAT-1 mediated urate reabsorption is likely enhanced by structural linkage

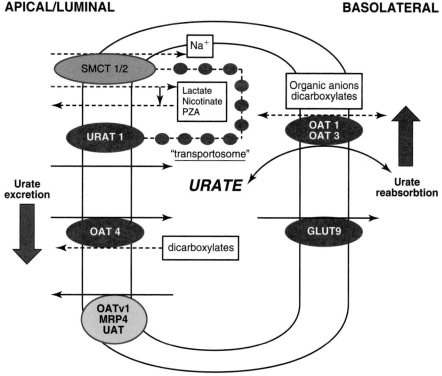

APICAL/LUMINAL   **BASOLATERAL**

Figure 5-3 Proximal tubule urate transport. *Solid lines* indicate the direction of urate transport; *dashed lines* show the movement of cotransported or countertransported ions. The urate anion transporter 1 (URAT-1) is a urate/dicarboxylate exchanger that provides most of the reabsorption for filtered uric acid. It is coupled by the PDZ domain containing scaffolding proteins (represented by the dotted box) to sodium/monocarboxylate cotransporter 1 and 2 (SMCT 1 and SMCT 2), which are Na, monocarboxylate cotransporters. This "urate transpososome" results in efficient monocarboxylate reabsorption and excretion, yielding net reabsorption of Na and urate. Organic anion transporter 4 (OAT-4) is a urate/dicarboxylate exchanger that may modestly contribute to urate reabsorption. OATv1 = Organic Anion Transporter variant 1, MRP4 = human Multi-drug Resistance Protein 4, and uric acid transporter (UAT), also located on the luminal membrane, are thought to contribute to the active excretion of uric acid (see text). On the basolateral membrane, OAT-1 and OAT-3 are bidirectional urate/dicarboxylate exchangers that provide the major pathway for reentry of uric acid into the circulation. Facilitative glucose transporter 9 (GLUT9) is a recently discovered fructose and uric acid transporter present on the basolateral membrane of proximal tubules and several other cell types.[76]

to sodium/monocarboxylate cotransporters SMCT-1 and SMCT-2.[72] Scaffolding proteins with PDZ protein binding motifs co-localize SMCT transporters and URAT-1. Monocarboxylate molecules entering the proximal tubular cell through SMCT transporters are then excreted, in exchange for urate, by URAT-1. The results of this channel pairing, called by some groups the "urate transportosome," are the local intracellular concentration of monocarboxlyates to drive urate reabsorption and the net reabsorption of sodium and urate in equal molar concentrations. Some experts have hypothesized that this indirect pairing of urate and sodium reabsorption led to an evolutionary advantage in times of a severely sodium-deficient diet and explains the loss of urate oxidase during hominid development.[3] URAT-1 can be inhibited by several pharmacologic agents, including benzbromarone, probenecid, losartan, and high-dose salicylate. The dominant role of URAT-1 in urate reabsorption is demonstrated by patients with hereditary renal hypouricemia in which mutations in URAT-1 lead to increased clearance and serum levels less than 2 mg/dL, which is as low as in animals with active urate oxidase.[73]

There are several other potential apical membrane urate transporters; however, their relative contribution to uric acid homeostasis is unclear. Organic anion transporter 4 (OAT-4) is an anion/dicarboxylate exchanger, structurally similar to URAT-1, that may participate in urate reabsorption. OAT-v1 is a voltage gated anion channel that may contribute to urate secretion into the tubular lumen.[74] Uric acid transporter (UAT) is a constitutively active urate channel expressed on the apical pole of proximal tubular cells that may also contribute to passive urate efflux. MRP-4 is an ATP-dependent urate transporter that may provide modifiable urate excretion.[64]

OAT-1 and OAT-3 are urate transporters located on the basolateral surface of proximal tubule cells. These dicarboxylate/urate exchangers provide the major pathway for reentry of uric acid into the circulation. It is as yet unknown if, or to what degree, these transporters are regulated.[64] Although tremendous strides in the understanding of proximal tubular urate handling have been made in the past 10 years, it remains incompletely understood and the focus of intense study.

Developmental Implications and Conclusions

In utero fetal uric acid concentrations are probably controlled by maternal metabolism; however, there are few data to confirm this hypothesis. The amount of uric acid generated by the mother is much greater than that of the fetus for reasons of body size and would be expected to equilibrate with the fetal circulation because urate readily crosses the placenta. Because fetal GFR is low, the vast majority of clearance occurs primarily in the maternal compartment. In the context of maternal hyperuricemia, particularly in severe preeclampsia or toxemia syndromes when maternal renal function may be impaired, the fetus would be expected to be exposed to higher levels of uric acid.

After delivery, the serum uric acid levels in neonates are largely regulated by changes in GFR. Premature newborns have serum uric acid levels that are essentially inversely proportional to their GFR, and the serum uric acid concentrations reach the nadir after 2 months of age.[74] The observed, very high fractional excretion of uric acid seen in premature patients suggests that the proximal tubule mechanisms for urate reabsorption are not yet fully developed, resulting in clearance that is largely a direct result of filtration. As children grow, the fractional excretion of urate and total urate clearance decreases dramatically, suggesting maturation of the proximal tubule reabsorptive capacity.[75] The nature of this maturational process is currently entirely unknown. Possible mechanisms include differential expression of luminal urate transporters, particularly URAT-1; changes in scaffolding of the transpososome; or even regulation of basolateral transporter expression.

There are several potential physiologic implications for the high urinary urate excretion in preterm neonates. The presence of relatively higher concentrations of urate in the urine of infants who also have moderate hypercalciuria may contribute to nephrocalcinosis and neonatal renal stone disease. Diuretics that increase calcium excretion, used by some clinicians in infants with bronchopulmonary dysplasia, are expected to exacerbate this process. Uric acid has been implicated in the progressive decline in GFR[38] in patients with normal as well as impaired renal function, and it is not clear if the effect is attributable to serum or urinary concentrations of uric acid or both.

Many questions regarding the renal metabolism of uric acid in neonates remain. In fact, despite dramatic advances defining the physiology of urate transport, few studies have been directed toward infants in the past 20 years. The data are sufficiently sparse that no evidence-based treatment guideline can be proposed. Investigations in the possibility of uric acid–mediated vascular or organ injury in our smallest patients are needed. Studies to define the developmental control of the generation and regulation of uric acid excretion should in the future improve the rational management of vulnerable neonates.

References

1. Sica D, Schoolwerth A. Renal handling of organic anions and cations: excretion of uric acid. In: BM B, ed. *The Kidney.* 6th ed. Philadelphia: WB Saunders; 2000:690-700.
2. Johnson RJ, Titte SR, Cade JR, et al. Uric acid, primitive cultures and evolution. *Semin Nephrol.* 2004;in press.
3. Watanabe S, Kang DH, Feng L, et al. Uric acid Hominoid Evolution and the Pathogenesis of Salt-sensitivity. *Hypertension.* 2002;40:355-360.
4. Yamanaka H. Gout and hyperuricemia in young people. *Curr Opin Rheumatol.* 2011;23:156-160.
5. Maesaka JK, Fishbane S. Regulation of renal urate excretion: a critical review. *Am J Kidney Dis.* 1998;32:917-933.
6. Johnson RJ, Feig DI, Herrera-Acosta J, Kang DH. Resurrection of uric acid as a causal risk factor in essential hypertension. *Hypertension.* 2005;45:18-20.
7. Rudd PT, Hughes EA, Placzek MM, Hodes DT. Reference ranges for plasma creatinine during the first month of life. *Arch Dis Child.* 1983;58:212-215.
8. Mahomed FA. On chronic Bright's disease , and its essential symptoms. *Lancet.* 1879;1:399-401.
9. Alper AB Jr, Chen W, Yau L, et al. Childhood uric acid predicts adult blood pressure: the Bogalusa Heart Study. *Hypertension.* 2005;45:34-38.
10. Dyer AR, Liu K, Walsh M, et al. Ten-year incidence of elevated blood pressure and its predictors: the CARDIA study. Coronary Artery Risk Development in (Young) Adults. *J Hum Hypertens.* 1999;13: 13-21.
11. Hunt SC, Stephenson SH, Hopkins PN, Williams RR. Predictors of an increased risk of future hypertension in Utah. A screening analysis. *Hypertension.* 1991;17:969-976.
12. Imazu M, Yamamoto H, Toyofuku M, et al. Hyperinsulinemia for the development of hypertension: data from the Hawaii-Los Angeles-Hiroshima Study. *Hypertens Res.* 2001;24:531-536.
13. Jossa F, Farinaro E, Panico S, et al. Serum uric acid and hypertension: the Olivetti heart study. *J Hum Hypertens.* 1994;8:677-681.
14. Masuo K, Kawaguchi H, Mikami H, et al. Serum uric acid and plasma norepinephrine concentrations predict subsequent weight gain and blood pressure elevation. *Hypertension.* 2003;42:474-480.
15. Nakanishi N, Okamato M, Yoshida H, et al. Serum uric acid and the risk for development of hypertension and impaired fasting glucose or type II diabetes in Japanese male office workers. *Eur J Epidemiol.* 2003;18:523-530.
16. Selby JV, Friedman GD, Quesenberry CP Jr. Precursors of essential hypertension: pulmonary function, heart rate, uric acid, serum cholesterol, and other serum chemistries. *Am J Epidemiol.* 1990;131: 1017-1027.
17. Sundstrom J, Sullivan L, D'Agostino RB, et al. Relations of serum uric acid to longitudinal blood pressure tracking and hypertension incidence. *Hypertension.* 2005;45:28-33.
18. Taniguchi Y, Hayashi T, Tsumura K, et al. Serum uric acid and the risk for hypertension and type 2 diabetes in Japanese men. The Osaka Health Survey. *J Hypertens.* 2001;19:1209-1215.
19. Forman JP, Choi H, Curhan GC. Plasma uric Acid level and risk for incident hypertension among men. *J Am Soc Nephrol.* 2007;18:287-292.
20. Mazzali M, Hughes J, Kim YG, et al. Elevated uric acid increases blood pressure in the rat by a novel crystal-independent mechanism. *Hypertension.* 2001;38:1101-1106.
21. Mazzali M, Kanellis J, Han L, et al. Hyperuricemia induces a primary renal arteriolopathy in rats by a blood pressure-independent mechanism. *Am J Physiol Renal Physiol.* 2002;282:F991-F997.
22. Mazzali M, Kim YG, Suga S, et al. Hyperuricemia exacerbates chronic cyclosporine nephropathy. *Transplantation.* 2001;71:900-905.
23. Kanellis J, Watanabe S, Li JH, et al. Uric acid stimulates monocyte chemoattractant protein-1 production in vascular smooth muscle cells via mitogen-activated protein kinase and cyclooxygenase-2. *Hypertension.* 2003;41:1287-1293.
24. Kang DH, Nakagawa T, Feng L, Johnson RJ. Nitric oxide modulates vascular disease in the remnant kidney model. *Am J Pathol.* 2002;161:239-248.
25. Kang DH, Nakagawa T, Feng L, et al. A role for uric acid in the progression of renal disease. *J Am Soc Nephrol.* 2002;13:2888-2897.
26. Nakagawa T, Hu H, Zharikov S, et al. A causal role for uric acid in fructose-induced metabolic syndrome. *Am J Physiol Renal Physiol.* 2006;290:F625-F631.

27. Feig DI, Kang DH, Johnson RJ. Uric acid and cardiovascular risk. *N Engl J Med.* 2008;359: 1811-1821.
28. Feig DI, Johnson RJ. Hyperuricemia in childhood primary hypertension. *Hypertension.* 2003;42: 247-252.
29. Feig DI, Soletsky B, Johnson RJ. Effect of allopurinol on blood pressure of adolescents with newly diagnosed essential hypertension: a randomized trial. *JAMA.* 2008;300:924-932.
30. Haig A. Gout. *In Uric Acid: A Factor in the Causation of Disease.* 4th ed. London: J & A Churchill; 1897, pp 512-548.
31. Nagahama K, Inoue T, Iseki K, et al. Hyperuricemia as a predictor of hypertension in a screened cohort in Okinawa, Japan. *Hypertens Res.* 2004;27:835-841.
32. Iseki K, Ikemiya Y, Inoue T, et al. Significance of hyperuricemia as a risk factor for developing ESRD in a screened cohort. *Am J Kidney Dis.* 2004;44:642-650.
33. Nagahama K, Iseki K, Inoue T, et al. Hyperuricemia and cardiovascular risk factor clustering in a screened cohort in Okinawa, Japan. *Hypertens Res.* 2004;27:227-233.
34. Sanchez-Lozada LG, Tapia E, Avila-Casado C, et al. Mild hyperuricemia induces glomerular hypertension in normal rats. *Am J Physiol Renal Physiol.* 2002;283:F1105-F1110.
35. Sanchez-Lozada LG, Tapia E, et al. Effects of febuxostat on metabolic and renal alterations in rats with fructose-induced metabolic syndrome. *Am J Physiol Renal Physiol.* 2008;294:F710-F718.
36. Sanchez-Lozada LG, Tapia E, et al. Effects of acute and chronic L-arginine treatment in experimental hyperuricemia. *Am J Physiol Renal Physiol.* 2007;292:F1238-F1244.
37. Sanchez-Lozada LG, Tapia E, Santamaria J, Herrera-Acosta J. Mild hyperuricemia increases arteriolopathy inducing renal cortical ischemia in 5/6 nephrectomy rats. *J Am Soc Nephrol.* 2003;13:618A.
38. Bellomo G, Venanzi S, Verdura C, et al. Association of uric acid with change in kidney function in healthy normotensive individuals. *Am J Kidney Dis.* 2010;56:264-272.
39. Kanbay M, Ozkara A, Selcoki Y et al. Effect of treatment of hyperuricemia with allopurinol on blood pressure, creatinine clearance, and proteinuria in patients with normal renal functions. *Int Urol Nephrol.* 2007;39:1227-1233.
40. Carnethon MR, Fortmann SP, Palaniappan L, et al. Risk factors for progression to incident hyperinsulinemia: the Atherosclerosis Risk in Communities Study, 1987-1998. *Am J Epidemiol.* 2003;158: 1058-1067.
41. Dehghan A, van Hoek M, Sijbrands EJ, et al. High serum uric acid as a novel risk factor for type 2 diabetes. *Diabetes Care.* 2008;31:361-362.
42. Lin KC, Tsai ST, Lin HY, Chou P. Different progressions of hyperglycemia and diabetes among hyperuricemic men and women in the kinmen study. *J Rheumatol.* 2004;31:1159-1165.
43. Boyko EJ, de Courten M, Zimmet PZ, et al. Features of the metabolic syndrome predict higher risk of diabetes and impaired glucose tolerance: a prospective study in Mauritius. *Diabetes Care.* 2000;23: 1242-1248.
44. Niskanen L, Laaksonen DE, Lindstrom J, et al. Serum uric acid as a harbinger of metabolic outcome in subjects with impaired glucose tolerance: the Finnish Diabetes Prevention Study. *Diabetes Care.* 2006;29:709-711.
45. Gersch MS, Mu W, Cirillo P, et al. Fructose, but not dextrose, accelerates the progression of chronic kidney disease. *Am J Physiol Renal Physiol.* 2007;293:F1256-F1261.
46. Ouyang X, Cirillo P, Sautin Y, et al. Fructose consumption as a risk factor for non-alcoholic fatty liver disease. *J Hepatol.* 2008;48:993-999.
47. Glushakova O, Kosugi T, Roncal C, et al. Fructose induces the inflammatory molecule ICAM-1 in endothelial cells. *J Am Soc Nephrol.* 2008;19:1712-1720.
48. Cirillo P, Gersch MS, Mu W, et al. Ketohexokinase-dependent metabolism of fructose induces proinflammatory mediators in proximal tubular cells. *J Am Soc Nephrol.* 2009;20:545-553.
49. Lee JE, Kim YG, Choi YH, et al. Serum uric acid is associated with microalbuminuria in prehypertension. *Hypertension.* 2006;47:962-967.
50. Ruggiero C, Cherubini A, Miller E 3rd, et al. Usefulness of uric acid to predict changes in C-reactive protein and interleukin-6 in 3-year period in Italians aged 21 to 98 years. *Am J Cardiol.* 2007;100: 115-121.
51. Kang DH, Johnson RJ. Uric acid induces C-reactive protein expression via upregulation of angiotensin type I receptor in vascular endothelial and smooth muscle cells. *J Am Soc Nephrol.* 2003:F-PO336.
52. Goicoechea M, de Vinuesa SG, Verdalles U, et al. Effect of allopurinol in chronic kidney disease progression and cardiovascular risk. *Clin J Am Soc Nephrol.* 2010;5:1388-1393.
53. Maynard SE, Min JY, Merchan J, et al. Excess placental soluble fms-like tyrosine kinase 1 (sFlt1) may contribute to endothelial dysfunction, hypertension, and proteinuria in preeclampsia. *J Clin Invest.* 2003;111:649-658.
54. Laughon SK, Catov J, Powers RW, et al. First trimester uric acid and adverse pregnancy outcomes *Am J Hypertens.* 2011;24:489-495.
55. Feig DI, Nakagawa T, Karumanchi SA, et al. Hypothesis: uric acid, nephron number and the pathogenesis of essential hypertension. *Kidney Int.* 2004;66:281-287.
56. Baldree LA, Stapleton FB. Uric acid metabolism in children. *Pediatr Clin North Am.* 1990;37: 391-418.
57. Guven AG, Koyun M, Baysal YE, et al. Urolithiasis in the first year of life. *Pediatr Nephrol.* 2010;25: 129-134.
58. Skinner CG, Thomas JD, Osterloh JD. Melamine toxicity. *J Med Toxicol.* 2010;6:50-55.
59. Gupta A, Kaliaperumal S, Setia S, et al. Retinopathy in preeclampsia: association with birth weight and uric acid level. *Retina.* 2008;28:1104-1110.

60. Park B, Park E, Cho SJ, et al. The association between fetal and postnatal growth status and serum levels of uric acid in children at 3 years of age. *Am J Hypertens.* 2009;22:403-408.
61. Ogihara T, Kim HS, Hirano K, et al. Oxidation products of uric acid and ascorbic acid in preterm infants with chronic lung disease. *Biol Neonate.* 1998;73:24-33.
62. Johnson RJ, Rideout BA. Uric acid and diet–insights into the epidemic of cardiovascular disease. *N Engl J Med.* 2004;350:1071-1073.
63. Cannella AC, Mikuls TR. Understanding treatments for gout. *Am J Manag Care.* 2005;11: S451-S458.
64. Fox IH, Kelley WN. Studies on the mechanism of fructose-induced hyperuricemia in man. *Metabolism.* 1972;21:713-721.
65. Ichida K. What lies behind serum urate concentration? Insights from genetic and genomic studies. *Genome Med.* 2009;1:118.
66. Schwartz GJ, Haycock GB, Edelmann CM Jr, Spitzer A. A simple estimate of glomerular filtration rate in children derived from body length and plasma creatinine. *Pediatrics.* 1976;58:259-263.
67. Tsukahara H, Kiyohara A, Kimura K, et al. Urinary uric acid excretion and renal function in newborn infants. *Eur J Pediatr.* 1996;155:834.
68. Vieux R, Hascoet JM, Merdariu D, et al. Glomerular filtration rate reference values in very preterm infants. *Pediatrics.* 2010;125:e1186-92.
69. Basu P, Som S, Choudhuri N, Das H. Urinary uric acid in preterm neonates. *Indian J Pediatr.* 2009;76:821-823.
70. Stapleton FB. Renal uric acid clearance in human neonates. *J Pediatr.* 1983;103:290-294.
71. Grivna M, Prusa R, Janda J. Urinary uric acid excretion in healthy male infants. *Pediatr Nephrol.* 1997;11:623-624.
72. Gubhaju L, Sutherland MR, Black MJ. Preterm birth and the kidney: implications for long-term renal health. *Reprod Sci.* 2011;18:322-333.
73. Anzai N, Kanai Y, Endou H. New insights into renal transport of urate. *Curr Opin Rheumatol.* 2007;19:151-157.
74. Endou H, Anzai N. Urate transport across the apical membrane of renal proximal tubules. *Nucleosides Nucleotides Nucleic Acids.* 2008;27:578-584.
75. Anzai N, Ichida K, Jutabha P, et al. Plasma urate level is directly regulated by a voltage-driven urate efflux transporter URATv1 (SLC2A9) in humans. *J Biol Chem.* 2008;283:26834-26838.
76. Doblado M, Moley KH. Facilitative glucose transporter 9, a unique hexose and urate transporter. *Am J Physiol Endocrinol Metab.* 2009;297:E831-E835.

5

CHAPTER 6

Perinatal Calcium and Phosphorus Metabolism

Ran Namgung, MD, PhD, Reginald C. Tsang, MBBS

- Body Distribution
- Regulation of Serum Calcium and Phosphorous Concentrations
- Clinical Disorders Associated with Abnormal Calcium and Phosphorus Homeostasis

Disturbances in mineral homeostasis, common in newborns, may be caused by altered responses to normal physiological transition from the intrauterine environment to neonatal independence. Mineral disturbances in newborns, either calcium (Ca) or phosphorus (P), may result from pathological intrauterine conditions, fetal immaturity, birth stress, inadequate mineral intakes, or genetic defects. Diagnosis requires understanding of unique perinatal, clinical, and biochemical features of newborn mineral metabolism. This chapter reviews Ca and P metabolism during fetal and neonatal periods with emphasis on neonatal transition followed by causes, pathophysiology, and treatment of mineral disturbances.

Body Distribution

Large amounts of Ca and P are needed to allow normal mineralization of the skeleton of developing fetuses and neonates. To meet the high mineral requirements of the developing skeleton, fetuses maintain higher blood Ca and P than maternal levels through active transport of Ca and P across placenta against a concentration gradient.

Calcium

At birth, term newborns contain approximately 30 g Ca in total body, 80% of which is accrued during the last trimester of pregnancy at a rate of 150 mg/kg fetal weight/day.[1] Fetal serum Ca (total and ionized) is higher than maternal serum Ca levels, primarily driven by transcellular active transport rather than passive paracellular pathways.[2]

At all ages, 99% of total body Ca is either in bone as hydroxyapatite or as noncrystalline, amorphous Ca phosphate form (predominant form in early life). One percent of total body Ca is in extracellular fluid (ECF) and soft tissues. Ca of mineral phase (at crystal surface) is in equilibrium with ECF; only about 1% is freely exchangeable with ECF.[3] Although this exchangeable pool is a small percentage of skeletal content, it approximates total Ca content in ECF and soft tissues and serves as a Ca reservoir. In children ages 3 to 16 years, total exchangeable Ca pool (TEP) size, by stable isotope technique, correlates with age independent of body weight variations. The bone Ca accretion rate (Vo^+) and Vo^+/TEP ratio are greater in children than adults, indicating increased bone flow of Ca in children compared with adults.[4]

Ca concentration in ECF is kept constant by a process that constantly feeds Ca into and withdraws Ca from this fluid compartment. Ca enters the plasma via intestinal absorption and bone resorption. In Ca balance, rates of Ca release from and uptake into bone are equal. In normal adults, total serum Ca ranges from 2.2 to 2.6 mmol/L (8.8–10.4 mg/dL) and is remarkably constant. Ionized Ca, although subject to changes directed by parathyroid hormone (PTH), calcitonin (CT), vitamin D, and blood pH, is also stable within individuals over prolonged periods and ranges from 1.2 to 1.3 mmol/L (4.8–5.2 mg/dL).[5]

At birth, abrupt termination of maternal-to-fetal Ca supply occurs. To maintain serum Ca homeostasis, an increase of 16% to 20% in Ca flux from bone to ECF is required unless sufficient exogenous Ca intake is achieved. In term newborns, cord blood total Ca is 2.6 mmol/L (10.2 mg/dL), and ionized Ca is 1.5 mmol/L (5.8 mg/dL). By 2 hours of age, serum total Ca declines by 5%, and by 24 to 36 hours, serum Ca reaches its nadir of total Ca of 2.3 mmol/L (9.0 mg/dL) and ionized Ca of 1.2 mmol/L (4.9 mg/dL). After a stabilization period, serum Ca slowly rises, reaching levels by 1 week of total Ca of 2.6 mmol/L (10.4 mg/dL) and ionized Ca of 1.4 mmol/L (5.5 mg/dL), similar to levels in childhood[6] (Fig. 6-1).

In preterm infants, mean cord serum ionized Ca is 1.45 mmol/L (95% confidence interval 1.29–1.61 mmol/L) [5.8 (5.74–5.86) mg/dL]), which decreases during the first 24 to 36 hours of life and rises at 6 days to values exceeding original cord blood. An early decrease in ionized Ca may be associated with parathyroid glandular unresponsiveness because of prematurity or hypomagnesemia, and severe hypo-calcemia may result.[7] Very low birth weight (VLBW) infants are likely to exhibit the lowest nadirs of ionized Ca; however, most are unassociated with tetany or decreased cardiac contractility[8,9] (see Fig. 6-1).

Cord serum Ca differs by season of birth (lower Ca in summer-born versus winter-born infants) and delivery mode, but is unaffected by gender, race, or weight appropriateness for gestation.[10-12]

Phosphorus

In term newborns, total body P is approximately 16 g (0.6% of body weight). As with Ca, approximately 80% of P in term newborns is accumulated during the last pregnancy trimester at a rate of 75 mg/kg fetal weight/day, closely linked to Ca accretion, with Ca/P ratio of 1.7 : 1; 75% of P is for bone mineralization and 25% is in other tissues.[1] Transplacental P transport is an active sodium-dependent process against the concentration gradient.[13]

About 85% of total body P is in bone, primarily as hydroxyapatite and as more loosely complexed amorphous forms of bone crystal.[3] P plays key structural roles in bone. In contrast to Ca, P is widely distributed in nonosseous tissues, as an inorganic form, and as a component of structural macromolecules. Unlike Ca, 15% of

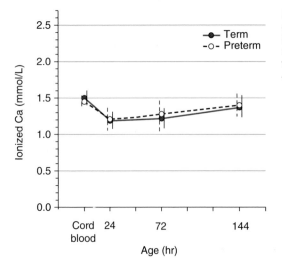

Figure 6-1 Serum ionized calcium concentrations during the first 7 days of life in term and preterm infants. (Adapted from Wandrup J, Kroner J, Pryds O, et al. Age-related reference values for ionized calcium in the first week of life in premature and full-term neonates. *Scand J Clin Invest.* 1988;48:255-260.)

total body P is in the ECF, largely as inorganic P ions. Soft tissue P is almost totally P esters. P is taken up from circulation into cells via type II and type III sodium phosphate co-transporters (NaPi) to facilitate cellular functions such as DNA and membrane lipid synthesis, generation of high-energy P esters (energy metabolism), and intracellular signaling. Intracellular P esters and phosphorylated intermediates are involved in important biologic processes and bone mineralization. Thus, P deficiency results in muscle weakness, impaired leukocyte function, and abnormal metabolism.[14]

Serum total P is higher in children than adults. Adult normal ranges are 1.24 to 1.86 mmol/L (3.0–4.5 mg/dL). In normal term infants, cord serum P does not differ by gender, race, season of birth, weight appropriateness for gestation, or mode of delivery.[10-12] P values in term infants range from 2.3 to 3.5 mmol/L (5.6–8.4 mg/dL) and in preterm infants from 1.7 to 3.3 mmol/L (4–8 mg/dL).[13] The relatively low initial birth values, 2.6 mmol/L (1.5–.4) (6.2 [3.7–8.1] mg/dL) increase shortly after birth, thought to be related to increased gluconeogenesis and endogenous P release or secondary to low glomerular filtration rate (GFR) and reduced P excretion. Mean serum P increases to 3.4 mmol/L (8.1 mg/dL) by 1 week and decreases to 1.7 mmol/L (4.1 mg/dL) in childhood.[15]

Regulation of Serum Calcium and Phosphorous Concentrations

Calcium

After birth, serum Ca is maintained at a nearly constant level primarily through interaction of three hormones, PTH, 1,25-dihydroxyvitamin D [1,25(OH)$_2$D], and CT; these hormones direct intestinal Ca absorption, renal Ca reabsorption or excretion, and transfer of Ca stores from bone. In the fetal period, both PTH and parathormone-related peptide (PTHrP) act in regulation of fetal mineral metabolism through regulation of placental Ca transfer and maintaining fetal blood Ca.[3,16]

Parathyroid Hormone

After birth, PTH is the main regulator of Ca and P homeostasis, acting in two main target tissues, kidney and bone, through the PTH/PTHrP receptor (PTHR1).[2] PTH elevates blood Ca. PTH secretion by parathyroid glands is regulated by circulating Ca ion, sensed by Ca-sensing receptors (CaSRs) in parathyroids. Increased serum Ca inhibits PTH secretion, and decreased serum Ca stimulates PTH secretion.[3] CaSR plays key roles in maintenance of a narrow range (4.4–5.2 mg/dL; 1.1–1.3 mM/L) of extracellular ionized Ca (Ca^{2+}). CaSR is expressed in target tissues for PTH, such as the kidneys, bone, and placenta, to sense alterations in Ca^{2+}, to respond with changes directed at normalizing blood Ca^{2+}.[17] Genetic mutations of the CASR gene, on the long arm of chromosome 3, result in either activation or suppression: CaSR is "reset" so that higher or lower than normal blood Ca^{2+} is sensed by the receptor as "normal." Whereas inactivating (loss-of-function) mutations of the CaSR cause hypercalcemia (hyperparathyroidism), activating (gain-of-function) mutations cause a hypocalcemic syndrome of varying severity (hypoparathyroidism).[18-20]

PTH acts directly on bone, stimulating resorption, thereby releasing Ca and P into circulation. PTH acts directly on the kidneys to increase urinary P excretion and decrease urinary Ca excretion. PTH indirectly enhances intestinal Ca absorption through effects on 1,25(OH)$_2$D synthesis. Thus, the net actions of PTH increase serum Ca.

After birth, the kidneys play an important role in Ca and P homeostasis by regulating mineral loss via urine. Under normal circumstances, nearly all (98%) filtered Ca is reabsorbed in the renal tubule, but Ca excretion is modified by local and systemic factors (e.g., PTH) to regulate extracellular Ca. Urinary Ca increases over the first 2 weeks of life.[21] Both in preterm and term neonates, the kidneys respond to exogenous PTH, as measured by increased production of nephrogenous cyclic AMP (cAMP), and improve with increasing postnatal age.[22]

Placental Transport

Active Ca transport is facilitated by CaSR that "senses" extracellular Ca. Placental CaSRs regulate Ca transport from mother to fetus. Thus, the fetus develops in a "hypercalcemic state" ($\approx$1 mg/dL higher Ca than maternal levels), and PTHrP (midregion fragment) is critical for maintaining this level. Cord PTH is low, presumably suppressed by hypercalcemia in utero.[23] The set point for fetal serum Ca is higher than the maternal set point.

Ca enters placental trophoblast at brush-border membrane (maternal–placental interface) primarily via the transient receptor potential (TRP) channel superfamily, especially TRPV6 channel (voltage-dependent Ca^{2+} channel). The time course of TRPV6 mRNA expression in wild-type fetuses reveals a 14-fold increase during the last trimester of pregnancy, coinciding with a period of maximal Ca transfer. Ca transport within trophoblast cells is facilitated by intracellular Ca-binding proteins (calbindinD9K) and actively transported into fetal circulation at the placental–fetal interface through a Ca pump, plasma membrane Ca^{2+} ATPase protein (PMCA3).[24]

Fetal PTH production is very low, especially at the end of gestation despite a stable serum ionized Ca.[25] In mice with homozygous ablation of transcriptional factor Hox 3, fetal parathyroids are not developed, with undetectable PTH production; serum ionized Ca is significantly lower in the Hox 3 ablated fetus than in maternal serum. Measures of placental Ca transfer are not changed, suggesting that fetal PTH has no effect on transplacental Ca transfer.[26] However, PTH-ablated mice show significant abnormalities in fetal bone formation, including decreased mineralization of cartilage matrix, suggesting an additional role.[27]

In mice with lack of PTHrP, ionized Ca is significantly low in fetuses and similar to maternal levels, suggesting abolition of the maternal–fetal gradient. Transplacental Ca transfer was restored by infusions of PTHrP(1–86) or midregion fragment (67–86) but not by PTHrP (1–34) nor by PTH (1–84).[28] However, in PTHrP ablated mice, using a different technique to assay placental Ca transfer (in situ artificially perfused placenta), surprisingly there is *increased* maternal–fetal Ca transfer, presumably related to significantly higher fetal Ca accretion, despite pronounced fetal hypocalcemia and abolition of fetomaternal Ca gradient. Thus, the influence of PTHrP on placental Ca transport is unclear, with data for facilitating and inhibiting effects.[29]

Serum Calcium and Calcium Homeostasis after Birth

In normal term infants, when serum Ca decreases after birth, PTH increases appropriately (two- to fivefold increase during 48 hours) and remains elevated for days. PTH secretion in term infants appears substantial and negatively correlates with Ca levels. Term neonates also show appropriate calcemic response when challenged with PTH. However, in extremely preterm infants, even with significant hypocalcemia as a stimulus, PTH remains low for the first 2 days. Transient hypocalcemia typically resolves within the first week and often requires no treatment.[8,9,30]

Vitamin D

Vitamin D is necessary for maintenance of normal Ca and P homeostasis. 1,25(OH)$_2$D is the major hormone affecting active intestinal Ca and P absorption. As a steroid, vitamin D binds to genomic receptors in intestinal epithelial cells and increases synthesis of Ca-binding proteins (calbindin), leading to increased Ca absorption. 1,25(OH)$_2$D acts on kidneys to conserve Ca and P. The overall result of this hormone is to increase serum Ca and P. 1,25(OH)$_2$D production by renal proximal tubule is enhanced by hypocalcemia, hypophosphatemia, PTH, and PTHrP and appears tightly regulated. 1,25(OH)$_2$D production is inhibited by elevated serum Ca and P.[3]

25-Hydroxyvitamin D (25OHD) crosses the placenta, and cord 25OHD correlates significantly with maternal 25OHD; fetal vitamin D pool depends entirely on the maternal vitamin D status (i.e., maternal sun exposure and dietary D intake). 1,25(OH)$_2$D is produced by the fetal kidneys and placenta, and vitamin D receptor is present in many fetal tissues, including the placenta.[25] The placenta synthesizes and metabolizes 1,25(OH)2D through activity of 25OHD-1α hydroxylase and 1,25(OH)2D-24 hydroxylase, two key enzymes for vitamin D metabolism.[31,32]

However, mice deficient in 1-α-hydroxylase are grossly normal at birth and until weaning.[33] Additionally, mice with null mutation of Vitamin D receptor (VDR) show no alteration in placental Ca transfer or fetal serum of Ca, P, or Mg despite significant maternal hypocalcemia.[34] The effect of 1,25(OH)$_2$D on placental Ca transfer, if any, could relate to expression of placental Ca transporter PMCA3 mRNA.[35]

Insufficiency of infant vitamin D arises from maternal vitamin D deficiency (sunshine deprivation with insufficient vitamin D intake), reduced production of active vitamin D metabolites caused by liver or renal disease, congenital deficiency of renal 1-α-hydroxylase, and 1,25(OH)$_2$D resistance. Deficiency of vitamin D or its metabolites causes decreased intestinal Ca absorption and renal Ca reabsorption and neonatal hypocalcemia.[36,37]

25-hydroxyvitamin D (25OHD), the major marker of vitamin D status, is lower in preterm than in term infants. However, conversion of 25OHD to 1,25(OH)$_2$D occurs normally in premature infants. In normal term infants, serum 1,25(OH)$_2$D is low at birth but increases to adult ranges by 24 hours, possibly reflecting a need for optimum intestinal Ca and P absorption.[38] In preterm infants, serum 1,25(OH)$_2$D at birth is comparable to that in healthy children and adults, increases significantly during the first few days, and is far above reference values between 3 and 12 weeks.[39] Cord serum 1,25(OH)2D is lower in small for gestational age infants compared with weight-appropriate infants, possibly reflecting decreased 1,25(OH)2D production from reduced uteroplacental blood flow.[40]

Calcitonin

CT is a Ca^{2+}-lowering hormone produced by thyroid parafollicular cells and acts as a physiologic antagonist to PTH. CT secretion is under direct control of blood Ca.[41] Elevation in Ca^{2+} stimulates CaSR and lowers Ca^{2+} by enhancing CT secretion; decreased Ca^{2+} causes a decrease in CT. After being secreted, CT has a circulatory half-life of 2 to 15 minutes. CT inhibits osteoclast-mediated bone resorption (decreasing Ca and P release) and secondarily increases renal Ca and P excretion (at high doses). The net consequence of CT is decreased serum Ca and P.[41]

CT is produced in fetal thyroid; fetal and newborn CT is higher than in the mother, related to chronic fetal hypercalcemia. Recently, ablation of CT and CT gene-related peptide (CT/CGRP-null mice) produced serum Ca and placental Ca transfer identical to wild-type littermates. There was a small, nonsignificant trend toward decreased serum P, but serum Mg was reduced by almost 50%.[42] Thus, the role of CT in fetuses is unclear.

Cord serum CT decreases with increasing gestational age. Infants less than 32 weeks' gestation have nearly three times term cord serum CT.[43] After birth, serum CT further increases in both preterm and term infants, peaking at 24 to 48 hours, followed by a decline to childhood values by 1 month.[43,44] The physiologic importance of this increase is unclear but may relate to CT counteracting PTH bone resorptive action.

Phosphorus

In contrast to regulation of Ca, the regulation of P homeostasis during the fetal and neonatal periods is less well understood.

Placental Transport

Similar to Ca, P is higher in fetuses compared with mothers, and PTHrP appears to help prevent additional elevation. Transplacental P transport is an active sodium-dependent process against concentration gradient.[13] Inorganic P enters placental trophoblast via NaPi-IIb, a family member of sodium-dependent inorganic P transporters critical for intestinal P transport.[45] NaPi-IIb is expressed in the embryonic endoderm and placental labyrinthine zone (where embryonic and maternal circulations are in closest contact), consistent with a role in placental P transfer.[46]

Fibroblast Growth Factor 23

Study of inherited disorders of P regulation, including X-linked hypophosphatemia (XLH) and autosomal recessive hypophosphatemia, has led to discovery of critical regulators of serum P, including P-regulating gene homologies to endopeptidases on the X chromosome (*PHEX*) and circulating hormone, fibroblast growth factor 23 (FGF23), produced by osteocytes[47,48] (Fig. 6-2).

Circulating P is determined by a balance between intestinal P absorption, storage in the skeleton, and P reabsorption from the kidneys. PTH increases renal P clearance and stimulates 1,25(OH)$_2$D synthesis. 1,25(OH)$_2$D stimulates intestinal P absorption. PTH acts through the G protein–coupled receptor, PTHR1, to increase osteoblast activity (and indirectly osteoclast activity). In turn, PTH synthesis and secretion are upregulated by low serum Ca and increased serum P and downregulated by increased serum Ca and 1,25(OH)$_2$D and possibly by increased FGF23. The net effect of these actions is increased serum Ca and decreased serum P.[14]

FGF23 is part of the newly recognized endocrine bone–parathyroid–kidney axis[49] modulated by PTH, 1,25(OH)$_2$D and dietary and serum P levels. Synthesis and secretion of FGF23 by osteocytes are upregulated by increased serum 1,25(OH)$_2$D and serum P and downregulated by *PHEX* and dentin matrix protein 1 (DMP1). In turn, FGF23 acts through FGF receptors, with Klotho as co-receptor, to inhibit renal P reabsorption, 1,25(OH)$_2$D synthesis, and possibly parathyroid PTH secretion.[50] FGF23 synergizes with PTH to increase renal P excretion by reducing expression of renal NaPi-IIa and NaPi-IIc in the proximal tubules. Its net effect is reduction in serum P and 1,25(OH)$_2$D, which may result in hypocalcemia.

1,25(OH)$_2$D expression is upregulated by PTH and downregulated by increased serum Ca, P, and FGF23. 1,25(OH)$_2$D acts through vitamin D receptor/RXR dimers to stimulate intestinal P absorption and FGF23 synthesis and secretion by osteocytes and possibly to inhibit parathyroid PTH secretion. Its net effect is increase in serum Ca and P.[48]

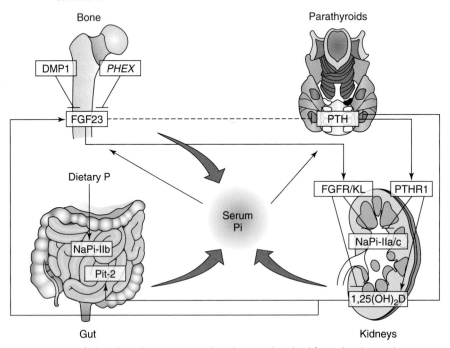

Figure 6-2. Regulation of phosphate homeostasis. Phosphate is absorbed from the diet in the gut, stored in the skeleton, and excreted by the kidneys. 1,25-Dihydroxyvitamin D [1,25(OH)$_2$D] stimulates absorption of phosphate from the diet. Fibroblast growth factor 23 (FGF23) increases renal phosphate clearance, suppresses synthesis of 1,25(OH)$_2$D, and may decrease parathyroid hormone (PTH) (*dashed line*). PTH increases renal phosphate clearance and stimulates synthesis of 1,25(OH)$_2$D. DMP1, dentin matrix protein 1; FGFR/KL, fibroblast growth factor receptor/klotho; NaPi, sodium–phosphate co-transporter; PTHR1, parathyroid hormone receptor 1. (From Bergwitz C, Jüppner H. Regulation of phosphate homeostasis by PTH, vitamin D, and FGF23. *Annu Rev Med.* 2010;61:91-104, with permission.)

Renal Excretion

The kidneys are the major determinant of plasma P. Because intestinal P absorption is very efficient and fairly unregulated (only 30% is regulated by $1,25(OH)_2D$), renal P excretion is important in maintaining balance.[14] Serum P is maintained at close to the tubular P threshold, or tubular P reabsorption maximum (TmP /GFR),[51] via an active and saturable reabsorption process.

Most filtered P is reabsorbed in the proximal tubule of the kidney through sodium-dependent transporter, the NaPi-II. Increased P intake (e.g., from formula with a high P content) leads to rapid downregulation of NaPi-II mRNA and protein in the brush-border membrane of the proximal tubule and increased P excretion.[52] Renal P reabsorption lies under tight hormonal control by PTH and FGF23 (which inhibits P reabsorption) and, to a lesser extent, insulin and hormones of the somatotropic pituitary axis.[46] In contrast, $1,25(OH)_2D$ synthesis, stimulated by decreased plasma P, has an indirect effect on renal P reabsorption via intestinal P absorption and bone P mobilization, resulting in increased serum P and suppression of PTH.

The role of FGF23 in early life remains to be established.[53] FGF23 principally functions as phosphaturic factor and counterregulates $1,25(OH)_2D$ production. Excess FGF23 secreted by osteocytes causes hypophosphatemia through inhibition of renal NaPi-II and suppresses $1,25(OH)_2D$ through inhibition of 25OHD-1α-hydroxylase and stimulation of 24-hydroxylase,which inactivates $1,25(OH)_2D$ in the proximal tubule. In contrast, deficiency of FGF23 results in hyperphosphatemia and elevated $1,25(OH)_2D$ production. In theory, downregulation of FGF23 could promote relative hyperphosphatemia and a relative increase in $1,25(OH)_2D$, promoting bone mineralization during early neonatal rapid growth.[49,54]

The kidneys contribute to positive P balance during growth by reabsorption of a relatively high fraction of filtered inorganic P (99% in newborns and 80% in adults). Growing infants, in particularly preterm infants, have high fractional excretion of P, reflecting their high P need. Age-related decrease in P reabsorption may relate to lower P needs with advancing age.[55]

Parathyroid Hormone

Wide variation in serum P concentrations corresponds to few direct regulatory mechanisms. PTH, which has greatest impact on serum P, primarily responds to changes in ionized Ca, not P. P is freely filtered at the glomerulus and presents to the renal tubules in high concentrations. The renal tubule reabsorbs P in both the proximal and distal nephrons. In states of low PTH, renal tubular cells reabsorb up to 95% to 97% of filtered P. In states of high PTH, P reabsorption in the proximal and distal tubules is inhibited, resulting in high urinary P excretion. Although markedly affected by PTH in the usual state, renal tubular cells have altered PTH responsiveness in severe P deficiency or overload. Hence, P is reabsorbed when there is severe P deficiency even in high PTH states, and P is excreted when serum P is high despite low PTH.[56]

During early postnatal life, whereas renal P response to PTH is blunted, PTH increases tubular Ca reabsorption. Together these actions result in retention of both Ca and P in infants, which is favorable for growth. Maternal smoking during pregnancy negatively influences Ca-regulating hormones, leading to relative hypoparathyroidism in both the mother and newborn and lower PTH and 25-OHD in the smoking mother and newborn despite higher serum P.[57]

Serum Phosphorous and Phosphorous Homeostasis after Birth

Absorbed P enters the extracellular P pool in equilibrium with bone and soft tissue. In adults with a neutral P balance, P excreted by the kidneys is equal to the net P absorbed by the intestine; in growing infants, it is less than net absorbed, owing to deposition of P in soft tissues and bone. In growing infants, P preferentially goes to soft tissue with a nitrogen-to-P (weight) ratio of 15 : 1 and to bone with a Ca-to-P (weight) ratio of 2.15 : 1. The residual P constitutes renal P load influencing plasma and urinary P. In limited P supply, bone mineral accretion may be limited, leading to significant Ca excretion associated with very low urinary P excretion.[3,51]

During P depletion, phosphaturia decreases before serum P declines through increased tubular reabsorption. Hypophosphatemic challenge results in (1) stimulation of kidney $1,25(OH)_2D$ synthesis, (2) enhanced mobilization of P and Ca from bone, and (3) a hypophosphatemia-induced increase in tubular maximum for P (TmP) and decreased renal P excretion. Increased circulating $1,25(OH)_2D$ increases P and Ca absorption in the intestine and stimulates P and Ca mobilization from the bone. The increased flow of Ca from the bone and intestine inhibits PTH secretion and lowers P excretion. The net result is a return of serum P to normal without a change in serum Ca.[51] FGF23 may possibly be downregulated in low serum P and may increase NaPi-II expression, leading to decreased renal P excretion.

Defense against hyperphosphatemia consists largely of reversal of these events. The principal humoral factor is PTH. An acute increase in serum P produces a transient decrease in serum ionized Ca and stimulation of PTH and possibly upregulates FGF23 expression, which reduces TmP/GFR by reducing renal NaPi-II expression, leading to increased renal P excretion and readjustment in serum P and Ca.[51]

Clinical Disorders Associated with Abnormal Calcium and Phosphorus Homeostasis

Neonatal Hypocalcemia

Definition

Hypocalcemia is generally defined as serum total Ca below 2 mmol/L (8.0 mg/dL) in term and below 1.75 mmol/L(7 mg/dL) in preterm infants or ionized Ca below 0.75 to 1.1 mmol/L (3.0–4.4 mg/dL). "Early-onset" neonatal hypocalcemia typically occurs during the first few days of life, with the lowest Ca at 24 to 48 hours, and "late-onset" hypocalcemia occurs toward the end of the first week of life.

Etiology and Pathophysiology

Early-onset neonatal hypocalcemia is commonly associated with prematurity, birth asphyxia, maternal insulin-dependent diabetes, gestational anticonvulsant exposure, and maternal hyperparathyroidism. Late-onset hypocalcemia, which is less frequent, is commonly associated with relatively high P-containing diets, disturbed maternal vitamin D metabolism, intestinal malabsorption of Ca, hypomagnesemia, and hypoparathyroidism.

Early-onset neonatal hypocalcemia represents exaggeration of normal serum Ca decrease during the first 24 to 48 hours of life; there is inadequate compensation for the sudden loss of placental Ca supply at birth (e.g., insufficient PTH release by immature parathyroids[8] or inadequate renal response to PTH). Preterm infants may or may not exhibit the surge in PTH secretion of term infants at birth, and restricted oral Ca intake aggravates the problem.[8,43] In asphyxiated infants, decreased Ca intake as a result of delayed feedings, increased endogenous P load, bicarbonate alkali therapy, and increased serum CT may contribute to the development of hypocalcemia. Hypocalcemia in infants of insulin-dependent diabetic mothers appears to be related to magnesium (Mg) insufficiency and consequent impaired PTH secretion. Mg is important in PTH secretion and action; chronic Mg deficiency causes impaired PTH secretion and PTH resistance at target organs.[7] Transient neonatal hypoparathyroidism occurs in infants exposed to maternal hypercalcemia in utero. Intrauterine hypercalcemia suppresses fetal parathyroids and apparently impairs PTH production response to hypocalcemia after birth.[58]

Late-onset hypocalcemia commonly results from dietary Ca and P imbalance and rarely may result from maternal hypercalcemia. Infants receiving cow's milk–derived formulas have lower serum ionized Ca and high serum P in the first week compared with breastfed infants, related to a higher absolute P amount of formula[59] or limited P excretion from low newborn GFR. P-containing enemas cause P overload and hypocalcemia.[60] Late hypocalcemia may relate to resistance of immature kidneys to PTH, leading to renal P retention and hypocalcemia; biochemical features resemble pseudohypoparathyroidism (defects in the *GNAS1* gene) but with normal nephrogenous cAMP responses to PTH.[61]

Congenital hypoparathyroidism is the most significant cause of late-onset hypocalcemia that has to be treated early. Congenital hypoparathyroidism may be a part of DiGeorge triad of hypoparathyroidism; T-cell incompetence (partial or absent thymus on chest radiograph); and conotruncal heart defects or aortic arch abnormalities, which suggest 22q11 syndrome (CARCH22 or DiGeorge sequence).[62]

Isolated hypoparathyroidism includes genetic defects that impair PTH synthesis (PTH gene defects)[63] or secretion (CASR gene defects) or parathyroid gland development (GCMB gene defects; parathyroid agenesis).[64] Gain-of-function (activating) mutations in the CASR gene encoding CaSR are the most common cause of mild isolated hypoparathyroidism (autosomal dominant hypocalcemia), associated with inappropriately low or low-normal serum PTH and relative hypercalciuria.[17-20]

Clinical Presentation

Neonates with hypocalcemia may be asymptomatic; the less mature the infant is, the more subtle and varied the clinical manifestations will be. Main clinical signs are jitteriness, tremors, twitching, and exaggerated startle responses or seizures (generalized or focal). Frank convulsions are seen more commonly with late hypocalcemia. Infants also may be lethargic, feed poorly, vomit, and have abdominal distension. Apnea, cyanosis, tachypnea, tachycardia, vomiting, or heart failure may also be seen. The classic signs of peripheral hyperexcitability of motor nerves (carpopedal spasm and laryngospasm) are uncommon in newborns.

Diagnosis

The diagnosis of hypocalcemia is based on serum ionized or total Ca levels, history, and physical examination; serum P, Mg and glucose, and serum pH are helpful. Functional atrioventricular block from electrocardiographic prolonged QTc interval (>0.4 sec) suggests hypocalcemia.[65]

When an infant is refractory to therapy or there are unusual findings, measurement of PTH, 25OHD, and 1,25(OH)$_2$D may be useful in establishing the less common causes (e.g., primary hypoparathyroidism, malabsorption, and vitamin D metabolism disorders) of hypocalcemia. Normal to moderately elevated 1,25(OH)$_2$D are consistent with hypoparathyroidism. Hypercalciuria (urinary Ca ≥4 mg/kg/day or urine Ca:creatinine ratio ≥0.2 [mg/mg]), associated with hypocalcemia support low PTH states.

Prolonged hypocalcemia should prompt investigation of permanent causes, such as hypoparathyroidism. DNA analysis for causal mutations may help confirm the diagnosis in proband and relatives.[66]

Therapeutic Approaches

Treatment of symptomatic hypocalcemia is by intravenous (IV) Ca infusion with a dosage of 30 to 75 mg/kg/day of elemental Ca, titrated to clinical and biochemical response, to maintain ionized Ca in the low-normal range. Clinical hypocalcemia signs are usually reversed rapidly by correcting serum Ca, which helps confirm the diagnosis.

During seizures (serum Ca usually <1.5 mmol/L [6 mg/dL]), emergency Ca (1–2 mL/kg of Ca gluconate 10%; ≈9–8 mg/kg of elemental Ca) is given IV over 10 minutes as heart rate is measured continuously to prevent bradycardia. If this complication occurs, Ca infusion should be discontinued temporarily. Another complication of Ca infusion is potential skin tissue injury from infusate extravasation. A follow-up bolus or intermittent infusions of Ca salts are avoided because of wide serum Ca excursions.

For less urgent purposes or for follow-up after initial seizure treatment, continuous IV administration of 75/kg/day of elemental Ca will maintain normocalcemia. Afterward, stepwise IV Ca reduction may help prevent rebound hypocalcemia (75 mg/kg/day for the first day, a half dose the next day, a half dose the third day, and discontinued the fourth day). Alternatively, if oral fluids are tolerated, the same dose of Ca gluconate can be given orally, divided among four to six doses per day after initial correction. Oral Ca may not be practical in sick infants because of bowel stimulation; proprietary oral Ca preparations are hypertonic (high osmolar) and are not used in infants at risk of necrotizing enterocolitis. Vitamin D metabolites are not useful for early hypocalcemia because of variable response and side effects.

With persistent hypocalcemia, serum Mg is measured because hypomagnesemic hypocalcemia cannot be corrected until hypomagnesemia is alleviated. Hypomagnesemia (serum Mg <0.6 mmol/L [1.5 mg/dL]) is treated with Mg sulfate 50% solution (500 mg or 4 mEq/mL), 0.1 to 0.2 mL/kg, IV or intramuscular (may cause local tissue necrosis) and repeated after 12 to 24 hours. Serum Mg is obtained before each dose (one or two doses may resolve transient hypomagnesemia).

Because most causes of neonatal hypocalcemia are transient, therapy duration varies with cause; commonly, as little as 2 to 3 days for early hypocalcemia is needed. Ca supplementation is usually required for long periods in hypocalcemia from malabsorption or hypoparathyroidism.

In neonates at risk, early hypocalcemia can be prevented by early oral feeding or parenteral Ca supplementation (75 mg/kg/day of elemental Ca continuously) to maintain total Ca above 2 mmol/L (8.0 mg/dL) and ionized Ca above 1 mmol/L (4.0 mg/dL). This may help prevent hypocalcemia in sick newborns with cardiovascular compromise requiring cardiotonic drugs or pressure support.

Most asymptomatic neonatal hypocalcemia resolves spontaneously with time, but hypocalcemia has potential adverse effects on the cardiovascular and central nervous systems, so treatment may be needed.[9] For asymptomatic ill infants and infants with severe hypocalcemia (serum total Ca <1.5 mmol/L [6.0 mg/dL] or ionized Ca <0.75 mmol/L [3 mg/dL]), either IV or oral therapy is usually required. In sick infants, judicious bicarbonate use and avoidance of respiratory alkalosis from excessive ventilation may reduce the risk of symptomatic hypocalcemia.

For late hypocalcemia, treatment goals are to reduce the P load and increase Ca absorption by using feedings with a Ca-to-P ratio of 4 : 1 or greater, such as use of low-P feedings (human milk or low-P formula) in conjunction with an oral Ca supplement.

Treatment of hypoparathyroidism is directed at maintaining plasma Ca to prevent symptoms without causing nephrocalcinosis. Hypoparathyroidism requires therapy with $1,25(OH)_2D$ (or 1 α-hydroxyvitamin D_3, a synthetic analog) and lifelong Ca supplementation. Infants with severe or persistent hypocalcemia may benefit from $1,25(OH)_2D$, IV or orally, 50 to 100 ng/kg per day in two or three divided doses. Close follow-up is required to monitor the serum Ca level. When serum Ca level is normalized, administration of $1,25(OH)_2D$ may be discontinued to prevent hypercalcemia.

Recombinant PTH (teriparatide)[67] has been tried as initial management of neonatal hypoparathyroidism. In infants with life-threatening seizures and persistent hypocalcemia despite aggressive management with high doses of $1,25(OH)_2D$ and Ca infusion, short-term use of teriparatide (5μg subcutaneously) can raise Ca levels faster (in <4 hours) than other commonly used methods, which take 1 day or longer.[68] Theoretically, teriparatide is safer and is a more physiologic means of correcting acute hypoparathyroid hypocalcemia; however, there is a concern regarding the risk of osteosarcoma related to long-term exposure.

Neonatal Hypercalcemia

Definition

Neonatal hypercalcemia is serum total Ca greater than 2.75 mmol/L (11 mg/dL) or ionized Ca greater than 1.4 mM/L (5.6 mg/dL)

Etiology and Pathophysiology

Hypercalcemia is uncommon in term infants but relatively common in preterm infants. The most common causes are relative deficiency in P supply and hypophosphatemia from inappropriate parenteral nutrition with or without excessive

Ca or human milk feeding in preterm infants (low P content relative to preterm needs).[69] Iatrogenic hypercalcemia results from excessive Ca or vitamin D for hypocalcemia or during exchange transfusion. Chronic maternal exposure to excessive vitamin D or metabolites, secondary to treatment of maternal hypocalcemic disorders, may cause hypercalcemia of the mother and neonate. Chronic diuretic therapy with thiazides during pregnancy may lead to maternal, fetal, and neonatal hypercalcemia.[70]

Other rarer causes include hyperparathyroidism (primary or secondary to maternal hypoparathyroidism) and hypercalcemia associated with subcutaneous fat necrosis, idiopathic infantile hypercalcemia, severe infantile hypophosphatasia, and a Bartter syndrome variant. Primary hyperparathyroidism is rare in neonates and children.

Elevated serum Ca in pathologic conditions with PTH or vitamin D overactivity implies increased Ca efflux into ECF from bone, intestine, or kidney. Hypophosphatemia increases circulating $1,25(OH)_2D$, which increases intestinal Ca absorption and bone resorption; Ca is not deposited in bone in the absence of P and contributes to hypercalcemia.[16]

Homozygous inactivating mutations of CaSR produce severe hypercalcemia, termed *neonatal severe primary hyperparathyroidism* (NSPHT). Heterozygous inactivating mutations of CaSR produce a "benign" hypercalcemia, termed *familial hypocalciuric hypercalcemia* (FHH), inherited as an autosomal dominant trait with high penetrance.[18,19] Mutations in Ca^{+2}-sensor lead to a dual defect in parathyroid cells (causing parathyroid hyperplasia) and renal tubules (causing hypocalciuria). FHH and NSHPT are associated with mutations in the *CASR* gene at 3q13.3-21 in nearly all affected subjects[19,20]; in some families, the disorder is linked to unknown genes on the long or short arms of chromosome 19.[71]

Hypercalcemia associated with subcutaneous fat necrosis occurs in asphyxiated, large for gestational age infants; possible mechanisms are increased prostaglandin E (PGE) activity, increased Ca release from fat and tissues, and unregulated production of $1,25(OH)_2D$ from macrophages infiltrating fat necrotic lesions.

Idiopathic infantile hypercalcemia (which may be part of Williams syndrome) is associated with mutations in the elastin gene on the long arm of chromosome 7; there may be a vitamin D hyperresponsive state and blunted CT response to Ca loading. Infantile hypophosphatasia is a rare autosomal recessive disorder that may be lethal in utero or shortly after birth because of inadequate bony support of the thorax and skull. Bartter variant–related hypercalcemia is associated with polyhydramnios and prematurity; in utero hypercalcemia may result in fetal hypercalciuria and polyuria, leading to early delivery; increased serum $1,25(OH)_2D$, normal serum PTH, and increased urinary PGE_2 are present.

Clinical Presentation

Clinical features of hypercalcemia depend on the underlying disorder, age, and degree of hypercalcemia. Its onset may be at birth or delayed for weeks or months. Neonates with hypercalcemia may be asymptomatic or have serious clinical signs (especially in hyperparathyroidism) requiring urgent treatment. Infants with mild increases in serum Ca (2.65–3.25 mmol/L [11–13 mg/dL]) often have no specific signs. Mild hypercalcemia may present as feeding difficulties or poor linear growth. Unrecognized hypercalcemia can result in significant morbidity or death.[72]

With moderate to severe hypercalcemia, nonspecific signs, such as anorexia, vomiting and constipation (rarely diarrhea), polyuria, and dehydration, may occur. Infants with chronic hypercalcemia may present with failure to thrive (poor growth). Severe hypercalcemia can affect the nervous system and cause lethargy, drowsiness, irritability, confusion, and seizure; in extreme cases, stupor and coma ensue. Thus, timely recognition and treatment of hypercalcemia are critical. In severely affected infants, hypertension, respiratory distress (caused by hypotonia and demineralization and deformation of the rib cage), nephrocalcinosis (from long-standing hypercalcemia), and band keratopathy of the limbus of the eye (rare) may be present. Associated features, such as elfin faces, cardiac murmur, and mental retardation (in

Williams syndrome) and bluish-red skin indurations (in subcutaneous fat necrosis), may be present on physical examination.

Diagnosis

The diagnosis may be made incidentally on routine chemistry screening. The workup may include serum total Ca, ionized Ca, P, Mg, alkaline phosphatase, pH, total protein, creatinine, electrolytes, PTH, and 25OHD; urine Ca, P, tubular reabsorption of P, and cAMP with renal function evaluation; and chest and hand x-ray radiography, abdominal ultrasonography, ophthalmologic evaluation, and electrocardiography (i.e., shortened QT interval) to determine the effect of hypercalcemia.

Very elevated serum Ca (>3.75 mmol/L [15 mg/dL]) usually indicates primary hyperparathyroidism or P depletion in VLBW infants. To differentiate parathyroid from nonparathyroid conditions, measurements include serum P (low in hyperparathyroidism, FHH, and rickets of prematurity), percent renal tubular P reabsorption (<85% in hyperparathyroidism; high in rickets of prematurity associated with hypophosphatemia), and serum PTH (elevated in hyperparathyroidism). A very low urinary Ca/urinary creatinine ratio [U_{ca}/U_{cr}] in the face of hypercalcemia suggests FHH.

The diagnosis of NSPHT is based on inappropriately normal or elevated PTH along with relative hypocalciuria in severe hypercalcemia (high Ca levels, 5–6 mmol/L [20–24 mg/dL]). Hyperparathyroidism causes erosion of bone (particularly along long bone subperiosteal margins; a "moth-eaten" appearance), which may be mistaken for rickets. In contrast to NSPHT, FHH infants usually remain asymptomatic. PTH is usually in the normal range, but inappropriately high for hypercalcemia. Urine Ca excretion is low, and nephrocalcinosis is not a problem. A family history of FHH or NSPHT in a sibling provides a strong confirmation. Care must be taken to distinguish these disorders from transient neonatal hyperparathyroidism associated with maternal hypocalcemia (e.g., in maternal pseudohypoparathyroidism or renal tubular acidosis).[73]

DNA analysis for FHH and NSPHT is available in few laboratories and requires molecular analysis of the entire *CASR* gene in a proband. Relatives of the patient's proband may be studied for genetic abnormalities and serum Ca.[66]

Bone radiographs identify demineralization, osteolytic lesions (hyperparathyroidism), or osteosclerotic lesions (occasionally with vitamin D excess).

A maternal dietary and drug history (e.g., excessive vitamin A or D, thiazides) or history of possible mineral disturbances or polyhydramnios during pregnancy should be sought. Family screening will depend on the primary diagnosis.[16]

Additional information concerning nephrocalcinosis from hypercalcemia or soft tissue calcification (e.g., in basal ganglia) can be obtained by ultrasonography or computed tomography. If hyperparathyroidism is diagnosed (rarely), localization of a parathyroid adenoma or hyperplasia by radionuclide scintigraphy may be useful.[66]

Therapeutic Approaches

Therapy includes correction of specific underlying causes and removal of iatrogenic or external causes (e.g., surgical removal of hyperparathyroid glands, stopping excessive Ca or vitamin D intake). Treatment of neonatal hyperparathyroidism depends on the severity. For mild asymptomatic hypercalcemia in a thriving infant, conservative management is appropriate. For moderate to severe hypercalcemia, prompt investigation and more aggressive therapy are instituted; stopping excessive dietary Ca and vitamin D intake and maintenance of adequate hydration are mainstays; and renal Ca excretion is enhanced by loop-acting diuretics. Reduced dietary Ca intakes by low Ca formula and inhibition of bone resorption by anti-bone resorptive agent may be used.

For short-term treatment of acute hypercalcemic episodes (symptomatic or serum Ca >3.5 mmol/L [14 mg/dL]), expansion of the ECF with 10 to 20 mL/kg of 0.9% sodium chloride IV followed by IV 1 mg/kg of furosemide every 6 to 8 hours may be effective by increasing urinary Ca excretion. Fluid and electrolyte imbalance is avoided by monitoring of fluid balance and serum Ca, P, Mg, sodium, potassium, and osmolarity; reduced GFR from dehydration can worsen hypercalcemia.

For restriction of dietary intakes of Ca and vitamin D, a low-Ca, low–vitamin D_3 infant formula containing trace Ca amounts (<10 mg/100 kcal versus standard formula, 78 mg/100 kcal) and no vitamin D (also low iron) is available for short- to medium-term management (CalciloXD, Ross Laboratories, Columbus, OH); iron supplement is needed. As hypercalcemia resolves, usual formula or human milk (≈10 mg/oz of Ca) can be mixed with the CalciloXD to increase Ca intake, closely monitoring serum and urine Ca to prevent rickets or hypocalcemia.

Adjuvant therapies in acute hypercalcemia are CT, glucocorticoids, bisphosphonate, and dialysis. Minimal information is available in neonatal hypercalcemia. Symptomatic infants with nonparathyroid hypercalcemia may require long-term CT or bisphosphonates. Short-term salmon CT (4–8 IU/kg every 6 to 12 hours subcutaneously or intramuscularly), prednisone (1–2 mg/kg/day), or a combination may be useful. The hypocalcemic effect of CT (a potent inhibitor of bone resorption) is transient and abates after a few days, which is not ideal for chronic therapy; effects may be prolonged with concomitant glucocorticoids, although there is limited experience in neonates.

High-dose glucocorticoids reduce intestinal Ca absorption and may decrease bone resorption; methylprednisolone (1–2 mg/kg/day IV), hydrocortisone (10 mg/kg/day IV), or the equivalent is effective, but is not recommended for long-term use because of many undesirable side effects. Although effective in several types of hypercalcemia, glucocorticoids are relatively ineffective in patients with primary hyperparathyroidism.

Bisphosphonate (an anti-bone resorptive agent) may be useful to treat hypercalcemia that is PTH mediated and for subcutaneous fat necrosis. Infants with NSPHT and marked hypercalcemia should be managed aggressively. In the past, treatment was urgent subtotal parathyroidectomy; more recent options include IV bisphosphonates (pamidronate 0.5–2.0 mg/kg) with parathyroidectomy delayed until the patient is clinically stable.[74,75] Bisphosphonate therapy seems safe in the short term and effective in controlling hypercalcemia even in very premature infants, allowing for planned surgery when feasible.

For severe and unremitting hypercalcemia, either hemodialysis (HD) if the patient is hemodynamically stable or peritoneal dialysis (PD) with a low-Ca dialysate (1.25 mM/L) may be helpful. To avoid iatrogenic mineral depletion, for HD or PD, supplemental P or Mg is given orally or IV, or sodium phosphate is added to PD solution (<0.75 mM); in PD, crystal formation in bags should be inspected hourly and fresh solutions changed every 8 hours.

Neonatal Hypophosphatemia

Definition

Hypophosphatemia is serum P below 1.65 mmol/L (4 mg/dL). Conventionally, hypophosphatemia is often graded as mild when serum P is below 1.45 mmol/L (<3.5 mg/dL), moderate when it is below 1.0 mmol/L (<2.5 mg/dL), and severe when it is below 0.4 mmol/L (<1.0 mg/dL).

Etiology and Pathophysiology

Hypophosphatemia occurs when there is decreased P intake (decreased intestinal absorption or increased intestinal loss) or excess renal wasting from a renal tubular defect or hyperparathyroidism. P deficiency is seen in preterm infants with rickets of prematurity resulting from inadequate Ca and P intakes.[3]

The pathophysiologic consequences of P deficiency are attributable to both direct and indirect effects of hypophosphatemia. P deficiency may directly enhance bone resorption and decrease matrix formation and bone mineralization. When serum P decreases, renal P excretion decreases and renal $1,25(OH)_2D$ production increases, which in turn increases intestinal Ca absorption and mainly stimulates bone resorption, releasing P and Ca (possibly compensatory mechanism in an attempt to maintain serum P for essential function).[76] The excess Ca results in hypercalcemia and hypercalciuria. Serum P remains low because P released from bone is used in intracellular metabolism. In VLBW infants, increased Ca absorbed from the gut or mobilized from the bone by 1,25(OH)$_2$D may not be used for bone mineralization and leads to "excess" filtered Ca being excreted in the urine.[76]

P deficiency is closely linked to metabolic bone disease in VLBW infants because P promotes bone formation and matrix production and limits bone resorption. In rats, P deficiency produces a histologic picture distinct from vitamin D deficiency.[77]

In preterm infants, a P depletion syndrome occurs in infants fed human milk,[76] with restricted enteral mineral intakes (mineral unfortified formula), and with chronic illnesses receiving prolonged parenteral nutrition without mineral supplements.[78] In the latter group, biochemical signs of extreme P deficiency are prominent, with rachitic bone changes; serum 1,25(OH)$_2$D increases with increased bone resorption and turnover (increased serum bone resorption marker, cross-linked carboxyterminal telopeptide of type I collagen and osteocalcin).[79]

Pathophysiologic results of P deficiency are inadequate supplies of energy-rich P and, in particular, inhibition of glyceraldehyde-3-phosphate dehydrogenase, which occupies a key position in glycolysis. The effect of P deficiency on energy metabolism is to reduce adenosine triphosphate (ATP) and 2,3-diphosphoglycerate, leading a shift of the oxygen-hemoglobin dissociation curve to the left, with decreased peripheral oxygen uptake and transport.[80]

Prolonged starvation, malabsorption, and chronic diarrhea cause hypophosphatemia related to decreased intestinal absorption. A chronically malnourished patient is often in a catabolic state, associated with muscle breakdown and subsequent loss of intracellular P.[81] When patients subsequently receive nutrition support, they may receive a P-depleted feed, especially with parenteral nutrition (PN), when large volumes of carbohydrate and amino acid solutions raise endogenous P requirements, and unbalanced amino acid solutions may induce further urinary P losses. If P replacement is insufficient, then hypophosphatemia will ensue.[82]

Diseases of vitamin D metabolism (vitamin D–dependent rickets) or renal P transport disorders (familial hypophosphatemic rickets) may lead to P deficiency in later infancy. Mutations in FGF23 are the cause of autosomal dominant hypophosphatemic rickets[83]; and in DMP1 are a cause of autosomal recessive hypophosphatemia.[84] Mutations in the P-regulating gene (PHEX) occur in XLH, the most frequent form of renal P wasting.[85] In addition, low serum P may also occur in extracellular to intracellular shifts from respiratory alkalosis. In the case of cellular shifts, total body P may not be depleted.

Clinical Presentation

P deficiency is accompanied by weakness, malaise, and anorexia. Bone pain, frequently occurred in growing children with hypophosphatemic rickets, is not present in neonates with hypophosphatemia. There are no easily recognizable symptoms. Signs of hypophosphatemia are usually only seen with moderate to severe hypophosphatemia. Severe hypophosphatemia has deleterious effects on muscular, cardiac, pulmonary, hematologic, and nervous system function, including muscle weakness, poor ventricular function, and difficulty weaning from a ventilator (poor tissue oxygenation), essentially because P depletion leads to a decrease in high-energy substrate availability and respiratory muscle function (impaired diaphragm contractility).[77,86] The mechanism of muscle weakness and red blood cell dysfunction caused by hypophosphatemia may relate to the role of P in intracellular signal transduction and synthesis of ATP or creatine phosphate.[14] Other manifestations are hemolysis; impaired platelet and white blood cell function; rhabdomyolysis; and in rare cases, neurologic disorders, peripheral neuropathy, convulsions, and coma.

Physical examination of VLBW infants with P deficiency is usually benign. Clinical evidence of osteopenia or rickets is present infrequently, and pathologic fractures of the ribs or limbs are late occurrences. The clinician is, therefore, dependent on biochemical tests and radiography to detect early bone disease.

Therapeutic Approaches

Because hypophosphatemia is the most prominent feature of P deficiency in preterm infants, extra P supplement has been given; however, hypocalcemia occurs after P supplementation alone, and about 66% of supplemented P is lost in urine. In addition, these infants are Ca deficient as well as P deficient; P-induced decreases in serum Ca may lead to secondary hyperparathyroidism; large amounts of supplemental P cannot be used and are wasted in urine. Thus, both P and Ca supplements (and not P alone) are necessary to avert hypocalcemia and to allow adequate bone mineral accretion.[77] Recent recommendation of enteral Ca supplementation is 120 to 200 mg/kg/day, and the recommendation for P is 70 to 120 mg/kg/day with vitamin D 400 IU/day, which allows normophosphatemia and normocalciuria with normal vitamin D status.[1]

Provision of P and Ca in total parenteral nutrition solution with a Ca-to-P ratio of 1.3 to 1.7 to 1 (500–600 mg of Ca/L and 400–450 mg of P/L of PN solution) allows optimal mineral retention for preterm infants, reaching intakes of Ca of 100 mg/kg/day and P of 65 mg/kg/day.[1,87] Sodium glycerophosphate (1 mmol/L organic P) improve solubility in PN.[88] P accumulation in preterm infants is correlated with a protein content: N-to-P ratio of 17 to 1 by weight (P retained = Ca retained/2.3 + N retained/17). Adequate supply of protein is also important for normal bone formation and mineralization. Considering optimal N retention of 350 to 400 mg/kg/day of N and provision of 100 mg/kg/day of Ca, the P supply must reach 65 mg/kg/day corresponding to a Ca-to-P ratio close to 1.5.[87]

In hypophosphatemia with high serum Ca, supplements of 0.5 to 1.0 mM//kg/day (16–31 mg/kg/day) of elemental phosphate in divided oral doses may normalize serum P and lower serum Ca; parenteral phosphate, however, should be avoided in severe hypercalcemia (serum total Ca>3 mmol/L [12 mg/dL]) unless hypophosphatemia is severe (<1.5 mg/dL) because extraskeletal calcification theoretically may occur.[69,89]

Neonatal Hyperphosphatemia

Definition

Hyperphosphatemia is a serum level greater than 3.3 mmol/L (8 mg/dL), which reflects P overload.

Etiology and Pathophysiology

Hyperphosphatemia occurs from medication errors,[90-92] increased intestinal absorption, decreased renal excretion, and cellular release or rapid intracellular to extracellular shifts. Increased tissue P release is commonly seen in profound catabolic states.

In steady state, serum P is maintained primarily by the ability of the kidneys to excrete dietary P, with efficient renal excretion. However, if acute P load is given over several hours, transient hyperphosphatemia will ensue.[90-92] In addition to absorption of excess P, volume contraction (caused by diarrhea) and renal insufficiency (caused by volume depletion and decreased renal perfusion) may contribute to hyperphosphatemia and hypocalcemia.[93]

Hyperphosphatemia is frequently the result of increased parenteral unbalanced administration of Ca, P, and Mg or a medication error (sodium phosphate instead of Ca gluconate).[90] Increased intestinal absorption is generally caused by a large oral P intake[91] and a vitamin D overdose in preterm infants or an erroneous medical prescription (oral phosphate Joulie's solution instead of alkaline solution) in newborn infants with renal insufficiency.[92]

Life-threatening hyperphosphatemia occurs after inadvertent administration of a hypertonic Fleet enema (60 mL of pediatric formula containing 105.4 mEq of P and 130.7 mEq of Na) in newborn infants, causing hyperphosphatemia and hypocalcemia; an osmotically active high P concentration in the enema solution results in excess retention and toxicity.[94] A P enema is particularly dangerous in renal insufficiency or bowel dysfunction (constipation), although even without predisposing factors, a P enema can result in severe toxicity if retained.[93]

Infants receiving cow's milk–derived formulas that contain high P (67–81 mg/dL of P) who have impaired renal excretion or hypoparathyroidism may develop hyperphosphatemia. Even in normal term infants, higher serum P and lower serum ionized Ca occur in the first week, versus breastfed infants, related to higher absolute P in formula and limited P excretion from low newborn GFR.[60] The biochemical features of high serum P and low serum Ca can resemble those of pseudohypoparathyroidism[61] because there may be resistance of the immature kidneys to PTH. Persistent hyperphosphatemia occurs almost exclusively in those with acute or chronic kidney disease.

Clinical Presentation

Acute hyperphosphatemia generally does not cause signs unless the patient has hypocalcemia. In patients given high bolus doses of P orally or rectally, symptomatic acute P intoxication occurs, presenting with severe life-threatening hyperphosphatemia and hypocalcemia; carpopedal spasm[92]; vomiting; apnea; cyanosis on mechanical ventilation; hypoactive, severe dehydration and shock[60]; depressed level of consciousness (lethargy); shallow, difficult respirations; and generalized seizure.[94] These patients are unresponsive to multiple doses of lorazepam, but responsive only to IV Ca. Clinical signs of chronic hyperphosphatemia include ectopic mineralization of muscular and subcutaneous tissues.

Therapeutic Approaches

P intoxication is a life-threatening condition. Treatment of P-induced hypocalcemia involves increasing urinary P excretion with diuretics and hydration (isotonic solution 20 mL/kg) and administrating IV Ca in symptomatic patients (avoiding lethal cardiac instability despite concern of Ca and P deposition in the kidneys) or oral Ca as an enteral P binder (promoting fecal excretion); enteral feedings with a low-P formula or human milk; and reducing parenteral P administration.[92,94]

Ca correction is required to prevent or treat potential severe adverse effects, including cardiovascular abnormalities (prolonged QT interval, specifically ST segment), tetany, and seizures.[92] Ca chloride (IV) is generally used for acute therapy in severe cases because it contains the highest concentration of ionized Ca compared with other Ca salts. However, in patients with limited or poor venous access, IV Ca gluconate is preferred because of the potential risk of peripheral extravasation. Ca should be administered with caution and only to alleviate clinical signs related to hypocalcemic toxicity. In the presence of severe hyperphosphatemia, Ca replacement can lead to extraskeletal calcification, especially in the renal tubule.[93]

Treatment of severe life-threatening hyperphosphatemia secondary to retention of an enema may include modalities to prevent further absorption (e.g., lavage).[60] Additionally, dialysis or hemofiltration can be used to rapidly lower the P concentration in renally impaired oliguric patients. Because PD strongly depends on total dialysate turnover, continuous flow-through PD, a closed PD system using two sterile polyvinylpyrrolidone short-term urethral catheters (6 Fr in and 8 Fr out) manufactured in Brazil, has been successfully applied in neonatal enema-induced hyperphosphatemia (8-day-old newborn) after achieving hemodynamic stability with vigorous fluid resuscitation and vasoactive drugs.[60]

In children with chronic renal failure, secondary hyperparathyroidism can be suppressed using mild dietary P reduction and high-dose P binders with small vitamin D supplementation. Ca carbonate is an effective P binder with no major side effects and is a drug of choice in correcting hyperphosphatemia and hyperparathyroidism in uremic children,[95] although neonatal use of Ca carbonate has not been reported.

References

1. Atkinson SA, Tsang RC. Calcium, magnesium, phosphorus, and vitamin D. In: Tsang RC, Uauy R, Koletzko B, Zlotkin SH, eds. *Nutrition of the Preterm Infant.* 2nd ed. Cincinnati, Ohio: Digital Education Publishing; 2005:245-276.
2. Mitchell DM, Jüppner H. Regulation of calcium homeostasis and bone metabolism in the fetus and neonate. *Curr Opin Endocrinol Diabetes Obes.* 2010;17:25-30.

3. Namgung R, Tsang RC. Neonatal calcium, phosphorus, and magnesium homeostasis. In: Polin RA, Fox WW, Abman HS, eds. *Fetal and Neonatal Physiology*. Philadelphia: WB Saunders; 2004:323-341.
4. Abrams SA. In utero physiology: role in nutrient delivery and fetal development for calcium, phosphorus, and vitamin D. *Am J Clin Nutr*. 2007;85(suppl):604S-607S.
5. Bowers GN Jr, Brassard C, Sena SF, et al. Measurement of ionized calcium in serum with ion-selective electrodes: a mature technology that can meet the daily service needs. *Clin Chem*. 1986;32: 1437-1447.
6. Wandrup J, Kroner J, Pryds O, et al. Age-related reference values for ionized calcium in the first week of life in premature and full-term neonates. *Scand J Clin Lab Invest*. 1988;48:255-260.
7. Loughead JL, Mimouni F, Tsang RC, et al. A role for Mg in neonatal parathyroid gland function. *J Am Coll Nutr*. 1991;10:123-126.
8. Venkataraman PS, Blick KE, Fry HD, et al. Postnatal changes in calcium-regulating hormones in very-low-birth-weight infants. *Am J Dis Child*. 1985;39:913-916.
9. Venkataraman PS, Wilson DA, Sheldon RE, et al. Effect of hypocalcemia on cardiac function in very-low-birth-weight preterm neonates: studies of blood ionized calcium, echocardiography, and cardiac effect of intravenous calcium therapy. *Pediatrics*. 1985;76:543-550.
10. Namgung R, Tsang RC, Specker BL, et al. Low bone mineral content and high serum osteocalcin and 1,25-dihydroxyvitamin D in summer- versus winter-born newborn infants: an early fetal effect? *J Pediatr Gastroenterol Nutr*. 1994;19:220-227.
11. Bagnoli F, Bruchi S, Garasi G, et al. Relationship between mode of delivery and neonatal calcium homeostasis. *Eur J Pediatr*. 1990;149:800-803.
12. Namgung R, Tsang RC, Specker BL, et al. Reduced serum osteocalcin and 1,25-dihydroxyvitamin D concentrations and low bone mineral content in small for gestational age infants: evidence of decreased bone formation rates. *J Pediatr*. 1993;122:269-275.
13. Williford AL, Pare LM, Carlson GT. Bone mineral metabolism in the neonate: calcium, phosphorus, magnesium, and alkaline phosphatase. *Neonat Net*. 2008;27:57-63.
14. Bergwitz C, Jüppner H. Disorders of phosphate homeostasis and tissue mineralization. In: Allgrove J, Shaw NJ, eds. *Calcium and Bone Disorders in Children and Adolescents*. Endocr Dev. vol 16. Basel, Karger AG. 2009:133-156.
15. David L, Anast CS. Calcium metabolism in newborn infants. The interrelationship of parathyroid function and calcium, magnesium, and phosphorus metabolism in normal, 'sick,' and hypocalcemic newborns. *J Clin Invest*. 1974;54:287-296.
16. Hsu SC, Levine MA. Perinatal calcium metabolism: physiology and pathophysiology. *Semin Neonatol*. 2004;9:23-36.
17. Bai M, Quinn S, Trivedi S, et al. Expression and characterization of inactivating and activating mutations in the human Ca_o^{2+o}-sensing receptor. *J Biol Chem*. 1996;271:19537-19545.
18. Pearce SH. Clinical disorders of extracellular calcium-sensing and the molecular biology of the calcium-sensing receptor. *Ann Med*. 2002;34:201-206.
19. Egbuna OI, Brown EM. Hypercalcemic and hypocalcemic conditions due to calcium-sensing receptor mutations. *Best Practice & Research Clin Rheumatol*. 2008;22:129-148.
20. Brown EM. The calcium-sensing receptor: physiology, pathophysiology and car-based therapeutics. *Subcell Biochem*. 2007;45:139-167.
21. Karlen J, Aperia A, Zetterstrom R. Renal excretion of calcium and phosphate in preterm and term infants. *J Pediatr*. 1985;106:814-819.
22. Mallet E, Basuyau JP, Brunelle P, et al. Neonatal parathyroid secretion and renal maturation in premature infants. *Biol Neonate*. 1978;33:304-308
23. Bass JK, Chan GM. Calcium nutrition and metabolism during infancy. *Nutrition*. 2006;22:1057-1066.
24. Belkacemi L, Bedard I, Simoneau L, et al. Calcium channels, transporters and exchangers in placenta: a review. *Cell Calcium*. 2005;37:1-8.
25. Kovacs CS, Kronenberg HM. Maternal-fetal calcium and bone metabolism during pregnancy, puerperium, and lactation. *Endocr Rev*. 1997;18:832-872.
26. Kovacs CS, Manley NR, Moseley JM, et al. Fetal parathyroids are not required to maintain placental calcium transport. *J Clin Invest*. 2001;107(8):1007-1015.
27. Miao D, He B, Karaplis AC, et al. Parathyroid hormone is essential for normal fetal bone formation. *J Clin Invest*. 2002;109:1173-1182.
28. Kovacs CS, Lanske B, Hunzelman JL, et al. Parathyroid hormone-related peptide (pthrp) regulates fetal-placental calcium transport through a receptor distinct from the PTH/pthrp receptor. *Proc Natl Acad Sci U S A*. 1996;93:15233-15238.
29. Bond H, Dilworth MR, Baker B, et al. Increased maternofetal calcium flux in parathyroid hormone-related protein-null mice. *J Physiol*. 2008;586:2015-2025.
30. Altirkawi K, Rozycki H. Hypocalcemia is common in the first 48 h of life in ELBW infants. *J Perinat Med*. 2008;36:348-353
31. Novakovic B, Sibson M, Ng HK, et al. Placenta-specific methylation of the vitamin D 24-hydroxylase gene: implications for feedback autoregulation of active vitamin D levels at the fetomaternal interface. *J Biol Chem*. 2009;284:14838-14848.
32. Avila E, Diaz L, Barrera D, et al. Regulation of vitamin D hydroxylase gene expression by 1,25-dihydroxyvitamin D3 and cyclic AMP in cultured human syncytiotrophoblasts. *J Steroid Biochem Mol Biol*. 2007;103:90-96.
33. Panda DK, Miao D, Tremblay ML, et al. Targeted ablation of the 25-hydroxyvitamin D 1alpha -hydroxylase enzyme: evidence for skeletal, reproductive, and immune dysfunction. *Proc Natl Acad Sci U S A*. 2001;98:7498-7503.

34. Kovacs CS, Woodland ML, Fudge NJ, et al. The vitamin D receptor is not required for fetal mineral homeostasis or for the regulation of placental calcium transfer in mice. *Am J Physiol Endocrinol Metab.* 2005;289:E133-E144.
35. Martin R, Harvey NC, Crozier SR, et al. Placental calcium transporter gene expression (PMCA3) predict intrauterine bone mineral accrual. *Bone.* 2007;40:1203-1208.
36. Holick MF. Vitamin D deficiency. *N Engl J Med.* 2007;357: 266-281.
37. Camadoo L, Tibott R, Isaza F. Maternal vitamin D deficiency associated with neonatal hypocalcemic convulsions. *Nutrition Journal.* 2007;6:23-24.
38. Steichen JJ, Tsang RC, Gratton TL, et al. Vitamin D homeostasis in the perinatal period: 1,25-dihydroxyvitamin D in maternal, cord and neonatal blood. *N Engl J Med.* 1980;302:315-319.
39. Markestad T, Aksnes L, Finne PH, et al. Plasma concentrations of vitamin D metabolites in premature infants. *Pediatr Res.* 1984;18:269-272.
40. Namgung R, Tsang RC, Specker BL, et al. Reduced serum osteocalcin and 1,25-dihydroxyvitamin D concentrations and low bone mineral content in small for gestational age infants: evidence of decreased bone formation rates. *J Pediatr.* 1993;122:269-275.
41. Austin LA, Heath H 3rd. Calcitonin: physiology and pathophysiology. *N Engl J Med.* 1981;304: 269-304.
42. McDonald KR, Fudge NJ, Woodrow JP, et al. Ablation of calcitonin/calcitonin gene-related peptide-alpha impairs fetal magnesium but not calcium homeostasis. *Am J Physiol Endocrinol Metab.* 2004;287:E218-E226.
43. Venkataraman PS, Tsang RC, Chen IW, et al. Pathogenesis of early neonatal hypocalcemia: studies of serum calcitonin, gastrin and plasma glucagon. *J Pediatr.* 1987;110:599-603.
44. Hillman LS, Rojanasathit S, Slatopolsky E, et al. Serial measurements of serum calcium, magnesium, parathyroid hormone, calcitonin, and 25-hydroxyvitamin D in premature and term infants during the first week of life. *Pediatr Res.* 1977;11:739744.
45. Sabbagh Y, O'Brien SP, Song W, et al. Intestinal Npt2b plays a major role in phosphate absorption and homeostasis. *J Am Soc Nephrol.* 2009;20:2348-2358.
46. Shibasaki Y, Etoh N, Hayasaka M, et al. Targeted deletion of the type IIb Na(+)-dependent Pi-cotransporter, NaPi-IIb, results in early embryonic lethality. *Biochem Biophys Res Commun.* 2009;381:482-486.
47. Bastepe M, Jüppner H. Inherited hypophosphatemic disorders in children and the evolving mechanisms of phosphate regulation. *Rev Endocr Metab Disord.* 2008;9:171-180.
48. Bergwitz C, Jüppner H. Regulation of phosphate homeostasis by PTH, vitamin D, and FGF23. *Annu Rev Med.* 2010;61:91-104.
49. Jüppner H, Myles Wolf, M, Salusky, I. FGF-23: More than a regulator of renal phosphate handling? *J Bone Miner Res.* 2010;25:2091-2097.
50. Urakawa I, Yamazaki Y, Shimada T, et al. Klotho converts canonical FGF receptor into a specific receptor for FGF23. *Nature.* 2006;444:770-774.
51. Favus MJ, Bushinsky DA, Lemann J Jr. Regulation of calcium, magnesium, and phosphate metabolism. In: Favus MJ, ed. *Primer on the Metabolic Bone Diseases and Disorders of Mineral Metabolism.* 6th ed. Washington DC: American Society for Bone and Mineral Research; 2006:76-83.
52. Tenenhouse HS. Regulation of phosphorus homeostasis by the type IIa Na/phosphate cotransporter. *Annu Rev Nutr.* 2005;25:197-214.
53. Garabedian M. Regulation of phosphate homeostasis in infants, children, and adolescents, and the role of phosphatonins in this process. *Curr Opin Pediatr.* 2007;19:488-491.
54. Tenenhouse HS. Phosphate transport: Molecular basis, regulation and pathophysiology. *J Steroid Biochem Mol Biol.* 2007;103:572-577.
55. Holtbäck U, Aperia AC. Molecular determinants of sodium and water balance during early human development. *Semin Neonatol.* 2003;8:291-299.
56. Gertner JM. Phosphorus metabolism and its disorders in childhood. *Pediatr Ann.* 1987;16:957-965.
57. Díaz-Gómez NM, Mendoza C, González-González NL, et al. Maternal smoking and the vitamin D-parathyroid hormone system during the perinatal period. *J Pediatr.* 2007;151:618-623.
58. Poomthavorn P, Ongphiphadhanakul B, Mahachoklertwattana P. Transient neonatal hypoparathyroidism in two siblings unmasking maternal normocalcemic hyperparathyroidism. *Eur J Pediatr.* 2008; 167:431-434.
59. Specker BL, Tsang RC, Ho ML, et al. Low serum calcium and high parathyroid hormone levels in neonates fed "humanized' cow's milk-based formula. *Am J Dis Child.* 1991;145:941-945.
60. Kostic D, Rodigues ABD, Leal A, et al. Flow-through peritoneal dialysis in neonatal enema-induced hyperphosphatemia. *Pediatr Nephrol.* 2010;25:2183-2186.
61. Lee CT, Tsai WY, Tung YC, et al. Transient pseudohypoparathyroidism as a cause of late-onset hypocalcemia in neonates and infants. *J Formos Med Assoc.* 2008;107:806-810.
62. Garcia-Garcia E, Camacho-Alonso J, Gomez-Rodriguez MJ, et al. Transient congenital hypoparathyroidism and 22q11 deletion. *J Pediatr Endocrinol Metab.* 2000;13:659-661.
63. Sunthorbthepvarakul T, Cheresigaew S, Ngowngarmratana S. A novel mutation of the signal peptide of the preproparathyroid hormone gene associated with autosomal recessive familial isolated hypoparathyroidism. *J Clin Endocrinol Metab.* 1999;84:3792-3796.
64. Ding CL, Buckingham B, Levine MA. Familial isolated hypoparathyroidism caused by a mutation in the gene for the transcription factor GCMB. *J Clin Invest.* 2001;108:1215-1220.
65. Stefanaki E, Koropuli M. Atrioventricular block in preterm infants caused by hypocalcemia: a case report and review of the literature. *Eur J Obstet Gynecol.* 2005;120:115-116.
66. Allgrove J. Disorders of calcium metabolism. *Current Pediatr.* 2003;13:529-535.

67. Puig-Domingo M, Diaz G, Nicolau J, et al. Successful treatment of vitamin D unresponsive hypoparathyroidism with multipulse subcutaneous infusion of teriparatide. *Eur J Endocrinol.* 2008;159: 653-657.
68. Newfiled RS. Recombinant PTH for initial management of neonatal hypocalcemia. *New Engl J Med.* 2007;356:1687.
69. Trindade CEP. Minerals in the nutrition of extremely low birth weight infants. *J Pediatr (Rio J).* 2005;81(1 suppl):S43-S51.
70. Mahomadi M, Bivins L, Becker KL. Effect of thiazides on serum calcium. *Clin Pharmacol Ther.* 1979;26:390-394.
71. Lloyd SE, Pannett AA, Dixon PH, et al. Localization of familial benign hypercalcemia, Oklahoma variant (FBHOk), to chromosome 19q13. *Am J Hum Genet.* 1999;64:189-195.
72. Ghirri P, Bottone U, Coccoli L, et al. Symptomatic hypercalcemia in the first months of life: calcium-regulating hormones and treatment. *J Endocrinol Invest.* 1999;22:349-353.
73. Rodriquez-Soriano J, Garcia-Fuentes M, Vallo A, et al. Hypercalcemia in neonatal distal renal tubular acidosis. *Pediatr Nephrol.* 2000;14:354-355.
74. Waller S, Kurzawinski T, Spitz L, et al. Neonatal severe hyperparathyroidism: genotype/phenotype correlation and the use of pamidronate as rescue therapy. *Eur J Pediatr.* 2004;163:589-594.
75. Fox L, Sadowsky J, Pringle KP, et al. Neonatal hyperparathyroidism and pamidronate therapy in an extremely premature infant. *Pediatrics.* 2007;120:e1350-e1354.
76. Lyon AJ, McIntosh N. Calcium and phosphorus balance in extremely low birthweight infants in the first six weeks of life. *Arch Dis Child.* 1984;59:1145.
77. Rowe JC, Carey DE. Phosphorus deficiency syndrome in very low birth weight infants. *Pediatr Adol Endocrinol.* 1987;34:997-1017.
78. Namgung R, Joo HJ, Lee EG, et al. Radiologic (rickets) and biochemical effects of calcium and phosphorus supplementation of parenteral nutrition in very low birth weight infants. *Pediatr Res.* 1993;33:308A.
79. Namgung R, Park KI, Lee C, et al. High serum osteocalcin and high serum cross-linked carboxyterminal telopeptide of type I collagen in rickets of preterm infants: evidence of increased bone turnover. *Pediatr Res.* 1994;35:317A.
80. Kalan G, Derganc M, Primo ic J. Phosphate metabolism in red blood cells of critically ill neonates. *Pflugers Arch.* 2000;440(5 Suppl):R109-R111.
81. Kimutai D, Maleche-Obimbo E, Kamenwa R, et al. Hypo-phosphatemia in children under five years with kwashiorkor and marasmic kwashiorkor. *East Afr Med J.* 2009;86:330-336.
82. Haglin L, Burman LA, Nilsson M. High prevalence of hypophosphatemia amongst patients with infectious diseases. A retrospective study. *J Intern Med.* 1999;246:45-52.
83. White KE, Evans WE, O'Riordan JLH, et al. Autosomal dominant hypophosphatemic rickets is associated with mutations in FGF23. *Nat Genet.* 2000;26:345-348.
84. Lorenz-Depiereux B, Bastepe M, Benet-Pages A, et al. DMP1 mutations in autosomal recessive hypophosphatemia implicate a bone matrix protein in the regulation of phosphate homeostasis. *Nat Genet.* 2006;38:1248-1250.
85. The HYP Consortium: A gene (PEX) with homologies to endopeptidases is mutated in patients with X-linked hypophosphatemic rickets. *Nat Genet.* 1995;11:130-136.
86. Takeda E, Taketani Y, Sawada N, et al. The regulation and function of phosphate in the human body. *BioFactors.* 2004;21:345-355.
87. Rigo J, De Curtis M, Pieltain C, et al. Bone mineral metabolism in the micropremie. *Clin Perinatol.* 2000;27:147-170.
88. Costello I, Powell C, Williams AF: Sodium glycerophosphate in the treatment of neonatal hypophosphatemia. *Arch Dis Child Fetal Neonatal Ed.* 1995;73:F44-F45.
89. Singer FR. Medical management of nonparathyroid hypercalcemia and hypocalcemia. *Otolaryngol Clin North Am.* 1996;29:701-710.
90. Biarent D, Brumagne C, Steppe M, et al. Acute phosphate intoxication in seven infants under parenteral nutrition. *J Parenter Enteral Nutr.* 1992;16:558-560.
91. Perlman M. Fatal hyperphosphatemia after oral phosphate overdose in a premature infant. *Am J Health Syst Pharm.* 1997;54:2488-2490.
92. Dissaneewate S, Vachvanichsanong P. Severe hyperphosphatemia in a newborn with renal insufficiency because of an erroneous medical prescription. *J Renal Nutr.* 2009;19:500-502.
93. Biebl A, Grillenberger A, Schmitt K. Enema-induced severe hyperphosphatemia in children. *Eur J Pediatr.* 2009;168:111-112.
94. Marraffa JM, Hui A, Stork CM. Severe hypophosphatemia and hypocalcemia following the rectal administration of a phosphate-containing Fleet(r) pediatric enema. *Pediatr Emerg Care.* 2004;7: 453-456.
95. Tamanaha K, Mak RHK, Rigden SPA, et al. Long-term suppression of hyperparathyroidism by phosphate binders in uremic children. *Pediatr Nephrol.* 1987;1:145-149.

6

CHAPTER 7

Acid–Base Homeostasis in the Fetus and Newborn

Istvan Seri, MD, PhD

- Regulation of Acid–Base Homeostasis
- Normal Acid–Base Balance and Growth
- Obstetric Management and Fetal and Neonatal Acid–Base Balance
- Summary

This chapter addresses the regulation of fetal and neonatal acid–base balance with a focus on the elimination of the acid load by the placenta, the lungs, and the kidneys; briefly discusses the impact of acid–base disturbance on fetal and postnatal growth; and describes the effect of selected obstetric management approaches on fetal and neonatal acid–base balance.

Hydrogen ion concentration is tightly regulated by the intra- and extracellular buffer systems and respiratory and renal compensatory mechanisms. The normal range of hydrogen ion concentration in the extracellular fluid (ECF) is between 35 and 45 mEq/L, which translates to a pH of 7.35 to 7.45. Under physiologic circumstances, volatile and fixed acids generated by normal metabolism are excreted, and the pH remains stable.[1] Carbonic acid is the most common volatile acid produced and is readily excreted by the lungs in the form of carbon dioxide. Fixed acids, such as lactic acid, ketoacids, phosphoric acid, and sulfuric acid, are buffered principally by bicarbonate in the extracellular compartment. The bicarbonate used in this process is then regenerated by the kidneys in a series of transmembrane transport processes linked to the excretion of hydrogen ions in the form of titratable acids (phosphate and sulfate salts) and ammonium. Several aspects of the regulation of acid–base homeostasis are developmentally regulated in fetuses and neonates and thus differ from those in children and adults. These developmentally regulated differences of acid–base homeostasis and their impact on fetal and postnatal growth are reviewed in this chapter.

Regulation of Acid–Base Homeostasis

Respiratory Acidosis

Unlike in fetal respiratory acidosis, in postnatal respiratory acidosis, immediate activation of the pulmonary compensatory mechanism leads to enhanced elimination of carbon dioxide, and the resulting decrease in carbon dioxide concentration increases the pH toward normal. *The rapid activation* of the respiratory compensatory mechanism is a result of the free movement of carbon dioxide across the blood–brain barrier,[2] leading to instantaneous changes in cerebrospinal fluid (CSF) and cerebral interstitial fluid hydrogen ion concentrations.

Correction of Fetal Respiratory Acidosis

Fetal respiratory acidosis develops when prolonged maternal hypoventilation occurs with maternal asthma, airway obstruction, narcotic overdosing, maternal anesthesia, and magnesium sulfate toxicity. Fetal breathing movements increase, and the fetal kidneys exert a maturation-dependent limited response by reclaiming more bicarbonate in an attempt to restore the physiologic 20 : 1 ratio of bicarbonate to carbonic acid, resulting in a return of the pH toward normal.[3] In fetuses, only the renal compensation has some limited physiologic significance when respiratory acidosis develops because of prolonged maternal hypoventilation.

Correction of Postnatal Respiratory Acidosis

In the clinical setting, acute neonatal respiratory acidosis develops most frequently in preterm infants with respiratory distress syndrome. Although stimulation of the respiratory center in the brain by elevated interstitial carbon dioxide concentration immediately increases the respiratory rate and depth, carbon dioxide elimination by the lungs is usually limited because of immaturity and parenchymal disease. As in fetuses, the kidneys reclaim more bicarbonate in response to respiratory acidosis. Especially during the first few weeks of postnatal life, however, renal compensation is limited by the developmentally regulated immaturity of renal tubular functions.

Metabolic Acidosis

As in respiratory acidosis, the pulmonary gas exchange serves as the *immediate* regulator of acid–base homeostasis when *metabolic acidosis* develops. However, because bicarbonate crosses the blood–brain barrier by active transport mechanisms[4] and because the central respiratory drive is triggered by the low steady-state values of CSF and not plasma bicarbonate,[2] a full activation of the respiratory acid–base regulatory system only occurs a few hours after the development of metabolic acidosis. This is different from the above-described truly immediate activation of the respiratory acid–base regulatory system by respiratory acidosis.

Fetoplacental Elimination of Metabolic Acid Load

Fetal respiratory and renal compensation in response to changes in fetal pH is limited by the level of maturity and the surrounding maternal environment. However, although the placentomaternal unit performs most compensatory functions,[3] the fetal kidneys have some, although limited, ability to contribute to the maintenance of fetal acid–base balance.

The most frequent cause of fetal metabolic acidosis is fetal hypoxemia owing to abnormalities of uteroplacental function or blood flow (or both). Primary maternal hypoxemia or maternal metabolic acidosis secondary to maternal diabetes mellitus, sepsis, or renal tubular abnormalities is an unusual cause of fetal metabolic acidosis.

Pregnant women, at least in late gestation, maintain a somewhat more alkaline plasma environment compared with that of nonpregnant control participants. This pattern of acid–base regulation in pregnant women is present during both resting and after maximal exertion and may serve as a protective mechanism from sudden decreases in fetal pH. Maintenance of the less acidic environment during pregnancy appears to be achieved through reduced plasma carbon dioxide and weak acid concentrations.[3,5]

The placenta plays an essential role in the maintenance of fetal acid–base balance when metabolic acidosis develops. As mentioned earlier, fetal metabolic acidosis most frequently occurs when abnormal uteroplacental function or blood flow results in fetal hypoxemia. Fetal hypoxemia then causes a shift to anaerobic metabolism, and large quantities of lactic acid accumulate. As hydrogen ions are buffered by the extracellular and intracellular buffering systems of the fetus, pH drops as plasma bicarbonate decreases. Because of the unhindered diffusion of carbon dioxide through the placenta,[3] restoration of normal fetal pH initially occurs through elimination of the volatile element of the carbonic acid–bicarbonate system via the maternal lungs. However, because lactate and other fixed acids cross the placenta more slowly,[3] the onset of maternal renal compensation of fetal metabolic acidosis is delayed. In addition, if fetal oxygenation improves, the products of anaerobic metabolism are also metabolized by the fetus.

Because there is no physiologic significance to respiratory compensation of metabolic acidosis in utero, the finding that the respiratory control system in fetuses is much less sensitive to changes in pH than in neonates[6] has little practical importance. Yet, a decrease in the fetal pH stimulates breathing movements in fetuses.[7,8]

Finally, as for the role of the *fetal kidneys* in the maintenance of acid–base balance, available evidence indicates that the fetal kidneys excrete both inorganic[9-11] and organic acids[12] and are also able to generate bicarbonate.[13,14] Studies in fetal sheep have found age-dependent increases in the glomerular filtration rate (GFR) and urinary titratable acid, ammonium, and net acid excretion.[9] A positive relationship also exists between changes in GFR and bicarbonate, sodium, and chloride excretions.[9,11] Yet, the adaptive capacity of the fetal kidneys to changes in fetal acid–base balance is limited. In fetal sheep, the hydrochloric acid infusion–induced metabolic acidosis results in increases in titratable acid, ammonium, and net acid excretion without significant changes in GFR or renal tubular bicarbonate absorption.[11] However, as mentioned earlier, under certain conditions such as volume depletion[13] or recovery from mild hypocapnic hypoxia,[14] the fetal kidney has the ability to increase bicarbonate reabsorption. It is also important to note that the vast majority of these data have been obtained in animal models and that there is only very limited information available concerning renal acidification by human fetuses.[15] In addition, the physiologic importance of the adaptive fetal renal responses is limited compared with that in the postnatal period because the acid load excreted in the fetal urine remains within the immediate fetal environment and needs to be eliminated by the placenta or metabolized by the fetus.

Indeed, *amniotic fluid* acid–base status and electrolyte composition have been shown to affect fetuses. When the effects of amnion infusion of physiologic saline to those of lactated Ringer solution were compared in fetal sheep, significant increases in fetal plasma sodium and chloride concentrations were noted only in the physiologic saline infusion group.[16] In addition, fetal arterial pH decreased in the physiologic saline group and the change in the fetal pH was directly related to the changes in plasma chloride concentrations. However, despite the significant changes in plasma sodium and chloride concentrations and pH, fetal plasma electrolyte composition and acid–base balance remained in the physiologic range, leaving these findings with little clinical significance.[16]

Postnatal Elimination of Metabolic Acid Load

The most frequent causes of increased anion gap (lactic acid) metabolic acidosis in neonates are hypoxemia and ischemia secondary to perinatal asphyxia; vasoregulatory disturbances or myocardial dysfunction caused by immaturity, sepsis, or asphyxia; severe lung disease with or without pulmonary hypertension; certain types of structural heart disease; and volume depletion. Severe metabolic acidosis caused by a neonatal metabolic disorder is rare but should always be considered. Preterm neonates frequently present with mild to moderate normal anion gap acidosis, which almost always is the consequence of the low renal bicarbonate threshold of the premature kidneys.[17-19] However, the use of carbonic anhydrase inhibitors and parenteral alimentation, as well as the maturation-related decreased sensitivity to aldosterone have also been suggested to contribute to the development of normal anion gap acidosis in neonates.[17,20,21]

As mentioned earlier, in metabolic acidosis caused by the accumulation of lactic acid, hydrogen ions are buffered by the intra- and extracellular buffering systems, and plasma bicarbonate concentration decreases and pH drops. Restoration of pH toward normal initially occurs through elimination of the volatile element of the carbonic acid–bicarbonate system *via the lungs*. This process may be severely compromised in sick preterm and term neonates with parenchymal lung disease.

The principle mechanism of the *renal compensation* is the regulation of renal tubular bicarbonate and acid secretion in response to changes in extracellular pH. Although full activation of this system requires at least 2 to 3 days, changes in renal acidification may be seen as early as a few hours after the development of the acid–base disturbance. Although renal compensation is the ultimate mechanism that

7

adjusts the hydrogen ion content of the body, this compensatory function is also affected by the immaturity of the neonatal kidneys.[19,22] Both *renal hemodynamic and tubular epithelial factors* play a role in the limited renal compensatory capacity of newborns.

Renal blood flow (RBF) significantly increases after the immediate postnatal period, and some of the renal vasodilatory mechanisms are functionally mature as early as the 24th week of gestation.[23] Similar to RBF, GFR is also low in the immediate postnatal period and increases as a function of both gestational and postnatal age.[24,25] Indeed, *low GFR is considered as the primary hemodynamic factor* limiting the ability of neonates to adequately handle an acid load.[19,22]

In addition, net renal acid excretion is regulated *by several tubular epithelial functions.*[19,26] In the proximal tubule, the following four transport mechanisms regulate active acid extrusion and transepithelial bicarbonate reabsorption: H^+-ATPase, the electrogenic $Na^+/3HCO_3^-$ cotransporter, the Na^+,K^+-ATPase-driven secondary active Na^+/H^+ antiporter, and the Na^+,K^+-ATPase-driven tertiary active Na^+-coupled organic ion transporter.[26] Because approximately 85% to 90% of the filtered bicarbonate is reabsorbed in the proximal tubule,[19,26] the function of these proximal tubular transporters determines the renal threshold for bicarbonate reabsorption. The bicarbonate threshold is 18 mEq/L in premature infants and 21 mEq/L in term infants, and it reaches adult levels (24–26 mEq/L) only after the first postnatal year.[17,18] In extremely low gestational age neonates, however, the renal bicarbonate threshold may be as low as 14 mEq/L. Because renal carbonic anhydrase is present and active during fetal life[27] and because its activity is similar in 26-week-old extremely immature neonates to that of adults,[28] a developmentally regulated immaturity of the function of the above-described proximal tubular transporters is most likely responsible for the low bicarbonate threshold during early development. Indeed, both the activity and the hormonal responsiveness of the proximal tubular Na^+,K^+-ATPase is decreased in younger compared with older animals.[29]

In addition to immaturity, medications used in critically ill neonates may also affect proximal tubular bicarbonate reabsorption. For example, via inhibition of the proximal tubular Na^+/H^+ antiporter,[30] dopamine may potentially decrease the low bicarbonate threshold of neonates.[31] Carbonic anhydrase inhibitors also decrease proximal tubular bicarbonate reabsorption by limiting bicarbonate formation and hydrogen ion availability for the Na^+/H^+ antiporter. By acting on several transport proteins along the nephron, furosemide directly increases urinary excretion of titratable acids (phosphate and sulfate salts) and ammonium.[32] On the other hand, by inhibition of the activation of aldosterone receptors, spironolactone indirectly decreases hydrogen ion excretion in the distal tubule.

Under physiologic circumstances, the distal nephron reabsorbs the remaining 10% to 15% of the filtered bicarbonate via transport mechanisms similar to those of the proximal tubule.[26] However, the distal tubule lacks the carbonic anhydrase enzyme.[26] Net hydrogen ion secretion in the distal nephron continues after the reabsorption of virtually all bicarbonate via active extrusion of hydrogen and the ability of the distal tubular epithelium to maintain large transepithelial concentration gradients for hydrogen and bicarbonate.[26] Aldosterone is one of the most important hormones influencing distal tubular acidification. By affecting the function of several different transport mechanisms, aldosterone stimulates net hydrogen ion excretion in the distal nephron. However, premature neonates have a developmentally regulated relative insensitivity to aldosterone.[17,21]

Hydrogen ions are excreted in the urine in the form of titratable acids (phosphate and sulfate salts) and as ammonium salts, which are formed by the combination of hydrogen with ammonia.[26] Because the major constituent of titratable acid in the urine is $H_2PO_4^-$, drugs that decrease proximal tubular phosphate reabsorption and thus increase the delivery of phosphate to the distal nephron may increase the renal acidification capacity of neonates. Indeed, by inhibiting proximal tubular phosphate reabsorption, dopamine has been shown to increase the excretion of titratable acids in preterm infants.[33] In addition, urinary excretion of titratable acid and ammonium increases as a function of gestational and postnatal age.[19] However, because effective urinary acidification is usually acquired by the age of 1 month even in premature infants, postnatal distal tubular hydrogen ion secretion is inducible independent of the gestational age at birth.[34]

In summary, the renal response to metabolic acidosis in the immediate postnatal period consists of attenuated increases in GFR, proximal tubular bicarbonate reabsorption, and distal tubular net acid secretion. However, a significant improvement in the overall renal response occurs after the first postnatal month even in premature infants.[22]

Respiratory Alkalosis

Correction of Fetal Respiratory Alkalosis

Rather than causing fetal respiratory alkalosis, acute maternal hyperventilation may lead to the development of fetal metabolic acidosis. The fetal acidosis under these circumstances is the consequence of the acute decrease in placental blood flow caused by the maternal hypocapnia-induced significant uterine vasoconstriction.[35] In these cases, restoration of maternal carbon dioxide levels rapidly corrects both the abnormal uterine blood flow and the acid–base abnormality in the fetus.

The *physiologic hyperventilation* of pregnant women causes a compensatory decrease in serum bicarbonate concentration to approximately 22 mm^3 without any apparent effect on the fetus (see above).

Correction of Postnatal Respiratory Alkalosis

Neonatal respiratory alkalosis occurs most often in febrile nonventilated neonates and in cases with iatrogenic hyperventilation of intubated preterm or term infants. Rarely, respiratory alkalosis may be the presenting sign of a urea cycle disorder during the first days of postnatal life because the rising ammonia level may initially stimulate the respiratory center in the brain. As for the renal compensation of respiratory alkalosis, both urinary bicarbonate reabsorption and distal tubular net acid excretion decrease, and thus extracellular pH tends to return toward normal. This renal compensation plays an important although somewhat limited role in neonatal respiratory alkalosis.

Metabolic Alkalosis

Correction of Fetal Metabolic Alkalosis

Although metabolic alkalosis is a very rare fetal condition, it may occur in hyperemesis gravidarum. As a result of the significant and lasting hydrogen chloride losses, maternal renal compensation results in retention of bicarbonate to maintain maternal anionic balance. Because bicarbonate is transported slowly across the placenta, the development of fetal metabolic alkalosis lags behind that of the mother. On the other hand, the maternal respiratory compensation (hypoventilation with the ensuing hypercapnia) tends to restore normal pH in the fetus as carbon dioxide is rapidly transported across the placenta.

Correction of Postnatal Metabolic Alkalosis

Metabolic alkalosis most frequently develops in preterm neonates receiving prolonged diuretic treatment for bronchopulmonary dysplasia. Although there is little evidence that chronic diuretic management results in an improved medium- or long-term pulmonary outcome, the majority of neonatologists use this treatment modality. If total-body chloride and potassium content is not appropriately maintained during chronic diuretic administration, severe metabolic "contraction" alkalosis may develop, which also results in poor growth. The respiratory response is a decrease in the rate and depth of breathing to increase carbon dioxide retention. This response may be interpreted as a sign of worsening pulmonary condition in a ventilated preterm neonate and may inappropriately trigger an increase in ventilatory support. Thus, respiratory compensation of metabolic alkalosis may be ineffective if the intubated neonate is subjected to iatrogenic overventilation on the mechanical ventilator. As for the neonatal renal compensation for metabolic alkalosis, urinary bicarbonate reabsorption and distal tubular net acid excretion decrease, resulting in a return of the extracellular pH toward normal.

Finally, metabolic alkalosis can also result from a nondiuretic administration–related loss of ECF containing disproportionally more chloride than bicarbonate. During the diuretic phase of normal postnatal adaptation, preterm and term newborns tend to retain relatively more bicarbonate than chloride.[36] The obvious benefits of allowing this physiologic extracellular volume contraction to occur clearly outweigh the clinical importance of a mild contraction alkalosis developing during postnatal adaptation. Thus, no specific treatment is needed in these cases, especially because with the stabilization of the extracellular volume status and the renal function with time, acid–base balance rapidly returns to normal.

Normal Acid–Base Balance and Growth

Growth is most accelerated during fetal life. The normal fetus grows from a weight of 0.22 g at 8 weeks' gestation to 3400 g at 40 weeks' completed gestation.[37] The estimated energy density of each gram of body weight gained (or lost) is 23 kJ (5.6 kcal). However, in premature infants, especially if they are critically ill or growth retarded, the energy density of the new tissue is estimated to be higher than 5.6 kcal/g.[38] For instance, in small for gestational age infants at approximately 5 weeks after birth, the total energy expenditure is estimated to be 20% greater than in appropriate for gestational age control participants.[39]

Fetal growth can be negatively affected by several fetal and placentomaternal conditions. Proven fetal conditions affecting fetal growth include certain genetic conditions and infection of the fetus.[40] Placentomaternal conditions with demonstrated influence on fetal growth are primary placental insufficiency and maternal diseases, nutritional status or substance abuse leading to secondary placental insufficiency, decreased fetal nutrient availability or direct fetal toxicity, or a combination of these harmful effects on fetal well-being.[40]

Although, there is little direct evidence available to demonstrate an impact of chronic fetal acid–base abnormality on fetal growth, a recent hypothesis implicates a *mild shift in the fetal acid–base status* as the primary pathologic factor for intrauterine growth restriction caused by placental insufficiency of any etiology.[41] From 18 weeks postconception, growth-retarded fetuses exhibit a greater degree of mild acidemia than their appropriately growing counterparts.[42] This acidemia is attributed to the reduced perfusion and mild hypoxemia the growth-retarded fetus faces as a result of the placental insufficiency. According to this hypothesis, the small initial reduction in the pH negatively affects nitric oxide production in the fetus, and the decreased availability of nitric oxide then plays a major role in the ensuing growth restriction.[41]

The following findings are in support of this hypothesis. Because locally formed nitric oxide regulates tissue perfusion and thus oxygen delivery and tissue growth itself, it has been suggested to play a pivotal role in regulation of growth in fetuses.[40,41] In addition to its effect on oxygen delivery to the tissues, nitric oxide is an anabolic factor. Indeed, it is necessary for normal growth of several tissues, including the bone and muscle, and for the action of different hormones, such as the parathyroid hormone, vitamin D, and estrogen, known to be of importance in fetal growth and development.[43,44]

Interestingly, the enzyme responsible for generating nitric oxide from L-arginine, constitutive nitric oxide synthase (cNOS), is sensitive to changes in pH, and its activity decreases even with a mild shift in the pH toward acidosis.[45] Thus, a vicious cycle may develop in growth-retarded fetuses because the initial decrease in blood flow and pH caused by placental insufficiency may lead to decreased cNOS activity and thus nitric oxide production. Decreased nitric oxide production, in turn, leads to further decreases in tissue perfusion and thus in pH, exacerbating the decrease in local nitric oxide production.[41]

In addition to being the source of locally generated nitric oxide, L-arginine also serves as the source polyamines and L-proline. These compounds are generated by the arginase enzyme and are important when growth and tissue repair processes predominate. The function of this enzyme is also pH dependent,[46] and the proposed decrease in its activity in growth-restricted fetuses may contribute to further impairment of fetal growth.

Based on this information, it seems that elevating the pH in the fetus toward normal and supplementing L-arginine to the mother may be a plausible approach to attenuating the impact on fetal growth of the placental insufficiency–induced decreased fetal oxygen delivery. However, because of the inherent difficulties associated with attempts to effectively control fetal pH, no clinical trial has as yet attempted this combined approach.

As for the neonate, the syndrome of late metabolic acidosis of prematurity is an example of how postnatal growth can be affected by alterations in the acid–base balance. This entity was first described in the 1960s, in which otherwise healthy premature infants after a few weeks developed mild to moderate anion gap acidosis and decreased growth rate. All of these infants were receiving high-protein cow's milk formulas and demonstrated increased net acid excretion compared with control participants. This type of late metabolic acidosis is now rarely seen, probably because of the use of special formulas for premature infants and the changes made to regular formulas now containing a decreased casein-to-whey ratio and lower fixed acid loads.

The diuretic administration–induced hypochloremic metabolic alkalosis is another example of the impact of acid–base balance on postnatal growth. This phenomenon is also associated with growth failure and may be a contributing factor of poor outcome in infants with bronchopulmonary dysplasia.[47] The growth failure is most likely caused by the decrease in cell proliferation and diminished DNA and protein synthesis in response to intracellular alkalosis.[48] Chronic decrease in total-body sodium resulting in a negative sodium balance may further hinder the growth of these infants.[49] Aggressive chloride and potassium supplementation with relatively limited sodium supplementation decreases the risk for the development of clinically significant severe contraction alkalosis associated with chronic diuretic use in these patients.

Obstetric Management and Fetal and Neonatal Acid–Base Balance

Evidence has recently accumulated on the impact of certain aspects of obstetric management of labor and delivery on fetal and neonatal acid–base homeostasis. These effects are transient, and it is unclear whether they have an independent impact on clinically relevant neonatal outcome measures.

Maternal betamethasone administration has been associated with a transient decrease in fetal movements, including fetal breathing[50] and fetal heart rate variability.[50,51] Although the exact pathomechanism of these effects of antenatal betamethasone administration is unclear, animal[52] and recent human[53] data suggest that transient fetal acidosis after maternal steroid administration may, at least in part, explain the findings. It has been suggested that the fetal acidosis is a consequence of the demonstrated fetal cardiovascular, endocrine, and metabolic effects of maternal steroid administration.[53,54]

The timing of umbilical cord clamping also appears to have an impact on neonatal acid–base balance immediately after delivery. The normally produced and accumulated anaerobic metabolites in nonvital organs during labor and delivery are washed out in a larger blood volume in neonates with delayed cord clamping, and thus they exert a smaller effect on blood pH in these infants.[55] Because the potential clinical relevance of fetal and immediate postnatal acidosis depends on the severity of hypoxemia and the associated acidosis, it may only have importance in neonates with prolonged labor and difficult delivery.[56]

Finally, the type of anesthesia during delivery via cesarean section also appears to have an impact on the fetal acid–base status. A recent prospective observational cohort study examined the relationship between the type of anesthesia provided during cesarean section and fetal acid–base balance and neonatal condition upon delivery in 900 women with uncomplicated singleton pregnancies.[57] The study found that epidural anesthesia was associated with higher venous cord pH (7.30 ± 7.26–7.34) than general (7.25 ± 7.21–7.26) or spinal (7.23 ± 7.19–7.26) anesthesia and that neonatal well-being was negatively affected primarily by general anesthesia.

Summary

This chapter has reviewed the available information and the gaps in our knowledge on how fetal and neonatal acid–base balance is regulated and the impact of alterations in acid–base balance on some aspects of fetal and postnatal growth as well as how selected obstetric management approaches affect fetal and neonatal acid–base balance. In the future, a better understanding of the role of growth factors and their interaction with fetal acid–base status may result in improved early management of growth-retarded fetuses. This, in turn, may decrease the negative impact of growth retardation on brain and other organ development.

References

1. Masoro EJ. An overview of hydrogen ion regulation. *Arch Intern Med.* 1982;142:1019.
2. Sorensen SC. The chemical control of ventilation. *Acta Physiol Scand.* 1971;361:1.
3. Blechner JN. Maternal-fetal acid-base, physiology. *Clin Obstet Gynecol.* 1993;36:3.
4. Vogh BP, Maren TH. Sodium, chloride, and bicarbonate movement from plasma to cerebrospinal fluid in cats. *Am J Physiol.* 1975;228:673.
5. Kemp JG, Greer FA, Wolfe LA. Acid-base regulation after maximal exercise testing in late gestation. *J Appl Physiol.* 1997;83:644.
6. Blechner JN, Meshia G, Barron DH. A study of the acid-base balance of fetal sheep and goats. *Q J Exp Physiol.* 1960;45:60.
7. Jansen A, Shernick V. Fetal breathing and development of control of breathing. *J Appl Physio.* 1991;70:143L.
8. Molteni RA, Melmed MH, Sheldon RE, et al. Induction of fetal breathing by metabolic acidemia and its effect on blood flow to the respiratory muscles. *Am J Obstet Gynecol.* 1980;136:609.
9. Kesby GJ, Lumbers ER. Factors affecting renal handling of sodium, hydrogen ions, and bicarbonate in the fetus. *Am J Physiol.* 1986;251:F226.
10. Hill KJ, Lumbers ER. Renal function in adult and fetal sheep. *Dev Physiol.* 1988;10:149.
11. Kesby GJ, Lumbers ER. The effects of metabolic acidosis on renal function of fetal sheep. *J Physiol.* 1988;396:65.
12. Elbourne I, Lumbers ER, Hill KJ. The secretion of organic acids and bases by the ovine fetal kidney. *Exp Physiol.* 1990;75:211.
13. Robillard JE, Sessions C, Burmeister L, Smith FG. Influence of fetal extracellular volume contraction on renal reabsorption of bicarbonate in fetal lambs. *Pediatr Res.* 1977;11:649.
14. Gibson KJ, McMullen JR, Lumbers ER. Renal acid-base and sodium handling in hypoxia and subsequent mild metabolic acidosis in fetal sheep. *Clin Exper Pharmacol Physiol.* 1977;27:67, 2000.
15. Blechner JN, Stenger VG, Eitzman DV, Prystowsky H. Effects of maternal metabolic acidosis on the human fetus and newborn infant. *Am J Obstet Gynecol.* 1967;9:46.
16. Shields LE, Moore TR, Brace RA. Fetal electrolyte and acid-base responses to amnioinfusion: lactated Ringer's versus normal saline in the ovine fetus. *J Soc Gynecol Invest.* 1995;2:602.
17. Sulyok E, Nemeth M, Tenyi I, et al. Relationship between maturity, electrolyte balance and the function of the renin-angiotensin-aldosterone system in newborn infants. *Biol Neonate.* 1979;35:60.
18. Avner ED. Normal neonates and the maturational development of homeostatic mechanisms. In Ichikawa I, ed. *Pediatric Textbook of Fluids and Electrolytes.* Baltimore: Williams & Wilkins; 1990;107-118.
19. Jones DP, Chesney RW. Development of tubular function. *Clin Perinatol.* 1992;19:33.
20. Brewer ED. Disorders of acid-base balance. *Pediatr Clin North Am.* 1990;37:429.
21. Stephenson G, Hammet M, Hadaway G, Funder JW. Ontogeny of renal mineralocorticoid receptors and urinary electrolyte responses in the rat. *Am J Physiol.* 1984;247:F665.
22. Guignard JP, John EG. Renal function in the tiny premature infant. *Clin Permatol.* 1986;13:377.
23. Seri I, Abbasi S, Wood DC, Gerdes JS. Regional hemodynamic effects of dopamine in the sick preterm infant. *J Pediatr.* 1998;133:728.
24. Fawer CL, Torrado A, Guignard J. Maturation of renal function in full-term and premature neonates. *Helv Paediatr Acta.* 1979;34:11.
25. Guignard JP, Torrado A, Da Cunha O, Gautier: Glomerular filtration rate in the first three weeks of life. *J Pediatr.* 1975;87:268.

26. Hamm LL Alpern RJ. Cellular mechanisms of renal tubular acidification. In Sedin DW, Giebisch G, eds. *The Kidney: Physiology and Pathophysiology*, 2nd ed. New York: Raven Press; 1992:2581-2626.
27. Robillard JP, Sessions C, Smith FG. In vivo demonstration of renal carbonic anhydrase activity in the fetal lamb. *Biol Neonate*. 1978 34:253.
28. Lonnerholm C, Wistrand PJ. Carbonic anhydrase in the human fetal kidney. *Pediatr Res*. 1983;17:390.
29. Fryckstedt J, Svensson LB, Linden M, Aperia A. The effect of dopamine on adenylate cyclase and Na+,K+-ATPase activity in the developing rat renal cortical and medullary tubule cells. *Pediatr Res*. 1993;34:308.
30. Felder CC, Campbell T, Albrecht F, Jose PA. Dopamine inhibits Na+/H+ exchanger activity in renal BBMV by stimulation of adenylate cyclase. *Am J Physiol*. 1990;259:F297.
31. Seri I. Cardiovascular, renal, and endocrine actions of dopamine in neonates and children. *J Pediatr*. 1995;126:333.
32. Hropot M, Fowler N, Karlmark B, Giebisch G. Tubular action of diuretics: distal effects on electrolyte transport and acidification. *Kidney Int*. 1985;28:477.
33. Seri I, Rudas G, Bors Zs, et al. Effects of low-dose dopamine on cardiovascular and renal functions, cerebral blood flow, and plasma catecholamine levels in sick preterm neonates. *Pediatr Res*. 1993;34:742.
34. Stonestreet BS, Rubin L, Pollak A. et al. Renal functions of low birth weight infants with hyperglycemia and glucosuria produced by glucose infusions. *Pediatrics*. 1980;66:561.
35. Moya F, Morishima HO, Shnider SM, James L. Influence of maternal hypoventilation on the newborn infant. *Am J Obstet Gynecol*. 1965;91:76.
36. Ramiro-Tolentino SB, Markarian K, Kleinman LI. Renal bicarbonate excretion in extremely low birth weight infants. *Pediatrics*. 1996;98:256-261.
37. Taeusch HW, Ballard RA, Gleason CA, eds. *Appendix 2. Avery's Diseases of the Newborn*. 8th ed. 2005:1574.
38. Davies PSW. Energy requirements for growth and development in infancy. *Am J Clin Nutr*. 1998;68:939S.
39. Davies PSW, Clough H, Bishop N, et al. Total energy expenditure in small-for-gestational-age infants. *Arch Dis Child*. 1996;74:F208.
40. Hay WW, Catz CS, Grave GD, Yaffe SJ. Workshop summary: fetal growth: its regulation and disorders. *Pediatrics*. 1997;99:585.
41. Stearns MR, Jackson CGR, Landauer JA, et al. Small for gestational age: a new insight? *Medical Hypotheses*. 1999;53:186.
42. Nicolaides KH, Economides DL, Soothill PW. Blood gasses, pH and lactate in appropriate- and small-for-gestational-age fetuses. *Am J Obstet Gynecol*. 1989;161:996.
43. Kaiser FE, Dirighi M, Muchnick J, et al. Regulation of gonadotropins and parathyroid hormone by nitric oxide. *Life Sci*. 1996;59:987.
44. Evans CH, Stefanovic-Racic M, Lancaster J. Nitric oxide and it role in orthopedic disease. *Clin Orthoped Rel Res*. 1995;312:275.
45. Fleming I, Hecker M, Busse R. Intracellular alkalinization induced by bradykinin sustains activation of the constitutive nitric oxide synthase in endothelial cells. *Circ Res*. 1994;74:1220.
46. Kuhn NJ, Ward S, Piponski M, Young TW. Purification of human hepatic arginase and its manganese (II)-dependent and pH-dependent interconversion between active and inactive forms: a possible pH-sensing function of the enzyme on the ornithine cycle. *Arch Biochem Biophys*. 1995;320:24.
47. Perlman JF, Moore V, Siegel MJ, Dawson J. Is chloride depletion an important contributing cause of death in infants with bronchopulmonary dysplasia? *Pediatrics*. 1986;77:212.
48. Heinly MM, Wassner SJ. The effect of isolated chloride depletion on growth and protein turnover in young rats. *Pediatr Nephrol*. 1994;8:555.
49. Sulyok E, Kovacs L, Lichardus B, et al. Late hyponatremia in premature infants: role of aldosterone and arginine vasopressin. *J Pediatr*. 1985;106:990.
50. Rotmensch S, Liberati M, Celentano C, et al. The effect of betamethasone on fetal biophysical activities and Doppler velocimetry of umbilical and middle cerebral arteries. *Acta Obstet Gynecol Scand*. 1999;78:768.
51. Senat MV, Minoui S, Multon O, et al. Effect of dexamethasone and betamethasone on fetal heart rate variability in preterm labour: a randomized study. *Br J Obstet Gynaecol*. 1998;105:749.
52. Bennett L, Kozuma S, McGarrigle HH, Hanson MA. (1999) Temporal changes in fetal cardiovascular, behavioral, metabolic and endocrine responses to maternally administered dexamethasone in the late gestation fetal sheep. *Br J Obstet Gynaecol*. 1999;106:331.
53. Shenhav S, Volodarsky M, Anteby EY, Gemer O. Fetal acid-base balance after betamethasone administration: relation to fetal heart rate variability. *Arch Gynecol Obstet*. 2008;278:333.
54. Derks JB, Mulder EJ, Visser GH. The effects of maternal betamethasone administration on the fetus. *Br J Obstet Gynaecol*. 1995;102:40.
55. Wiberg N, Källén K, Olofsson P. Delayed umbilical cord clamping at birth has effects on arterial and venous blood gases and lactate concentrations. *BJOG*. 2008;115:697.
56. Hutchon DJ. Immediate cord clamping may increase neonatal acidaemia. *BJOG*. 2008; 115:1190.
57. Tonni G, Ferrari B, De Felice C, Ventura A. Fetal acid-base and neonatal status after general and neuraxial anesthesia for elective cesarean section. *Int J Gynaecol Obstet*. 2007;97:143.

The Kidney: Normal Development and Hormonal Control

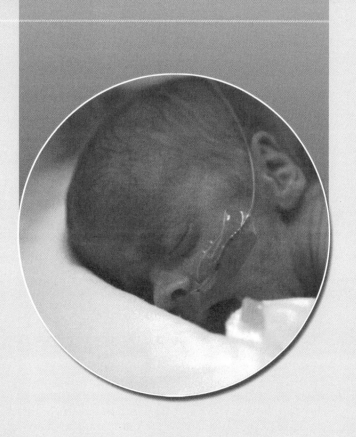

CHAPTER 8

Glomerular Filtration Rate in Neonates

Jean-Pierre Guignard, MD, Jean-Bernard Gouyon, MD

- ● Development of Glomerular Filtration
- ● Assessment of Glomerular Filtration Rate
- ● Conditions and Factors that Impair Glomerular Filtration Rate
- ● Prevention of Oliguric States Caused by Low Glomerular Filtration Rate

Ultrafiltration of plasma across permselective capillaries is the first step in urine formation. This process starts with the development of the metanephros around the 10th week of gestation. The glomerular filtration rate (GFR) increases progressively throughout fetal and postnatal life, reaching the "adult" mature levels by 1 year of life. During the period of maturation, the function of the kidney is characterized by elevated renal vascular resistance (RVR), low arterial renal perfusion pressure, and low renal blood flow (RBF). The ultrafiltration process is maintained by a delicate balance between vasoconstrictor and counteracting vasodilator forces. This balance can be easily disturbed by various factors, resulting in a transient or permanent impairment in GFR. This chapter briefly reviews the maturation of glomerular filtration, discusses the techniques available to assess GFR in neonates, and describes factors and agents that can impair or protect maturing glomerular filtration.

Development of Glomerular Filtration

Glomerular ultrafiltration depends on the net ultrafiltration pressure, which is the difference between the hydrostatic and oncotic pressures across glomerular capillaries. The low perfusion pressure and low glomerular plasma flow account, at least in part, for the low levels of GFR present during gestation. For any given ultrafiltration pressure, GFR will depend on the rate at which plasma flows through the glomerular capillaries as well as on the ultrafiltration coefficient (K_f). K_f is a function of the total capillary surface area and of the permeability per unit of surface area.

During gestation, GFR increases in parallel with gestational age (GA), up to the end of nephrogenesis around the 35th week of gestation.[1] This pattern of development reflects both an increase in the number of nephrons and the growth of existing nephrons. From the 35th week of gestation, the development of GFR slows down up to the time of birth (Fig. 8-1). Postnatal maturation of renal function is characterized by a striking increase in GFR, the value of which doubles within the first 2 weeks of life (Fig. 8-2).[1] The velocity of this increase is somewhat slower in the most premature infants. An increase in both the net filtration pressure and the K_f accounts for the large postnatal increase in GFR. The increase in the glomerular capillary surface area represents the main factor responsible for the increase in the K_f.[2] Additional maturational changes that may contribute to the postnatal maturation of GFR include an increase in pore size and glomerular hydraulic permeability and a decrease in both the afferent and efferent arteriolar resistance.

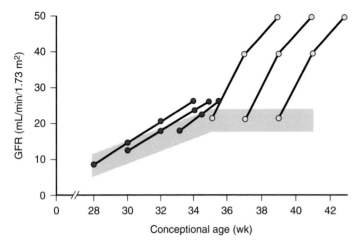

Figure 8-1 Development of glomerular filtration rate (GFR) as a function of conceptional age during the last 3 months of gestation and the first month of postnatal life. The *shaded area* represents the range of normal values. The postnatal increase in GFR observed in preterm (•–•) and term neonates (o–o) is schematically represented. (Modified from Guignard JP, John EG. Renal function in the tiny, premature infant. *Clin Perinatol.* 1986;13:377.)

Vasoactive Factors

Several vasoactive agents and hormones modulate GFR and RBF.[2] By acting on the arcuate arteries, the interlobular arteries, and the afferent and efferent arterioles, they regulate the glomerular hydrostatic pressure and the glomerular transcapillary hydraulic pressure gradient. These agents can also modify the ultrafiltration coefficient by two mechanisms: a change in the capillary filtration area by contracting the mesangial cells and a change in hydraulic conductivity by decreasing the number or size (or both) of the filtration slit pores. The main vasoactive forces modulating single-nephron GFR (SNGFR) are listed in Table 8-1. Two vasoactive systems, the renin–angiotensin system and the prostaglandins (PGs) (Fig. 8-3), play key roles in the protection of the stressed kidney.

Angiotensin II

Angiotensin II (ATII) is a very potent vasoconstrictor of the afferent and efferent arterioles, acting on two types of receptors, the AT_1 and the AT_2 receptor subtypes. The AT_1 receptors are widely distributed and appear to mediate most of the biologic effects of ATII. The exact role of the AT_2 receptors remains uncertain. ATII acts on both pre- and postglomerular resistance, but appears to predominantly vasoconstrict the efferent arteriole, thereby increasing the glomerular capillary hydrostatic pressure

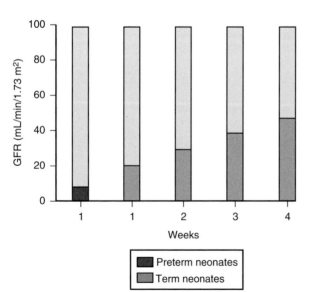

Figure 8-2 Postnatal increase in glomerular filtration rate (GFR) in term and preterm infants. The upper part of each column represents the deficit between the neonate's GFR and mature levels (100 mL/min/1.73 m²). Note that at the end of the first month of life, human neonates are in a state of relative renal insufficiency compared with adults. (Modified from Guignard JP, John EG. Renal function in the tiny, premature infant. *Clin Perinatol.* 1986;13:377.)

Table 8-1 VASOACTIVE FACTORS REGULATING THE GLOMERULAR MICROCIRCULATION

Vasoconstrictors	Vasodilators
Circulating hormones	Circulating hormones
• Catecholamines	• Dopamine
• Angiotensin II	
• Vasopressin	
• Glucocorticoids	
Paracrine + autocoïds	Paracrine + autocoïds
• Endothelin	• Nitric oxide
• Thromboxane A_2	• Acetylcholine
• Leukotrienes	• PGI_2 + PGE_2
• Adenosine	• Bradykinin
	• Adenosine

PG, prostaglandin.

while decreasing the glomerular plasma flow rate.[3] This mechanism serves to maintain GFR when the renal perfusion pressure decreases to low levels. The action of ATII on the efferent arteriole is counterbalanced by intrarenal adenosine, an agent modulating the tubuloglomerular feedback mechanism. When both ATII and adenosine are overstimulated, their combined action results in afferent vasoconstriction.[4]

Prostaglandins

The renal PGs are potent vasoactive metabolites of arachidonic acid.[5,6] Under normal conditions, the renal PGs are present in low concentrations and exert only minor effects on the renal circulation and GFR. However, the vasodilator PGs are of major importance in protecting renal perfusion and GFR when vasoconstrictor forces are activated as, for instance, during hypotensive, hypovolemic, and sodium depletion states or during congestive heart failure. The PGs protect GFR by vasodilating the afferent arterioles and by dampening the renal vasoconstrictor effects of ATII, endothelin, and sympathetic nerve stimulation on the afferent arteriole.

Maturational Aspects of the Renin–Angiotensin and Prostaglandins Systems

The Renin–Angiotensin System

Renin is found as early as the 5th week in the mesonephros and by the 8th week in the metanephros. The plasma renin concentration and activity generated by the fetal kidney are elevated.[7] The presence of an intact functional renin–angiotensin

Figure 8-3 The physiologic regulation of glomerular filtration rate (GFR) depends on two main factors: the afferent vasodilator prostaglandins and the efferent vasoconstrictor angiotensin II. RBF, renal blood flow.

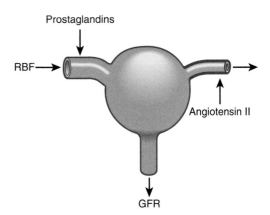

system is a key factor for the maintenance of blood pressure and RBF during fetal life. Acting through its AT_1 receptors, ATII is indeed the promoter of the postnatal expression of postglomerular capillaries and organization of vasa recta bundles, which are necessary for development of normal RBF.[8] Mutations in the genes encoding any of the components of the renin–angiotensin system result in severe tubular dysgenesis.[9] The plasma renin activity further increases after birth before slowly decreasing through infancy. The factors controlling renin release (macula densa, baroreceptor, sympathetic nervous system, and hormonal mechanisms) are active in fetuses.[7]

Elevated levels of ATII are present in fetuses and remain high in the neonatal period. Although AT_2 receptors predominate during embryonic and fetal life, they rapidly decline after birth.[10] AT_1 receptors predominate after birth and are found in glomeruli, macula densa and mesangial cells, resistance arteries, and vasa recta.[11] In addition to its AT_1-mediated vasoconstrictor effects, ATII promotes growth of the renal vasculature.[10] Blockade of the AT_1 receptors with losartan during fetal life interferes with normal renal development and results in vascular malformations, cystic dilatation of the tubules, and a decrease in the number of glomeruli.[12] Blockade of AT_1 receptor by losartan in newborn rabbits induces a decrease in GFR without affecting RBF,[13] thus illustrating the major role of ATII in regulating and protecting GFR in kidneys perfused at low systemic arterial pressures.

The Prostaglandins

Cyclooxygenases 1 and 2 (COX-1 and COX-2) are expressed in the fetal renal vasculature, glomeruli, and collecting ducts. COX-2 activity is highest after birth.[13] Renal cortical COX2-derived prostanoids, particularly PGI_2 and PGE_2, play critical roles in maintaining blood pressure and renal function in volume-contracted states.[14] Interference with PG synthesis during fetal life leads to renal dysgenesis with cortical dysplasia, cystic tubular dilatation, and impaired nephrogenesis.[15] COX-2 is probably involved in this pathogenesis.[16] Although the PGs do probably not regulate GFR in normal conditions, interference with PG synthesis may have deleterious effects in conditions associated with renal hypoperfusion.

Assessment of Glomerular Filtration Rate

Different methods using various markers have been used to assess GFR in neonates. The most common measurement of GFR is based on the concept of "clearance," which relates the quantitative urinary excretion of a substance per unit of time to the volume of plasma that, if "cleared" completely of the same contained substance, would yield a quantity equivalent to that excreted in the urine. The clearance C of a substance x is expressed by the formula:

$$C = U_X \bullet V/P_X$$

where U_X represents the urinary concentration of the substance, V the urine flow rate, and P_X the plasma concentration. For its clearance to be equal to the rate of glomerular filtration, a substance must have the following properties: (1) it must be freely filterable through the glomerular capillary membranes, that is, not be bound to plasma proteins or sieved in the process of ultrafiltration; (2) it must not be excreted by an extrarenal route; and (3) it must be biologically inert and neither reabsorbed nor secreted by the renal tubules. Several substances, endogenous or exogenous, have been claimed to have these properties: inulin, creatinine, iohexol, ethylenediaminetetra-acetic acid (EDTA), diethylenetriaminepenta-acetic acid (DTPA), and sodium iothalamate. The experimental evidence that this is true has been produced only for inulin.

Glomerular Markers

Several endogenous or exogenous markers have been used to assess GFR (Table 8-2). The markers used in neonates are described below.

Table 8-2 CHARACTERISTICS OF THE GLOMERULAR MARKERS

	Inulin	Creatinine	Iohexol	DTPA	EDTA	Iothalamate
Molecular weight (Da)	5200	113	811	393	292	637
Elimination half-life (min)	70	200	90	110	120	120
Plasma protein binding (%)	0	0	<2	5	0	<5
Space of distribution	EC	TBW	EC	EC	EC	EC

DTPA, diethylenetriaminepenta-acetic acid; EC, extracellular space; EDTA, ethylenediaminetetra-acetic acid; TBW, total body water.

Inulin

Inulin, an exogenous starchlike fructose polymer extracted from Jerusalem artichokes, has an Einstein-Stokes radius of 1.5 nm, and a molecular weight (MW) of approximately 5.2 kDa. It diffuses, as would a spherical body of such radius. Inulin is inert, it is not metabolized, not reabsorbed and not secreted by the renal tubular cells. Its clearance, consequently, reflects the rate of filtration only. Estimates of inulin clearance provide the basis for a standard reference against which the route or mechanisms of excretion of other substances can be ascertained.

Inulin as a Marker of Glomerular Filtration Rate in Neonates

The hypothesis that inulin may not be freely filtered by the immature glomerular barrier has never been confirmed, neither in animal nor in human studies.[17] Inulin has been used as a marker of GFR in human neonates using three different techniques to measure or estimate its clearance: (1) the urinary UV/P clearance (where U is the urine concentration, V is the urine flow rate, and P is the plasma concentration), (2) the constant infusion technique without urine collection, and (3) the single-injection (plasma disappearance curve) technique.

Creatinine

Creatinine, the normal metabolite of creatine phosphate present in skeletal muscle, has a MW of 113 Da. The renal excretion of endogenous creatinine is fairly similar to that of inulin in humans and several animal species. However, in addition to being filtered through the glomerulus, creatinine is secreted in part by the renal tubular cells.

Overestimation of GFR by creatinine clearance (eC$_{creat}$) is usually more evident at low GFRs. As GFR decreases progressively during the course of renal disease, the renal tubular secretion of creatinine contributes an increasing fraction to urinary excretion, so that eC$_{creat}$ may substantially exceed the actual GFR. Secretion of creatinine into the gut plays a role in this phenomenon.

Although creatinine has been used for decades, the methods available for its chemical determination are still biased by various interfering substances.[18] The coloric method described by Jaffe is still widely used in clinical laboratories. Its major drawback is the interference by noncreatinine chromogens such as bilirubin, pyruvate, uric acid, cotrimoxazole, and cyclosporins. The use of enzymatic methods has increased the specificity of creatinine determination.[19] Further improvement in measuring creatinine has been achieved by the use of newer techniques such as high-performance liquid chromatography (HPLC), gas chromatography isotope dilution mass spectrometry (Gc-IDSM), and the HPLC-IMSD coupled technique.[18] Gas chromatography isotope dilution mass spectrometry (Gc-IDMS) is now considered the method of choice for measuring true creatinine. It has an excellent specificity and low relative SD (<0.3%).[18] A method coupling HPLC with IDMS for the direct determination of creatinine has been developed recently.[20] The procedure is simple and speedy. It appears to offer the same advantage as the Gc-IDMS technique.

Although accurate and reproducible assessment of creatinine is mandatory, the calibration of its measurement is not yet standardized to a gold standard in most places, leading to substantial variations among laboratories.[18]

Creatinine as a Marker of GFR in the Neonate

The handling of creatinine by immature kidneys is unique, with creatinine apparently undergoing glomerular filtration and partial tubular reabsorption. In newborn rabbits, the urinary clearance of creatinine underestimates the concomitantly measured clearance of inulin with creatinine-to-inulin ratios below 1 in the first days of life[21] (Fig. 8.4). Such ratios indicate that creatinine is actually reabsorbed at this stage of renal development. As the animals mature, the ratios increase above 1, reflecting filtration *and* secretion of creatinine. Reabsorption of creatinine is only present in the first postnatal days and is probably explained by the passive reabsorption of the filtered creatinine across immature leaky tubules. When water is reabsorbed along the nephron, the concentration of filtered creatinine rises so that creatinine back-diffuses into the blood according to its concentration gradient, thus raising its plasma concentration. The clearance of creatinine has also been shown to underestimate true GFR in very low birth weight (VLBW) human neonates, thus suggesting the occurrence of the same phenomenon in human immature kidneys.[22]

The use of creatinine as a marker of GFR in neonates is not only hampered by its specific handling by the immature kidney but also, as previously mentioned, by the interference of noncreatinine chromogens, sometimes leading to spurious overestimation of the true plasma creatinine.

Iohexol

Iohexol is a nonionic agent with a MW of 821 Da that appears to be eliminated exclusively by glomerular filtration. A significant correlation has been observed between the urinary clearance of inulin and both the urinary clearance of iohexol or its plasma disappearance clearance in a limited number of children.[23,24] Large studies to validate iohexol as a true glomerular marker are not yet available. Iohexol has not been validated in neonates.

Iothalamate Sodium

Iothalamate sodium has a MW of 637 Da. It can be used as ^{125}I-radiolabeled or without radioactive label, its plasma concentration then being assessed by X-ray

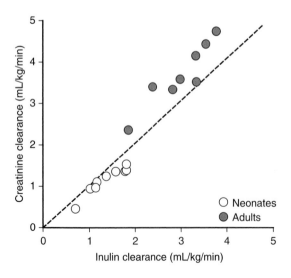

Figure 8-4 The relationship between the clearances of creatinine and inulin in newborn and adult rabbits with comparable plasma levels of creatinine. (Modified from Matos P, Duarte-Silva M, Drukker A, et al. *Pediatr Res.* 1998;44:639.)

fluorescence or by HPLC or, more recently, by capillary electrophoresis. It is only minimally bound to proteins, and its renal handling has some similarities with that of inulin. Critical studies have, however, unequivocally demonstrated that iothalamate is actively secreted by the renal tubules and perhaps also undergoes tubular reabsorption in humans and animal species.[25] The agreement between iothalamate and inulin clearances appears to be a fortuitous cancellation of errors between tubular excretion and protein binding of the agent. The substance does not consequently appear suitable for accurate estimation of GFR. The use of iothalamate has not been properly validated in neonates. Radiolabeled iothalamate should not be used in the first month of life.

^{99m}Tc-DTPA and ^{51}Cr-EDTA

The use of radiolabeled markers is not recommended during the neonatal period. This group of markers is thus not discussed here.

Techniques Used to Assess Glomerular Filtration Rate in Neonates

The Plasma Concentration

The use of the plasma creatinine (P_{creat}) concentration to estimate GFR presents specific problems in neonates. Neonates' plasma creatinine level is elevated at birth, reflecting the maternal plasma creatinine concentration. A near perfect equilibrium between the maternal and fetal plasma creatinine concentrations has indeed been shown to occur throughout gestation (Fig. 8-5).[22] In preterm infants, the elevated plasma creatinine further increases transiently to reach a peak value between the second and fourth days of postnatal life (Fig. 8-6).[26,27] Peak plasma creatinine concentrations as high as 195 to 247 μmol/L in 23 to 26 weeks' GA neonates and 99 to 140 μmol/L in 33 to 40 weeks' GA neonates have been recorded (Table 8-3).[27] This transient increase in the VLBW neonates' postnatal plasma creatinine concentration is probably the result of creatinine reabsorption across leaky tubules. This phenomenon accounts for the observation that when measured during the first week of life, the P_{creat} is highest in the most premature infants.[28] Reference ranges for P_{creat} have been established from a cohort of 161 extremely premature infants followed

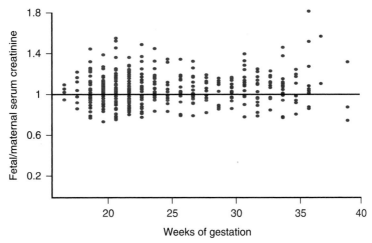

Figure 8-5 Relationship between fetal cord and maternal serum creatinine during gestation. The ratio of the fetal to maternal serum creatinine remains close to 1 throughout gestation, indicating free diffusion of creatinine across the placental barrier. (Modified from Guignard JP, Drukker A. Why do newborn infants have a high plasma creatinine? *Pediatrics.* 1999;103(4):e49.)

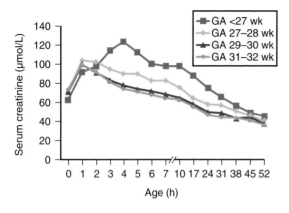

Figure 8-6 Changes in serum creatinine in preterm neonates during the first 52 hours of postnatal life. Peak increases are observed on day 4 in the most premature infants. GA, gestational age. (Modified from Gallini F, Maggio L, Romagnoli C, et al. Progression of renal function in preterm neonates with gestational age ≤ 32 weeks. *Pediatr Nephrol.* 2000;15:119.)

during the first 8 weeks of life[29](Fig. 8-7). Normal values for P_{creat} (as measured by an enzymatic assay during the first year of life are also available.[19] Factors affecting P_{creat} at birth and during the first postnatal weeks have been defined recently.[30] Hypertensive disease of pregnancy, ibuprofen-treated patent ductus arteriosus, and low GA were prominent factors influencing P_{creat} at birth and later. In infants with hemodynamically significant patent ductus arteriosus (PDA), P_{creat} levels before ibuprofen were significantly higher than those recorded in GA-matched control participants without PDA.

Urinary Clearance
Inulin

The method based on the urinary clearance of inulin is the reference method for GFR. Measurement of the urinary clearance of this exogenous marker is cumbersome, however, because it requires its constant intravenous infusion to maintain a steady state and the precise timed collection of urine. The method has been used in early developmental studies[1] to define the maturation of GFR in relation to gestational and postnatal age (Figs. 8-1 and 8-2).

Creatinine

The urinary clearance of creatinine has been claimed to approximate the urinary clearance of inulin in both preterm and term neonates. In premature infants, a creatinine-to-inulin clearance ratio below 1 has often been observed, suggesting that tubular reabsorption of creatinine also occurs in premature humans, as it does in immature animals.[21] Developmental studies based on the urinary clearance of creatinine have produced valuable information on the maturation of GFR.[28,31,32]

Table 8-3 CHANGES IN PLASMA CREATININE OVER TIME FOR DIFFERENT GESTATION GROUPS

Group Gestation Age (wk)	Birth Creatinine (µmol/L)*	Peak Plasma Creatinine (µmol/L)*	Time to Peak Plasma Creatinine (h)*
23–26	67–92	195–247	40–78
27–29	65–89	158–200	28–51
30–32	60–69	120–158	25–40
33–45	67–79	99–140	8–23

*Range intervals. From Miall LA, Henderson MJ, Turner, AJ, et al. Plasma creatinine rises dramatically in the first 48 hours of life in preterm infants. *Pediatrics.* 1999;6:104.

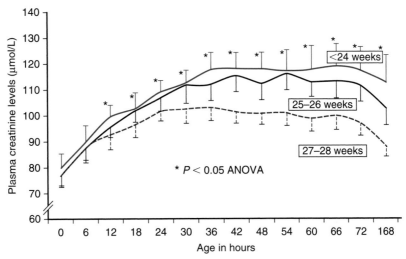

Figure 8-7 Mean plasma creatinine level (95% confidence interval) and gestational age during the first week of life. (From Thayyil S, Sheik S, Kempley ST, et al. *J Perinatol.* 2008;28:226.)

Reference values for the urinary clearance of creatinine during the first month of life of premature infants with GA ranging from 29 to 31 weeks has been published recently.[33] The postnatal increase in C_{creat} observed in these preterm infants is illustrated in Figure 8.8. Regression lines for calculating the normal values of C_{creat} as a function of GA and postnatal day are given in Table 8-4.[34]

The Constant Infusion Technique without Urine Collection

The constant infusion technique[34] assumes that the rate of infusion of a marker (x) needed to maintain constant its plasma concentration is equal to the rate of its excretion. After equilibration of the marker in its distribution space, the excretion rate must thus be equal to the rate of infusion (IR), hence the derived clearance formula:

$$C_x = U_x \cdot V/P_x = IR_x \cdot P_x$$

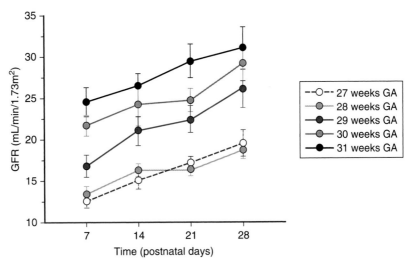

Figure 8-8 Glomerular filtration rate (GFR) according to gestational age (GA) in the first month of life (n = 275). Data are means + SEM. (From Vieux R, Hascoet JM, Merdariu D, et al. *Pediatrics.* 2010;125:e1186.)

Table 8-4 REGRESSION LINES TO CALCULATE THE REFERENCE MEDIAN NORMAL VALUE OF GLOMERULAR FILTRATION RATE AS A FUNCTION OF GESTATIONAL AGE (IN WEEKS) AND POSTNATAL DAY

Postnatal day	Median GFR
7	$63.57 + 2.85 \times GA$
14	$60.73 + 2.85 \times GA$
21	$58.97 + 2.85 \times GA$
28	$55.93 + 2.85 \times GA$

GA, gestational age. (Modified from Vieux R, Hascoet JM, Merdariu D, et al. Glomerular filtration rate reference values in very preterm infants. *Pediatrics*. 2010;124:e1186.)

The flow rate of the test solution containing the marker is expressed in mL/min per 1.73 m^2; so is the clearance C of the marker x.

The constant infusion technique without urine collection is attractive and has been used in newborn infants. The results obtained in short-term (a few hours) infusion studies have produced conflicting results. When inulin was constantly infused for 24 hours, the results obtained by this technique were in reasonable agreement with those obtained by the traditional urinary clearance.[35,36] As a whole, the infusion technique has the advantage of avoiding the need for urine collection, but presents with the main disadvantage of requiring careful time-consuming supervision of the long-duration infusion of inulin.

The Single-Injection (Plasma Disappearance Curve) Technique

The mathematical model for this technique is an open two-compartment system. The glomerular marker is injected in the first compartment, equilibrates with the second compartment, and is excreted from the first compartment by glomerular filtration. The plasma disappearance curve of the marker follows two consecutive patterns. In the first phase, the agent diffuses in its distribution space, and its plasma concentration falls rapidly. In the second phase, when the equilibration has been reached, the slope of the decline of the plasma concentration of the marker basically reflects its urinary excretion rate.

The plasma disappearance curve method has occasionally been used in neonates. A large overestimation of GFR by the single-injection technique has been repeatedly observed; it was ascribed to incomplete equilibration of inulin in its distribution space during the study period.[36,37]

Estimation of Creatinine Clearance from Its Plasma Concentration without Urine Collection

The concentration of endogenous markers, such as creatinine, increases when GFR decreases. The increase in plasma creatinine is not linear, however. Several attempts have thus been made to develop reliable methods that will allow a correct estimate of eC_{creat} from its plasma concentration alone without urine collection. A formula has been developed for children,[38,39] which allows an estimate of eC_{creat} derived from the patient's creatinine plasma concentration and body length:

$$eCcreat = k \cdot Length/P_{creat}$$

where k is a constant, L represents the body length and P_{creat} the plasma creatinine concentration. This formula is based on the assumption that creatinine excretion is proportional to body length and inversely proportional to plasma creatinine.[39] The value of the constant k can be obtained from the formula $k = eC_{creat} \cdot P_{creat}/Length$. When length is expressed in cm and P_{creat} in mg (%), the resulting eC_{creat} is expressed in mL/min per 1.73 m^2. Under steady state conditions, k should be directly proportional to the muscle component of body weight, which corresponds reasonably well to the daily urinary creatinine excretion rate.

The Schwartz formula has been used in neonates.[39] The mean value of k, calculated in 118 low birth weight infants with corrected ages of 25 to 105 weeks, was 0.33 ± 0.01. It rose to 0.45 in full-term infants up to 18 months.[39] Despite a large scatter of normal values, the formula was claimed to be useful because it correlated well with the inulin single-injection technique.[39] It is only unfortunate that the $k \bullet Length/P_{creat}$ formula has not been validated in neonates by comparing its results with those given by the standard $U \bullet (V/P)$ inulin clearance. The accuracy of the $k \bullet Length/P_{creat}$ formula, as an estimate of GFR, has indeed been questioned. In a study in infants younger than 1 year of age, the k value ranged from 0.17 to 0.82 (15–72 when P_{creat} in $\mu mol/L$), and factor k was found to vary markedly with the state of hydration.[40] The $k \bullet Length/P_{creat}$ formula may be more informative clinically than P_{creat} alone because the creatinine value, in addition to renal function, is critically dependent on the percentage of muscle mass. Caution should be exercised, however, when using the formula as an estimate of GFR in studies aimed at defining renal pathophysiologic mechanisms in neonates.

The Special Case of Cystatin C: A Nonclassical Glomerular Marker!

Cystatin C, a nonglycosated 13-kDa basic protein, is a proteinase inhibitor involved in the intracellular catabolism of proteins.[41] It is produced by all nucleated cells, freely filtered across the glomerular capillaries, almost completely reabsorbed, and catabolized in the renal proximal tubular cells.[42] Being reabsorbed, cystatin C is not a classical marker of glomerular filtration, as strictly defined (see Assessment of Glomerular Filtration Rate). When using the particle-enhanced immunonephelometry assay for its determination in blood, no interference from bilirubin, hemoglobin, triglycerides, and rheumatoid factor could be observed.[43] Cystatin C has been claimed to be a reliable marker of GFR independent of inflammatory conditions, muscle mass, and gender.[44,45] In children ages 1.8 to 18.8 years with various levels of GFR, serum cystatin C has been claimed to be broadly equivalent[46] or even superior[47] to P_{creat} as an estimate of GFR. A very large recent study of 8058 inhabitants of Groeningen questions, however, the advantages of cystatin C.[48] In this study, male gender, older age, greater weight, higher serum C-reactive protein levels, and cigarette smoking were all independently associated with higher cystatin C levels after adjusting for eC_{creat}. Cystatin C has also been shown to be a poor marker of GFR in pregnancy,[49] in renal transplant patients, and in patients receiving corticosteroids[50-52] as well as in intensive care unit patients.[53] In a recent study in children, cystatin C has also been shown to be less reliable than the Schwartz formula in distinguishing impaired from normal GFR.[54]

Cystatin C as a Marker of Glomerular Filtration Rate in Neonates

The handling of cystatin C by immature kidneys is not known. Cystatin C does not appear to cross the placental barrier, and there is no correlation between maternal and neonatal serum cystatin C levels.[55] Serum cystatin C concentrations are highest at birth and then decrease to stabilize after 12 months of age[55] (Fig. 8-9). Cystatin C is significantly higher in premature infants than in term infants.[44,56] Serum cystatin C values ranging from 1.24 to 2.84 mg/L have been recorded on the first day of life of premature neonates with a mean GA of 32.5 ± 2.6 weeks (x $\pm$ SD).[57] In the study by Randers et al,[45] mean values of 1.63 ± 0.26 mg/L (x $\pm$ SD) were recorded during the first month of life, 0.95 ± 0.22 mg/L during months 1 to 12, and 0.72 ± 0.12 mg/L after the first year of life.

The claim has been made that the concentration of cystatin C offers a greater sensitivity and reliability than creatinine in detecting an abnormal GFR in newborn infants and "that unlike creatinine, cystatin C can be used to assess GFR of the newborn and even the fetus."[58] Such a statement is somewhat ill-founded, and there are numerous reasons to refute this conclusion:

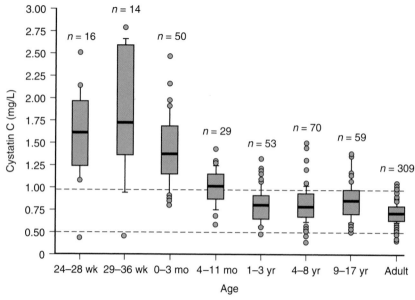

Figure 8-9 Box plot distributions showing plasma cystatin C values across the age groups. *Dotted lines* indicate 95% confidence interval of the adult range. Preterm babies born between 24 and 36 weeks of gestation were 1 day old. (Modified from Finney H, Newman DJ, Thakkar H, et al. Reference ranges for plasma cystatin C and creatinine measurements in premature infants, neonates, and older children. *Arch Dis Child*. 2000;82:71.)

1. The handling of cystatin C by the immature kidney is not known.
2. The scatter of the serum cystatin C concentrations in neonates is very large, so it is unlikely that a useful formula will be established to reliably estimate GFR at this age.
3. Because cystatin C is filtered and then reabsorbed and catabolized by the proximal tubular cells, its plasma concentration is obviously influenced by changes in the rate of degradation of cystatin C by injured renal proximal tubular cells.
4. The claim that cystatin C is a valuable marker of GFR has not been validated by comparison to the gold standard, either in neonates or in children.
5. The production and concentration of cystatin C may be influenced by factors other than GFR, such as the serum C-reactive protein levels, thyroid dysfunction, or corticosteroid administration.
6. Measurement of cystatin C is considerably more expensive than that of creatinine, by a factor of at least 12.[58]

Assessment of Renal Function in Neonates: Which Method for Which Purpose?

Developmental Investigative Studies

When the purpose of performing clearance studies is to obtain basic information on the physiological maturation of GFR, the use of reliable methods is mandatory. The urinary clearance of inulin remains the method of choice. This method requires constant inulin infusion to maintain steady state and timed urine collection by bladder catheterization or bag. The urinary clearance of creatinine also requires timed collection of urine and blood sampling in the middle of the urinary collection period. Valuable information has been obtained by this technique. The need for urine collection can be avoided by using the constant inulin infusion technique. In this case, inulin needs to be constantly infused for at least 24 hours, requiring careful supervision. When respecting the protocol strictly,[35,36] useful information can be obtained by this technique.

Other nonvalidated methods for measuring GFR should be avoided because they are unnecessarily complex without providing indisputable data.

Clinical Purposes

Simpler techniques can be used to estimate GFR for clinical purposes. When interpreted with caution, the serum creatinine concentrations can provide crude but valid information on the neonate's renal function. The transient "physiologic" increase in plasma concentrations occurring during the first days of very premature infants should be taken into account when interpreting such concentrations. The data published by Miall et al[27] and Gallini et al[26] should be used as reference values for creatinine levels in VLBW infants. In doing so, sequential measurements of the plasma concentration of creatinine can provide useful information on the putative presence of renal insufficiency.

When a rough estimate of eC_{creat} is needed, the Schwartz formula adapted for neonates[39] can be used. The formula is simple and only requires measurement of the neonate's plasma creatinine and body length. The formula has indeed been shown to provide useful data on the level of GFR. The value of 0.33 ± 0.01 for constant k (when creatinine is expressed in mg%, and 29 when it is expressed in μmol/L) will, of course, only be valid if the reference values for creatinine are the same in the laboratory where creatinine is tested and in the laboratory where the value of factor k has been calculated.[40] Ideally, each laboratory should define its own value for constant k in a selected group of patients.

The use of more sophisticated techniques for clinical purpose is not justified. Such is the case for the single-injection technique of inulin or iothalamate and for the plasma cystatin C concentration. The information they give is not accurate enough to justify their complexity. They do not provide information that cannot be obtained by the simple Schwartz formula.

Conditions and Factors That Impair Glomerular Filtration Rate

In human neonates, the major risk factors for developing acute renal insufficiency are severe respiratory disorders and perinatal exposure to PGs synthase inhibitors.[59-62]

Perinatal Asphyxia

Perinatal asphyxia is defined as a condition leading to progressive hypoxemia, hypercapnia, and metabolic acidosis with multiorgan failure, including the kidney. The pathogenesis of the hypoxia-induced vasomotor nephropathy has been studied in newborn rabbits and lambs. In the rabbit model, isolated hypoxemia induces intense renal vasoconstriction with a consequent decrease in GFR and in the filtration fraction (FF) and to a lesser extent in RBF. The observed decrease in FF suggests efferent arteriolar vasodilation, presumably as a consequence of intrarenal activation of adenosine,[63] an endogenous vasoactive agent known to vasodilate the efferent arteriole and to decrease the intraglomerular pressure. The hypothesis that adenosine plays a key role in mediating the hypoxemic renal vasoconstriction was supported by the fact that theophylline, a nonspecific antagonist of adenosine cell surface receptors, prevented the decrease in GFR induced by hypoxemia in newborn rabbits.[64] Such an effect was not observed when enprofylline, a xanthine devoid of adenosine antagonistic properties, was administered instead of theophylline.[64] Clinical studies using prophylactic theophylline in high-risk asphyxiated neonates seem to confirm the putative beneficial effect of theophylline in protecting GFR (see Theophylline below).

Nonsteroidal Antiinflammatory Agents

Exposure to PGs synthesis inhibitors during fetal development can lead to severe renal dysgenesis. Increased activity of the vasodilator PGs present during development is necessary to protect the function of immature kidneys. By blunting the effect of vasodilator PGs on the afferent arteriole, PGs synthesis inhibitors can impair GFR in both fetuses and neonates. Indomethacin is sometimes used in pregnant women with polyhydramnios to reduce fetal urine output and consequently the production of amniotic fluid.[65] It should be realized that this "obstetric" benefit is achieved by producing a state of renal insufficiency in the fetus. Decreased GFR has been demonstrated in neonates whose mothers had been administered indomethacin shortly before birth[66] as well as in neonates administered indomethacin for the closure of PDA.[67] This deleterious effect is usually transient, with renal function normalizing within 30 days,[68] but may have deleterious consequences for the elimination of drugs such as vancomycin, aminoglycosides, and digoxin, which are excreted mainly by glomerular filtration.

Ibuprofen, a COX nonselective inhibitor like indomethacin, has been claimed to be safer than the latter for newborn kidneys.[69] The efficacy and renal side effects of ibuprofen and indomethacin have been compared in two recent meta-analyses.[70,71] Although the efficacy of the two drugs in closing the PDA was similar, ibuprofen appeared to have fewer renal side effects than indomethacin. Ibuprofen-treated neonates presented with higher urine output (+0.74 mL/kg/min) and a lower increase of serum creatinine concentration (+0.44 ± 0.10 μmol/L). In contrast, in a recent well-controlled clinical study, the prophylactic administration of either acetylsalicylic acid (4×11 mg/kg per day for 2 days) or ibuprofen (10 mg/kg and 5 mg/kg at 24 h and 48 h, respectively) was associated with similar decreases in the clearance of amikacin administered concomitantly[72,73] (Fig. 8-10). Amikacin is eliminated almost exclusively by glomerular filtration, so that a decrease in its clearance indicates a decrease in GFR. This observation casts doubt on the renal innocuousness of ibuprofen. This doubt is supported by experimental studies failing to demonstrate a difference between various nonsteroidal antiinflammatory drugs, including the nonspecific COX inhibitors aspirin, indomethacin, and ibuprofen. All agents acutely decreased GFR and RBF when administered to newborn rabbits.[74,75]

Differences in the renal side effects of indomethacin and ibuprofen, if they do exist, may depend on the ratio of their respective activities on the two COX isoenzymes COX-1 and COX-2, with indomethacin inhibiting COX-1 more than COX-2. This hypothesis does not fit well, however, with the observation made in newborn rabbits that the preferential COX-2 inhibitor nimesulide induced the same renal vasoconstriction as the nonselective inhibitors.[76] If real, the potential advantage of using ibuprofen may have to be counterbalanced by a slight increase in the occurrence of chronic lung disease at 28 days of age.[71] The warning that COX-2 selective inhibitors are also unsafe for human immature kidneys is supported by the occurrence of severe renal failure in several neonates born from mothers treated by nimesulide during pregnancy.[77,78]

Angiotensin-Converting Enzyme Inhibitors and Angiotensin II Receptor Antagonists

Angiotensin-converting enzyme (ACE) inhibitors and ATII receptor antagonists (ARAs) are potent hypotensive agents that act by interfering with the formation or the action of ATII. When administered to mothers with hypertension early in

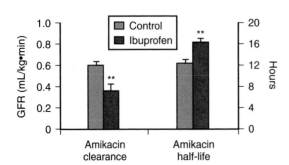

Figure 8-10 Effect of prophylactic ibuprofen on the pharmacokinetics of amikacin. The decrease in amikacin clearance and the increase in amikacin half-life reflect the decrease in glomerular filtration rate (GFR) induced by ibuprofen. (Modified from Allegaert K, Cossey V, Langhendries JP, et al. Effects of co-administration of ibuprofen-lysine on the pharmacokinetics of amikacin in preterm infants during the first days of life. *Biol Neonate.* 2004;86:207.)

pregnancy, they can induce renal dysgenesis.[79] When administered later in pregnancy or to a neonate after birth, these agents can induce neonatal renal failure.[80-82] Renal abnormalities after brief intrauterine exposure to enalapril during late gestation have been detected in an adolescent girl.[83] In high-risk hypertensive neonates with bronchopulmonary dysplasia, whose renin-angiotensin system is overstimulated beyond the neonatal period, the administration of captopril has resulted in dramatic decreases in blood pressure and episodes of prolonged oliguria and seizures.[84] ACE inhibitors and ARAs must not be administered to pregnant mothers and should be administered with great caution to sick neonates.

Prevention of Oliguric States Caused by Low Glomerular Filtration Rate

Furosemide in Oliguric Neonates

Loop diuretics (furosemide, bumetanide) are commonly used to increase urine output in oliguric neonates, with the hope of improving GFR. This hope is based on the fact that furosemide stimulates the production of vasodilator PGs. When a diuretic response actually occurs following the administration of loop diuretics, it may give the illusory impression that GFR has been improved by the diuretic agent. This is evidently rarely the case, since increased urine output usually induces hypovolemia with consequent vasoconstriction of the kidney and depression of GFR.

Loop diuretics are discussed in Chapter 14.

Dopaminergic Agents (Dopamine, Dopexamine) in Oliguric Neonates

Low doses of dopamine, the so-called "renal" doses (0.5–2.5 µg/kg/min) have been widely used in the hope that its selective actions on DA_1 dopaminergic receptors in the vascular bed would induce renal vasodilation and improve GFR in newborn infants. In initial clinical observations, increases in urine output, sodium excretion, and eC_{creat} have been described after the administration of renal doses of dopamine to normotensive oliguric neonates[85] or to oliguric indomethacin-treated neonates treated.[86] These beneficial effects of low-dose dopamine on GFR have, however, not been confirmed by a critical review of neonatal clinical studies[87] or by the meta-analysis of randomized trials, either in infants[88] or in adults.[89,90]

Theophylline

Intrarenal adenosine is a physiologic regulator of GFR acting on the glomerular arteriolar tone.[91] When overstimulated, as for instance in hypoxemic states, adenosine dilates the efferent arteriole, thus decreasing the effective filtration pressure and GFR. Low-dose theophylline (0.5–1 mg/kg), a xanthine derivative with strong adenosine antagonistic properties, has been shown to prevent the hypoxemia-induced vasoconstriction in both newborn and adult rabbits.[62] It probably does so by blunting the efferent arteriolar adenosine-mediated vasodilation induced by hypoxia. A marked improvement in both urinary water excretion and GFR after theophylline administration was first observed in high-risk neonates with oliguric renal insufficiency (Fig. 8.11).[92] Well-controlled studies in severely asphyxiated term-neonates have shown that a single dose of theophylline (5 or 8 mg/kg) given in the first hours of life significantly improved renal function and eC_{creat}[93-96] without affecting the central nervous system. An improvement in urine output and eC_{creat} has also been observed in a controlled study in preterm neonates with respiratory distress syndrome (RDS) given low-dose theophylline (1 mg/kg) for 3 days.[97] Interestingly enough, in the neonatal rabbit model, the specific adenosine A_1 receptor antagonist DPCPX does not offer the same protection as theophylline during hypoxemic stress.[98]

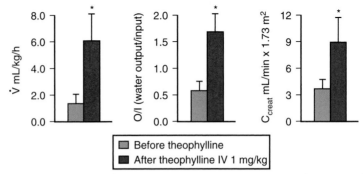

Figure 8-11   Changes in urine flow rate (V), water input/output ratio, and creatinine clearance (C_{creat}) after theophylline administration in high-risk neonates with compromised renal function. IV, intravenous. (Modified from Huet F, Semama D, Grimaldi M, et al. Effects of theophylline on renal insufficiency in neonates with respiratory distress syndrome. *Intensive Care Med.* 1995;21:511.)

Although the use of the nonspecific adenosine antagonist theophylline appears to offer significant protection for the stressed kidney, additional studies are required before recommending the routine use of theophylline for preventive or curative purposes in neonates with perinatal asphyxia or RDS.

References

1. Guignard JP, John EG. Renal function in the tiny, premature infant. *Clin Perinatol.* 1986;13:377.
2. Turner AJ, Brown RD, Carlström A, et al. Mechanisms of neonatal increase in glomerular filtration rate. *Am J Physiol Regul Integr Comp Physiol.* 2008;295:916.
3. Arendshorst WJ, Brännström K, Ruan X. Actions of angiotensin II on the renal microvasculature. *J Am Soc Nephrol.* 1999;10:S149.
4. Guignard JP, Gouyon JB, John E. Vasoactive factors in the immature kidney. *Pediatr Nephrol.* 1991;5:443.
5. Morris JL, Rosen DA, Rosen KR. Nonsteroidal anti-inflammatory agents in neonates. *Paediatr Drug.* 2003;5:385.
6. Hao CM, Breyer MD. Physiological regulation of prostaglandins in the kidney. *Ann Rev Physiol.* 2008;70:357.
7. Gomez RA, Pupilli C, Everett AD. Molecular and cellular aspects of renin during kidney ontogeny. *Pediatr Nephrol.* 1991;5:80.
8. Madsden K, Marcussen N, Pedersen M, et al. Angiotensin II promotes development of the renal microcirculation through its AT1 receptors. *J Am Soc Nephrol.* 2010;21:448.
9. Gubler MC, Antignac C. Renin-angiotensin system in kidney development: renal tubular dysgenesis. *Kidney Int.* 2010;77:400.
10. Norwood VF, Craig MR, Harris JM, et al. Differential expression of angiotensin II receptors during early renal morphogenesis. *Am J Physiol.* 1997;272:R662.
11. Tufro-McReddie A, Harrison JK, Everett AD, et al. Ontogeny of type 1 angiotensin II receptor gene expression in the rat. *J Clin Invest.* 1993;91:530.
12. Tufro-McReddie A, Romano LM, Harris JM, et al. Angiotensin II regulates nephrogenesis and renal vascular development. *Am J Physiol.* 1995;269:F110.
13. Prévot A, Mosig D, Guignard JP. The effects of losartan on renal function in the newborn rabbit. *Pediatr Res.* 2002;51:728.
14. Khan KN, Paulson SK, Verburg KM, et al. Pharmacology of cyclooxygenase-2 inhibition in the kidney. *Kidney Int.* 2002;61:1210.
15. Kömoff M, Wang JL, Cheng HF, et al. Cyclooxygenase-2-selective inhibitors impair glomerulogenesis and renal cortical development. *Kidney Int.* 2000;57:14.
16. Norwood VF, Morham SG, Smithies O. Postnatal development and progression of renal dysplasia in cyclooxygenase-2 null-mice. *Kidney Int.* 2000;58:2291.
17. Coulthard MG, Ruddock V. Validation of inulin as a marker for glomerular filtration in preterm babies. *Kidney Int.* 1983;23:407.
18. Myers GL, Miller WG, Coresh J, et al. Recommendations for improving serum creatinine measurement: a report from the Laboratory Working Group of the National Kidney Disease Education Program. *Clin Chem.* 2006;52:169.
19. Boer DP, de Rijke YB, Hop WC, et al. Reference values for serum creatinine in children younger than 1 year of age. *Pediatr Nephrol.* 2010;25:2010.
20. Stokes P, O'Connor G. Development of a liquid chromatography-mass spectrometry method for high-accuracy determination of creatinine in serum. *J Chromatogr B Analyt Technol Biomed Life Sci.* 2003;794:125.

21. Matos P, Duarte-Silva M, Drukker A, Guignard JP. Creatinine reabsorption by the newborn rabbit kidney. *Pediatr Res.* 1998;44:639.
22. Guignard JP, Drukker A. Why do newborn infants have a high plasma creatinine? *Pediatrics.* 1999;103:e49.
23. Lindblad HG, Berg HB. Comparative evaluation of iohexol and inulin clearance for glomerular filtration rate determinations. *Acta Paediatr.* 1994;83:418.
24. Berg UB, Bäck R, Celsi G, et al. Comparison of plasma clearance of iohexol and urinary clearance of inuline for measurement of GFR in children. *Am J Kidney Dis.* 2011;57:55.
25. Odlind B, Hallgren R, Sohtell M, et al. Is 125I iothalamate an ideal marker for glomerular filtration? *Kidney Int.* 1985;27:9.
26. Gallini F, Maggio L, Romagnoli C, et al. Progression of renal function in preterm neonates with gestational age ≤32 weeks. *Pediatr Nephrol.* 2000;15:119.
27. Miall LS, Henderson MJ, Turner AJ, et al. Plasma creatinine rises dramatically in the first 48 hours of life in preterm infants. *Pediatrics.* 1999;6:104.
28. Bueva A, Guignard JP. Renal function in preterm neonates. *Pediatr Res.* 1994;36:572.
29. Thayyil S, Sheik S, Kempley ST, et al. A gestation- and postnatal age- based reference chart for assessing renal function in extremely premature infants. *J Perinatol.* 2008;28:226.
30. Iacobelli S, Bonsante F, Ferdinus C, et al. Factors affecting postnatal changes in serum creatinine in preterm infants with gestational <32 weeks. *J Perinatol.* 2009;29:232.
31. Stonestreet BS, Bell EF, Oh W. Validity of endogenous creatinine clearance in low birthweight infants. *Pediatr Res.* 1979;13:1002.
32. Coulthard MG, Hey EN, Ruddock V. Creatinine and urea clearances compared to inulin clearance in preterm and mature babies. *Early Hum Dev.* 1985;11:11.
33. Vieux R, Hascoet JM, Merdariu D, et al. Glomerular filtration rate reference values in very premature infants. *Pediatrics.* 2010;125:e1186.
34. Cole BR, Giangiacomo J, Ingelfinger JR, et al. Measurement of renal function without urine collection. A critical evaluation of the constant-infusion technique for determination of inulin and para-aminohippurate. *N Engl J Med.* 1972;287:1109.
35. vd Heijden AJ, Grose WF, Ambagtsheer JJ, et al. Glomerular filtration rate in the preterm infant: the relation to gestational and postnatal age. *Eur J Pediatr.* 1988;148:24.
36. Coulthard MG. Comparison of methods of measuring renal function in preterm babies using inulin. *J Pediatr.* 1983;102:923.
37. Fawer CL, Torrado A, Guignard JP. Maturation of renal function in full-term and premature neonates. *Helv Paediatr Acta.* 1979;34:11.
38. Counahan R, Chantler C, Ghazali S, et al. Estimation of glomerular filtration rate from plasma creatinine concentration in children. *Arch Dis Child.* 1976;51:875.
39. Schwartz GJ, Brion LP, Spitzer A. The use of plasma creatinine concentration for estimating glomerular filtration rate in infants, children, and adolescents. *Pediatr Clin North Am.* 1987;34:571.
40. Haenggi MH, Pelet J, Guignard JP. Estimation of glomerular filtration rate by the formula GFR = K × T/Pc. *Arch Pediatr.* 1999;6:165.
41. Olafsson I. The human cystatin C gene promotor: functional analysis and identification of heterogeneous mRNA. *Scand J Clin Lab Invest.* 1995;55:597.
42. Tenstad O, Roald AB, Grubb A. Renal handling of radiolabelled human cystatin C in the rat. *Scand J Clin Lab Invest.* 1996;56:409.
43. Erlandsen EJ, Randers E, Kristensen JH. Evaluation of the N Latex Cystatin C assay on the Dade Behring Nephelometer II system. *Scand J Clin Lab Invest.* 1999;59:1.
44. Finney H, Newman DJ, Thakkar H, et al. Reference ranges for plasma cystatin C and creatinine measurements in premature infants, neonates, and older children. *Arch Dis Child.* 2000;82:71.
45. Randers E, Krue S, Erlandsen EJ, et al. Reference interval for serum cystatin C in children. *Clinical Chemistry.* 1999;45:1856.
46. Stickle D, Cole B, Hock K, et al. Correlation of plasma concentrations of cystatin C and creatinine to inulin clearance in a pediatric population. *Clin Chem.* 1998;44:1334.
47. Bökenkamp A, Domanetzki M, Zinck R, et al. Reference values for cystatin C serum concentrations in children. *Pediatr Nephrol.* 1998;12:125.
48. Knight EL, Verhave JC, Spiegelman D, et al. Factors influencing serum cystatin C levels other than renal function and the impact on renal function measurement. *Kidney Int.* 2004;65:777.
49. Akbari A, Lepage N, Keely E, et al. Cystatin-C and beta trace protein as markers of renal function in pregnancy. *BJOG.* 2005;112:575.
50. Podraacka L, Feber J, Lepage N, et al. Intra-individual variation of cystatin C and creatinine in pediatric solid organ transplant recipients. *Pediatr Transplant.* 2005;9:28.
51. Mendiluce A, Bustamante J, Martin D, et al. Cystatin C as a marker of renal function in kidney transplant patients. *Transplant Proc.* 2005;37:3844.
52. Bökenkamp A, van Wijk JAE, Lentze MJ, et al. Effects of corticosteroid therapy on serum cystatin C and beta 2-microglobulin concentrations. *Clin Chem.* 2002;48:1123.
53. Wulkan R, den Hollander J, Berghout A. Cystatin C unsuited to use as a marker of kidney function in the intensive care unit. *Crit Care.* 2005;9:531.
54. Martini S, Prévot A, Mosig D, Guignard JP. Glomerular filtration rate: measure creatinine and height rather than cystatin C! *Acta Paediatr.* 2003;92:1052.
55. Cataldi L, Mussap M, Bertelli N, et al. Cystatin C in healthy women at term pregnancy and in their infant newborns: relationship between maternal and neonatal serum levels and reference values. *Am J Perinatol.* 1999;16:287.

56. Harmoinen A, Ylinen E, Ala-Houhala M, et al. Reference intervals for cystatin C in pre-and full-term infants and children. *Pediatr Nephrol.* 2000;15:105.
57. Armangil D, Yurka M, Canpolat FE, et al. Determination of reference values for plasma cystatin C and comparison with creatinine in premature infants. *Pediatr Nephrol.* 2008;23:2081.
58. Filler G, Bökenkamp A, Hofmann W, et al. Cystatin C as a marker of GFR: history, indications, and future research. *Clin Biochem.* 2005;38:1.
59. Toth-Heynh P, Drukker A, Guignard JP. The stressed neonatal kidney: from pathophysiology to clinical management of neonatal vasomotor nephropathy. *Pediatr Nephrol.* 2000;14:227.
60. Gouyon JB, Guignard JP. Management of acute renal failure in newborns. *Pediatr Nephrol.* 2000;14:1037.
61. Choker G, Gouyon JB. Diagnosis of acute renal failure in very preterm infants. *Biol Neonate.* 2004;86:212.
62. Cataldi L, Leone R, Moretti U, et al. Potential risk factors for the development of acute renal failure in preterm newborn infants: a case-control study. *Arch Dis Child Fetal Neonatal Ed.* 2005;90:F514.
63. Gouyon JB, Guignard JP. Theophylline prevents the hypoxemia-induced renal hemodynamic changes in rabbits. *Kidney Int.* 1988;33:1078.
64. Gouyon JB, Arnaud M, Guignard JP. Renal effects of low-dose aminophylline and enprofylline in newborn rabbits. *Life Sci.* 1988;42:1271.
65. Abhyankar S, Salvi VS. Indomethacin therapy in hydrammios. *J Postgrad Med.* 2000;46:176.
66. vd Heijden AJ, Provoost AP, Nauta J, et al. Renal function impairment in preterm neonates related to intrauterine indomethacin exposure. *Pediatr Res.* 1988;24:644.
67. Catterton Z, Sellers B, Gray B. Inulin clearance in the premature infant receiving indomethacin. *J Pedriatr.* 1980;96:737.
68. Akima S, Kent A, Reynolds GJ, et al. Indomethacin and renal impairment in neonates. *Pediatr Nephrol.* 2004;19:490.
69. Van Overmeire B, Smets K, Lecoutere D, et al. A comparison of ibuprofen and indomethacin for closure of patent ductus arteriosus. *N Engl J Med.* 2000;343:674.
70. Thomas RL, Parker GC, Van Overmeire B, et al. A meta-analysis of ibuprofen versus indomethacin for closure of patent ductus arteriosus. *Eur J Pediatr.* 2005;164:135.
71. Ohlsson A, Walia R, Schah S. Ibuprofen for the treatment of patent ductus arteriosus in preterm and/or low birth weight infants. *Cochrane Database Syst Rev.* 2003;2:CD003481.
72. Allegaert K, Cossey V, Langhendries JP, et al. Effects of co-administration of ibuprofen-lysine on the pharmacokinetics of amikacin in preterm infants during the first days of life. *Biol Neonate.* 2004;86:207.
73. Allegaert K, Vanhole C, de Hoon J, et al. Nonselective cyclo-oxygenase inhibitors and glomerular filtration rate in preterm neonates. *Pediatr Nephrol.* 2005;20:1557.
74. Guignard JP. The adverse renal effects of prostaglandin-synthesis inhibitors in the newborn rabbit. *Semin Perinatol.* 2002;26:398.
75. Chamaa NS, Mosig D, Drukker A, et al. The renal hemodynamic effects of ibuprofen in the newborn rabbit. *Pediatr Res.* 2000;48:600.
76. Prevot A, Mosig D, Martini S, et al. Nimesulide, a cyclooxygenase-2 preferential inhibitor, impairs renal function in the newborn rabbit. *Pediatr Res.* 2004;55:254.
77. Peruzzi L, Gianoglio B, Porcellini M, et al. Neonatal end-stage renal failure associated with maternal ingestion of cyclo-oxygenase type I selective inhibitor nimesulide as tocolytic. *Lancet.* 1999;354:9190.
78. Ali US, Khubchandani S, Andankar P, et al. Renal tubular dysgenesis associated with in utero exposure to nimesulide. *Pediatr Nephrol.* 2006;21:274.
79. Cunniff C, Jones KL, Phillipson J, et al. Oligohydramnios sequence and renal tubular malformation associated with maternal enalapril use. *Am J Obstet Gynecol.* 1990;162:187.
80. Guignard JP, Burgener F, Calame A. Persistent anuria in a neonate: a side effect of captopril? *Int J Pediatr Nephrol.* 1981;2:133.
81. Vendemmia M, Garcia-Méric P, Rizzoti A, et al. Fetal and neonatal consequences of antenatal exposure to type 1 angiotensin II receptor-antagonists. *J Matern Fetal Neonatal Med.* 2005;18:137.
82. Gersak K, Cvijic M, Cerar LK. Angiotensin II receptor blockers in pregnancy: a report of five cases. *Reprod Toxicol.* 2009;28:109.
83. Guron G, Mölne J, Swerkersson S, et al. A 14-year-old girl with renal abnormalities after brief intrauterine exposure to enalapril during late gestation. *Nephrol Dial Transplant.* 2006;21:522.
84. Tack ED, Perlman JM. Renal failure in sick hypertensive premature infants receiving captopril therapy. *J Pediatr.* 1988;112:805.
85. Lynch SK, Lemley KV, Polak MJ. The effect of dopamine on glomerular filtration rate in normotensive, oliguric premature neonates. *Pediatr Nephrol.* 2003;18:649.
86. Seri I, Abbasi S, Wood DC, et al. Regional hemodynamic effects of dopamine in the indomethacin-treated preterm infant. *J Perinatol.* 2002;22:300.
87. Prins I, Plötz FB Cuno SPM, et al. Low-dose dopamine in neonatal and pediatric intensive care: a systematic review. *Intensive Care Med.* 2001;27:206.
88. Barrington K, Brion LP. Dopamine versus no treatment to prevent renal dysfunction in indomethacin-treated preterm newborn infants. *Cochrane Database Syst Rev* 2002;3:CD003213.
89. Lauschke A, Teichgraber UK, Frei U, Eckhardt KU. "Low-dose" dopamine worsens renal perfusion in patients with acute renal failure. *Kidney Int.* 2004;65:1416.
90. Kellum JA, Decker J. Use of dopamine in acute failure: a meta-analysis. *Crit Care Med.* 2001;29(8):1526-1531.
91. Gouyon JB, Guignard JP. Adenosine in the immature kidney. *Dev Pharmacol Ther.* 1989;13:113.

92. Huet F, Semama D, Grimaldi M, et al. Effects of theophylline on renal insufficiency in neonates with respiratory distress syndrome. *Intensive Care Med.* 1995;21:511.

93. Jenik AG, Ceriani Cernadas JM, Gorenstein A, et al. A randomized, double blind, placebo-controlled trial of the effects of prophylactic theophylline on renal function in term neonates with perinatal asphyxia. *Pediatrics.* 2000;105(4):e45.

94. Bakr AF. Prophylactic theophylline to prevent renal dysfunction in newborns exposed to perinatal asphyxia—a study in a developing country. *Pediatr Nephrol.* 2005;20:1249.

95. Bhat MA, Shah ZA, Makhdoomi MS, Mufti MH. Theophylline for renal function in term neonates with perinatal asphyxia: a randomized, placebo-controlled trial. *J Pediatr.* 2006;149:e180-e184.

96. Eslami Z, Shajari A, Kheirandish M, et al. Theophylline for prevention of kidney dysfunction in neonates with severe asphyxia. *Iran J Kidney Dis.* 2009;3:222.

97. Cattarelli D, Spandrio M, Gasparoni A, et al. A randomized, double blind, placebo controlled trial of the effect of theophylline in prevention of vasomotor nephropathy in very preterm neonates with respiratory distress syndrome. *Arch Dis Child Fetal Neonatal Ed.* 2006;91:F80.

98. Prévot A, Mosig D, Rijtema M, et al. Renal effects of adenosine A1-receptor blockade with 8-cyclopentyl-1, 3-dipropylxanthine in hypoxemic newborn rabbits. *Pediatr Res.* 2003;54:400.

8

SECTION D

Special Problems

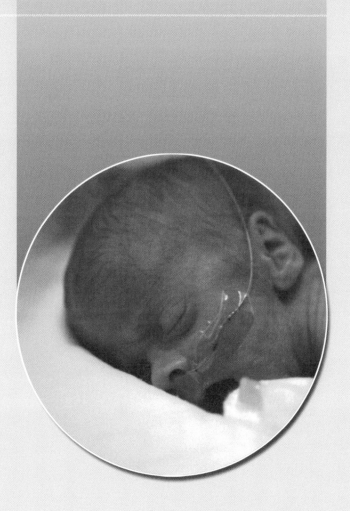

CHAPTER 9

The Developing Kidney and the Fetal Origins of Adult Cardiovascular Disease

Farid Boubred, MD, Christophe Buffat, PharmD, Daniel Vaiman, PhD, Umberto Simeoni, MD

- Developmental Origins of Health and Disease
- Developing Kidney and Long-Term Consequences
- Molecular Mechanisms Involved in the Developmental Origins of Cardiovascular Disease
- Conclusion

Since the pioneering work of David Barker and colleagues,[1] worldwide epidemiologic studies have demonstrated that low birth weight (LBW) is associated with an increased risk of death from coronary heart disease.[2-4] The link between early development and adult disease has been shown to involve arterial hypertension and metabolic disorders, such as insulin resistance and hyperlipidemia, the elements of "metabolic syndrome" or "X syndrome."[5,6] Although with less evidence, the risk of chronic kidney disease (CKD), defined by proteinuria, decreased glomerular filtration rate (GFR), and end-stage renal disease (ESRD), has been related to LBW.[7-10] The concept of the developmental origins and programming of adult disease is now widely understood because evidence of the relationship between early growth and development of disease occurring in the long term is growing.

Studies on blood pressure and early growth show that in both children and adults, there is an inverse relationship between birth weight and arterial blood pressure: blood pressure increases 1 to 3 mm Hg per birth weight reduction of 1 kg.[11] Such findings have been replicated in various animal models of intrauterine growth restriction (IUGR) in guinea pigs,[12] sheep,[13] and particularly rats.[14-16] Although evidence of the early programming of cardiovascular function and disease is provided by studies including subjects with IUGR, recent studies raised the issue of the long-term consequences of premature birth. Premature birth has been shown to be associated with elevated arterial blood pressure in adulthood independently of birth weight. Blood pressure levels are inversely related to gestational age (GA).[17-20]

The pathophysiologic and molecular mechanisms involved in the early programming of health and disease are multiple and only partially understood. It is well established that the developmental programming of arterial hypertension involves renal factors.[21-23] The kidney has been shown to be one key organ involved in the programming of hypertension in adulthood through the definitive reduction in the total number of nephrons. Reduced nephron number is a characteristic of LBW.[24-26]

The aim of this review is to summarize current knowledge on the physiologic, structural and molecular mechanisms by which the kidneys are involved in the developmental origins of arterial hypertension and to discuss the potential impact of such findings on the care and follow-up of LBW subjects and patients.

Developmental Origins of Health and Disease

The concept of the developmental programming of disease implies that a stimulus or an insult, acting during a unique, narrow window of sensitivity in the prenatal and early postnatal periods of life, induces silent physiologic alterations that translate into disease during adulthood. In this paradigm, initial adaptive responses during fetal life or early infancy conditions, such as IUGR, preterm birth, or intrauterine exposure to diabetes in pregnancy, prove to be durable and later become harmful as a mismatch between the predicted restrictive environment and the real environment develops. Adaptive responses are the expression of developmental plasticity, the process that allows a single genotype to develop into different phenotypes according to environmental influences.[27-29]

Birth Weight and Developmental Origins of Adult Cardiovascular and Renal Diseases

The early origins of adult diseases hypothesis has been developed by David Barker and colleagues[1] after they characterized a relationship between increased coronary heart disease mortality rates and decreasing birth weight in a cohort of men and women in Hertfordshire, United Kingdom whose characteristics at birth were known.[1] LBW is now recognized as a risk factor for hypertension, type 2 diabetes, and other metabolic dysfunctions. Such association has been demonstrated in various epidemiologic studies from different countries and validated with animal studies from various animal species. However, attentive analysis of the relationship between birth weight and adult diseases is U shaped. Large birth weight infants with body weight greater than 4 kg have a slight but significantly higher risk than normal BW infants to develop cardiovascular, metabolic, and probably renal diseases. Such U-shaped relationship suggest that different fetal environments may permanently alter the structure and function of various systems. Exposure to maternal diabetes during pregnancy, known to induce large birth weight infants, may be another fetal environmental factor involved in the developmental programming of adult health and disease.

Emerging evidence suggests that LBW is a risk factor of early CKD.[30] In a population-based study, it has been shown that the estimated GFR (eGFR) at adulthood is correlted with birth weight. It has been estimated that a 1-kg increase in birth weight is associated with an increase in eGFR of about 2.6 to 7 mL/min.[31-33] In a case control study, Lackland et al[34] have shown in a population from the state of South Carolina, in USA, that the odds ratio for ESRD was 1.4 (95% confidence interval [CI], 1.1–1.8) in adults with birth weight below 2.5 kg. Such result have been recently confirmed in a Norwegian study (the Medical Birth Registry and the Norwegian Renal Registry) in which patients with birth weight below the 10th percentile had a relative risk for ESRD of 1.7 (95% CI, 1.4–2.2).[10] In the Dutch famine cohort, adults exposed to maternal famine during midgestation, at a time of active nephrogenesis, had albuminuria, a sign of glomerular injury associated with nephron number reduction.[35] Finally, LBW is associated with more rapid progression of various kidney diseases such as membranous and IgA nephropathies, nephrotic syndrome, or kidney disease related to obesity and metabolic disorders.[36-38] In all of these studies, GA is mostly unknown, which raises the question of the relationship of long-term renal disease with preterm birth. Preterm birth may be a risk factor for CKD. Patients from the Dutch POPS cohort of preterm, less than 32 weeks GA, have been investigated at young adult age.[9] Renal function measurements showed that the urinary microalbumin-to-creatinine ratio and plasma creatinine levels at adulthood were inversely proportional to birth weight in this population. However, data from other studies show conflicting results.[39-41] Such discrepancies may be attributable to the eligible population, the association with IUGR, the degree of immaturity, and the age at which renal and vascular functions were evaluated (late infancy, young adulthood). The lack of very long-term follow-up prevents definitive conclusions. Data are scarce regarding renal structure. Recently, Hodgin et al[42] have reported six adults born preterm, with a mean age of 32 years, in whom renal biopsies have been done for proteinuria. Renal histology showed focal segmental glomerular sclerosis with unknown causes identified, unlike premature birth. eGFR was unaffected.

Postnatal Growth and Developmental Origins of Adult Cardiovascular and Renal Diseases

Longitudinal as well as nutritional intervention studies in LBW premature babies suggest that postnatal growth, especially accelerated weight gain, may play an important role in the late programming of cardiovascular diseases.[43-50] But the role of postnatal growth on adult chronic renal diseases is still unknown.

Infants with LBW often show accelerated rates of growth in infancy and early childhood, a phenomenon coined as catch-up growth. The critical "window" when catch-up growth contributes to higher blood pressure in adulthood is still debated. Many studies have shown that increased weight gain in early childhood (5–7 years) is independently associated with increased blood pressure levels in adulthood, but others have suggested that body mass index in pre-adolescents (11–15 years), which is predicted by early postnatal growth, contributes to cardiovascular disease in adults. Late infancy seems a key period in programming the risk of adult disease by switching from poor growth early in life to more favorable nutrition. Low weight at birth but also at the age of 1 year has been shown to be associated with higher rates of cardiovascular mortality.[2] Studies in Finland show that LBW associated with later catch-up growth after the age of 2 years is associated with increased rates of death from coronary heart disease, hypertension, and type 2 diabetes.[43] Interestingly, in this cohort, postnatal growth restriction after normal birth weight is a risk factor for hypertension and stroke.

The role of weight gain in the first months of postnatal life is a matter of considerable interest. In a nutritional intervention study, Singhal et al[49] have shown that increased weight gain during the first 2 weeks of postnatal life was associated with elevated diastolic blood pressure in adolescents born preterm. In some populations, reduced infant growth seems to confer additional cardiovascular risk that is predicted by birth weight and may independently affect blood pressure in adulthood. In a young adult population study in Hong Kong, those who were thinner and, independently, those who had gained less body mass between 6 and 18 months had higher systolic blood pressure.[50] The authors suggested that the poor infant growth may be attributable to living disadvantages and a higher burden of infectious diseases. Similar results have been observed in 11- to 12-year-old Jamaican children who were stunted in early infancy (6–24 months).[48] However, such a relationship has not been observed in other studies.[44,45]

The role of postnatal nutrition on programming later systemic hypertension and CKD has been confirmed by animal models.[51-55] Rapid neonatal catch-up growth and high caloric diet in peripubertal IUGR offspring affect long-term vascular and renal function. We and others have shown that early postnatal caloric overfeeding, obtained by reduction of litter size and limited to the suckling period, induces obesity and cardiovascular, metabolic, and renal diseases in aging adult rat offspring born with normal birth weight (Fig. 9-1). Such effects are enhanced when postnatal overfeeding occurs after IUGR.[53,54] Indeed, early postnatal overfeeding superimposed on IUGR offspring clearly allows rapid postnatal catch-up growth during the neonatal period, but accelerates the occurrence of programmed hypertension and the development of early CKD. It has been demonstrated that rapid catch-up growth after IUGR accelerates renal senescence with shortening telomere.[56] On the other hand, such maternal nutritionally programmed cardiovascular, metabolic, and renal diseases may be prevented by slow postnatal growth.[53,57] Such influence of neonatal growth on long-term diseases in rats has been observed in other species. Peripubertal nutrition and growth influence adult metabolic and vascular function as well. In 100- to 125-day-old IUGR rat offspring (obtained by a 30% reduction of global maternal diet) Vickers et al[51] showed that blood pressure, fasting insulin, and leptin levels were amplified by a hypercaloric diet applied in weaning offspring. Similar findings have been reported by other authors when IUGR offspring displayed spontaneous catch-up growth at the time of evaluation of cardiovascular or renal functions confirming the determinant role of postnatal growth.[55]

D

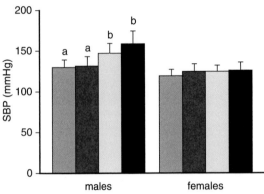

A

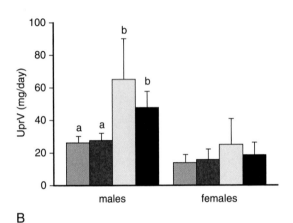

B

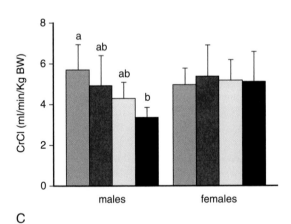

C

Figure 9-1 Early postnatal overfeeding (OF) induces long-term hypertension and early impaired renal function in intrauterine growth restricted (IUGR) male offspring. Systolic blood pressure (SBP; **A**), proteinuria (UprV; **B**), and clearance of creatinine (CrCl; **C**) in 12-month-old normal birth weight (NBW) offspring (*pink bars*), IUGR (*red bars*), NBW + OF (*light pink bars*), and IUGR + OF (*black bars*) offspring, according to gender are shown. Values are means + standard deviation; n = 8–10. Significant differences (P <.05) across groups are indicated by different letters; for example, a is different from b but not different from ab. (From Boubred F, Daniel L, Buffat C, et al. Early postnatal overfeeding induces early chronic renal dysfunction in adult male rats. *Am J Physiol Renal Physiol.* 2009;29:946.)

According to this concept, environmental factors, particularly nutrition, act early during fetal and postnatal life to program the risk for later cardiovascular and renal diseases in adulthood. Common risk factors, such as arterial hypertension, hyperlipidemia, obesity, type 2 diabetes and the components of the metabolic syndrome, and factors associated with lifestyle (e.g., high caloric nutrition, tobacco, sedentarity) are at least partly associated with environmental conditions in early life. The early programming of durable physiologic alterations and risk of disease is likely to occur at critical periods of early life during a sensitive window covering fetal life and infancy. Such critical periods allow developmental plasticity (i.e., the ability of a single genotype to produce different phenotypes) to take place.[58] The fact that an impairment of fetal growth or growth during early infancy followed by an accelerated postnatal growth may contribute to elevated blood pressure in adulthood suggests that postnatal adaptations in growth are responsible for higher levels of blood pressure later.

Biologic Mechanism of Developmental Programming of Adult Disease

The development of fetuses is complex and depends in part on maternal constraint, which includes maternal nutrition, physiology and disease, and placental functions. The thrifty phenotype hypothesis has been the principal mechanistic frame proposed to explain that an adverse fetal environment results in an adaptive response designed to protect key fetal organs and systems, such as the brain and the heart, to the detriment of others, such as the kidneys and muscles. Such an adaptive response to fetal chronic stress results in a physiologic programming that then enables the newborn to adapt and thrive under scarce environmental conditions, but also favors the development of disease when the postnatal environment is abundant instead of restricted.[59] It is speculated that the adaptive fetal response to adverse environment results in reduced muscle mass and nephron number, which is responsible for the development of insulin resistance and altered kidney functions, respectively. Such changes may promote type 2 diabetes mellitus, hypertension, and CKD. Immediate fetal and neonatal survival advantage is thus balanced by unfavorable long-term consequences. However, the thrifty phenotype theory may show its limits when taking into account that not only LBW caused by IUGR but also by preterm birth, large birth weight, and fetal exposure to various drugs and toxics are associated with long-term functional alterations. New paradigms are needed because premature birth most frequently is not associated with chronic fetal distress.

Being born small may reflect a process that involves adaptive responses. However, small size at birth may also induce responses that intervene as consequences of the process and are defective in nature. For example, LBW, whether attributable to IUGR or to preterm birth, is associated with a reduction in the constitutive nephron endowment. As far as its consequences are known, congenital nephron number reduction is not likely to reflect an adaptive response but simply an arrest in nephron development that may induce long-term renal and vascular physiologic changes of utmost importance.

Developing Kidney and Long-Term Consequences

The kidney has been identified early as a key player in the pathogenesis of developmentally programmed hypertension through the pathway of reduced congenital nephron endowment.[21,25] Low nephron number characterizes perinatal conditions such as LBW or maternal diabetes in pregnancy and is considered to be involved in the development of both increased arterial blood pressure and altered renal function on the long term in such conditions.[21,24,55]

Experimental studies and human findings provide evidence for a pathogenic link between low nephron number and systemic hypertension and renal function deterioration. In animals as well as in humans, a reduction in nephron number leads to the development of hypertension and progressive renal failure. It has been shown that in some individuals born with a solitary kidney or with severe degrees of oligomeganephronia, hypertension and renal disease develop.[60] Interestingly, in a recent autopsy study, patients with essential hypertension had a significantly lower nephron number and higher glomerular volume than sex and age-matched normotensive patients.[26] Such findings have been reproduced in recent experimental studies of reduced nephron mass. Reduction of nephron mass by nephrectomy during nephrogenesis is associated with arterial hypertension and alteration of GFR in adulthood.[61,62]

Nephrogenesis and Environment

Nephrogenesis is achieved prenatally in the human, most nephrons being formed between 28 and 34 weeks of gestation. This process results at around 34 to 36 weeks of gestation in a finite nephron number endowment acquired by each individual for life; it is generally admitted that no additional nephrons are formed after the end of nephrogenesis. The average nephron number per kidney is ±750,000 with a wide interindividual range (250,000–1,500,000).[26,63] The glomerular volume is inversely correlated to the nephron number. Such variability may be related to fetal environment, maternal constraint, and genetic factors. In rats, it has been demonstrated that nephron number can be "programmed" through an intergenerational process. Reduced nephron number associated with IUGR persists in the second generation without any subsequent modification of fetal environment and birth weight.[64]

Birth weight is the principal factor associated with nephron number endowment, but is certainly not the only predicting factor. It has been estimated that the number of nephrons per kidney increases by an average of 250,000 per kilogram increase in birth weight.[63] And for a given birth weight, the nephron number can vary with a factor of 2 to 3. Studies on necropsies of human fetuses and newborns and experimental studies in various animal species have shown that the total number of nephrons is proportional to birth weight and is reduced by approximately 30% to 40% when IUGR is present.[24,65] Animal models in various species have shown that IUGR (maternal low protein diet or global diet restriction, uterine arteries ligation), maternal gestational administration of glucocorticoids or other drugs (aminosides, ampicillin), maternal vitamin A and iron deficiency, fetal exposure to alcohol, and maternal gestational diabetes lead to a reduced nephron number.[24]

However, little is known regarding glomerulogenesis in preterm infants. It has been postulated that nephrogenesis may be impaired when part of it has to develop "ex utero," contributing to the susceptibility of preterm infants to hypertension in adulthood. Ultrasound measurement of kidney size during postnatal growth in humans has shown that even at the age of 8 years, kidney size is lower in children who were born preterm.[66,67] In an autopsy study of 56 extremely premature infants, whose birth weights were, in the majority, appropriate for GA, Rodriguez et al[68] found that nephrogenesis was considerably decreased compared with term control participants and that radial glomerular count number correlated with GA. However, markers of active glomerulogenesis were absent in extremely preterm infants who had survived for a longer time. Signs of impaired nephrogenesis were furthermore accentuated in patients with renal failure. Various postnatal factors, including nephrotoxic drugs, undernutrition, and stress (infection, oxidative stress), may impair extrauterine nephrogenesis.[55]

Such findings emphasize that LBW is one, but certainly not the only, predictor of nephron endowment and suggest that the relationship between reduced nephron endowment and the risk of developing adult-onset disease is still valid among normal birth weight individuals and depends partly on the fetal environment.

Recent experimental evidence suggests that fetal environment leads to subtle renal changes. It has been shown that fetal environment may program sensibility to the renin–angiotensin system (RAS), higher activity of the renal nerve system, and tubular sodium handling, but the expression of the principal components of the RAS is extinguished in the developing kidneys of IUGR rat pups and overexpression of the renal RAS proteins and mRNAs can be observed as soon as at 4 weeks in a similar model.[69,70] Increased expression of the renal tubular Na^+, K^+, $2Cl^-$ co-transporter (NKCC2) and loss of the Na^+, K^+, ATPase $\alpha 1$ subunit from the inner medulla have been evidenced in low-protein maternal rat offspring, suggesting that altered renal sodium handling is also programmed prenatally.[71] Such changes result in sodium sensitivity of fetal programmed hypertension in this model. Interestingly, salt sensitivity of arterial blood pressure has been documented in LBW children.[72] The importance of the fetal programming of tubular functions and of salt-sensitive hypertension has been also evidenced in the offspring exposed to maternal diabetes.[73] It is of note that such mechanisms have been described in young adult IUGR animals with reduced endowment of nephron.

Long-Term Vascular and Renal Disease: Role of Nephron Number

As postulated by Brenner and coworkers,[25] nephron deficit as a result of IUGR leads to reduced filtration surface area and glomerular single-nephron hyperfiltration, which is responsible over a long time for glomerular injury, long-term proteinuria, glomerulosclerosis, progressive deterioration of renal function, and finally arterial hypertension (Fig. 9-2). Reduced filtration surface area results in an initial salt retention, increased volume stroke, and resetting in pressure-natriuresis mechanisms that contribute to a slight increase in blood pressure. Compensatory glomerular hemodynamic changes associated with increased single-nephron GFR (SNGFR) initiate and perpetuate injury after inborn nephron deficit. In response to reduced nephron number, remaining nephrons undergo an adaptation in structure and function, including nephron hypertrophy (an increase in glomerular volume) and increases in SNGFR to meet excretory demands. Such compensatory adaptation, which at first appears beneficial, may have a harmful long-term effect. In general, hypertension occurs because of reduced GFR and the inability of the kidney to maintain sodium and water balance at a normal blood pressure. Recent experimental studies have shown that other mechanisms may be involved in such adaptive changes. Both renal expression of and responsiveness to the RAS are upregulated during early adulthood in IUGR rats, further increasing the systemic blood pressure needed to maintain sodium and water balance.[74] Experimental and clinical data confirm the role of nephron number on the pathophysiology of hypertension and CKD. In sheep and rodents, uninephrectomy during active nephrogenesis leads to elevated blood pressure, impaired renal function and renal damage, and elevated peripheral vascular resistance during adulthood, which enhance with age.[61,62] Rats genetically programmed to develop hypertension (SHR strain) had a reduced nephron number and a particular susceptibility to glomerular sclerosis.[75] In humans, patients with congenital renal agenesia develop hypertension and CKD during adulthood and uninephrectomized adults, while children, are prone to develop hypertension and early CKD compared with the general population.[76] Recently, in an autopsy case control study, Keller et al[26] demonstrated that young adults with a history of hypertension had an average 50% decrease in nephron number compared with age-match controlled adults. Aside from reduced nephron endowment, hypertension can be caused by an alteration in tubular handling of sodium with increased sodium reabsorption, overactivity of the sympathetic nerve to the kidney, and oxidative stress.

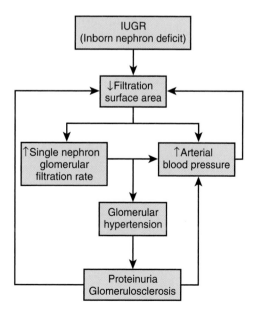

Figure 9-2 Pathogenesis of elevated blood pressure and reduced glomerular function associated with decreased birth weight and nephron endowment. (After Brenner BM, Garcia DL, Anderson S. Glomeruli and blood pressure. Less of one, more the other? *Am J Hypertens.* 1988;1:335-347.)

Reduction of nephron endowment is not systematically associated with long-term hypertension, especially when the reduction is moderate. In humans, Hughson et al[77] did not find a relationship between a moderate nephron number reduction and hypertension. In contrast with congenital renal agenesis, adult renal transplant donors have a lower risk of hypertension and renal disease.[78] In animal models, renal mass reduction does not lead in all cases to hypertension and renal disease in adulthood.[79] Similar findings have been observed in adult offspring exposed prenatally to maternal protein diet restriction and to maternal administration of glucocorticoids.[55]

All of these findings suggest that a moderate reduction of nephron number alone is not sufficient to mediate long-term "fetal-programmed" cardiovascular and renal diseases. Nephron number and postnatal environment have to be taken into account. The risk of hypertension may be correlated to the severity of nephron deficit: the lower the nephron number, the higher the blood pressure.[25]

Developing Kidney, Postnatal Factors, and Long-Term Vascular and Renal Diseases

When nephron number is moderately reduced, hypertension and CKD may develop with additional factors such as rapid postnatal catch-up growth, and increase in sodium or protein intakes[26,53,55,80,81]. Postnatal factors may play a determinant role, since nephron number varies widely for a given birth weight and is moderately decreased in IUGR offspring as compared with congenital renal hypoplasia.

Postnatal factors, especially postnatal growth and/or nutrition, may act early in infancy and induce/enhance the adaptive single nephron glomerular hyperfiltration and renal hypertrophy. Such factors may thus enhance the vulnerability of a kidney with a deficit in the number of nephrons. The effects on renal function of accelerated weight gain, favored by high caloric and protein intakes, are not completely known, but they may contribute to an alteration in renal function in adulthood. We have shown in IUGR rat offspring that early postnatal overfeeding induces rapid catch-up growth in young adult offspring, sustained proteinuria and long term CKD (glomerular sclerosis and impaired glomerular filtration function). It has been known for a long time that a high protein intake in rats is associated with an adaptive, elevated GFR and renal hypertrophy, which result over a long time in glomerular damage, especially when renal mass is reduced. Similar renal effects have been observed in adult IUGR rat offspring when exposed neonatally to a high protein diet. In the same way, *increased* sodium intakes enhance renal injury through oxidative mechanism in IUGR adult rat offspring.[82] The role of early growth/nutrition in humans has to be evaluated. Increases in protein and caloric diet are proposed for LBW infants to enhance growth, to avoid postnatal growth restriction, with the aim to promote long term neurocognitive functions.

As demonstrated in epidemiologic studies, lifestyle, tobacco, alcohol, obesity, diabetes, hypercholesterolemia, and hypertension are known risk factors for cardiovascular and renal diseases. Such postnatal factors affect vascular and renal structure and function through different pathways and may enhance the early programming of adult disease. Vascular changes (endothelial dysfunction and microvascular hypertrophy), hormonal dysregulation (hyperletinemia, up regulation of the renin angiotensin system and the hypothalamopituitary axis), and increase in SNGFR have been associated with diabetes, obesity, or hypertension. It is of note that parts of such postnatal factors are "programmed" early in development. Finally, a vicious circle takes place with initiation of glomerular damage during early development and worsening of such damages through additional deleterious effects of hypertension and metabolic diseases programmed themselves prenatally and postnatally: the kidney is both the underlying pathophysiologic mechanism and the target organ of programmed diseases (Fig. 9-3).

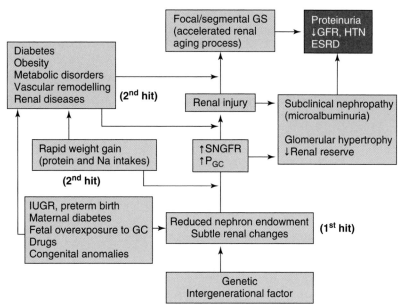

Figure 9-3   "Multi-hits" hypothesis of adult hypertension and chronic kidney disease (CKD). Early growth and nutrition (e.g., caloric, protein, sodium intake) may enhance the adaptive renal mechanisms associated with nephron number deficit and lead to metabolic and hormonal changes, which in turn promote the development of hypertension and CKD through different pathways. ESRD, end-stage renal disease; GC, glucocorticoids; GFR, glomerular filtration rate; HTN, hypertension; IUGR, intrauterine growth restriction; P_{GC}, glomerular capillary pression; SNGFR, single-nephron glomerular filtration rate. (Reproduced with permission from Simeoni U, Ligi I, Buffat C, Boubred F. Adverse consequences of accelerated neonatal growth: cardiovascular and renal issues. *Pediatr Nephrol.* 2011;26(4):493-508.)

Molecular Mechanisms Involved in the Developmental Origins of Cardiovascular Disease

Fetal Environment and Altered Kidney Gene Expression

Nephron formation during embryonic and fetal life occurs through the epithelial differentiation of mesenchymal cells within the nephrogenic blastema induced by the adjacent ureteric bud branch division. It is thus not surprising that the expression of genes involved in kidney development is altered in conditions of an adverse intrauterine environment such as IUGR. Altered genes involved in early stages of nephrogenesis are likely to markedly reduce nephron number endowment. RAS components, mRNA, and protein expression are downregulated in rats born with IUGR, further confirming the role of renin as a renal growth factor.[83] Vitamin A deficiency has been shown to alter nephron development in rats and may be a key factor in nephron mass reduction because of IUGR. Indeed, a 50% reduction in maternal retinol circulating concentration leads to a 20% reduction in nephron number in the offspring, but overall fetal development was not affected, a fact confirmed in cultured explanted metanephroi.[24] Genes of specific growth factors, such as midkine, a retinoic acid responsive gene to a heparin-binding growth factor, have been shown to interfere with nephron development alteration because of retinoic acid deficiency. The regulation cascade of all-transretinoic acid control of nephron development involves C-ret because both C-ret mRNA and protein are significantly altered in conditions of retinoic acid deficiency in vitro. Altered expression of specific genes such as *Pax 2* and *GDNF* have been shown in metanephroi cultured in vitro of kidneys from fetuses exposed to maternal gestational administration of glucocorticoids and to maternal protein diet restriction.[84,85] Various genes are modified in the kidney of IUGR fetuses. We found in a study of renal transcriptome, that expression of around 20% of the genome is altered in IUGR newborn rats exposed in utero to a low-protein maternal diet. In particular, the expression of genes involved in cell maintenance mechanisms and signal transduction was reduced, and that of the prothrombotic pathway in blood coagulation, that of the complement components, and that of apoptosis were considerably enhanced. This induction of coagulation cascades in the kidneys of low birth-weight rats and provides a possible rationale for the thromboendothelial disorders observed in IUGR human newborns.[86]

Imprinted Genes and Programming

The concept of developmental "programming" of adult diseases can be referred to as developmental plasticity to convey the ability to change structure and function in an irreversible fashion during a critical time window in response to a pre- or postnatal environment.[58,87] The environment has a great influence on the phenotypic expression with the aim of adapting to the conditions of existence. Adaptation of species follows the line of evolution, which operates over very long periods and many generations, giving rise to genetic variation in populations and ultimately new species driven by mutation, gene flow, and genetic drift. Populations adapt on an intermediate scale within one or a few life spans, and individuals adapt in fractions of a life span. Adaptation by mutation cannot parallel short-term environmental alterations, and the necessary flexibility comes from regulation of gene expression. This may occur by moment-to-moment control via transcriptional activators and repressors, which respond through a sequence of signal transduction mechanisms to external stimuli such as nutrients and sunlight, also named labile regulation.[88] A second mechanism is by epigenetic regulation.[88,89] Epigenetics comprise the stable and heritable (or potentially heritable) changes in gene expression that do not entail a change in DNA sequence.

One molecular background of epigenetic changes is by alteration of chromatin structure through modification of histones by methylation, acetylation, phosphorylation, and ubiquitylation, all together giving rise to what is referred to as the epigenotype. But the best characterized epigenetic modifications concern DNA and consist of the methylation of cytosine residues within CpG dinucleotides.[90] DNA methylation is of particular importance for gene regulation and is strongly implicated in fetal development. Even minor changes to the degree of gene methylation can have severe consequences. An accurate quantification of the methylation status at any given position within the genome is a powerful diagnostic indicator.

Genomic Imprinting and Nutrient Supply to the Fetus

Nutrition can modify gene expression through epigenetic modifications, as for instance in the case of folate. Folate, a water-soluble B group vitamin, is essential for the transfer of one-carbon units.[91] It is indispensable to the methionine cycle and therefore to the synthesis of S-adenosylmethionine, the common methyl donor for DNA methylation. The status of folate and of other substrates and co-factors in one-carbon metabolism may consequently be expected to influence phenotype, an abnormal status or imbalances being able to cause diseases such as neurologic disorders, cancer, and endocrine and cardiovascular diseases. Folate deficiency leads to a decrease in S-adenosylmethionine and an increase in homocysteine. Abnormalities in folate metabolism and DNA methylation have been associated with Down syndrome, and aberrant DNA methylation has been implicated in the pathogenesis of neurologic disorders, including Alzheimer, Parkinson, and Huntington diseases.[92] Altered DNA methylation has been extensively documented in tumorigenesis.[91]

Nutritional anomalies, either during the entire pregnancy period or at critical ontogenetic stages, are likely to have major and persistent effects on the fetal epigenotype and thereby the expression or depression of genes that may cause diseas in later life. Nutrition, via nutrient–gene interaction, may in this way at least partially determine phenotypic characteristics, and this phenotype may subsequently be transmitted to future generations, given that the epigenome can to some extent be conveyed as well. The epigenetic makeup may constitute a link between LBW and cardiovascular disease and many other complex diseases during adulthood.[90]

Several research studies focused on the classes of elements in the genome that are particularly sensitive to nutritional regulation during early life. There is a growing body of evidence from studies of in vitro embryo culture that the methylation status of genomically imprinted genes, including *IGF2*, *H19*, *IGF2R*, and so on, can be altered with consequences for subsequent organ growth and function.[90,93,94] Importantly, the epigenetic lability of imprinted genes is not limited to the preimplantation period and includes the early postnatal period in rodents.[95] Recent studies have also demonstrated that retrotransposons are elements within the genome that may also be epigenetically labile to early nutrition.[96,97]

Directional effects on fetal growth of maternally and paternally expressed genes have been documented in a number of mouse knockouts. Whereas paternally expressed genes involved in fetal growth tend to increase fetal size, maternally expressed genes decrease fetal size. Imprinted genes are epigenetically regulated and play important roles in development such as fetal growth, placental development and function, and behavior after birth.[98,99] The control of fetal growth by imprinted genes can be exerted at the level of cell proliferation, apoptosis, and extracellular fluid composition in fetuses.

To prove that such mechanisms are at work in kidney development, asymmetric IUGR has been induced through bilateral uterine artery ligation in pregnant rats by Pham et al.[100] Uteroplacental insufficiency reduced glomeruli number while increasing TUNEL (terminal deoxynucleotidyl transferase dUTP nick end labeling) staining and caspase-3 activity in the IUGR kidney, both indicating increased apoptosis. Furthermore, a significant decrease in Bcl-2 mRNA and a significant increase in Bax and p53 mRNA have been observed.

Genomic imprinting is thought to have evolved as a result of genetic conflict between paternal and maternal genomes over the allocation of maternal resources, leading to the prediction that imprinted genes have substantial control over size at birth. This is confirmed by recent studies, from which we have suggested that imprinted genes have central roles in the genetic control of both the fetal demand for and the placenta supply of maternal nutrients. Constancia et al[101] have recently provided the demonstration that dysregulation of an imprinted gene, specifically in the placenta, affects fetal growth by showing that placental-specific *Igf2* is an important modulator for fetal growth in the mouse. The *Igf2* gene combines and balances the genetic control of supply (through expression in the placenta) with the genetic control of demand (through expression in the fetus) for nutrients. This hypothesis can be extended to other imprinted genes. Paternally expressed genes in the fetus increase the demand for nutrients, and maternally expressed genes in the fetus decrease demand for nutrients. Alterations in demand may create a signal to the placenta to alter supply. Knowledge of how nutrient supply and demand are genetically regulated is crucial for understanding the mechanisms of fetal growth restriction. The role of human imprinted genes in fetal growth restriction, however, remains poorly understood, largely through the difficulties of human experimentation.

Conclusion

Increasing clinical and experimental data support the concept that renal function in adulthood seems partly "programmed" in utero or in the early postnatal period (or both), independently of the eventual occurrence of congenital or acquired kidney disease. Such developmental programming of function and disease in adulthood is related to LBW, whether because of IUGR or premature birth. Large birth weight infants and those exposed to maternal diabetes have to be considered at increased risk as well. The consequent glomerular hyperfiltration contributes to the increased arterial blood pressure and CKD in adulthood. Despite this clear pathophysiologic rationale, a number of points still need to be addressed to allow the design of effective preventive strategies. Blood pressure, nutrition, growth status, and renal (microalbuminuria) and metabolic functions should be monitored carefully and prospectively in infants at higher risk. The long-term influence of postnatal nutrition, especially protein intake, on the development of renal function, especially in conditions of altered perinatal renal development, is still unknown. Rapid postnatal catch-up growth may amplify fetal-programmed adult diseases, particularly CKD. Epigenetic changes are likely to be key molecular factors in the long-term memory that characterizes long-term consequences of altered perinatal growth and development. Future research should clarify the optimal perinatal nutritional approach and define relevant biomarkers for follow-up. The prophylactic measures to be applied to infants at increased risk of developmentally programmed adult disease should also be defined.

References

1. Barker DJ, Winter PD, Osmond C, et al. Weight in infancy and death from ischaemic heart disease. *Lancet*. 1989;2:577-580.
2. Osmond C, Barker DJ, Winter PD, et al. Early growth and death from cardiovascular disease in women. *BMJ*. 1993;307:1519-1524.
3. Stein CE, Fall CH, Kumaran K, et al. Fetal growth and coronary heart disease in south India. *Lancet*. 1996;348:1269-1273.
4. Eriksson JG, Forsen T, Tuomilehto J, et al. Early growth and coronary heart disease in later life: longitudinal study. *BMJ*. 2001;322:949-953.
5. Hales CN, Barker DJ, Clark PM, et al. Fetal and infant growth and impaired glucose tolerance at age 64. *BMJ*. 1991;303:1019-1022.
6. Barker DJ, Hales CN, Fall CH, et al. Type 2 (non-insulin-dependent) diabetes mellitus, hypertension and hyperlipidaemia (syndrome X): relation to reduced fetal growth. *Diabetologia*. 1993;36:62-67.
7. Hoy WE, Douglas-Denton RN, Hughson MD, et al. A stereological study of glomerular number and volume: preliminary findings in a multiracial study of kidneys at autopsy. *Kidney Int Suppl*. 2003; S31-S37.
8. Lackland DT, Bendall HE, Osmond C, et al. Low birth weights contribute to high rates of early-onset chronic renal failure in the Southeastern United States. *Arch Intern Med*. 2001;160: 1472-1476.
9. Keijzer-Veen MG, Finken MJ, Nauta J, et al. Microalbuminuria and lower glomerular filtration rate at young adult age in subjects born very premature and after intrauterine growth retardation. *J Am Soc Nephrol*. 2005;16:2762-2768.
10. Vikse BE, Irgens LM, Leivestad T, et al. Low birth weight increases risk for end-stage renal disease. *J Am Soc Nephrol*. 2008;19:151-157.
11. Huxley RR, Shiell AW, Law CM. The role of size at birth and postnatal catch-up growth in determining systolic blood pressure: a systematic review of the literature. *J Hypertens*. 2000;18: 815-831.
12. Persson E, Jansson T. Low birth weight is associated with elevated adult blood pressure in the chronically catheterized guinea-pig. *Acta Physiol Scand*. 1992;145:195-196.
13. Moritz K, Butkus A, Hantzis V, et al. Prolonged low-dose dexamethasone, in early gestation, has no long-term deleterious effect on normal ovine fetuses. *Endocrinology*. 2002;143:1159-1165.
14. Langley-Evans SC, Gardner DS, Welham SJ. Intrauterine programming of cardiovascular disease by maternal nutritional status. *Nutrition*. 1998;14:39-47.
15. Woodall SM, Johnston BM, Breier BH, Gluckman PD. Chronic maternal undernutrition in the rat leads to delayed postnatal growth and elevated blood pressure of offspring. *Pediatr Res*. 1996; 40:438-443.
16. Ozaki T, Nishina H, Hanson MA, Poston L. Dietary restriction in pregnant rats causes gender-related hypertension and vascular dysfunction in offspring. *J Physiol*. 2001;530:141-152.
17. Kistner A, Jacobson L, Jacobson SH, et al. Low gestational age associated with abnormal retinal vascularization and increased blood pressure in adult women. *Pediatr Res*. 2002;51:675-680.
18. Kistner A, Celsi G, Vanpee M, Jacobson SH. Increased systolic daily ambulatory blood pressure in adult women born preterm. *Pediatr Nephrol*. 2005;20:232-233.
19. Keijzer–Veen MG, Finken MJ, Nauta J, et al. Is blood pressure increased 19 years after intrauterine growth restriction and preterm birth? A prospective follow-up study in The Netherlands. *Pediatrics*. 2005;116:725-731.
20. Irving RJ, Belton NR, Elton RA, Walker BR. Adult cardiovascular risk factors in premature babies. *Lancet*. 2000;355:2135-2136.
21. Brenner BM, Chertow GM. Congenital oligonephropathy and the etiology of adult hypertension and progressive renal injury. *Am J Kidney Dis*. 1994;23:171-175.
22. Vehaskari VM, Woods LL. Prenatal programming of hypertension: lessons from experimental models. *J Am Soc Nephrol*. 2005;16:2545-2556.
23. McMillen IC, Robinson JS. Developmental origins of the metabolic syndrome: prediction, plasticity, and programming. *Physiol Rev*. 2005;85:571-633.
24. Merlet-Benichou C, Gilbert T, Vilar J, et al. Nephron number: variability is the rule. Causes and consequences. *Lab Invest*. 1999;79:515-527.
25. Brenner BM, Garcia DL, Anderson S. Glomeruli and blood pressure. Less of one, more the other? *Am J Hypertens*. 1988;1:335-347.

26. Keller G, Zimmer G, Mall G, et al. Nephron number in patients with primary hypertension. *N Engl J Med*. 2003;348:101-108.
27. Kuzawa CW. Fetal origins of developmental plasticity: are fetal cues reliable predictors of future nutritional environments? *Am J Hum Biol*. 2005;17:5-21.
28. Bateson P. Developmental plasticity and evolutionary biology. *J Nutr*. 2007;137:1060-1062.
29. Gluckman PD, Hanson MA, Cooper C, Thornburg KL. Effect of in utero and early-life conditions on adult health and disease. *N Engl J Med*. 2008;359:61-73.
30. White SL, Perkovic V, Cass A, et al. Is low birth weight an antecedent of CKD in later life? A systematic review of observational studies. *Am J Kidney Dis*. 2009;54:248-261.
31. Fagerudd J, Forsblom C, Pettersson-Fernholm K, et al. Low birth weight does not increase the risk of nephropathy in Finnish type 1 diabetic patients. *Nephrol Dial Transplant*. 2006;21:2159-2165.
32. Li S, Chen SC, Shlipak M, et al. Low birth weight is associated with chronic kidney disease only in men. *Kidney Int*. 2008;73:637-642.
33. Hallan S, Euser AM, Irgens LM, et al. Effect of intrauterine growth restriction on kidney function at young adult age: the Nord Trondelag Health (HUNT 2) Study. *Am J Kidney Dis*. 2008;51: 10-20.
34. Lackland DT, Bendall HE, Osmond C, et al. Low birth weights contribute to high rates of early-onset chronic renal failure in the Southeastern United States. *Arch Intern Med*. 2000;160: 1472-1476.
35. Painter RC, Roseboom TJ, van Montfrans GA, et al. Microalbuminuria in adults after prenatal exposure to the Dutch famine. *J Am Soc Nephrol*. 2005;16:189-194.
36. Zidar N, Avgustin Cavic M, Kenda RB, Ferluga D. Unfavorable course of minimal change nephrotic syndrome in children with intrauterine growth retardation. *Kidney Int*. 1998;54:1320-1323.
37. Zidar N, Cavic MA, Kenda RB, et al. Effect of intrauterine growth retardation on the clinical course and prognosis of IgA glomerulonephritis in children. *Nephron*. 1998;79:28-32.
38. Plank C, Ostreicher I, Dittrich K, et al. Low birth weight, but not postnatal weight gain, aggravates the course of nephrotic syndrome. *Pediatr Nephrol*. 2007;22:1881-1889.
39. Rodriguez-Soriano J, Aguirre M, Oliveros R, Vallo A. Long-term renal follow-up of extremely low birth weight infants. *Pediatr Nephrol*. 2005;20:579-584.
40. Rakow A, Johansson S, Legnevall L, et al. Renal volume and function in school-age children born preterm or small for gestational age. *Pediatr Nephrol*. 2008;23:1309-1315.
41. Kistner A, Celsi G, Vanpee M, Jacobson SH. Increased blood pressure but normal renal function in adult women born preterm. *Pediatr Nephrol*. 2000;15:215-220.
42. Hodgin JB, Rasoulpour M, Markowitz GS, D'Agati VD. Very low birth weight is a risk factor for secondary focal segmental glomerulosclerosis. *Clin J Am Soc Nephrol*. 2009;4:71-76.
43. Barker DJ, Osmond C, Forsen TJ, et al. Trajectories of growth among children who have coronary events as adults. *N Engl J Med*. 2005;353:1802-1809.
44. Law CM, Shiell AW, Newsome CA, et al. Fetal, infant, and childhood growth and adult blood pressure: a longitudinal study from birth to 22 years of age. *Circulation*. 2002;105:1088-1092.
45. Adair LS, Cole TJ. Rapid child growth raises blood pressure in adolescent boys who were thin at birth. *Hypertension*. 2003;41:451-456.
46. Cruickshank JK, Mzayek F, Liu L, et al. Origins of the 'black/white' difference in blood pressure: roles of birth weight, postnatal growth, early blood pressure, and adolescent body size: the Bogalusa heart study. *Circulation*. 2005;111:1932-1937.
47. Eriksson J, Forsen T, Tuomilehto J, et al. Fetal and childhood growth and hypertension in adult life. *Hypertension*. 2000;36:790-794.
48. Walker SP, Gaskin P, Powell CA, et al. The effects of birth weight and postnatal linear growth retardation on blood pressure at age 11–12 years. *J Epidemiol Community Health*. 2001;55: 394-398.
49. Singhal A, Cole TJ, Lucas A. Early nutrition in preterm infants and later blood pressure: two cohorts after randomised trials. *Lancet*. 2001;357:413-419.
50. Cheung YB, Low L, Osmond C, et al. Fetal growth and early postnatal growth are related to blood pressure in adults. *Hypertension*. 2000;36:795-800.
51. Vickers MH, Breier BH, Cutfield WS, et al. Fetal origins of hyperphagia, obesity, and hypertension and postnatal amplification by hypercaloric nutrition. *Am J Physiol Endocrinol Metab*. 2000;279: E83-E87.
52. Plagemann A, Heidrich I, Gotz F, et al. Obesity and enhanced diabetes and cardiovascular risk in adult rats due to early postnatal overfeeding. *Exp Clin Endocrinol*. 1992;99:154-158.
53. Boubred F, Daniel L, Buffat C, et al. Early postnatal overfeeding induces early chronic renal dysfunction in adult male rats. *Am J Physiol Renal Physiol*. 2009;297:F943-F951.
54. Boubred F, Buffat C, Feuerstein JM, et al. Effects of early postnatal hypernutrition on nephron number and long-term renal function and structure in rats. *Am J Physiol Renal Physiol*. 2007; 293:F1944-F1949.
55. Simeoni U, Ligi I, Buffat C, Boubred F. Adverse consequences of accelerated neonatal growth: cardiovascular and renal issues. *Pediatr Nephrol*. 2011;26(4):493-508.
56. Jennings BJ, Ozanne SE, Dorling MW, Hales CN. Early growth determines longevity in male rats and may be related to telomere shortening in the kidney. *FEBS Lett*. 1999;448:4-8.
57. Hoppe CC, Evans RG, Moritz KM, et al. Combined prenatal and postnatal protein restriction influences adult kidney structure, function, and arterial pressure. *Am J Physiol Regul Integr Comp Physiol*. 2007;292:R462-R469.

9

58. Gluckman PD, Hanson MA. Living with the past: evolution, development, and patterns of disease. *Science.* 2004;305:1733-1736.
59. Hales CN, Barker DJ. Type 2 (non-insulin-dependent) diabetes mellitus: the thrifty phenotype hypothesis. *Diabetologia.* 1992;35:595-601.
60. Mei-Zahav M, Korzets Z, Cohen I, et al. Ambulatory blood pressure monitoring in children with a solitary kidney—a comparison between unilateral renal agenesis and uninephrectomy. *Blood Press Monit.* 2001;6:263-267.
61. Woods LL. Neonatal uninephrectomy causes hypertension in adult rats. *Am J Physiol.* 1999;276:R974-R978.
62. Moritz KM, Wintour EM, Dodic M. Fetal uninephrectomy leads to postnatal hypertension and compromised renal function. *Hypertension.* 2002;39:1071-1076.
63. Hughson M, Farris AB, Douglas-Denton R, et al. Glomerular number and size in autopsy kidneys: the relationship to birth weight. *Kidney Int.* 2003;63:2113-2122.
64. Harrison M, Langley-Evans SC. Intergenerational programming of impaired nephrogenesis and hypertension in rats following maternal protein restriction during pregnancy. *Br J Nutr.* 2009;101:1020-1030.
65. Hinchliffe SA, Lynch MR, Sargent PH, et al. The effect of intrauterine growth retardation on the development of renal nephrons. *Br J Obstet Gynaecol.* 1992;99:296-301.
66. Schmidt IM, Chellakooty M, Boisen KA, et al. Impaired kidney growth in low-birth-weight children: distinct effects of maturity and weight for gestational age. *Kidney Int.* 2005;68:731-740.
67. Drougia A, Giapros V, Hotoura E, et al. (2009) The effects of gestational age and growth restriction on compensatory kidney growth. *Nephrol Dial Transplant.* 2009;24:142-148.
68. Rodriguez MM, Gomez AH, Abitbol CL, et al. Histomorphometric analysis of postnatal glomerulogenesis in extremely preterm infants. *Pediatr Dev Pathol.* 2004;7:17-25.
69. Sahajpal V, Ashton N. Renal function and angiotensin AT1 receptor expression in young rats following intrauterine exposure to a maternal low-protein diet. *Clin Sci (Lond).* 2003;104:607-614.
70. Vehaskari VM, Stewart T, Lafont D, et al. Kidney angiotensin and angiotensin receptor expression in prenatally programmed hypertension. *Am J Physiol Renal Physiol.* 2004;287:F262-F267.
71. Alwasel SH, Ashton N. Prenatal programming of renal sodium handling in the rat. *Clin Sci (Lond).* 2009;117:75-84.
72. Simonetti GD, Raio L, Surbek D, et al. Salt sensitivity of children with low birth weight. *Hypertension.* 2008;52:625-630.
73. Nehiri T, Duong Van Huyen JP, et al. Exposure to maternal diabetes induces salt-sensitive hypertension and impairs renal function in adult rat offspring. *Diabetes.* 2008;57:2167-2175.
74. Vehaskari VM, Stewart T, Lafont D, et al. Kidney angiotensin and angiotensin receptor expression in prenatally programmed hypertension. *Am J Physiol Renal Physiol.* 2004;287:F262-F267.
75. Kreutz R, Kovacevic L, Schulz A, et al. Effect of high NaCl diet on spontaneous hypertension in a genetic rat model with reduced nephron number. *J Hypertens.* 2000;18:777-782.
76. Zucchelli P, Cagnoli L. Proteinuria and hypertension after unilateral nephrectomy. *Lancet.* 1985;2:212.
77. Hughson MD, Douglas-Denton R, Bertram JF, Hoy WE. Hypertension, glomerular number, and birth weight in African Americans and white subjects in the southeastern United States. *Kidney Int.* 2006;69:671-678.
78. Gossmann J, Wilhelm A, Kachel HG, et al. Long-term consequences of live kidney donation follow-up in 93% of living kidney donors in a single transplant center. *Am J Transplant.* 2005;5:2417-2424.
79. Griffin KA, Picken MM, Churchill M, et al. Functional and structural correlates of glomerulosclerosis after renal mass reduction in the rat. *J Am Soc Nephrol.* 2000;11:497-506.
80. Stewart T, Ascani J, Craver RD, Vehaskari VM. Role of postnatal dietary sodium in prenatally programmed hypertension. *Pediatr Nephrol.* 2009;24:1727-1733.
81. Hammond KA, Janes DN. The effects of increased protein intake on kidney size and function. *J Exp Biol.* 1998;201:2081-2090.
82. Stewart T, Jung FF, Manning J, Vehaskari VM. Kidney immune cell infiltration and oxidative stress contribute to prenatally programmed hypertension. *Kidney Int.* 2005;68:2180-2188.
83. Woods LL, Ingelfinger JR, Nyengaard JR, Rasch R. Maternal protein restriction suppresses the newborn renin-angiotensin system and programs adult hypertension in rats. *Pediatr Res.* 2001;49:460-467.
84. Welham SJ, Riley PR, Wade A, et al. Maternal diet programs embryonic kidney gene expression. *Physiol Genomics.* 2005;22:48-56.
85. Singh RR, Moritz KM, Bertram JF, Cullen-McEwen LA. Effects of dexamethasone exposure on rat metanephric development: in vitro and in vivo studies. *Am J Physiol Renal Physiol.* 2007;293:F548-F554.
86. Buffat C, Boubred F, Mondon F, et al. Kidney gene expression analysis in a rat model of intrauterine growth restriction reveals massive alterations of coagulation genes. *Endocrinology.* 2007;148:5549-5557.
87. Stewart RJ, Sheppard H, Preece R, Waterlow JC. The effect of rehabilitation at different stages of development of rats marginally malnourished for ten to twelve generations. *Br J Nutr.* 1980;43:403-412.
88. Jiang YH, Bressler J, Beaudet AL. Epigenetics and human disease. *Annu Rev Genomics Hum Genet.* 2004;5:479-510.

89. Abdolmaleky HM, Smith CL, Faraone SV, et al. Methylomics in psychiatry: modulation of gene-environment interactions may be through DNA methylation. *Am J Med Genet B Neuropsychiatr Genet.* 2004;127:51-59.
90. Waterland RA, Jirtle RL. Early nutrition, epigenetic changes at transposons and imprinted genes, and enhanced susceptibility to adult chronic diseases. *Nutrition.* 2004;20:63-68.
91. Lucock M. Folic acid: nutritional biochemistry, molecular biology, and role in disease processes. *Mol Genet Metab.* 2000;71:121-138.
92. Mattson MP. Methylation and acetylation in nervous system development and neurodegenerative disorders. *Ageing Res Rev.* 2003;2:329-342.
93. Young LE. Imprinting of genes and the Barker hypothesis. *Twin Res.* 2001;4:307-317.
94. Young LE, Fernandes K, McEvoy TG, et al. Epigenetic change in IGF2R is associated with fetal overgrowth after sheep embryo culture. *Nat Genet.* 2001;27:153-154.
95. Waterland RA, Garza C. Early postnatal nutrition determines adult pancreatic glucose-responsive insulin secretion and islet gene expression in rats. *J Nutr.* 2002;132:357-364.
96. Waterland RA, Jirtle RL. Transposable elements: targets for early nutritional effects on epigenetic gene regulation. *Mol Cell Biol.* 2003;23:5293-5300.
97. Wolff GL, Kodell RL, Moore SR, Cooney CA. Maternal epigenetics and methyl supplements affect agouti gene expression in Avy/a mice. *Faseb J.* 1998;12:949-957.
98. Reik W, . Walter J. Genomic imprinting: parental influence on the genome. *Nat Rev Genet.* 2001;2:21-32.
99. Tycko B, Morison IM. Physiological functions of imprinted genes. *J Cell Physiol.* 2002;192:245-258.
100. Pham TD, MacLennan NK, Chiu CT, et al. Uteroplacental insufficiency increases apoptosis and alters p53 gene methylation in the full-term IUGR rat kidney. *Am J Physiol Regul Integr Comp Physiol.* 2003;285:R962-R970.
101. Constancia M, Hemberger M, Hughes J, et al. Placental-specific IGF-II is a major modulator of placental and fetal growth. *Nature.* 2002;417:945-948.

CHAPTER 10

Renal Modulation: The Renin–Angiotensin–Aldosterone System

Aruna Natarajan, MD, DCh, PhD, Pedro A. Jose, MD, PhD

10

- **Components of the Renin–Angiotensin–Aldosterone System**
- **Ontogeny**
- **Current Concepts and Controversies**

The renin–angiotensin–aldosterone system (RAAS) plays a critical role in the maintenance of salt and water homeostasis by the kidneys, particularly in hypovolemic and salt-depleted states. The unopposed activation of this system results in sodium retention, potassium loss, and an increase in blood pressure.[1]

Components of the Renin–Angiotensin–Aldosterone System

Angiotensin Generation

Renin (Fig. 10-1) is synthesized in the juxtaglomerular (JG) cells (smooth muscle cells in the walls of the afferent arteriole as it enters the glomerulus) (Fig. 10-2) and is stored as prorenin.[2-5] It is released as renin, which enzymatically causes the formation of angiotensin I (Ang I) from angiotensinogen, its only substrate. In the classical pathway, Ang I is acted upon by angiotensin-converting enzyme (ACE) to form angiotensin II (Ang II). The rate-limiting step in this sequence of events in humans is the release of renin, which is the most well-regulated component of all constituents of the renin–angiotensin system (RAS). Renin secretion or release in the kidney is increased by three primary pathways: (1) stimulation of renal baroreceptors by a decrease in afferent arterial stretch (pressure)[6,7]; (2) stimulation of renal β_1-adrenergic receptors, partly through increased renal sympathetic nerve activity[8-10]; and (3) a decrease in sodium and chloride delivery to and transport by the macula densa.[11,12] Renin secretion can also be regulated by several endocrine and paracrine hormones.[13]

Renin–Angiotensin System Outside Juxtaglomerular Cells

Recent research has revealed ramifications of this canonical system. The RAS has been demonstrated in tissues other than the kidney. Synthesis of certain components of the RAAS occurs to a greater extent in some organs relative to others, such as ACE in the lung, aldosterone in the adrenal glands, angiotensinogen in the liver, and renin in the kidney, which function together as an endocrine system. Some or all of its components are expressed in the brain, heart, vasculature, adipose tissue, pancreas, placenta, and kidney, among others, exerting autocrine, intracrine, and paracrine effects. This adds complexity to our understanding of the modulatory effects of the RAAS in maintaining homeostasis.[5] Extraglomerular sites of prorenin synthesis include the adrenal gland zona glomerulosa, eye (retina and vitreous humor),[14] Muller cells, renal collecting duct cells, mast cells, ovary,[15] uterus, placenta, chorionic villi, submandibular gland,[16] adipocytes,[17,18] and testes[19]; the extraglomerular sites of synthesis are species specific.[20] Angiotensinogen is produced in extrahepatic sites

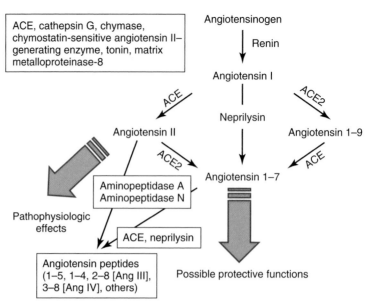

Figure 10-1 Pathways of angiotensin (Ang) generation showing the generation of Ang peptides. Both angiotensin-converting enzyme (ACE) and ACE2 are involved in the production of the biologically active peptides Ang II and Ang (1–7) from Ang I. Inappropriately elevated levels of Ang II are detrimental to the function of the heart and kidney. Ang (1–7) may function as a key peptide involved in cardioprotection and renoprotection. The main products of angiotensin I in the heart and kidney are Ang (1–9) and Ang II.[223,224] Genetic experiments suggest that ACE and ACE2 have complementary functions by negatively regulating different RAS products. The fine details of their regulatory function may differ depending on the local RAS environment. (Adapted from Danilczyk U, Penninger JM. Angiotensin-converting enzyme II in the heart and the kidney. *Circ Res.* 2006;98(4):463-471.)

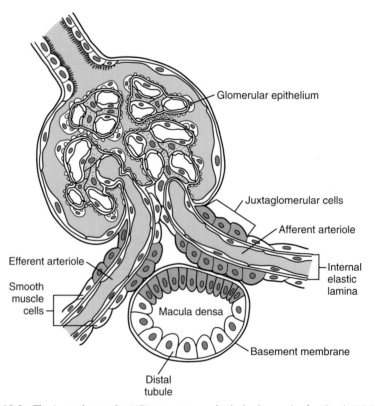

Figure 10-2 The juxtaglomerular (JG) apparatus and tubuloglomerular feedback (TGF). TGF is achieved because of the anatomy of the nephron and JG apparatus. TGF is a phenomenon that occurs when changes in tubular fluid concentrations of Na^+ and Cl^- are sensed by the macula densa via the luminal Na^+, K^+, $2Cl^-$ cotransporter. Increases or decreases in luminal uptake of these ions cause reciprocal changes in glomerular filtration rate by alterations in vascular tone, mainly in the afferent arteriole.[125] (From Guyton AC, Hall JE. The kidneys and body fluids. In *Guyton and Hall Textbook of Medical Physiology*. St. Louis, WB Saunders, 2000, p. 292).

such as the adrenal gland, cardiac atrium, brain, kidney, large intestine, lung, mesentery, ovary, spinal cord, stomach, and spleen and is also expressed in the ventricle and conduction tissue of the heart.[5,21] ACE is ubiquitously expressed. However, the conversion of circulating Ang I to Ang II by ACE occurs mainly in the lung. ACE2 has been identified in the human heart, kidney, and testis and may be present in other tissues as well.[21,22]

Effects of Angiotensin-Converting Enzyme and Non–Angiotensin-Converting Enzyme Other Than the Production of Angiotensin II

ACE acts on Ang I (Ang 1–10) to cleave off the active octapeptide, Ang II (Ang 1–8), which is a more potent vasoconstrictor than Ang I[23] (Fig. 10-1). Ang II can also be formed by non-ACE enzymes and non-renin enzymes, such as cathepsin G, chymase, chymostatin-sensitive Ang II-generating enzyme, tonin, and matrix metalloproteinase-8.[24] This assumes greater significance in the organs where not all components of the RAAS are expressed, providing alternate means of generation of Ang II, and cardiovascular sequelae. For example, mast cells produce renin and have chymases, which help form Ang II and may play a role in heart failure and generation of arrhythmias.[25] Mast cell chymases limit the cardiac efficacy of ACE inhibitors[26] and may also have a role in progression of the atherosclerotic plaques.[27]

ACE2 is a human homolog of ACE, sharing about 42% sequence homology. ACE2 is relatively abundant in the kidney, specifically in the proximal tubule, and may be an important regulator of the balance between Ang II and Ang (1–7) in the kidney, with a potential for being a therapeutic target in renal diseases.[28] In neonatal rat cardiomyocytes, aldosterone increases the expression of ACE, but the opposite is observed for ACE2.[29] ACE2 is a carboxypeptidase and the main catabolic enzyme of Ang II, generating Ang (1–7). Ang (1–7), probably by occupying the Mas receptor, has natriuretic, vasodilator, and antiproliferative properties and counteracts the effects of Ang II. ACE2 also decreases the level of Ang II by converting Ang I to Ang (1–9), which is inactive.[30,31] Thus, ACE and ACE2 exert opposing roles on the effects of the RAS; a decrease in ACE2 may account for increased levels of Ang II, and the opposite occurs with ACE. Sympathetic vasoconstriction in systemic disorders of vascular regulation may be related to ACE2 deficiency, leading to a decrease in Ang (1–7).[32] The ACE2-Ang (1–7)–Mas axis plays a role in the pathogenesis of hypertension, regulation of renal function, and progression of renal disease, including diabetic nephropathy. A decrease in the expression or function of this system may play a critical role in the progression of cardiovascular diseases as elucidated below.[33]

The processing of angiotensins is tissue specific. The effects of angiotensin metabolites are also tissue specific.

Cardiovascular System

Ang I can be converted to Ang (1–9) by ACE and carboxypeptidase A or carboxypeptidase A-like enzymes. The main products of Ang 1 due to ACE are Ang (1–9) and Ang II in the heart[34], and Ang (1–9) but not Ang II in platelets.[35] Circulating Ang (1–9) levels are increased after myocardial infarction[36] and inhibit cardiac hypertrophy.[37] Whereas Ang (1–9)[38] is prethrombotic, Ang (1–7) is antithrombotic.[39]

Adipocytes

In adipocytes, Ang (1–7) derived from Ang (1–9) is the main degradation product, and Ang III inhibits insulin-regulated amino peptidase.[17]

Renal

In rat glomeruli, Ang I is converted to Ang (2–10) via aminopeptidase A and Ang (1–7) via neprilysin.[40]

Mesenteric Bed

In mesenteric arteries, the main angiotensin processing enzymes are carboxypeptidase A-like enzymes.[41]

10

Angiotensin II and Its Metabolites

Aminopeptidases cleave Ang II at different sites. Aminopeptidase A acts on Ang II to form the heptapeptide Ang III, which participates, along with Ang II, in the classical effects on body fluid and electrolyte homeostasis, such as drinking behavior, vasopressin release, and sodium appetite in brain centers.[5,42] Ang III has been shown to exert a natriuretic effect via its interaction with the AT_2 receptor.[43] Ang IV is a hexapeptide (Ang 3–8), formed by the action of aminopeptidase N on Ang II.[44,45] Ang IV negatively regulates aminopeptidase A and thus influences the generation of Ang III.[43]

The RAS in the brain has been well studied. It helps regulate central blood pressure by stimulating sympathetic nerve activity, which causes vasoconstriction, influencing neurohormonal regulation of salt and water balance and exerting behavioral effects on salt and water intake. These effects are mediated by Ang II via the AT_1 receptor. Although renin levels in the brain are low, this could be compensated by the high expression of the prorenin receptor (PRR).[46,47]

In summary, the RAS is now accepted to be present in many tissues and composed of two distinct and opposing arms: the first, composed of ACE, which generates Ang II, acting via the AT_1 receptors to subserve the biologic effects of vasoconstriction and increase in renal sodium transport, and the second comprising the monocarboxypeptidase ACE2, which generates an endogenous antagonist to Ang II, namely Ang (1–7) activating the oncogene Mas receptor protein to subserve vasodilatory and antiproliferative effects on the vasculature and decreased epithelial ion transport. In the brain, ACE2 activation also opposes the effects of Ang II exerted via the AT_1 receptor.

Aldosterone

Ang II stimulates aldosterone synthesis and secretion by zona glomerulosa cells of the adrenal gland.[48] Extra-adrenal sites of aldosterone synthesis include brain neurons, where it stimulates thirst, and cardiac myocytes, where it plays a role in the ventricular remodeling associated with salt retention.[49] In these areas, the effects of aldosterone oppose those of glucocorticoids.[50] Recent research suggests that aldosterone and glucocorticoids are not synthesized in the heart, but the abundance of receptors to both hormones in the cardiac interstitium generates a response to the circulating aldosterone. Both act by unique pathways; whereas steroids enhance cardiac contractility and increase coronary flow,[51] aldosterone promotes salt and water retention by stimulating sodium transport mediated by epithelial sodium channel (ENaC) in the distal nephron. Aldosterone is also reported to regulate sodium transport in the renal proximal tubule by stimulation of the type I Na^+/H^+ exchanger, NHE1.[52]

Gene Targeting of Angiotensin Synthesis: Lessons from Genetically Manipulated Rodents

Tissue-specific targeted ablation helps to elucidate the paracrine and autocrine effects of tissue RAS. Glial-specific deletion of angiotensinogen in mice results in lowered blood pressure,[53] supporting the notion that the central nervous system contributes to the regulation of blood pressure via the RAS. Introduction of the mouse Ren-2 gene into normotensive rats creates a transgenic strain that expresses Ren-2 mRNA in the adrenal gland and the kidney.[54] This transgenic rat is a monogenic model for a form of sodium-dependent malignant hypertension. The Ren-2 transgenic rat has hyperproreninemia, low plasma and renal renin, high adrenal renin, and increased adrenal corticosteroid production. Blockade of the ET_A receptor in young Ren-2 transgenic rats decreases blood pressure and ameliorates end-organ damage, suggesting potential application in the management of hypertension in newborn babies.[55]

ACE-deficient mice have decreased blood pressure and severe renal disease characterized by vascular hyperplasia of the intrarenal arteries, perivascular infiltrates, a paucity of renal papillae,[56] and impaired concentrating ability, highlighting the role of ACE in the development of the kidneys.[57] Inhibitors of ACE have been identified in hypoallergenic infant milk formulas containing hydrolyzed milk proteins, which could potentially affect renal function later in life.[58] ACE inhibition in young rats has been reported to cause retardation of glomerular growth (see below).

ACE2-deficient mice develop dilated cardiomyopathy and have a hypertensive response to Ang II.[59,60] A decrease in ACE2 receptor expression has been implicated in the delayed hypertension observed in sheep treated antenatally with betamethasone,[61] which needs further elucidation in humans given the widespread use of antenatal steroids to enhance lung maturity in premature labor.

Angiotensin Receptors

The effects of the angiotensin ligands Ang II, Ang III, and Ang IV are mediated by their occupation of specific angiotensin receptors. Ang II interacts mainly with two receptors, AT_1 and AT_2. Whereas Ang II and Ang III are full agonists at the AT_1 receptor, Ang IV binds to this receptor with low affinity.[54,57,62-65] The conversion of Ang II to Ang III is necessary for its interaction with the AT_2 receptor to cause natriuresis.[66]

The human AT_1 receptor gene is located in chromosome 3q21-q25. The human AT_2 receptor is located in chromosome Xq22-q23. AT_1 and AT_2 receptors belong to the seven-transmembrane class of G protein-coupled receptors.[5,49,50,67] Adult human renal vasculature, glomeruli, and tubules (proximal and distal convoluted tubule, ascending limb of Henle, and collecting duct) express AT_1 receptors; AT_2 receptors are expressed in the vasculature and glomeruli, but not in the tubules.[64] In rodents, AT_2 receptors are expressed in most segments of the nephron.

The current understanding that AT_2 receptor expression is higher in fetal life than in newborns or adults has been challenged by recent observations in rats wherein AT_2 receptor protein expression is lower and AT_1 receptor protein expression is higher in the fetal and neonatal brain and kidneys than in adults, but expression of AT_2 receptor is higher in the fetal and neonatal liver compared with adults.[68]

Occupation of the AT_1 receptor by Ang II triggers the generation of various second messengers via heterotrimeric G-proteins, mainly $G_{q/11}$. Phospholipase C (PLC) $\beta1$ is activated, leading to the formation of 1,4,5-inositol trisphosphate (IP_3) and diacylglycerol (DAG) from the hydrolysis of phosphatidylinositol-4,5-bisphosphonate (PIP_2). IP_3 activates IP_3 receptors in the endoplasmic reticulum, releasing Ca^{2+}. Ca^{2+} released from the endoplasmic reticulum causes the Ca^{2+}-sensing stromal interaction molecule (STIM1) protein to interact with Orai1 in the plasma membrane. This interaction, together with the activation of IP_3 receptors at the plasma membrane, allows the influx of extracellular calcium.[69,70] The increase in intracellular calcium and the stimulation of protein kinase C (PKC) by DAG lead to vasoconstriction.[71] Activation of the AT_1 receptor stimulates growth factor pathways such as tyrosine phosphorylation and PLCγ activation, leading to activation of downstream proteins, including mitogen-activated protein (MAP) kinases, and signal transducers and activators of transcription (STAT protein). These cellular proliferative pathways, mediated by the AT_1 receptor, have been implicated in the proliferative changes seen in cardiovascular and renal diseases.[72] AT_1 receptor signaling may also be affected by reactive oxygen species (ROS) and reactive nitrogen species, but nitric oxide (NO) may decrease AT_1 receptor signaling by cysteine modification of the nuclear transcription factor, NFκB.[73]

The AT_1 and AT_2 receptors are differentiated based on their affinity for various nonpeptide antagonists.[74] The AT_2 receptor shares 32% to 34% amino acid homology with the AT_1 receptor, but activates second messenger systems with opposite effects via various signal transduction systems, mainly G_i and G_o proteins.[75] Stimulation of the AT_2 receptor leads to activation of various phosphatases, resulting in inactivation of extracellular signal-regulated kinase (ERK), opening of K^+ channels, and inhibition of T-type Ca^{2+} channels. The AT_2 receptor has a higher affinity for Ang III than Ang II; indeed, Ang III may be the preferred ligand for the AT_2 receptor, exerting its natriuretic effect in the kidney.[66] Whereas AT_1 receptors mediate increased ion transport, vasoconstriction, inflammation, and immunity and decreased longevity, AT_2 receptors may mediate antiproliferative effects, apoptosis, differentiation, and possibly vasodilatation, offering therapeutic targets for the treatment of cardiovascular diseases.[76] An increase in the concentration of AT_1 receptors and a decrease in the concentration of AT_2 receptors are associated with more hypertensive renal injury in rodents.[77]

Gene Targeting of Angiotensin Receptors
Other Angiotensin II Receptors

There are two other receptors for Ang II. The AT_3 receptor represents an angiotensin-binding site identified in a mouse neuroblastoma cell line.[65] The AT_3 receptor has a high affinity for Ang II but a low affinity for Ang III. The AT_4 receptor is an angiotensin-binding site with a high affinity for Ang IV.[44,62,78] Unlike the AT_1 and AT_2 receptors, the AT_4 receptor is not coupled to heterotrimeric G proteins and has been identified as an insulin-regulated transmembrane aminopeptidase (IRAP). A unique binding site for the heptapeptide Ang 1–7 (formed by the action of ACE2 on Ang I), Mas receptor, has also been identified.

Renin Receptors

The recent discovery of the renin receptors has added another layer of complexity to our understanding of the scope and extent of the RAAS. Circulating levels of prorenin are 10 times higher than levels of renin. The PRR, so called because it binds to renin and prorenin, regulates intracellular profibrotic and cyclooxygenase genes independent of Ang II. The binding affinity of prorenin for the PRR is two to three times the affinity of renin for the PRR.[79] The PRR appears to have catalytic (generation of Ang II) and noncatalytic signal transduction effects (which lead to hypertension and glomerulosclerosis). Furthermore, the myriad intracellular signaling pathways mediated by this receptor may hold the key to the mechanisms underlying important developmental processes and the progression of diseases such as hypertension and diabetes.[80] For example, ablation of the prorenin *ATP6ap2* gene results in embryonic lethality.[81,82] By associating with vacuolar H+-ATPase, the PRR is essential for the Wnt/ß catenin signaling molecular pathways, now known to be responsible for neural and renal embryonic development (Fig. 10-3).[83-85]

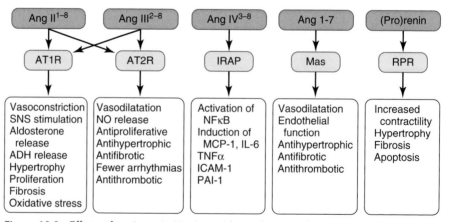

Figure 10-3 Effects of angiotensin (Ang) peptides and renin and prorenin mediated by their corresponding receptors.[230]
ADH, antidiuretic hormone; ICAM-1, intercellular adhesion molecule 1; IRAP, insulin-regulated aminopeptidase; MAS; MCP, monocyte chemotactic protein; NO, nitric oxide; PAI-1, plasminogen activator inhibitor 1; RPR, prorenin receptor; SNS, sympathetic nervous system; TNF-α, tumor necrosis factor α. (From Fyhrquist F, Saijonmaa O. Renin-angiotensin system revisited. *J Intern Med.* 264(3):224-236, 2008.)

Physiologic Effects of Angiotensin II

Via the Angiotensin$_1$ Receptor

Ang II exerts most of its physiologic effects via the AT$_1$ receptor. Ang II has pleiotropic actions,[86] including direct and indirect vasopressor effects. In response to sodium depletion, hypotension, or hypovolemia, Ang II is formed, which causes immediate vasoconstriction of arteries and veins and activates the sympathetic nervous system, increasing peripheral vascular resistance and venous return, respectively, and raising blood pressure. The effect of Ang II on blood pressure secondary to increased ion transport by the renal tubule is more gradual. Ang II increases sodium and chloride reabsorption directly in several segments of the nephron. In the proximal tubule, low concentrations of Ang II play a central role in ion transport by increasing the activity of luminal NHE, Na-glucose co-transporter,[87] sodium phosphate co-transporter (NaPi-II),[88] and basolateral Na$^+$, K$^+$-ATPase[89,90] and Na$^+$-HCO3$^-$ co-transporter.[91] AT$_1$ receptors stimulate NHE3[92-94] but not NHE2[95] activity in brush-border membranes of renal proximal tubules. High concentrations of Ang II can inhibit proximal tubule sodium transport via the stimulation of PLA2- and cytochrome P450–dependent metabolites of arachidonic acid.[91,95-99] Ang II also affects ion transport in the medullary thick ascending limb of the loop of Henle in a biphasic manner.[100] In this nephron segment, low concentrations of Ang II increase sodium, potassium, and chloride transport by stimulating NHE3 and Na$^+$, K$^+$, 2Cl$^-$ co-transporter activities.[101] The inositol 1,4,5-triphosphate receptor-binding protein released with inositol 1,4,5-trisphosphate is important in the stimulatory effect of Ang II in renal proximal tubules.[102] Ang II stimulates NHE1 activity in the macula densa.[103] Ang II also stimulates amiloride-sensitive Na$^+$ transport (ENaC) in the collecting duct[104] and NHE2 in the distal convoluted tubule, but not in the proximal tubule.[95] All of these effects are mediated by the AT$_1$ receptors.

Via the Angiotensin$_2$ Receptor

The role of AT$_2$ receptors in influencing sodium transport is not well established. AT$_2$ receptors may inhibit sodium transport. As mentioned previously, the natriuresis mediated by the AT$_2$ receptor occurs because of its interaction with Ang III.[66] AT$_2$ receptors are coupled to the sodium/hydrogen exchanger type 6 (NHE6),[105] but NHE6 is not involved in sodium reabsorption.[106] Ang (1–7) has been reported to inhibit Na$^+$, K$^+$-ATPase in pig outer cortical nephrons[107] and Na$^+$-HCO$_3^-$ exchanger in mouse renal proximal tubules.[108] However, an increase in sodium transport via AT$_2$ receptors in rat proximal tubules has also been reported.[109] These discrepancies may be related to the condition of the animal. For example, AT$_2$ receptors inhibit Na$^+$, K$^+$-ATPase activity in renal proximal tubules of obese but not lean rats[110] and during AT$_1$ receptor blockade.[111]

Ang II indirectly increases sodium transport, partly by stimulating the synthesis of aldosterone in the zona glomerulosa of the adrenal cortex. Aldosterone increases ENaC activity by inducing the transcription of α-ENaC and redistribution of α-ENaC in the connecting tubule and collecting duct from a cytoplasmic to an apical location. However, Ang II can stimulate the expression of α, β, and γ ENaC independent of aldosterone.[112] Aldosterone also activates Na$^+$, K$^+$-ATPase in the basolateral membrane of the principal cells of the collecting duct. Aldosterone, similar to Ang II, can act in an autocrine and paracrine manner. Aldosterone has been reported to be produced by aldosterone-producing cells other than the adrenal glomerulosa, such as neuronal glial cells and cardiac myocytes.[113] Aldosterone can also stimulate NHE1 activity in the renal proximal tubule of spontaneously hypertensive (SHR), but not normotensive Wistar-Kyoto rats.[52] Evidence suggests that aldosterone and Ang II may act in ligand-independent ways to affect cell signaling, cell–cell communication, and growth. Some components of the RAS may have effects opposite those of aldosterone and among the products of the RAS and their receptors.[114] Although the AT$_1$ receptors can be stimulated by stretch, independent of Ang II,[115,116] Ang II can have intracellular effects independent of the AT$_1$ receptors.[117]

Concepts and Controversies in Our Current Understanding of the Renal Effects of the Renin–Angiotensin–Aldosterone System in Maintaining Fluid and Electrolyte Homeostasis and Blood Pressure

Feedback mechanisms in the kidney contribute to the maintenance of renal blood flow (RBF) and glomerular filtration rate (GFR) in the face of fluctuations in blood pressure. This phenomenon of renal autoregulation was first recognized as early as 1931.[118] In some animals, autoregulation of RBF is negligible at birth.[119] In primates, in the immediate neonatal period, autoregulation of RBF is present, but autoregulation of blood flow to other organs, such as the brain, myocardium, and intestines, is not observed.[120] Autoregulation of RBF is observed in canine puppies as young as 14 days of age.[121] However the set point is lower, and the efficiency of autoregulation is less in younger than in older puppies.

Autoregulation is achieved by the interplay of two mechanisms: (1) tubuloglomerular feedback (TGF), which involves a flow-dependent signal from the macula densa and alteration of afferent arteriolar tone that is mediated by adenosine, adenosine triphosphate (ATP), or both,[122-125] and (2) myogenic response, which involves direct vasoconstriction of the afferent arteriole in response to increased transmural pressure.[124] These two mechanisms act in concert to prevent acute fluctuations in RBF and GFR in response to changes in blood pressure (Fig. 10-2).

Recent studies challenge preexisting concepts and merit discussion. Glomerulotubular balance (GTB) is a negative feedback loop that occurs when proximal tubular reabsorption of sodium and water increases in response to increased GFR[126] and vice versa. Thus, GTB affects distal sodium delivery and, consequently, TGF. TGF and GTB may be more critical in the regulation of renal function in neonates than in adults because sodium intake is low in newborns and therefore sodium balance must be tightly regulated to achieve the net positive balance required for growth. Recent advances in our understanding of GTB, specifically in neonates, are discussed next.

Ontogeny

Development of the Renin–Angiotensin–Aldosterone System: Structure of the Kidney and Urinary Tract

Studies in Humans

In humans, Ang-related genes are activated at stage 11 of the developing embryo,[127] which corresponds to 23 to 24 days of gestation. AT_1 and AT_2 receptors are expressed very early (24 days of gestation), indicating that Ang II may play a role in organogenesis. Whereas the AT_1 receptor is expressed in the glomeruli, the AT_2 receptor is found in the undifferentiated mesonephros that surrounds the primitive tubules and glomeruli. The AT_2 receptor is maximally expressed at about 8 weeks of gestation followed by decreasing but persistent expression until about 20 weeks of gestation.[128] At stage 12 to 13, which corresponds to 25 to 29 days of gestation, angiotensinogen is expressed in the proximal part of the primitive tubule, and renin is expressed in glomeruli and JG arterioles. ACE is detected in the mesonephric tubules at stage 14. By 30 to 35 days, all components of the RAAS are expressed in the human embryonic mesonephros. Expression of these proteins in the future collecting system occurs later, at about 8 weeks of gestation.

ACE has a role in fetal growth and development. ACE inhibitor–induced fetopathy, consisting of oligohydramnios, IUGR, hypocalvaria, renal dysplasia, anuria, and death, has been described in mothers exposed to ACE inhibitors during the second and third trimesters of pregnancy.[129] These effects were initially believed to arise from a decrease in organ perfusion.[130] More recent evidence indicates that ACE inhibition has teratogenic effects during development. Fetuses exposed to ACE inhibitors during the first trimester have an increased risk of congenital malformations, with an incidence of 7.1%, compared with those with no maternal exposure to antihypertensive medications during the same time period. The congenital anomalies are major and include cardiovascular defects such as atrial septal defect, patent ductus arteriosus, ventricular septal defect, and pulmonary stenosis; skeletal malformations, including polydactyly, upper limb defects, and craniofacial anomalies; gastrointestinal malformations such as pyloric stenosis and intestinal atresia; central nervous system malformations such as hydrocephalus, spina bifida, and microcephaly; and genitourinary malformations, including renal malformations.[131] Angiotensin receptor blockers (ARBs) have also been reported to be fetotoxic.[132] Inhibition of the activity of the RAAS in pregnancy may have effects on the fetus that manifest later on in life, such as hypertension, which are addressed later.

The expression patterns of the RAS components in the embryonic kidney are similar in rodents and humans.[127,133] In rodents, mutations of genes encoding renin, angiotensinogen, ACE, or the AT_1 receptor are associated with skull ossification defects[134] as well as autosomal recessive renal tubular dysgenesis.[135-137] AT_1 receptor–deficient mice do not develop a renal pelvis.[135] AT_2 receptor deficient mice have congenital abnormalities of the kidney and urinary tract, such as multicystic dysplastic and aplastic kidneys.[137] The more dramatic phenotypes seen in mice with deficient AT_2 receptor compared with humans with similar defects are attributed to the fact that human nephrogenesis is completed in utero, but maturation of rodent nephrons continues for up to 10 days after birth. However, the phenotypes of AT_1 receptor gene deficiency are similar in rodents and humans. As indicated earlier, mutations in Ang-related genes in humans are associated with renal tubular dysgenesis[136] characterized by early onset and persistent fetal anuria leading to oligohydramnios and the Potter sequence. Whereas increased renin production is noted in the kidneys of patients with mutations in the genes encoding angiotensinogen, ACE, or AT_1 receptor, the effect of defects in the human renin gene (*REN*) on renin production is variable with loss of function mutation associated with absence of renin production, and *REN* missense mutations are associated with increased renin production.[138] These studies demonstrate the importance of the RAAS in the development and maturation of the kidneys and collecting systems.[139] The importance of the PRR in embryonic development has been discussed previously.

Postnatal Changes in Renin–Angiotensin–Aldosterone System Structure and Function in Humans

The RAAS is more active in the neonatal period and infancy than later in childhood.[140] Plasma renin activity and plasma aldosterone levels are markedly increased in preterm human infants in the first 3 weeks of life.[141] Although fetal ACE levels remain stable during gestation in rats,[142] serum ACE activity has been reported by some to be higher in late fetal than in early neonatal life in humans,[142-144] lambs, and guinea pigs.[145,146] In contrast, renal ACE activity may increase with age, at least in pigs and horses.[147,148] A similar pattern may be found in humans based on measurement of urine ACE isoforms.[149] One study reported that plasma Ang II levels are similar among human infants with normal and low birth weights. However, at 7 days of life, plasma Ang II levels are markedly increased in very low birth weight infants.[150] Small for gestational age boys (8–13 years) may have increased circulating Ang II and ACE activity relative to those with birth weights appropriate for gestational age.[151] High serum aldosterone levels are seen at 2 hours of age and gradually decrease over the first year of life.[152]

Sodium Homeostasis in the Neonatal Period

Sodium intake is low in infants compared with adults because milk is a poor source of sodium. However, a positive balance of sodium in neonates is needed to sustain growth in contrast to normal adults, who are in neutral sodium balance. The kidney of a full-term infant filters 4% to 5% of the volume of plasma filtered by an adult (120 mL/min/1.73m^2). Despite the relative paucity of sodium transporters, full-term neonates do retain sodium, partly because of the low GFR.[3] Although the expression of renal sodium transporters is reduced, neonates cannot excrete a sodium load compared with adults. This has been attributed to the increased activity of agents that increase sodium reabsorption in the neonatal period, including the RAAS and α-adrenergic receptors.[153] Endogenous Ang II inhibits the natriuresis of acute volume expansion in neonatal rats.[154] The decreased effects of natriuretic factors (e.g., atrial natriuretic peptide, dopamine, NO) in term neonates compared with adults may also impair the ability to excrete a sodium load.[155-157] Water transport across the proximal tubule also differs in adults and neonates. The renal tubules transport water via water channels called aquaporins (which belong to the category of nonsolute carrier-related genes). There are at least 13 members of the aquaporin family. These are present in very low concentrations in the neonatal nephron. However, water is transported effectively in the neonatal nephron by paracellular and transmembrane mechanisms and by passage through non-aquaporin channels to maintain GTB (see later discussion).[158] The expression of some aquaporins (e.g., aquaporin 2) increases with age, an effect that is mediated by glucocorticoids,[159] while the expression of others, such as aquaporin 3 and aquaporin 4, is not developmentally regulated).[160]

Development of Tubuloglomerular Feedback

Growth and maturation affect the influence of distal ion delivery on the sensors of the macula densa in producing a vascular response. TGF responses are operative in neonatal rats as early as 3.5 weeks of age.[158] However, the inflection point for TGF is different between younger and older rats. Connexin 40, which is important in the formation of gap junctions facilitating intercellular communication in vascular tissue, has been shown to mediate the TGF contribution to the autoregulation of RBF.[161] Extracellular fluid volume and dietary protein affect the TGF response profoundly. The effect of dietary protein on the TGF response varies in different studies, with high-protein diets stimulating or blunting the TGF response.

Despite a lower GFR, urinary sodium losses are highest in the most premature babies, and fractional sodium excretion (FE_{Na}) is inversely related to gestational age. The renal sodium loss in prematurity appears partly to result from the immaturity of the TGF mechanism. Postnatal age has been shown to have an independent effect on FE_{Na} but not on GFR. These findings indicate that in infants of greater than 33 weeks' gestation, sodium conservation is possible because of adequate TGF. The rapid increase in sodium reabsorption in the first few days of postnatal life seems to be attributable to maturation of distal tubular function. Although this was initially attributed to aldosterone,[162] the decreased amount of transporters that are targets of aldosterone makes this mechanism unlikely. An increase in maturation of the Na^+, K^+-ATPase in the distal tubule and a decrease in extracellular fluid volume may be contributory factors to the postnatal increase of sodium transport in the distal tubule.

Development of Glomerulotubular Balance

The essential regulatory mechanisms of tubule transport include GTB and neural and hormonal factors such as sympathetic innervation, Ang II, endothelin, parathormone, and other mediators. As defined earlier, GTB is the capacity of each segment of the nephron to reabsorb a constant fraction of the GFR and is influenced by peritubular and intratubular capillary pressures and GFR.[163] The capacity of the proximal tubule to reabsorb sodium, chloride and water, bicarbonate, glucose, and organic substances is adjusted to GFR: the higher the GFR, the greater the reabsorption. The underlying physical mechanism of GTB is a flow-dependent reabsorption of ions and water across the renal proximal tubular luminal membrane in response to changes in GFR that is independent of neural and hormonal systems. Maintenance of GTB is influenced by flow rate, substrate delivery, and other unknown systems. It is signaled by the hydrodynamic torque (bending movement) on epithelial microvilli.[164] Increases in luminal diameter have the effect of blunting the impact of flow velocity on microvillous shear stress and thus on microvillous torque. Variations in microvillous torque produce nearly identical fractional changes in sodium reabsorption. Furthermore, the flow-dependent sodium transport is enhanced by increasing luminal fluid viscosity, diminished in NHE3 knockout mice, and abolished by nontoxic disruption of the actin cytoskeleton. These data suggest that the "brush-border" microvilli serve a mechanosensory function wherein fluid dynamic torque is transmitted to the actin cytoskeleton to modulate sodium absorption in renal proximal tubules.

Clinical studies have been conducted to study GTB in term and preterm human infants, which suggest that GTB is operational from about 33 weeks of gestational age.[163] In a study of 70 infants of gestational ages 27 to 40 weeks and postnatal ages 3 to 68 days, 24-hour sodium balance studies and creatinine clearance measurements showed that intrauterine and extrauterine existence independently increased the maturation of this function. The incidence of hyponatremia was associated with a negative sodium balance, which varied directly with the degree of prematurity. Indeed, no babies born after 36 weeks were in negative sodium balance. Thus, it appears that GTB is maintained during development by proportional maturation of GFR and tubular reabsorptive mechanisms.[165]

Current Concepts and Controversies

The changes in preglomerular resistance that regulate RBF and GFR in the face of changing blood pressure are attributed to TGF and the renal myogenic response acting in concert, as mentioned earlier. This is the classic paradigm. However, over the past 20 years, the importance of TGF and renal autoregulation in the regulation of renal function has been amended, and the role of the myogenic response as a renoprotective mechanism to prevent renal damage caused by increased blood pressure has been demonstrated. There is also purported to be a "third mechanism" that constitutes a feedback loop occurring in response to increased sodium delivery to the connecting tubule (connecting tubule glomerular feedback [CTGF]) and causing renal afferent arteriolar dilatation to enhance glomerular filtration.[166,167]

Evidence indicates that renal protection against changes in pressure and flow is lost when autoregulation fails.[168,169] The changes in glomerular capillary pressure to maintain GFR at a relatively constant level in the face of increasing or decreasing blood pressure are different from the vascular response needed to reduce GFR to limit pressure-induced increases, which cause renal injury. Thus, TGF and the myogenic response occur at different levels and may have different goals in the balance between renal autoregulation and renal protection. Classic studies in the two-kidney, one-clip model of hypertension[170,171] were followed by studies in the uninephrectomized deoxycorticosterone acetate (DOCA) salt model of malignant nephrosclerosis,[172] confirming the damage engendered by a dilated renal vascular bed in the face of hypertension. In a 5/6 ablation model of chronic kidney disease, the loss of autoregulation increases susceptibility to hypertensive renal injury.

There are different requirements for protection versus regulation. The myogenic response, which constricts the afferent arteriole, occurs within 3 to 4 seconds of a change in blood pressure. A TGF response takes up to 20 seconds because it involves the sequence of increased distal delivery, sensing by the macula densa, release of mediator (now presumed to be adenosine or ATP), and generation of arteriolar afferent response.[173] There is a third slower mechanism that is not well defined. Thus, very brief perturbations of blood pressure have insignificant effects on RBF and GFR. Such brief episodes should alter the myogenic response. However, there have been no studies on the effects of spikes in systolic versus spikes in mean arterial blood pressure in generating a renal myogenic response. A delay in the onset of pressure-induced vasoconstriction has been reported in intact kidneys,[174] with a longer delay in vasodilatation induced by decreasing blood pressure in intact kidneys and an even longer delay in hydronephrotic kidneys.

The advocates for TGF as the dominant mechanism argue that because GFR is influenced by several factors, including plasma colloid pressure, proximal tubular pressure, and the filtration coefficient,[175] a vascular response to changes in pressure alone may not be adequate for regulation. TGF, with its response to alteration in distal sodium delivery, may thus play the stronger autoregulatory role; its immediate renoprotective role may be less important.

D

Differentiating these two closely aligned mechanisms is difficult. In Fawn-Hooded rats, Brown-Norway rats, and Dahl salt-sensitive rats, the genetic defect in autoregulation seems to involve the myogenic response, with an intact or even enhanced TGF.[176-178] Studies of renal injury in these models may shed more light on this issue. We do know that humans with uncomplicated, essential hypertension and intact renal autoregulation do not exhibit renal injury.[168,169]

Recent studies have used transfer function analysis from arterial pressure to RBF in the frequency domain to evaluate the independent contributions of the myogenic response and TGF. This method allows the studying of the mechanisms underlying dynamic autoregulation of RBF in physiologic and pathologic conditions.[179]

If autoregulation is essential for volume homeostasis, one would expect an unequivocal relationship between the two. However, there is little evidence that impaired autoregulation leads to impaired volume homeostasis. Hypertension is not clearly linked to loss of autoregulation. In Brown-Norway rats, administration of DOCA or NaCl has little effect on blood pressure, but is more susceptible to hypertension-induced kidney damage.[180] In ecto-5′ nucleotidase/CD73-deficient mice without the TGF mechanism, no overt volume disturbances are noted.[181] Similarly, if distal delivery is manipulated, such as by the chronic use of loop diuretics, the effects should be catastrophic because these also suppress TGF. However after an initial loss of volume, steady-state adaptations occur within 3 to 4 days. GTB helps in this adjustment.

What is the Physiologic Basis and Purpose, If Any, of the "Third Mechanism?"

Recent research reveals the presence of an in vivo feedback mechanism sensed by the connecting tubule (CTGF), the segment of the nephron between the distal convoluted tubule and the collecting duct, which is close to the vascular pole of the kidney and accompanies the afferent arteriole for varying distances. This mechanism causes afferent arteriolar dilatation in response to increased sodium delivery mediated by ENaC, thus acting in opposition to TGF. Its purpose is speculated to be protection of the kidney from relative ischemia secondary to enhanced metabolic activity during salt loading. In this situation, renal arteriolar dilatation would enhance RBF and prevent ischemia while also enhancing the natriuresis that occurs in response to a salt load. However, this mechanism could also be harmful, as in diabetes mellitus, when the connecting tubule TGF response to osmotic diuresis may increase intraglomerular pressure and perhaps increase glomerular damage.[182]

Mediators and Modulators of Tubuloglomerular Feedback

There are several mediators of the TGF mechanism, which is critical to autoregulation. As defined earlier, TGF is a phenomenon that occurs when changes in tubular ion transport by the macula densa cause reciprocal changes in GFR by alterations in vascular tone, mainly in the afferent arteriole.[125] The initial step in the TGF mechanisms is the sensing of the luminal signal by the Na^+, K^+, $2Cl^-$ co-transporter (NKCC2) at the macula densa (NKCC2A and NKCC2B). The activation of the NKCC2 generates adenosine, which stimulates A_1 adenosine (A_1) receptors, resulting in increased cytosolic calcium. Some investigators have suggested that ATP, activating P2X1 receptors, triggers the increase in cytosolic calcium. The calcium signal is propagated to extraglomerular mesangial cells, constricting vascular smooth muscle cells of the afferent arteriole and decreasing GFR. Renin secretion is also inhibited, which allows recovery of arteriolar flow and GFR. TGF is absent in A_1 receptor knockout mice.[183] In contrast, TGF response persists in mice in which ACE, AT_1 receptor, NOS1, or the thromboxane receptor gene is disrupted.[184] Whereas vasoconstrictors, such as Ang II, increase the sensitivity of the TGF response, vasodilators, such as NO blunt the response.[125] These studies indicate that TGF is modulated by Ang II, arachidonic acid metabolites, and NO; the primary mediators are adenosine, ATP, or both.

Adenosine

Studies in cd73-/- mice, which cannot generate ATP or adenosine, suggest that a humoral factor, adenosine, mediates the TGF response.[181] Thus, a lack of adenosine abrogates the change in GFR engendered by TGF, but does not affect distal reabsorption of sodium and water along the tubule, likely mediated by aldosterone.[185] The cells of the macula densa are important in the TGF mechanism by sensing increased NaCl delivery to the distal tubule and activation of NKCC2 activity to reduce GFR with adenosine via the A_1 adenosine receptor most likely being the mediator of this response. Indeed, TGF is absent in A_1 adenosine receptor knockout mice[183-185] and enhanced by vascular overexpression of the A_1 adenosine receptor.[122] In anesthetized wild-type and A_1 adenosine receptor knockout mice, GFR and RBF were measured before and after reducing renal perfusion pressure by a suprarenal aortic clamp. A reduction in blood pressure produced a significantly greater decrease in GFR in A_1 adenosine receptor knockout mice compared with the wild type, indicating reduced regulatory responses in the knockout mice. This suggests that deficient autoregulation in the absence of the effector adenosine or A_1 adenosine receptor is mediated by abrogation of the TGF response. The administration of the highly selective adenosine 1 receptor antagonist CVT-124 results in marked diuresis and natriuresis, which are accompanied by a reduction in absolute proximal tubular reabsorption.[186] There is no corresponding decrease in GFR, indicating a blunted response of the macula densa to increased distal delivery of sodium chloride. These data provide additional support for adenosine being the mediator of the TGF response.

While adenosine can mediate the TGF response via activation of A_1 adenosine receptors in the afferent arteriole, both A_1 and A_2 adenosine receptors can regulate preglomerular resistance. A_2 adenosine receptors modulate the response by opposing the effects of the A_1 adenosine receptors. A_{2A} adenosine receptors counter the TGF response by the stimulation of the activity of endothelial NO synthase (eNOS or NOS3).[187,188] The lack of regulation of proximal tubular transport in A_1 adenosine receptor knockout mice and with A_1 adenosine receptor blockade could be indicative of adenosine being also a player in GTB in addition to the known and accepted peritubular, luminal, and oncotic factors that regulate it. Although the mechanism underlying the increased formation of adenosine, in response to an increase in NKCC2 activity, remains to be determined, it is evident from studies of genetically altered mice that transcellular sodium transport regulates the generation of adenosine, which together with Ang II causes the vasoconstriction that is the hallmark of TGF.[189]

Adenosine Triphosphate

Nishiyama and Navar[190] present evidence implicating ATP as the mediator of the TGF response. Their conclusion is based up on the finding that ATP selectively affects renal afferent arteriolar tone, the presence of ATP-specific receptors P2X1 in the renal afferent arteriole, the absence of the TGF response in mice lacking the P2X1 receptor, and the ability of ATP to stimulate directly the L-type voltage gated calcium channel, leading to calcium influx and vascular smooth muscle cell contraction.[191] More recent studies support ATP as the mediator of TGF based on the finding that an ATP conducting maxi-anion channel in the basolateral cells of the macula densa, likely a chloride channel, opens in response to increasing levels of luminal sodium chloride.[192] ATP may also mediate efferent arteriolar TGF through its metabolite adenosine in the presence of calcium ions.[193]

Nitric Oxide

NO, derived from arginine, modulates TGF. Neuronal NOS (nNOS, NOS1) is expressed in the macula densa.[194] Other NOS isoforms may be expressed in the mesangium and glomerular microvessels. These enzymes are strategically positioned to influence each step of the TGF process.[195] However, micropuncture studies using NOS antagonists have shown that NO does not mediate TGF. Instead, local NOS blockade causes the TGF curve to shift leftward and become steeper. Changes in

NO production in the macula densa may underlie the resetting of TGF, which is needed to maintain the TGF curve so that it adapts to different conditions of ambient tubular flow to accommodate physiologic circumstances and maintain homeostasis. Also, macula densa NO production may be substrate limited and dissociated from NOS protein content. The importance of NO to TGF resetting and the substrate dependence of NO production have both been found during changes in dietary salt.[196] Changes in nNOS or NOS1 function have been shown to occur in the JGA of the SHR.[197] NOS inhibition has a reduced effect on TGF in the SHR.[194] The study of salt-sensitive splice variants of nNOS suggests that increased levels of nNOS-β increase macula densa NO and are responsible for the attenuated TGF response during high salt intake.[198]

Reactive Oxygen Species

ROS and ongoing oxidative stress are increasingly implicated in the pathophysiology of vascular changes in many diseases, including hypertension. AT$_1$ receptors increase the sensitivity of the TGF response that could also be related to ROS. Although the superoxide anion may lead to vasoconstriction and an increase in myogenic tone, directly, it also influences vasoconstriction and vasodilatation via many signaling pathways as a consequence of TGF. These effects occur because of changes in macula densa cell function in response to changes in sodium chloride delivery to the distal tubule. The macula densa expresses nNOS[194,199] which is activated during sodium chloride reabsorption and has a vasodilatory effect; this blunts the vasoconstriction caused by the TGF in response to increased sodium chloride transport. Oxygen radicals enhance the TGF response and limit NO signaling from the macula densa.[200] ROS react with NO, producing peroxynitrite, which impairs vasorelaxation and promotes hypertrophy.[201-203] Therefore, ROS effectively counteracts the vasodilatory effects of NO. The vasoconstrictor effect of ROS is presumably exerted by superoxide because increasing its dismutation by superoxide dismutase mimetics prevents the vasoconstrictor effect.[125] However, the role of other ROS on TGF remains to be clarified. H$_2$O$_2$ can have both vasodilatory and vasoconstrictor effects.

The interaction between NO and superoxide anion has been studied in microperfusion experiments. The infusion of a NO precursor into the macula densa caused a graded reduction in the TGF-mediated afferent arteriolar vasoconstriction; this response was more pronounced in normotensive WKY rats than SHR rats.[204] The thick ascending limb of the loop of Henle also produces NO because it expresses eNOS/NOS3.[195,198] NO decreases net absorption of chloride and bicarbonate in the isolated thick ascending limb,[204] thus indirectly decreasing the TGF response by increasing their delivery to the distal tubule. Superoxide anion activates 5′-nucleotidase, thereby increasing adenosine (a mediator of TGF) generation in the kidney. These studies support the notion that superoxide enhances the sensitivity of TGF.[125]

Sodium Transporters

Sodium Potassium 2 Chloride Co-transporters

TGF begins with sodium chloride entry through the macula densa cells, which express two NKCC2 isoforms (NKCC2A and NKCC2B). These isoforms for NKCC2, with high or low affinity for chloride, enable the TGF response to be spread over a wider range of sodium chloride concentrations.[189] The coexpression of NKCC2A and NKCC2B in the macula densa facilitates salt sensing.[205] Intracellular signaling pathways of salt sensing during low salt are mediated by NKCC2, including the activation of AMP-activated protein kinases in macula densa cells.[206]

Na$^+$, K$^+$-ATPase

Rabbit macula densa cells lack Na$^+$, K$^+$-ATPase; rather, they express colonic H$^+$, K$^+$-ATPase in the apical macula densa. Because H$^+$, K$^+$-ATPase is ouabain sensitive, it may function as Na$^+$, K$^+$-ATPase.[207,208] However, mice lacking ouabain-sensitive α-1 Na$^+$, K$^+$-ATPase do not have TGF response.[209] Moreover, deletion of colonic H-K-ATPase in mice does not impair TGF.[209] Whether or not these discrepancies are attributable to species variation remains to be determined.

Calcium Wave

Intracellular calcium modulates vascular smooth muscle tone and is a negative regulator of renin release. There is evidence for a calcium wave that spreads through the mesangial cell field and constricts the afferent arteriolar smooth muscle cells. It appears that both gap junctional communication (e.g., connexin 40)[162] and extracellular ATP are integral components of the TGF calcium wave. The finding that the calcium wave is generated by ATP but not by adenosine offers a new model for a direct effect of ATP, not necessarily mediated by adenosine, as the final common pathway of changes in vascular tone in response to signals from the JGA and macula densa. A recent study demonstrates this using ratiometric calcium imaging of the in vitro microperfused isolated rabbit JGA–glomerular complex.[210]

New Directions

Unconventional Behavior of Renin–Angiotensin System Components

Although the canonical scheme of activation of the RAS components from renin to Ang II and its effects on Ang receptors is well recognized, recent evidence of other effects merits discussion. Both Ang I and Ang II may lead to effects that are independent of, or even antagonistic to, the accepted effects of the RAS.[114] ACE may also function as a "receptor" that initiates intracellular signaling and influences gene expression.[211] AT$_1$ and AT$_2$ receptors have been shown to form heterodimers with other 7-transmembrane receptors and influence signal transduction pathways.[212-215] Intracellular Ang II affects cell communication, cell growth, and gene expression via the AT$_1$ receptor, but also has independent effects.[115,116,216]

Molecular Mechanisms Underlying Salt Sensing by the Macula Densa

The generation of the prohypertensive agent renin by the cells of the macula densa is the primary event necessary for TGF, and its molecular basis has been elucidated in a recent study. The macula densa responds to changes in intracellular milieu by the accumulation of tubular succinate, which acts via a newly identified receptor GPR91 to initiate the intracellular signaling that ultimately results in renin release and may be the integral event in homeostasis engendered by the RAS.[217]

Fetal Programming for Hypertension: Failure of Renoprotection?

The association of low birth weight with the development of hypertension later in life has been validated epidemiologically[218] and, more recently, has been demonstrated experimentally in animal models.[219] A suboptimal fetal environment may lead to maladaptive responses, including failure of renal autoregulation and the development of hypertension. A reduction in nephron number during development may contribute to a reduction in GFR, but this is not always borne out in experimental studies. Multiple factors may contribute to the development of hypertension, but this review is restricted to the role of renal hemodynamics. The RAAS may play a more important role than other factors because it is expressed early and associated with nephrogenesis. Blockade of the AT$_1$ receptor during the nephrogenic period after birth in rats led to a decrease in nephron number, a reduction in renal function, and hypertension.[220] The consequences of impairment of the RAS in utero and during development have been discussed earlier. Protein-restricted diets have also been shown to increase ACE levels in pregnant ewes.[221] A general stimulation of all components of the systemic RAS, in response to protein restriction, is blocked by treatment with an ACE inhibitor or an AT$_1$ receptor blocker. Thus, the adverse environment in utero, which programs the fetus to develop hypertension, could be critically linked to abnormalities in the RAS.[222] Recent research in fetal programming

D

for atherosclerosis implicates mitochondrial dysfunction as a possible trigger leading to the generation of ROS, which leads to the predisposition to hypertension and atherosclerosis.[223]

Clinical Aspects

As discussed earlier, the development of the kidney occurs during the first 35 days postconception in humans. The integrity of the RAAS is essential for normal development, and Ang II is essential for normal structural development of the kidney and collecting system. The complex interplay of GTB and TGF increases with gestational age. The excretory function of the kidney begins soon after clamping of the umbilical cord at birth. It follows that the neonate is exquisitely sensitive to stressors, which activate the RAAS, and lead to profound oligoanuric states. Disruption of the production or action of Ang II by genetic manipulation or pharmacologic blockade results in renal tubular agenesis and anemia in fetuses. More recently, the recognition of ACE2 as an important player in vasodilation by generation of alternative metabolites of Ang II, has led to the discovery that blunting of ACE2 effect is responsible for the postural orthostatic tachycardia syndrome, a syndrome of widespread vasoconstriction. This is probably the first human illness that is directly related to ACE2 and is applicable to the wider field of disordered vasoregulation, extending to fetal and neonatal life.[32] The recognition of the importance of renin receptor in hypertension has paved the way for the use of new antihypertensive drugs based on their ability to block the renin receptor.[224,225] Ischemia and asphyxia generate renin by sympathetic stimulation. Drugs, such as furosemide, that increase distal delivery of sodium and water, decrease NKCC2 activity and should decrease renin secretion. However, decreased co-transporter activity impairs TGF and in the face of continued ion and water excretion may result in hypovolemia and activation of the RAS and may result in oliguria. Indomethacin, used to treat patent ductus arteriosus in neonates, could lead to altered renal vasoregulation.[226] Congenital abnormalities in steroid synthesis that lead to deficiencies in aldosterone production cause profound salt wasting.[227] In type 1 pseudohypoaldosteronism, mutations in the sodium channel may cause profound neonatal salt wasting.[228] To counter the heightened activity of the RAAS in neonates, adenosine receptor antagonists may offer new avenues of therapy. The association between maternal ACE inhibition and renal abnormalities in fetuses was described earlier in this chapter. Recent observations of increased fetal renin levels in hydronephrosis lend credence to the developmental significance of an intact RAAS in developing embryos.[229]

In summary, the RAAS is an important developmental and physiologic system that contributes to RBF and GFR autoregulation, involving TGF and myogenic response. Together with the myogenic response, TGF serves to maintain volume homeostasis in sodium and volume-depleted states and renoprotection in hypertensive states. The third mechanism (CTGF) of sensing of salt and water balance by the connecting tubule is an important negative modulator of the RAAS, leading to renal afferent artery vasodilatation. Central and peripheral sympathetic inputs influence all aspects of renal autoregulation. The elucidation of molecular events that underlie salt sensing by the macula densa and JG cell offers new avenues for further investigation in the developing kidney. A better understanding of these mechanisms would translate to better care for premature and full-term newborns with renal dysregulation, hyponatremia, and oligoanuric renal failure.

References

1. Guyton AC, Hall JE. Dominant role of the kidney in long-term regulation of arterial pressure and in hypertension: the integrated system for pressure control. In *Textbook of Medical Physiology Tenth Edition*. Philadelphia: W.B. Saunders Company; 2001;201-203.
2. Gomez RA, McReddie TA, Everett AD, et al. Ontogeny of renin and AT1 receptor in the rat. *Pediatr Nephrol*. 1993;7(5):635-638.
3. Chevalier RL. The moth and the aspen tree: sodium in early postnatal development. *Kidney Int*. 2001;59(5):1617-1625.
4. Persson AE, Ollerstam A, Liu R, et al. Mechanisms for macula densa cell release of renin. *Acta Physiol Scand*. 2004;181(4):471-474.

5. Lavoie JL, Sigmund CD. Minireview: overview of the renin-angiotensin system—an endocrine and paracrine system. *Endocrinology*. 2003;144(6):2179-2183.
6. Krieger MH, Moreira ED, Oliveira EM, et al. Dissociation of blood pressure and sympathetic activation of renin release in sinoaortic-denervated rats. *Clin Exp Pharmacol Physiol*. 2006; 33(5-6):471-476.
7. Schweda F, Segerer F, Castrop H, et al. Blood pressure-dependent inhibition of renin secretion requires A1 adenosine receptors. *Hypertension*. 2005;46(4):780-786.
8. Milavec-Krizman M, Evenou JP, Wagner H, et al. Characterization of beta-adrenoceptor subtypes in rat kidney with new highly selective beta 1 blockers and their role in renin release. *Biochem Pharmacol*. 1985;34(22):3951-3957.
9. DiBona GF. Neural regulation of renal tubular sodium reabsorption and renin secretion. *Fed Proc*. 1985;44(13):2816-2822.
10. Goldsmith SR. Interactions between the sympathetic nervous system and the RAAS in heart failure. *Curr Heart Fail Rep*. 2004;1(2):45-50.
11. Bell PD, Lapointe JY, Peti-Peterdi J. Macula densa signaling. *Annu Rev Physiol*. 2003;65:481-500.
12. Lorenz JN, Greenberg SG, Briggs JP. The macula densa mechanism for control of renin secretion. *Semin Nephrol*. 1993;13(6):531-542.
13. Bie P, Damkjaer M. Renin secretion and total body sodium: pathways of integrative control. *Clin Exp Pharmacol Physiol*. 2010;37(2):e34-42.
14. Danser AH, van den Dorpel MA, Deinum J, et al. Renin, prorenin, and immunoreactive renin in vitreous fluid from eyes with and without diabetic retinopathy. *J Clin Endocrinol Metab*. 1989;68(1):160–167.
15. Itskovitz J, Sealey JE, Glorioso N, et al. Plasma prorenin response to human chorionic gonadotropin in ovarian-hyperstimulated women: correlation with the number of ovarian follicles and steroid hormone concentrations. *Proc Natl Acad Sci USA*. 1987;84(20):7285–7289.
16. Krop M, Danser AH. Circulating versus tissue renin-angiotensin system: on the origin of (pro)renin. *Curr Hypertens Rep*. 2008;10(2)112–118.
17. Weiland F, Verspohl EJ. Local formation of angiotensin peptides with paracrine activity by adipocytes. *J Pept Sci*. 2009;15(11):767–776.
18. Gálvez-Prieto B, Bolbrinker J, Stucchi P, et al. Comparative expression analysis of the renin-angiotensin system components between white and brown perivascular adipose tissue. *J Endocrinol*. 2008;197(1):55–64.
19. Sealey JE, Goldstein M, Pitarresi T, et al. Prorenin secretion from human testis: no evidence for secretion of active renin or angiotensinogen. *J Clin Endocrinol Metab*. 1988;66(5):974–978.
20. Danser AH, Deinum J. Renin, prorenin and the putative (pro)renin receptor. *Hypertension*. 2005;46(5):1069–1076.
21. Gavras I, Gavras H. Angiotensin II as a cardiovascular risk factor. *J Hum Hypertens*. 2002;16(Suppl 2):S2-S6.
22. Danilczyk U, Penninger JM. Angiotensin-converting enzyme II in the heart and kidney. *Circ Res*. 2006;98(4):463-471.
23. Erdos EG. Conversion of angiotensin I to angiotensin II. *Am J Med*. 1976;60:749-759.
24. Urata H, Nishimura H, Ganten D. Mechanisms of angiotensin II formation in humans. *Eur Heart J*. 1995;16(Suppl N):79-85.
25. Le TH, Coffman TM. A new cardiac MASTer switch for the renin-angiotensin system. *J Clin Invest*. 2006;116(4):866-869.
26. Wei CC, Hase N, Inoue Y, et al. Mast cell chymase limits the cardiac efficacy of Ang I-converting enzyme inhibitor therapy in rodents. *J Clin Invest*. 2010;120(4):1229-1239.
27. Bot I, Bot M, van Heiningen SH, van Santbrink, et al. Mast cell chymase inhibition reduces atherosclerotic plaque progression and improves plaque stability in ApoE-/- mice. *Cardiovasc Res*. 2011;89(1):244-252.
28. Burns KD. The emerging role of angiotensin-converting enzyme-2 in the kidney. *Curr Opin Nephrol Hypertens*. 2007;16(2):116-121.
29. Yamamuro M, Yoshimura M, Nakayama M, et al. Aldosterone, but not angiotensin II, reduces angiotensin converting enzyme 2 gene expression levels in cultured neonatal rat cardiomyocytes. *Circ J*. 2008;72(8):1346-1350.
30. Chappel MC, Ferrario CM. ACE and ACE2: their role to balance the expression of angiotensin II and angiotensin-(1-7). *Kidney Int*. 2006;70(1):34-41.
31. Donoghue M, Hsieh F, Baronas E, et al. A novel angiotensin-converting enzyme-related carboxypeptidase (ACE2) converts angiotensin I to angiotensin 1-9. *Circ Res*. 2000;87(5):E1-E9.
32. Stewart JM, Ocon AJ, Clarke D, et al. Defects in cutaneous angiotensin-converting enzyme 2 and angiotensin-(1-7) production in postural tachycardia syndrome. *Hypertension*. 2009;53(5): 767-774.
33. Ferrario CM. ACE2: more of Ang-(1-7) or less Ang II? *Curr Opin Nephrol Hypertens*. 2010;20(1):1-6.
34. Kokkonen JO, Saarinen J, Kovanen PT. Regulation of local angiotensin II formation in the human heart in the presence of interstitial fluid. Inhibition of chymase by protease inhibitors of interstitial fluid and of angiotensin-converting enzyme by Ang-(1-9) formed by heart carboxypeptidase A-like activity. *Circulation*. 1997;95(6):1455-1463.
35. Snyder RA, Watt KW, Wintroub BU. A human platelet angiotensin I-processing system. Identification of components and inhibition of angiotensin-converting enzyme by product. *J Biol Chem*. 1985;260(13):7857-7860.

10

36. Ocaranza MP, Godoy I, Jalil JE, et al. Enalapril attenuates downregulation of Angiotensin-converting enzyme 2 in the late phase of ventricular dysfunction in myocardial infracted heart. *Hypertension.* 2006;48(4):572-578.
37. Ocaranza MP, Lavandero S, Jalil JE, et al. Angiotensin-(1-9) regulates cardiac hypertrophy in vivo and in vitro. *J Hypertens.* 2010;28(5):1054-1064.
38. Kramkowski K, Mogielnicki A, Leszczynska A, et al. Angiotensin-(1-9), the product of angiotensin I conversion in platelets, enhances arterial thrombosis in rats. *J Physiol Pharmacol.* 2010;61(3): 317-324.
39. Kucharewicz I, Pawlak R, Matys T, et al. Antithrombotic effect of captopril and losartan is mediated by angiotensin-(1-7). *Hypertension.* 2002;40(5):774-779.
40. Velez JC, Ryan KJ, Harbeson CE, et al. Angiotensin I is largely converted to angiotensin (1-7) and angiotensin (2-10) by isolated rat glomeruli. *Hypertension.* 2009;53(5):790-797.
41. Pereira HJ, Souza LL, Salgado MC, et al. Angiotensin processing is partially carried out by carboxy-peptidases in the rat mesenteric arterial bed perfusate. *Regul Pept.* 2008;151(1-3):135-138.
42. Veerasingham SJ, Raizada MK. Brain renin-angiotensin system dysfunction in hypertension: recent advances and perspectives. *Br J Pharmacol.* 2003;139(2):191-202.
43. Padia SH, Howell NL, Kemp BA, et al. Intrarenal aminopeptidase N inhibition restores defective angiotensin II type 2-mediated natriuresis in spontaneously hypertensive rats. *Hypertension.* 2010; 55(2):474-480.
44. Chai SY, Fernando R, Peck G, et al. The angiotensin IV/AT4 receptor. Cell Mol; *Life Sci.* 2004;61(21): 2728-2737.
45. Saavedra JM, Ando H, Armando I, et al. Brain angiotensin II, an important stress hormone: regula-tory sites and therapeutic opportunities. *Ann N Y Acad Sci.* 2004;1018:76-84.
46. Grobe JL, Grobe CL, Beltz TG, et al. The brain renin-angiotensin system controls divergent efferent mechanisms to regulate fluid and energy balance. *Cell Metab.* 2010;12(5):431-442.
47. Cuadra AE, Shan Z, Sumners C. A current view of brain renin-angiotensin system: Is the (pro)renin receptor the missing link? *Pharmacol Ther.* 2010;125(1):27-38.
48. Romero DG, Plonczynski M, Vergara GR, et al. Angiotensin II early regulated genes in H295R human adrenocortical cells. *Physiol Genomics.* 2004;19(1):106-116.
49. Delcayre C, Swynghedauw B. Molecular mechanisms of myocardial remodeling. The role of aldo-sterone. *J Mol Cell Cardiol.* 2002;34(12):1577-1584.
50. Colombo L, Dala Valle L, Fiore C, et al. Aldosterone and the conquest of land. *J Endocrinol Invest.* 2006;29(4):373-379.
51. Chai W, Hofland J, Jansen PM, et al. Steroidogenesis vs. steroid uptake in the heart: do corticoste-roids mediate effects via cardiac mineralocorticoid receptors? *J Hypertens.* 2010;28(5):1044-1053.
52. Pinto V, Pinho MJ, Hopfer U, et al. Oxidative stress and the genomic regulation of aldosterone-stimulated NHE1 activity in SHR renal proximal tubular cells. *Mol Cell Biochem.* 2008;310(1-2): 191-201.
53. Sherrod M, David DR, Zhou X, et al. Glial-specific ablation of angiotensinogen lowers arterial pres-sure in renin and angiotensin transgenic mice. *Am J Physiol Regul Integr Comp Physiol.* 2005;289(6): R1763-R1769.
54. Wagner J, Thiele F, Ganten D. The renin-angiotensin system in transgenic rats. *Pediatr Nephrol.* 1996;10(1):108-112.
55. Vernerová Z, Kujal P, Kramer HJ, et al. End-organ damage in hypertensive transgenic Ren-2 rats: influence of early and late endothelin receptor blockade. *Physiol Res.* 2009;58(Suppl 2):S69-S78.
56. Esther CR Jr, Howard TE, Marino EM, et al. Mice lacking angiotensin-converting enzyme have low blood pressure, renal pathology, and reduced male fertility. *Lab Invest.* 1996;74(5):953-965.
57. Bernstein KE. Views of the renin-angiotensin system: brilling, mimsy and slithy tove. *Hypertension.* 2006;47(3):509-514.
58. Martin M, Wellner A, Ossowski I, et al. Identification and quantification of inhibitors for angiotensin-converting enzyme in hypoallergenic infant milk formulas. *J Agric Food Chem.* 2008;56(15): 6333-6338.
59. Yamamoto K, Ohishi M, Katsuya T, et al. Deletion of angiotensin-converting enzyme 2 accelerates pressure overload-induced cardiac dysfunction by increasing local angiotensin II. *Hypertension.* 2006;47(4):718-726.
60. Crackower MA, Sarao R, Oudit GY, et al. Angiotensin-converting enzyme 2 is an essential regulator of heart function. *Nature.* 2002;417(6891):822-828.
61. Shaltout HA, Figueroa JP, Rose JC, et al. Alterations in circulatory and renal angiotensin-converting enzyme and angiotensin-converting enzyme 2 in fetal programmed hypertension. *Hypertension.* 2009;53(2):404-408.
62. Davis CJ, Kramár EA, De A, et al. AT4 receptor activation increases intracellular calcium influx and induces a non-N-methyl-D-aspartate dependent form of long-term potentiation. *Neuroscience.* 2006;137(4):1369-1379.
63. Crowley SD, Tharaux PL, Audoly LP, et al. Exploring type I angiotensin (AT1) receptor functions through gene targeting. *Acta Physiol Scand.* 2004;181(4):561-567.
64. Mifune M, Sasamura H, Nakazato Y, et al. Examination of Ang II type 1 and type 2 receptor expres-sion in human kidneys by immunohistochemistry. *Clin Exp Hypertens.* 2001;23(3):257-266.
65. Chaki S, Inagami T. Identification and characterization of a new binding site for angiotensin II in mouse neuroblastoma neuro-2A cells. *Biochem Biophys Res Commun.* 1992;182(1):388-394.
66. Padia SH, Kemp BA, Howell NL, et al. Conversion of renal angiotensin II to angiotensin III is critical for AT2 receptor-mediated natriuresis in rats. *Hypertension.* 2008;51(2):460-465.

67. Dellis O, Dedos SG, Tovey SC, et al. Ca2+ entry through plasma membrane IP3 receptors. *Science.* 2006;313:229-233.
68. Yu L, Zheng M, Wang W, et al. Developmental changes in AT1 and AT2 receptor-protein expression in rats. *J Renin Angiotensin Aldosterone Syst.* 2010;11(4):214-221.
69. Gill DL, Spassova MA, Soboloff J. Signal transduction. Calcium entry signals–trickles and torrents. *Science.* 2006;313(5784):183-184.
70. Sandberg K, Ji H. Comparative analysis of amphibian and mammalian angiotensin receptors. *Comp Biochem Physiol A Mol Integr Physiol.* 2001;128(1):53-75.
71. Wynne BM, Chiao CW, Webb RC. Vascular smooth muscle cell signaling mechanisms for contraction to angiotensin ii and endothelin-1. *J Am Soc Hypertens.* 2009;3(2):84-95.
72. Kalantarinia K, Okusa MD. The renin-angiotensin system and its blockade in diabetic renal and cardiovascular disease. *Curr Diab Rep.* 2006;6(1):8-16.
73. Nishida M, Kitajima N, Saiki S. Regulation of angiotensin II receptor signaling by cysteine modification of NF-κB. *Nitric Oxide.* 2011;25(2):112-117.
74. De Gasparo M, Catt KJ, Inagami T, et al. International union of pharmacology XXIII. The angiotensin II receptors. *Pharmacol Rev.* 2000;52:415-472.
75. Zhang J, Pratt RE. The AT2 receptor selectively associates with Giα2 and Giα3 in the rat fetus. *J Biol Chem.* 1996;271(25):15026-15033.
76. Stegbauer J, Coffman TM. New insights into angiotensin receptor actions: from blood pressure to aging. *Curr Opin Nephrol Hypertens.* 2011;20(1):84-88.
77. Landgraf SS, Wengert M, Silva JS, et al. Changes in angiotensin receptors expression play a pivotal role in the renal damage observed in spontaneous hypertensive rats. *Am J Physiol Renal Physiol.* 2011;300(2):F499-F510.
78. Albiston AL, McDowall SG, Matsacos D, et al. Evidence that the angiotensin IV (AT4) receptor is the enzyme insulin-regulated aminopeptidase. *J Biol Chem.* 2001;276(520):48623-48626.
79. Batenburg WW, Krop M, Garrelds IM, et al. Prorenin is the endogenous agonist of the (pro)renin receptor. Binding kinetics of renin and prorenin in rat vascular smooth muscle cells overexpressing the human (pro)renin receptor. *J Hypertens.* 2007;25(12):2441–2453.
80. Nguyen G. The (pro)renin receptor: pathophysiological roles in cardiovascular and renal pathology. *Curr Opin Nephrol Hypertens.* 2007;16(2):129–133.
81. Amsterdam A, Nissen RM, Sun Z, et al. Identification of 315 genes essential for early zebrafish development. *Proc Natl Acad Sci USA.* 2004;101(35):12792–12797.
82. Burckle C, Bader M. Prorenin and its ancient receptor. *Hypertension.* 2006;48(4):549–551.
83. Ille F, Sommer L. Wnt signaling: multiple functions in neural development. *Cell Mol Life Sci.* 2005;62(10):1100–1108.
84. Falk S, Wurdak H, Ittner LM, et al. Brain area-specific effect of TGF-beta signaling on Wnt-dependent neural stem cell expansion. *Cell Stem Cell.* 2008;2(5):472-483.
85. Schmidt-Ott KM, Barasch J. WNT/beta-catenin signaling in nephron progenitors and their epithelial progeny. *Kidney Int.* 2008;74(8):1004-1008.
86. Hunyadi L, Catt KJ. Pleiotropic AT1 receptor signaling pathways mediating physiological and pathogenic actions of Ang II. *Mol Endocrinol.* 2006;20(5):953-970.
87. Garvin JL. Angiotensin stimulates glucose and fluid absorption by rat proximal straight tubules. *J Am Soc Nephrol.* 1990;1(3):272-277.
88. Xu L, Dixit MP, Chen R, et al. Effects of angiotensin II on NaPi-IIa co-transporter expression and activity in rat renal cortex. *Biochim Biophys Acta.* 2004;1667(2):114-121.
89. Yingst DR, Massey KJ, Rossi NF, et al. Angiotensin II directly stimulates activity and alters the phosphorylation of Na-K-ATPase in rat proximal tubule with a rapid time course. *Am J Physiol Renal Physiol.* 2004;287(4):F713-F721.
90. Shah S, Hussain T. Enhanced angiotensin II-induced activation of Na+- K+- ATPase in the proximal tubules of obese Zucker rats. *Clin Exp Hypertens.* 2006;28(1):29-40.
91. Horita S, Zheng Y, Hara C. Biphasic regulation of Na+HCO3- cotransporter by angiotensin II type 1A receptor. *Hypertension.* 2002;40(5):707-712.
92. Noonan WT, Woo AL, Nieman ML, et al. Blood pressure maintenance in NHE3-deficient mice with transgenic expression of NHE3 in small intestine. *Am J Physiol Regul Integr Comp Physiol.* 2005;288(3):R685-R691.
93. Kolb RJ, Woost PG, Hopfer U, et al. Membrane trafficking of angiotensin receptor type-1 and mechanochemical signal transduction in proximal tubule cells. *Hypertension.* 2004;44(3):352-359.
94. Quan A, Chakravarty S, Chen JK, et al. Androgens augment proximal tubule transport. *Am J Physiol Renal Physiol.* 2004;287(3):F452-F459.
95. Dixit MP, Xu L, Xu H, et al. Effect of angiotensin II on renal Na+/H+ exchanger-NHE3 and NHE2. *Biochim Biophys Acta.* 2004;1664(1):38-44.
96. Good DW, George T, Wang DH, et al. Angiotensin II inhibits HCO3 absorption via a cytochrome P450 dependent pathway in MTAL. *Am J Physiol.* 1999;276(5pt2):F726-F736.
97. Han HJ, Park SH, Koh HJ, et al. Mechanism of regulation of Na+ transport by angiotensin II in primary renal cells. *Kidney Int.* 2000;57(6):2457-2467.
98. Romero MF, Madhun ZT, Hopfer U, et al. An epoxygenase metabolite of arachidonic acid 5,6 epoxy-eicosatrienoic acid mediates angiotensin-induced natriuresis in proximal tubular epithelium. *Adv Prostaglandin Thromboxane Leukot Res.* 1991;21A:205-208.
99. Romero MF, Hopfer U, Madhun ZT, et al. Angiotensin II actions in the rabbit proximal tubule. Angiotensin II mediated signaling mechanisms and electrolyte transport in the rabbit proximal tubule. *Ren. Physiol Biochem.* 1991;14(4-5):191-207.

100. Houillier P, Chambrey R, Achard JM, et al. Signaling pathways in the biphasic effect of angiotensin II on apical Na/H antiport activity in proximal tubule. *Kidney Int.* 1996;50(5):1496-1505.

101. Kwon TH, Nielsen J, Kim H, et al. Regulation of sodium transporters in the thick ascending limb of rat kidney: response to angiotensin II. *Am J Physiol Renal Physiol.* 2003;285(1): F152-F165.

102. He P, Klein J, Yun CC. Activation of Na+/H+ exchanger NHE3 by angiotensin II is mediated by inositol 1,4,5-triphosphate (IP3) receptor-binding protein released with IP3 (IRBIT) and Ca2+/calmodulin-dependent protein kinase II. *J Biol Chem.* 2010;285(36):27869-27878.

103. Bell PD, Peti-Peterdi J. Angiotensin II stimulates macula densa basolateral sodium/hydrogen exchange via type 1 angiotensin II receptors. *J. Am Soc Nephrol.* 1999;10(Suppl 11):S225-S229.

104. Wang T, Geibisch G. Effects of angiotensin II on electrolyte transport in the early and late distal tubule in rat kidney *Am J Physiol.* 1996;271(1 Pt 2):F143-F149.

105. Pulakat L, Cooper S, Knowle D, et al. Ligand-dependent complex formation between the Angiotensin II receptor subtype AT2 and Na+/H+ exchanger NHE6 in mammalian cells. *Peptides.* 2005; 26(5):863-873.

106. Bobulescu IA, Di Sole F, Moe OW. Na+/H+ exchangers; physiology and link to hypertension and organ ischemia. *Curr Opin Nephrol Hypertens.* 2005;14(5):485-494.

107. Lara Lda S, Cavalcante F, Axelband F, et al. Involvement of Gi/o/cGMP/PKG pathway in the AT2-mediated inhibition of outer cortex proximal tubule Na+-ATPase by Ang-(1-7). *Biochem J.* 2006; 395(1):183-190.

108. Haithcock D, Jiao H, Cui XL, et al. Renal proximal tubular AT2 receptor: signaling and transport. *J Am Soc Nephrol.* 1999;10(Supp 11):S69-S74.

109. Quan A, Baum M. Effect of luminal angiotensin II receptor antagonists on proximal tubule transport. *Am J Hypertens.* 1999;12(5):499-503.

110. Hakam AC, Hussain T. Angiotensin II type 2 receptor agonist directly inhibits proximal tubule sodium pump activity in obese but not in lean Zucker rats. *Hypertension.* 2006;47(6):1117-1124.

111. Padia SH, Howell NL, Siragy HM, et al. Renal angiotensin type 2 receptors mediate natriuresis via angiotensin III in the angiotensin II type 1 receptor-blocked rat. *Hypertension.* 2006;47(3): 537-544.

112. Beutler KT, Masilamani S, Turban S, et al. Long-term regulation of ENaC expression in kidney by angiotensin II. *Hypertension.* 2003;41(5):1143-1150.

113. Davies E, McKenzie SM. Extra adrenal production of corticosteroids. *Clin Exp Pharmacol Physiol.* 2003;30(7):437-445.

114. Kurdi M, De Mello WC, Booz GW. Working outside the system: an update on the unconventional behavior of the renin-angiotensin system components. *Int J Biochem Cell Biol.* 2005;37(7):1357-1367.

115. Zou Y, Akazawa H, Qin Y, et al. Mechanical stress activates angiotensin II type 1 receptor without the involvement of angiotensin II. *Nat Cell Biol.* 2004;6(6):499-506.

116. Yatabe J, Sanada H, Yatabe MS, et al. Angiotensin II type 1 receptor blocker attenuates the activation of ERK and NADPH oxidase by mechanical strain in mesangial cells in the absence of angiotensin II. *Am J Physiol Renal Physiol.* 2009;296(5):F1052-F1060.

117. Baker KM, Kumar R. Intracellular Ang II induces cell proliferation independent of AT1 receptor. *Am J Physiol Cell Physiol.* 2006;291(5):C995-C1001.

118. Rein H. Vasomotorische regulationen. *Ergebn de Physiol.* 1931;32:28-72.

119. Buckley NM, Brazeau P, Frasier ID. Renal blood flow autoregulation in developing swine. *Am J Physiol.* 1983;245(1):H1-H6.

120. Paton JB, Fisher DE. Organ blood flows of fetal and infant baboons. *Early Hum Dev.* 1984;10(1-2): 137-144.

121. Jose PA, Slotkoff LM, Montgomery S, et al. Autoregulation of renal blood flow in the puppy. *Am J Physiol.* 1975;229(4):983-988.

122. Oppermann M, Qin Y, Lai EY, et al. Enhanced tubuloglomerular feedback in mice with vascular overexpression of A1 adenosine receptors. *Am J Physiol Renal Physiol.* 2009;297(5):F1256-F1264.

123. Inscho EW, Cook AK, Imig JD, et al. Physiological role for P2X1 receptors in renal microvascular autoregulatory behavior. *J Clin Invest.* 2003;112(12):1895-1905.

124. Vallon V, Miracle C, Thomson S. Adenosine and kidney function: potential implications in patients with heart failure. *Eur J Heart Fail.* 2008;10(2):176-187,

125. Wilcox CS. Redox regulation of the afferent arteriole and tubuloglomerular feedback. *Acta Physiol Scand.* 2003;179(3):217-223.

126. Thomson SC, Blantz RC. Glomerulotubular balance, tubuloglomerular feedback, and salt homeostasis. *J Am Soc Nephrol.* 2008;19(12):2272-2275.

127. Schütz S, Le Moullec JM, Corvol P, et al. Early expression of all the components of the renin-angiotensin system in human development. *Am J Pathol.* 1996;149(6):2067-2079.

128. Niimura F, Kon V, Ichikawa I. The renin-angiotensin system in the development of congenital anomalies of the kidney and urinary tract. *Curr Opin Pediatr.* 2006;18(2):161-166.

129. Tabacova S, Little R, Tsong Y, et al. Adverse pregnancy outcomes associated with maternal enalapril antihypertensive treatment. *Pharmacoepidemiol Drug Saf.* 2003;12(8):633-646.

130. Buttar HS. An overview of the influence of ACE inhibitors on fetal-placental circulation and perinatal development. *Mol Cell Biochem.* 1997;176(1-2):61-67.

131. Cooper WO, Harnandez-Diaz S, Arbogast PG, et al. Major congenital malformations after first-trimester exposure to ACE inhibitors. *N Engl J Med.* 2006;354(23):2443-2451.

132. Schaefer C. Angiotensin II-receptor-antagonists: further evidence of fetotoxicity but not teratogenicity. *Birth Defects Res A Clin Mol Teratol.* 2003;67(8):591-594.

133. Niimura F, Okubo S, Fogo A, et al. Temporal and spatial expression pattern of the angiotensinogen gene in mice and rats. *Am J Physiol.* 1997;272(1 pt 2):R142-R147.

134. Kumar D, Moss G, Primhak R, et al. Congenital renal tubular dysplasia and skull ossification defects similar to teratogenic effects of angiotensin converting enzyme (ACE) inhibitors. *J Med Genet.* 1997;34(7):541-545.

135. Gribouval O, Gonzales M, Neuhaus T, et al. Mutations in genes in the renin-angiotensin system are associated with autosomal recessive renal tubular dysgenesis. *Nat Genet.* 2005;37(9):964-968.

136. Lacoste M, Cai Y, Guicharnaud L, et al. Renal tubular dysgenesis, a not uncommon autosomal recessive disorder leading to oligohydramnios: role of the renin-angiotensin system. *J Am Soc Nephrol.* 2006;17(8):2253-2263.

137. Nishimura H, Yerkes E, Hohenfellner K, et al. Role of the angiotensin type 2 receptor gene in congenital anomalies of the kidney and urinary tract, CAKUT, of mice and men. *Mol Cell.* 1999;3(1):1-10.

138. Gubler MC, Antignac C. Renin-angiotensin system in kidney development: renal tubular dysgenesis. *Kidney Int.* 2010;77(5):400-406.

139. Yosypiv IV, El-Dahr SS. Role of the renin-angiotensin system in the development of the ureteric bud and renal collecting system. *Pediatr Nephrol.* 2005;20(9):1219-1229.

140. Fiselier T, Monnens L, van Munster P, et al. The renin-angiotensin-aldosterone system in infancy and childhood in basal conditions and after stimulation. *Eur J Pediatr.* 1984;143(1):18-24.

141. Sulyok E, Nemeth M, Tenyi I, et al. Relationship between the postnatal development of the renin-angiotensin- aldosterone system and electrolyte and acid-base status of the NaCl-supplemented premature infants. In: Spitzer A, ed. *The Kidney during Development Morphogenesis and Function.* New York: Masson Publishing USA Inc; 1982:273-281.

142. Peleg E, Peleg D, Yaron A, et al. Perinatal development of angiotensin-converting enzyme in the rat's blood. *Gynecol Obstet Invest.* 1988;25(1):12-15.

143. Walther T, Faber R, Maul B, et al. Fetal, neonatal cord and maternal plasma concentrations of angiotensin converting enzyme (ACE). *Prenat Diagn.* 2002;22(2):111-113.

144. Bender JW, Davitt MK, Jose P. Angiotensin-1-converting enzyme activity in term and premature infants. *Biol Neonate.* 1978;34(1-2):19-23.

145. Forhead AJ, Melvin R, Balouzet V, et al. Developmental changes in plasma angiotensin—converting enzyme concentration in fetal and neonatal lambs. *Reprod Fertil Dev.* 1998;10(5):393-398.

146. Raimbach SJ, Thomas AL. Renin and angiotensin converting enzyme concentrations in the fetal and neonatal guinea-pig. *J Physiol.* 1990;423-441-451.

147. Forhead AJ, Gulati V, Poore KR, et al. Ontogeny of pulmonary and renal angiotensin-converting enzyme in pigs. *Mol Cell Endocrinol.* 2001;185(1-2):127-133.

148. O'Connor SJ, Fowden AL, Holdstock N, et al. Developmental changes in pulmonary and renal angiotensin-converting enzyme concentration in fetal and neonatal horses. *Reprod Fertil Dev.* 2002;14(7-8):413-417.

149. Hattori MA, Del Ben GL, Carmona AK, et al. Angiotensin I-converting enzyme isoforms (high and low molecular weight) in urine of premature and full-term infants. *Hypertension.* 2000;35(6):1284-1290.

150. Miyawaki M, Okutani T, Higuchi R, et al. Plasma angiotensin II levels in the early neonatal period. *Arch Dis Child Fetal Neonatal Ed.* 2006;91(5):F359-F362.

151. Franco MC, Casarini DE, Carneiro-Ramos MS, et al. Circulating renin-angiotensin system and catecholamines in childhood: is there a role for birthweight? *Clin Sci (Lond).* 2008;114(5):375-380.

152. Sippell WG, Dörr HG, Bidlingmaier F, et al. Plasma levels of aldosterone, corticosterone, 11-deoxycorticosterone, progesterone, 17-hydroxyprogesterone, cortisol, and cortisone during infancy and childhood. *Pediatr Res.* 1980;14(1):39-46.

153. Felder RA, Pelayo JC, Calcagno PL, et al. Alpha adrenoreceptors in the developing kidney. *Pediatr Res.* 1983;17(2):177-180.

154. Chevalier RL, Thornhill BA, Belmonte DC, et al. Endogenous angiotensin II inhibits natriuresis after acute volume expansion in the neonatal rat. *Am J Physiol.* 1996;270(2 Pt 2):R393-R397.

155. Pelayo JC, Fildes RD, Jose PA. Age-dependent renal effects of intrarenal infusion dopamine infusion. *Am J Physiol.* 1984;247(1 Pt 2):R212-R216.

156. Muchant DG, Thornhill BA, Belmonte DC, et al. Chronic sodium loading augments natriuretic response to acute volume expansion in the preweaned rat. *Am J Physiol.* 1995;269(1 Pt2):R15-R22.

157. Solhaug MJ, Dong XO, Adelman RD, et al. Ontogeny of neuronal nitric oxide synthase NOS1, in the developing porcine kidney. *Am J Physiol Regul Integr Comp Physiol.* 2000;278(6):R1453-R1459.

158. Mulder J, Baum M, Quigley R. Diffusional water permeability (PDW) of adult and neonatal rabbit renal brush border membrane vesicles. *J Membr Biol.* 2002;187(3):167-174.

159. Mulder J, Chakravarty S, Haddad MN, et al. Glucocorticoids increase osmotic water permeability (Pf) of neonatal rabbit renal brush border membrane vesicles. *Am J Physiol Regul Integr Comp Physiol.* 2005;288(5):R1417-R1421.

160. Bonilla-Felix M. Development of water transport in the collecting duct. *Am J Physiol Renal Physiol.* 2004;287(6):F1093-F2001.

161. Dilley JR, Arendshorst WJ. Enhanced tubuloglomerular feedback activity in rats developing spontaneous hypertension. *Am J Physiol.* 1984;274(4Pt2):F672-F679.

162. Just A, Kurtz L, de Wit C, et al. Connexin 40 mediates the tubuloglomerular feedback contribution to renal blood flow autoregulation. *J Am Soc Nephrol.* 2009;20(7):1577-1585.

10

163. Al-Dahhan J, Haycock GB, Chantler C, et al. Sodium Homeostasis in term and preterm neonates. I. Renal aspects. *Arch Dis Child.* 1983;58(5):335-342.

164. Du Z, Duan Y, Yan Q, et al. Mechanosensory function of microvilli of the kidney proximal tubule. *Proc Natl Acad Sci USA.* 2004;101(35):13068-13073.

165. Kon V, Hughes ML, Ichikawa I. Physiological basis for the maintenance of glomerulotubular balance in young growing rats. *Kidney Int.* 1984;25(2):391-396.

166. Seeliger E, Wronski T, Ladwig M, et al. The renin-angiotensin system and the third mechanism of renal blood flow autoregulation. *Am J Physiol Renal Physiol.* 2009;296(6):F1334-F1345.

167. Wang H, Garvin JL, D'Ambrosio MA, et al. Connecting tubule glomerular feedback (CTGF) antagonizes tubuloglomerular feedback (TGF) in vivo. *Am J Physiol Renal Physiol.* 2010;299(6): F1374-F1378.

168. Palmer BF. Impaired renal autoregulation: implications for the genesis of hypertension and hypertension-induced renal injury. *Am J Med Sci.* 2001;321(6):388-400.

169. Bidani AK, Griffin KA, Williamson G, et al. Protective importance of the myogenic response in the renal circulation. *Hypertension.* 2009;54(2):393-398.

170. Wilson C, Byrom FB. Renal changes in malignant hypertension. *Lancet.* 1939;1:136-139.

171. Wilson C, Byrom FB. The vicious circle in chronic Bright's disease. Experimental evidence from the hypertensive rat. *Q J Med.* 1941;10(2):65-93.

172. Hill GS, Heptinstall RH. Steroid-induced hypertension in the rat. A microangiographic and histologic study on the pathogenesis of hypertensive vascular and glomerular lesions. *Am J Pathol.* 1968;52(1):1-40.

173. Loutzenhiser R, Griffin K, Williamson G, et al. Renal autoregulation: new perspectives regarding the protective and regulatory roles of the underlying mechanisms. *Am J Physiol Regul Integr Comp Physiol.* 2006;290(5):R1153-1167.

174. Just A, Arendshorst WJ. Dynamics and contribution of mechanisms mediating renal blood flow autoregulation. *Am J Physiol Regul Integr Comp Physiol.* 2003;285(3):R619-R631.

175. Navar LG. Renal autoregulation: perspectives from whole kidney and single nephron studies. *Am J Physiol.* 1978;234(5):F357-F370.

176. Ochodnický P, Henning RH, Buikema HJ, et al. Renal vascular dysfunction precedes the development of renal damage in the hypertensive Fawn-Hooded rat. *Am J Physiol Renal Physiol.* 2010; 298(3):F625-F633.

177. Takemaka T, Forster H, De Micheli A, et al. Impaired myogenic responsiveness of renal microvessels in Dahl salt-sensitive rats. *Circ Res.* 1992;71(2):471-480.

178. Karlsen FM, Leyssac PP, Holstein-Rathlou NH. Tubuloglomerular feedback in Dahl rats. *Am J Physiol Renal Physiol.* 1998;274(6 Pt 2):F1561-F1569.

179. Saeed A, Dibona GF, Marcussen N, et al. High-NaCl intake impairs dynamic autoregulation of renal blood flow in ANG II-infused rats. *Am J Physiol Regul Integr Comp Physiol.* 2010;299(5): R1142-R1149.

180. Churchill PC, Churchill MC, Bidani AK, et al. Genetic susceptibility to hypertension-induced renal damage in the rat. Evidence based on kidney-specific genome transfer. *J Clin Invest.* 1997;100(6): 1373-1382.

181. Castrop H, Huang Y, Hashimoto S, et al. Impairment of tubuloglomerular feedback regulation of GFR in ecto-5'-nucleotidase/CD73-deficient mice. *J Clin Invest.* 2004;114(5):634-642.

182. Wang H, Garvin JL, D'Ambrosio MA, et al. Connecting tubule glomerular feedback antagonizes tubuloglomerular feedback in vivo. *Am J Physiol Renal Physiol.* 2010;299(6):F1374-F1378.

183. Brown R, Ollerstam A, Johansson B, Skott O, et al. Abolished tubuloglomerular feedback and increased plasma renin in adenosine A1 receptor-deficient mice. *Am J Physiol Regul Integr Comp Physiol.* 2001;281(5):R1362-R1367.

184. Vallon V. Tubuloglomerular feedback in the kidney: insights from gene-targeted mice. *Pflugers Arch.* 2003;445(4):470-476.

185. Hashimoto S, Huang Y, Briggs J, et al. Reduced autoregulatory effectiveness in adenosine 1 receptor-deficient mice. *Am J Physiol Renal Physiol.* 2006;290(4):F888-F891.

186. Wilcox CS, Welch WJ, Schreiner GF, et al. Natriuretic and diuretic actions of a highly-selective adenosine A1 receptor antagonist. *J Am Soc Nephrol.* 1990;10(4):714-720.

187. Carlström M, Wilcox CS, Welch WJ. Adenosine A2 receptors modulate tubuloglomerular feedback. *Am J Physiol Renal Physiol.* 2010;299(2):F412-F417.

188. Carlström M, Wilcox CS, Welch WJ. Adenosine A2A receptor activation attenuates tubuloglomerular feedback responses by stimulation of endothelial nitric oxide synthase. *Am J Physiol Renal Physiol.* 2001;300(2):F457-F464.

189. Schnermann J, Briggs JP. Tubuloglomerular feedback: mechanistic insights from gene-manipulated mice. *Kidney Int.* 2008;74(4):418-426.

190. Nishiyama A, Navar LG. ATP mediates tubuloglomerular feedback. *Am J Physiol Regul Integr Comp Physiol.* 2002;283(1):R273-R275.

191. Inscho EW. PX2 receptors in regulation of renal microvascular function. *Am J Physiol Renal Physiol* 2001;280:F927-F944.

192. Bell PD, Komlosi P, Zhang ZR. ATP as a mediator of macula densa cell signalling. *Purinergic Signal.* 2009;5(4):461-471.

193. Ren Y, Garvin JL, Liu R, et al. Possible mechanism of efferent arteriole (Ef-Art) tubuloglomerular feedback. *Kidney Int.* 2007;71(9):861-866.

194. Tojo A, Madsen KM, Wilcox CS, et al. Expression of immunoreactive nitric oxide synthase isoforms in rat kidney. Effects of dietary salt and losartan. *Jpn Heart J.* 1995;36(3):389-398.

D

195. Wilcox CS, Welch WJ, Murad F, et al. Nitric oxide synthase in macula densa regulates glomerular capillary pressure. *Proc Natl Acad Sci USA*. 1992;89(24):11993-11997.

196. Welch WJ, Wilcox CS, Thomson SC. Nitric oxide and tubuloglomerular feedback. *Semin Nephrol*. 1999;19(3):251-262.

197. Welch WJ, Tojo A, Lee Ju, et al. Nitric oxide synthase in the JGA of the SHR: expression and role in tubuloglomerular feedback. *Am J Physiol*. 1999;277(1 Pt 2):F130-F138.

198. Thorup C, Persson AE. Impaired effect of nitric oxide synthesis inhibition on tubuloglomerular feedback in hypertensive rats. *Am J Physiol*. 1996;271(2 Pt 2) F246-F252.

199. Lu D, Fu Y, Lopez-Ruiz A, et al. Salt-sensitive splice variant of nNOS expressed in the macula densa cells. *Am J Physiol Renal Physiol*. 2010;298(6):F1465-F1471.

200. Welch WJ, Tojo A, Wilcox CS. Roles of NO and oxygen radicals in tubuloglomerular feedback in SHR. *Am J Physiol Renal Physiol*. 2000;278(5):F769-F776.

201. Chen YF, Li PL, Zuo AP. Oxidative stress enhances the production and actions of adenosine in the kidney. *Am J Physiol Regul Integr Comp Physiol*. 2001;281(6):R1808-R1816.

202. McIntyre M, Bohr DF, Dominiczak AF. Endothelial function in hypertension: the role of superoxide anion. *Hypertension*. 1999;34(4 Pt 1):539-545.

203. Yang ZZ, Zhang AY, Yi FX, et al. Redox regulation of HIF-1alpha levels and HO-1 expression in renal medullary interstitial cells. *Am J Physiol Renal Physiol*. 2003;284(6):F1207-F1215.

204. Ortiz PA, Garvin JL. Role of nitric oxide in the regulation of nephron transport. *Am J Physiol Renal Physiol*. 2002;282(5):F777-F784.

205. Castrop H, Schnermann J. Isoforms of renal Na-K-2Cl cotransporter NKCC2: expression and functional significance. *Am J Physiol Renal Physiol*. 2008;295(4):F859-F866.

206. Cook N, Fraser SA, Katerelos M, et al. Low salt concentrations activate AMP-activated protein kinase in mouse macula densa cells. *Am J Physiol Renal Physiol*. 2009;296(4):F801-F809.

207. Peti-Peterdi J, Bebok Z, Lapointe JY, Bell PD. Novel regulation of cell [Na+] in macula densa cells: apical Na+ recycling by H-K-ATPase. *Am J Physiol Renal Physiol*. 2002;282(2):F324-F329.

208. Rajendran VM, Sangan P, Geibel J, et al. Ouabain-sensitive H,K-ATPase functions as Na,K-ATPase in apical membranes of rat distal colon. *J Biol Chem*. 2000;275(17):13035-13040.

209. Lorenz JN, Dostanic-Larson I, Shull GE, et al. Ouabain inhibits tubuloglomerular feedback in mutant mice with ouabain-sensitive alpha1 NaKATPase. *J Am Soc Nephrol*. 2006;17:2457–2463.

210. Peti-Peterdi J. Calcium wave of tubuloglomerular feedback. *Am J Physiol Renal Physiol*. 2006;291(2):F473-F480.

211. Kohlstedt K, Brandis RP, Muller-Esterl W, et al. Angiotensin-converting enzyme is involved in outside-in signaling in endothelial cells. *Circ Res*. 2002;94(1):60-67.

212. Zeng C, Wang Z, Hopfer U, et al. Rat strain effects of AT1 receptor activation on D1 dopamine receptors in immortalized renal proximal tubule cells. *Hypertension*. 2005;46(4):799-805.

213. Zeng C, Hopfer U, Asico LD, et al. Altered AT1 receptor regulation of ETB receptors in renal proximal tubule cells of spontaneously hypertensive rats. *Hypertension*. 2005;46(4):926-931.

214. AbdAlla S, Lother H, Quitterer U. AT1-receptor heterodimers show enhanced G-protein activation and altered receptor sequestration. *Nature*. 2000;407(6800):94-98.

215. Abadir PM, Periasamy A, Carey RM, et al. Angiotensin II type 2 receptor-bradykinin B2 receptor functional heterodimerization. *Hypertension*. 2006;48(2):316-322.

216. Zhuo JL. Intracrine renin and angiotensin II: a novel role in cardiovascular and renal cellular regulation. *J Hypertens*. 2006;24(6):1017-1020.

217. Vargas SL, Toma I, Kang JJ, et al. Activation of the succinate receptor GPR91 in macula densa cells causes renin release. *J Am Soc Nephrol*. 2009;20(5):1002-1011.

218. Barker DJ, Osmond C, Golding J, et al. Growth in utero, blood pressure in childhood and adult life, and mortality from cardiovascular disease. *BMJ* 1989;298(6673):564-567.

219. Alexander BT. Fetal programming of hypertension. *Am J Physiol Regul Integr Comp Physiol*. 2006;290(1):R1-R10.

220. Woods LL, Rasch R. Perinatal ANG II programs adult blood pressure, glomerular number, and renal function in rats.. *Am J Physiol*. 1998;275(5 Pt 2):R1593-R1599.

221. Gilbert JS, Lang AL, Grant AR, et al. Maternal nutrient restriction in sheep: hypertension and decreased nephron number in offspring at 9 months of age. *J Physiol*. 2005;565(Pt 1):137-147.

222. Leduc L, Levy E, Bouity-Voubou M, et al. Fetal programming of atherosclerosis: possible role of the mitochondria. *Eur J Obstet Gynecol Reprod Biol*. 2010;149(2):127-130.

223. Rao MS. Inhibition of the renin angiotensin aldosterone system: focus on aliskiren. *J Assoc Physicians India*. 2010;58:102-108.

224. Nguyen G. Renin and prorenin receptor in hypertension: What's new? *Curr Hypertens Rep*. 2011;13(1):79-85.

225. Drukker A, Guignard JP. Renal aspects of the term and preterm infant: a selective update. *Current Opin Pediatr*. 2002;14(2):175-182.

226. Merke DP, Bornstein SR. Congenital adrenal hyperplasia. *Lancet*. 2005;365(9477):2125-2136.

227. Chang SS, Grunder S, Hanukoglu A, et al. Mutations in subunits of the epithelial sodium channel cause salt wasting with hyperkalemic acidosis, pseudohypoaldosteronism type 1. *Nat Genet*. 1996;12(3):248-533.

228. Stipsanelli A, Daskalakis G, Koutra P, et al. Renin-angiotensin system dysregulation in fetuses with hydronephrosis. *Eur J Obstet Gynecol Reprod Biol*. 2010;150(1):39-41.

229. Danilczyk U, Penninger JM. Angiotensin-converting enzyme II in the heart and the kidney. *Circ Res*. 2006;98(4):463-471.

230. Fyhrquist F, Saijonmaa O. Renin-angiotensin system revisited. *J Intern Med*. 2008;264(3):224-236.

10

CHAPTER 11

Renal Modulation: Arginine Vasopressin and Atrial Natriuretic Peptide

Marco Zaffanello, MD, Andrea Dotta, MD, Francesco Emma, MD

- ● **Arginine Vasopressin**
- ● **Atrial Natriuretic Peptide**

Total body water (TBW) is distributed in compartments divided by semipermeable membranes. In postnatal life, approximately two-thirds of TBW is located in the intracellular space, and one-third is located in the extracellular space. The latter is further divided with a 3:1 ratio in the interstitial and plasma compartments.

Passive equilibration of solutes between body compartments is driven by electrochemical gradients and is mediated by a complex system of transport mechanisms that includes pumps, channels, facilitated carriers, and selective paracellular pathways. With few exceptions, water diffuses rapidly across epithelia and cell membranes following osmotic gradients. High transcellular water transport cannot occur through pure lipid bilayers because these have low osmotic water permeability (≈ 0.002 cm/sec).[1] Water diffusion through cell membranes is therefore mediated by specific water channels, termed aquaporins (AQPs), which enhance osmotic water permeability by 10- to 1000-fold. Because solutes diffuse less rapidly than their solvents, the relative water content of body compartments is primarily regulated by their solute distribution. This allows the organism to adjust its TBW distribution by regulating the activity of solute transporters located in biologic membranes that separate body compartments.

During early fetal life, TBW represents approximately 90% of body mass. As pregnancy progresses, TBW decreases progressively, to reach 75% to 80% of body mass at the end of gestation. These changes are primarily attributable to a decline in extracellular water, while intracellular water increases. In the first 24 to 48 hours after birth, the extracellular compartment further decreases as a result of a negative fluid balance in the immediate postnatal period.[2]

Fetuses constantly regulate their TBW by salt and water exchanges through the placental membrane. After birth, uptake of water and solutes is limited to gastrointestinal intakes, and insensible fluid losses increase dramatically. Newborns need, therefore, to activate mechanisms that are aimed at controlling water and salt losses. Most of these mechanisms involve the secretion of hormones, which act directly on the kidney. To be efficient, these mechanisms require that sensors, hormone secretion pathways, and target organs have reached an appropriate level of maturity.

Water excretion or retention is primarily modulated through the regulation of arginine vasopressin (AVP) secretion. Stimulation of thirst has only limited value in newborns because of their restricted access to free water and the immaturity of the central nervous system (CNS).

Salt retention by the kidney is predominantly achieved by activation of the renin–angiotensin–aldosterone system, which is potentiated by endothelins and adrenergic renal nerve activity. Conversely, renal salt losses are stimulated by natriuretic peptides (NPs), prostaglandins, kinins, nitric oxide (NO), and adrenomedullin.

In this chapter, the roles of AVP and NPs in the regulation of body fluid composition during the prenatal and perinatal periods are briefly reviewed. It is important to notice, however, that their action is part of a complex network in which all of the above-mentioned pathways are synergistically activated or inhibited to maintain body homeostasis.

Arginine Vasopressin

Normal Arginine Vasopressin Physiology

Arginine Vasopressin Synthesis

AVP is a cyclic nonapeptide that constitutes the principal antidiuretic hormone (ADH) for regulation of free water excretion by the kidney. It is composed of an intrachain disulfide bridge and has a structure similar to oxytocin, which acts primarily as a vasoconstrictor hormone with marginal antidiuretic effects.[3] AVP-induced vasoconstriction, on the other hand, is elicited only at nonphysiologic plasma concentrations in humans.[3]

AVP is encoded by the pre-pro-vasopressin gene (PPV), which is translated into protein as a prohormone. The PPV peptide undergoes two posttranslational modifications, which generate equimolar quantities of AVP and neurophysin II peptides.[3] Both AVP and oxytocin are synthesized in cell bodies of neurosecretory axons located in the neurohypophysis. After being synthesized, they are packaged in granules together with their neurophysin carrier protein and stored in nerve terminals.[4] Neurons containing AVP originate primarily from the supraoptic and paraventricular nuclei of the hypothalamus and are surrounded by a rich network of capillaries scattered throughout the neurohypophysis.[5]

Recently, the apelinergic system, which includes apelin and its G protein–coupled receptor, has been shown to play a crucial role in regulating AVP synthesis and release. Human and animal studies have linked the activity of the apelinergic system to regulation of body fluid homeostasis,[6] to central AVP response to osmotic stimuli, and to the renal response to AVP.[7]

Sensor Mechanisms for Arginine Vasopressin Secretion

AVP secretion can be stimulated by several mechanisms (Fig. 11-1). The two prominent stimuli are changes in plasma osmolality and changes in blood pressure or volume.[8] Other triggers for AVP secretion include emetic stimuli, hypoglycemia, pain, thermic stresses, hypoxia, hypercapnia, acidosis, and angiotensin II (ATII) stimulation.[9]

Under physiologic conditions, serum AVP levels are chiefly dependent on plasma osmolality, which is detected by osmoresponsive cells located near the supraoptic nuclei. These cells act as set-point receptors that inhibit AVP secretion below a given plasma osmolality and gradually stimulate AVP secretion above this set point.[3] Normal subjects differ considerably on a genetic basis, in their osmoreceptor sensitivity, and in their set point for AVP secretion.[10] Some subjects respond to changes in plasma osmolality as small as 0.5 mOsm/kg/H_2O, but other subjects require changes as high as 5 mOsm/kg/H_2O.[11] The set point for AVP secretion can range from 275 mOsm/kg/H_2O to 290 mOsm/kg/H_2O.[11] In addition to the genetic background, other factors such as age, sex, blood volume, and serum calcium levels, can also modify the set point.[11] To date, there is very little information on the ontogenicity of osmoreceptors. In particular, it has not been clearly established if the sensitivity of osmoreceptors is fully mature at birth.

The second most important stimuli for AVP secretion are blood pressure and blood volume. Changes lower than 10% in blood volume or blood pressure have little effect on serum AVP levels.[12] Above these values, AVP secretion increases rapidly.[13] Because these changes are not physiologic, AVP levels are primarily regulated by osmoreceptors under normal conditions. Blood volume and pressure changes do not override osmoreceptors, but produce a shift in the set point for AVP secretion.[10] Hemodynamic sensors that mediate AVP secretion are chiefly located in baroreceptor cells of the cardiac atria, carotid sinus, and aorta.[13]

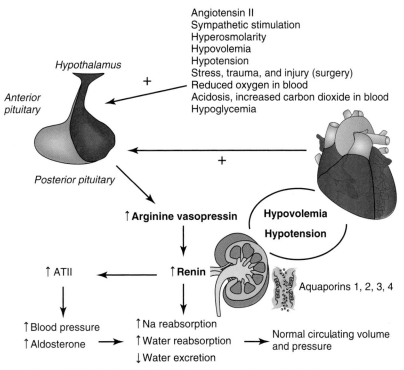

Figure 11-1   Pituitary/renal AVP response to hypovolemia/hypotension.

In adults, the ability to regulate water intake and excretion exceeds by far physiologic needs, which allows the maintenance of serum sodium and plasma osmolality within a very narrow range. In contrast, renal immaturity limits the ability of neonatal kidneys to dilute or concentrate the urine, and water intake is poorly regulated by activation of thirst in newborns. Consequently, serum sodium levels and plasma osmolality are less stable in neonates, particularly in premature infants.

Arginine Vasopressin Receptors and Signal Transduction

AVP receptors are members of the rhodopsin subfamily of G protein–coupled receptors.[14] Classically, two types of AVP receptors, V1 and V2, have been identified. The V2 receptor is the primary target of AVP in the kidneys and is primarily expressed on the basolateral membranes of collecting duct tubular cells. The V2 receptor is composed of seven transmembrane domains that come together to form a groove for ADH binding in the extracellular region and contains a binding site for a G_s protein in its intracellular domain.[15]

V1 receptors are mainly located in vascular endothelial cells and are subdivided in V1a (vascular or hepatic) and V1b (anterior pituitary) subtypes, according to their location and genetic sequence.[16] In addition, it is now well established that V1 receptors are also expressed in renal tubular cells, where they modulate AVP action.[17] Unlike V2 receptors, V1 receptors are generally coupled to the inositol triphosphate pathway, which causes a vasoconstrictive response induced by increased cytosolic calcium levels.[18] Through the activation of vasopressin V1a and V2 receptors, AVP regulates body fluid homeostasis, vascular tone, and cardiac contractility.[19] In neonatal murine cardiomyocytes, AVP stimulates protein synthesis and increases cell surface area through activation of V1a receptors that are expressed in the neonatal heart; the activity of AVP is in part counterbalanced by increased expression of atrial natriuretic peptide (ANP) in hypertrophic cardiomyocytes.[20]

Renal Arginine Vasopressin Action and Aquaporin 2 Water Channels

Basolateral binding of AVP to V2 receptors in collecting duct cells activates cytosolic adenylate cyclase, leading to increased intracellular cyclic AMP (cAMP) concentrations. This stimulates protein kinase A (PKA), which in turn promotes phosphorylation of AQP2 proteins and their translocation into the apical membrane.[21] In vitro, membrane insertion of AQP2 increases cell water permeability from approximately 0.005 cm/sec to approximately 0.1 cm/sec.[22] AQP2 is a member of the AQP superfamily, which to date contains 12 different human water channels.[23] AQPs are 26- to 34-kD glycosylated proteins sharing 50% to 85% homology. They contain 6 transmembrane-spanning domains and are organized in homotetramers. AQPs differ between them by their water transport properties, solute selectivity, and tissue expression.

In the kidney, whereas AQP1 is mostly expressed in water-permeable proximal tubular cells and capillaries, water transport in the collecting duct is mediated basolaterally by AQP3 and AQP4 and by AVP-dependent insertion of AQP2 on the apical aspects of cells.

AVP stimulation also decreases glomerular capillary ultrafiltration and renal medulla blood flow, increases sodium reabsorption in cortical collecting ducts and in the thick ascending limb of Henle, promotes urea reabsorption in medullary collecting ducts, and stimulates prostaglandin synthesis in medullary interstitial cells.[24] Most of these actions increase the osmotic gradient for renal water reabsorption.

Extrarenal actions of AVP include limited vasoconstrictive action, platelet activation (release of von Willebrand factor), and regulation of several CNS functions, including learning and memory abilities, neuroendocrine reactions, social behaviors, circadian rhythm, thermoregulation, and autonomic functions.[24] The clinical relevance of these effects remains uncertain.

Modulation of Arginine Vasopressin Action

Renal responses of AVP can be blunted in several conditions. These conditions may have significant clinical relevance because they may interfere with normal mechanisms of body water regulation.

Chronic water loading in animals, for example, produces vasopressin-independent inhibition of V2 receptor mRNA transcription.[25,26] This phenomenon is referred to as *ADH escape*. Similarly, ADH escape can be induced by hypercalciuria secondary to inhibition of cAMP production through activation of the calcium-sensing receptor,[27] by chronic hypokalemia,[28] or through acute water loading.[25] AQP2 and AQP3 expression are also downregulated in experimental nephrotic syndrome.[29] Conversely, prolonged fasting increases AVP-independent collecting duct renal water reabsorption.[30]

Several hormones and molecules modulate AVP action. Estrogens, for example, can directly increase renal fluid reabsorption,[31] but endothelin-1 decreases the sensitivity to AVP of collecting ducts.[32] Lithium also produces water diuresis by inhibiting AVP-stimulated translocation of AQP2 through inhibition of adenylate cyclase, and prolonged indomethacin treatment can induce AVP escape by modulating the intrarenal synthesis of prostaglandins.[33,34]

Developmental Differences Between Fetuses and Newborn Infants

Role of Arginine Vasopressin in the Placenta

Normal fetal growth depends on constant exchanges of fluids at the level of the placenta. V1a receptors are expressed in the placenta, particularly during the first half of the pregnancy.[35] In sheep, the time of maximal placental expression of V1a receptor correlates with the time of maximal placental growth, suggesting that AVP stimulation through V1a receptors may play a role in placental growth and differentiation.[35] The expression of V1a receptors in the placenta also suggests that AVP may exert a vasoconstrictor effect on the placental circulation, although no definitive evidence has been produced to date.

Low levels of placenta V2 receptor expression are also found throughout gestation. Fetal infusion of AVP in sheep, however, produces no changes in placenta adenylate cyclase activity, bringing into question the physiologic relevance of V2 receptor expression in this organ.[36] No evidence indicating a physiologic role of maternal AVP on placenta water permeability or solute transport has been reported.[37,38] In particular, maternal or fetal infusion of AVP, at least in experimental ovine models, has no effect on placental fluid exchanges.[38]

Several water channels are expressed in human and ovine placentas. AQP1 is primarily expressed in the placental vasculature and fetal membranes, AQP3 and AQP8 in trophoblast epithelial cells, and AQP9 in the amnion and allantoid.[39-42] No expression of AQP2 has been documented to date.

The relationship between maternal AVP levels and maternal plasma osmolality or maternal renal water clearance is not significantly modified in pregnant animals.[43]

In humans, maternal serum AVP levels decrease progressively in the third trimester of pregnancy as TBW increases.[44] Despite decreased plasma AVP concentrations, maternal urinary AQP2 excretion increases during pregnancy, indicating an AVP-independent mechanism of renal AQP2 stimulation.[44] Because maternal AVP does not cross the placental membrane, maternal AVP levels do not influence fetal plasma osmolality.[45,46]

Amniotic fluid contains AVP of fetal origin.[47] Assays using reverse-transcription polymerase chain reaction (PCR) have shown no evidence of AVP gene expression in placentas, which reasonably excludes that amniotic AVP is produced by the placental membranes.[48] Intraamniotic infusion of AVP, on the other hand, produces a sharp increase in fetal serum AVP levels, indicating fast equilibration of AVP concentrations across the amniotic membranes, and that amniotic AVP levels reflect fetal concentrations.[49]

Increased concentrations of AVP in the amniotic fluid have been shown to correlate with fetal growth retardation in rats and with fetal stress, particularly fetal acidosis, in humans.[50]

Arginine Vasopressin in Fetal Life

In humans, AVP and V1b receptors are detectable in the fetal pituitary gland at 11 to 12 weeks of gestation.[48,51] AVP concentrations increase rapidly thereafter until the second trimester of pregnancy.[48] Several experimental models support early activation of the AVP system in fetuses. In fetal ewes, for example, hypothalamic neurons are activated during maternal water deprivation, resulting in higher AVP concentrations in the fetal circulation; consequently, maternal water deprivation increases fetal serum sodium and osmolality, decreases fetal urine output, and increases fetal urine osmolarity.[52] A similar effect is obtained by maternal infusion of mannitol to early pregnant ewes (<120 days), which increases fetal AVP secretion in response to increased fetal plasma osmolality.[36,38] In sheep, the expression of pituitary V1b receptors decreases progressively during pregnancy despite increased AVP responsiveness to glucocorticoid, indicating maturation of the feedback mechanisms that regulate AVP secretion throughout gestation.[51]

As mentioned previously, ATII is a potent stimulator of AVP secretion. In ovine fetuses, both AT1 and AT2 receptors are expressed in the fetal brain at the end of gestation, suggesting that ATII stimulation contributes to AVP secretion near term; accordingly, ATII-induced fetal AVP secretion has been shown to be mediated through stimulation of AT1 receptors in this experimental model.[53] Interactions between the renin–angiotensin–vasopressin systems are also bidirectional; inhibition of V1 receptors, for example, inhibits ATII-induced blood pressure changes, indicating that AVP plays a role in blood pressure regulation during fetal life in conjunction with ATII.[54]

Although renal V1a and V2 receptors in rats have been shown to be significantly expressed since day 16 days of gestation,[55] AVP probably has little involvement in modulating urine concentration during fetal life under physiologic conditions because of the relative renal unresponsiveness to this hormone.

Overall, fetal serum AVP concentrations are relatively stable during normal pregnancy in humans, but correlate poorly with fetal urine production.[36] Only limited correlation has been reported between amniotic fluid volume and fetal AVP levels.[56] This clinical evidence is substantiated by experimental data showing that AVP infusion in different fetal animal models often produces marginal changes in urine osmolarity or plasma osmolarity, although a certain degree of maturation of these responses during gestation has been documented.[36,38,54,57] The effective role of AVP in regulating fetal urine osmolarity in pathologic fetal conditions remains unclear.

Arginine Vasopressin in Newborns

AVP is released during labor in term newborns, as demonstrated by high levels of the hormone in the umbilical cord.[58] Conflicting data exist on the influence of the mode of delivery on AVP secretion. In some studies, AVP concentrations have been reported to be similar in infants born by cesarean section or by natural delivery, calling into question the physiologic relevance of AVP during labor and raising questions on the exact mechanisms that stimulate AVP secretion.[59] Conversely, other data indicate that AVP concentrations in the umbilical cord are lower in infants born by cesarean section, suggesting that birth stress stimulates fetal AVP secretion, which may contribute to the postnatal hemodynamic adaptation, particularly to the redistribution of fetal blood flow, leading to delayed voiding after birth.[60]

In humans, the urine concentration ability develops progressively during the first year of life and reaches full maturity around 18 months of age.[61,62]

Functional impairment of neonatal kidneys to respond to AVP has been established by several investigators by direct injection of ADH or pituitary extracts to neonates.[63,64] Renal AVP unresponsiveness does not appear to be related to lack of receptors. Murine V2 receptor expression, for example, increases rapidly after the first weeks of life, reaching adult levels by the fifth week,[65] demonstrating an adequate number of binding sites for AVP during renal development.

Several investigators have dissected the mechanisms involved in the maturation of cortical collecting ducts' water permeability (reviewed by Bonilla-Felix[55]). Overall, these data show that transduction pathways for AVP are limited by prostaglandin E2–mediated inhibition of cAMP synthesis and by increased degradation of cAMP secondary to high phosphodiesterase activity.[66-69] Water movement across collecting ducts is also limited by low medullary tonicity, which is caused primarily by the immaturity of the salt reabsorption machinery in the thick ascending limb of Henle and of the urea recycling mechanisms.[66] Low dietary protein intake may also play a limiting role in urea generation. In addition, the performance of the countercurrent system is limited by the physical length of the loop of Henle, which increases progressively with renal growth after birth.[70]

Finally, it has been proposed that renal concentration ability is limited during the first year of life by expression of AQPs because AQP2 expression increases progressively after birth in humans and animal models.[66] Several investigators have failed, however, to demonstrate alterations in AQP2 expression at birth, both in preterm and term infants[71] and in animal models.[72] Urinary AQP2 excretion decreases postnatally from day 1 to 4, then remains stable during the first 4 weeks of life, and increases rapidly between weeks 4 to 6,[71] but the correlation between urinary AQP2 excretion, AVP levels, and renal water concentration ability in the early postnatal period is relatively poor.[73]

Experimental studies have also shown that AQP2 synthesis in immature kidneys can be efficiently stimulated by intravenous (IV) AVP or dehydration, which is not followed by an increase in urine osmolality.[74]

Altogether, these data indicate that AQP2 expression is probably not a limiting factor for the urinary concentration ability of neonates and that low levels of AQP2 expression are related to low stimulation of their synthesis in collecting duct cells. Similarly, the expression of AQP1, AQP3, and AQP4 increases progressively during fetal and early postnatal life and does not limit water reabsorption in the kidneys.[55,75,76]

Role of Arginine Vasopressin in Pathologic Conditions of Neonates

Diabetes Insipidus

Genetic forms of diabetes insipidus are caused by a lack of AVP secretion (central diabetes insipidus [CDI]) or by insensibility of the kidney to AVP (nephrogenic diabetes insipidus [NDI]). Whereas CDI is caused by autosomal dominant mutations of the PPV gene (*PPV*),[77] NDI is caused by X-linked mutations of the V2 receptor gene or autosomal recessive mutations of the AQP2 gene.[78] Exceptionally, these later mutations can be transmitted following an autosomal dominant pattern.[79] In addition to genetic forms, CDI develops in association with malformations of the CNS, particularly midline defects, or is caused by tumor processes that disrupt the neurohypophysis and its connections.[80] Acquired forms of NDI are generally secondary to the renal toxic effects of drugs such as lithium, antibiotics, antifungals, antineoplastic agents, and antivirals.[81] Maternal lithium treatment for bipolar disorders aggravates neonatal unresponsiveness to AVP.[33]

Because AVP has a limited role in prenatal and neonatal fluid balance, CDI and NDI do not cause polyhydramnios, and newborns are generally asymptomatic. Although genetic defects are present at birth, infants do not develop classic symptoms, including failure to thrive, polyuria, dehydration, and hypernatremia, because human milk has relatively low salt and protein content and therefore generates a low urine osmolar load. Symptoms usually begin after the first months of life when infants are switched to formulas, which generate twice the osmolar load of breast milk and are nearly always present when cow's milk and solid foods are introduced.[78]

Syndrome of Inappropriate Secretion of Antidiuretic Hormone

Inappropriate secretion of ADH causes hyponatremia with extracellular volume expansion. Protracted high AVP levels upregulate AQP2 water channel expression in the collecting ducts, which further stimulates water reabsorption leading to hyponatremia.[82] In older children, the syndrome of inappropriate secretion of ADH (SIADH) is caused by neurologic lesions, pulmonary diseases or tumors, or treatment with drugs that increase ADH release such as barbiturates, clofibrate, isoproterenol, or vincristine.[83]

In SIADH, the urine is inappropriately concentrated compared with plasma osmolality. Because newborns cannot efficiently concentrate their urine, excessive AVP secretion is generally asymptomatic in the neonatal period and SIADH does not develop. Therefore, the association of hyponatremia with extracellular volume expansion in newborns is nearly invariably caused by excessive IV infusion of dextrose solutions or, less frequently, by decreased renal clearance of free water caused by congenital or acquired renal diseases.

Arginine Vasopressin Secretion in Neonatal Pathologic Conditions

AVP is a hormone released during conditions of stress. Increased AVP secretion has been reported in numerous clinical conditions, including cardiomyopathy, intracardiac shunts, congestive heart failure, respiratory distress, mechanical ventilation, systemic infections, meningitis, gastroenteritis, pneumonia, and botulism.[84-88] Here again, the relative unresponsiveness of neonatal kidneys to AVP calls into question the clinical relevance of this secretion. Furthermore, infants undergoing general anesthesia are at higher risk of developing postoperative hyponatremia because of AVP excess; after surgery, AVP production may increase in response to several stimuli, including pain, stress, nausea, vomiting, use of narcotic drugs, hypotension, and third spacing.[89]

11

Atrial Natriuretic Peptide

Normal Physiology of Atrial Natriuretic Peptide and Related Natriuretic Peptides

Introduction to Natriuretic Peptides

The existence of NPs has been suspected since 1956 after the observation that saline infusion released circulating factors that increased natriuresis.[90] It was not until 1981 that de Bold et al[91] demonstrated for the first time that extracts of rat atrial cells contained peptides, which inhibited renal sodium reabsorption.

NPs are a family of peptides encoded by three different genes. Type A ANP was first isolated in 1984 from cardiac atrial cells.[92] Soon after, two other NPs were isolated from brain cells, namely, BNP and CNP.[93,94] Although initially isolated from brain tissue, BNP is primarily expressed by cardiac myocytes and CNP by endothelial cells.[95,96] CNP has important functions of regulating chondrocyte proliferation and differentiation, as demonstrated by CNP knock-out mice with severe dwarfism.[97]

Synthesis of Natriuretic Peptides

Similarly to AVP, oxytocin, and adrenocorticotropic hormone, NPs are short peptides[28-32] that differ in a few residues within a 17–amino acid ring that is closed by a disulfide bridge and are synthesized as prohormones that undergo a series of posttranslational modifications. The major site of synthesis of NPs is the heart.

Unlike its BNP and CNP analogues, posttranslational processing of the pre-pro-ANP gene generates three additional peptides, namely, long-acting NP (LANP), the vessel dilator peptide, and the kaliuretic peptide, which are released into the circulation and enhance ANP activity.[98]

Corin, a transmembrane serine protease identified in the heart, converts pro-ANP (pro-ANP) to active ANP. Lack of Corin protease prevents the conversion of pro-ANP to ANP and causes salt-sensitive hypertension in mice.[99] Posttranslational processing of the ANP gene in the kidneys also results in a 4–amino acid longer ANP molecule, termed *urodilatin*.[100] Locally secreted urodilatin in the kidney regulates sodium and water reabsorption.[96] Since very early in life, urodilatin excretion highly correlates with sodium excretion, but not with body weight loss; in full-term infants as in adults, urodilatin appears to have a distinct physiologic role in the kidney from ANP.[101]

NPs' mRNA has also been documented in several tissues, including the aorta, brain, lungs, kidneys, adrenal glands, intestine, and adipose tissue.[96,98] Gene expression in these tissues, however, is far lower than in the heart.[86] Therefore, the majority of circulating NPs acting on the cardiovascular and renal systems are of cardiac origin. Nonetheless, extracardiac synthesis of NPs has important local effects. In hypothalamic neurons, for example, regional ANP production is thought to regulate AVP secretion and sympathetic nerve activity.[102]

Sensor Mechanisms for Atrial Natriuretic Peptide Secretion

Both ANP and BNP are stored in secretory granules of atrial and to a lesser degree ventricular myocytes.[95] The major triggers for ANP release are increased cardiac wall stretch and increased blood pressure.[91,95,100] In the first case, ANP release is triggered by changes in the central venous return and dilatation of the atrial chambers. The second type of stimulation is brought about by sustained hemodynamic and neuroendocrine stimuli and involves, at least in part, a separate pertussis toxin-sensitive pathway.[103] Various hormones, including glucocorticoids, AVP, ATII, and catecholamines, modulate the rate of ANP release.[102]

Natriuretic Peptide Receptors and Signal Transduction

To date, three different membrane receptors for NPs have been identified. ANP and BNP bind to a specific guanyl cyclase receptor type A, termed NPR-A, and increase intracellular cyclic guanosine monophosphate (cGMP) levels, similar to NO and endothelium-derived relaxing factor.[104,105] cGMP in turn activates cGMP-gated channels, cGMP-dependent phosphodiesterases, and the cGMP-dependent protein kinases cGKI and cGKII.[96,105,106] CNP binds to another guanyl cyclase receptor, named NPR-B, which activates similar pathways.[96,105,106] The third receptor, NPR-C, is expressed in target organs in similar or even greater amounts than receptors A and B.[10] Unlike its other two homologues, NPR-C has no guanyl cyclase activity and has been reported to decrease cAMP levels.[107] Its most major role is to internalize and degrade NPs in order to modulate their activity in various tissues.[10] The predominant clearance function of NPR-C is well documented in NPR-C knockout mice, which exhibit hypotension and reduced urinary concentration ability as a result of increased bioavailability of both ANP and BNP.[108]

Biologic Action of Natriuretic Peptides

ANP and BNP are potent natriuretic, diuretic, and vasodilator hormones that act primarily on the cardiovascular and renal systems (Fig. 11-2). In the kidneys, the type A receptors are expressed throughout the nephron. The highest levels of ANP-stimulated accumulation of cGMP are found in the inner medulla collecting ducts and, at higher concentrations of the hormone, in the glomerulus.[109,110] Both ANP and BNP increase the glomerular filtration rate by promoting vasodilatation of the afferent arteriole and vasoconstriction of the efferent arteriole, an effect opposed to the action of ATII.[111] Glomerular podocytes also express NP receptors and respond to ANP stimulation similarly to NO by upregulating their cGMP synthesis. The podocyte foot processes contractile apparatus seems to be an obvious target for this signaling cascade.[112]

In collecting duct cells, low concentrations of ANP can reduce Na reabsorption by as much as 50% even in the presence of AVP.[108,113-117] Additionally, ANP has been shown to inhibit water permeability by 40% to 50% in non–AVP-stimulated renal collecting ducts.[118] In other tubular segments, the action of AVP is more controversial. Decreased ATII-stimulated sodium reabsorption, in the presence of ANP, has been reported in proximal tubular cells and in the thick ascending limb of Henle,[117,119] but these data have not been confirmed by other authors.[120-122] Urodilatin, which is locally synthesized in the kidneys, is secreted directly in the renal tubules, where it has similar actions to the cardiac-derived ANP.[123]

The above-mentioned ATII antagonist effect of ANP is further reinforced by direct inhibition of renin secretion and aldosterone secretion.[124-126] At the

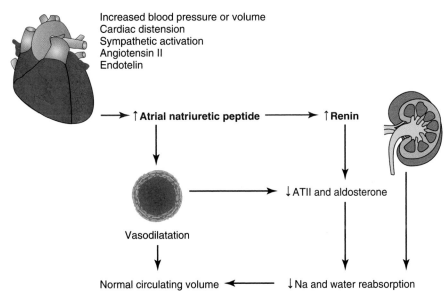

Figure 11-2   ANP and the RAS response.

D

cardiovascular level, stimulation of type A receptors induces vessel dilatation, increased endothelial permeability, and inhibition of the sympathetic system, which add to the inhibition of the renin–ATII--aldosterone axis.[10,97]

The essential role of NPs in blood pressure regulation is best demonstrated by experiments in transgenic animals, where targeted deletion of the ANP gene or of the type A receptor gene leads to severe arterial hypertension, but overexpression of the same genes induces hypotension.[95] Deletion of the NPR-A gene limited to vascular smooth muscle cells, on the other hand, does not cause hypotension under normal conditions, but abolishes the vasodilatatory response after acute volume loading, demonstrating the complexity of the biologic activities that are mediated by NPs.[127]

In conditions of chronic volume expansion or hypertension, ANP also exerts an antihypertrophic effect, and BNP exerts an antifibrotic effect by inhibiting myocyte and fibroblast proliferation, respectively.[96,128-130]

In humans, whereas heterozygous mutations located in the promoter of the NPR-A gene cause hypertension and heart failure, homozygous mutations of the NPR-B gene cause short-limbed dwarfism, termed Moroteaux acromesomelic dysplasia[131]).

Modulation of Atrial Natriuretic Peptide Action

The above-discussed data shows that NPs counteract the renal and cardiovascular effects of a combined secretion of ATII and AVP. These various systems are heavily interdependent and can influence each other significantly. ATII receptor blockade during heart failure, for example, mitigates renal hyporesponsiveness to ANP.[132] These interactions occur at different levels, including reciprocal modulation of gene transcription, of sensor mechanisms that trigger hormone secretion, of receptor expression and activity on second messengers.[133] Inhibition of PKA, for example, increases NPR-A activity, which results in increased generation of cGMP after ANP stimulation.[134] Conversely, activation of cGMP-coupled phosphodiesterases by ANP decreases intracellular cAMP levels,[96,106] which is the second messenger for AVP activity in the kidneys, where it activates PKA (see above).

In summary, ANP signals via cGMP, which is inhibited by phosphodiesterases. High intrarenal phosphodiesterase activity in pregnant rats blunts the natriuretic response to ANP, which may contribute to physiologic fetal volume expansion.[135]

These various levels of interaction have a critical role in creating a dynamic balance between different hormonal pathways, allowing the preservation of TBW and blood pressure control. Other hormones also modulate the activity of NPs at different levels. The neutral endopeptidase (NEP), for example, is a zinc-metallopeptidase that degrades biologically active peptides. In the kidneys, NEP is heavily expressed in the brush border of renal proximal epithelial cells[136] and in mesangial cells, where it is thought to have an important role in modulating renal hemodynamics, partly by inactivation of NPs.[137] Endothelin 1, on the other hand, promotes gene expression of NP in ventricular myocytes,[138] and bradykinin counteracts the ANP-stimulated sodium and water excretion by acting directly on the kidney.[139,140]

Developmental Differences Between Fetuses and Newborn Infants
Role of Atrial Natriuretic Peptide in the Placenta

Pregnancy is characterized by a state of physiologic maternal vasodilatation and renal sodium and water retention despite activation of the renin–angiotensin system. Maternal ANP levels increase steadily during pregnancy from week 12 and decline significantly in the postpartum period.[141] In a simple view, higher ANP activity contributes to the systemic vasodilatation and vascular resistance to ATII of pregnant women.[142] More accurately, ANP is part of a complex hormonal system of regulation that mediates changes in systemic hemodynamics, in blood pressure, and in renal excretion, which are essential to maternal adaptation to pregnancy.[143]

Currently, no evidence suggests that ANP or other NPs cross the placenta. In 20-days pregnant rats, for example, no active or passive transport of intact radiolabeled ANP across the placenta has been documented.[144] Because ANP plays a major role in the regulation of vascular tone, several investigators have studied the role of ANP in regulating placenta hemodynamics. In particular, because the placenta lacks an autonomic innervation, it has been hypothesized that locally produced vasoactive factors, such as NPs, contribute to placental vascular tone control.[145] This hypothesis has now been confirmed by several studies showing that NPs and their receptors are expressed in the placenta.

Placental synthesis of ANP has been documented by immunocytochemistry and reverse transcription PCR in human extravillous trophoblasts and to a lesser degree in decidual cells, but villous trophoblasts do not appear to express significant amounts of ANP.[145] ANP and BNP synthesis has also been documented in vitro in cultured human umbilical vein endothelial cells and human amnion cells, respectively.[146,147] In mice, strong expression of CNP and, to a lesser degree, of BNP, has been shown early during gestation in the decidua, but placental synthesis of ANP remains controversial.[148-150]

The presence of NP receptors was demonstrated using binding assays in nonvillous microsomal placental extracts even before their isolation and molecular characterization.[151] Subsequently, the expression of NPR-A and NPR-B was confirmed in human uterine tissues, including decidua, chorion, and myometrium, and in the placenta itself.[147] ANP receptors in the human placenta have been found to be significantly more expressed in its fetal components than in the maternal microvillous membranes.[152] The human placental artery has also been found to be the site of expression of large amounts of ANP and BNP receptors and expresses the clearance receptor (NPR-C).[153]

Clearance receptors are downregulated in fetoplacental artery endothelial cells toward the end of gestation, which increases the local concentrations of ANP and corresponds to increased generation of cGMP.[154] This is thought to be, at least in part, secondary to increased placental secretion of basic fibroblast growth factor during the last trimester of pregnancy.[154] On this basis, it has been postulated that ANP and other NPs are critical for maintaining adequate blood flow in the placental and uterine tissues and that in pathologic conditions, such as preeclampsia, these hormones play an important role.

In fact, the number of guanyl cyclase–coupled receptors in the placental vasculature, maternal ANP plasma levels, and fetal ANP plasma levels are increased during preeclampsia.[155-160] Increased ANP and ANP receptor expression in this condition may represent a local defense mechanism to prevent further increases in maternal blood pressure by promoting arterial vasodilatation and natriuresis.[156] Accordingly, infusion of ANP in human placenta inhibits arterial vasoconstriction induced by L-arginine, ATII, and to a lesser extent endothelin-1.[155,161-163] These effects are not mediated by NO and may also extend to thromboxane-induced vasoconstriction at higher nonphysiologic ANP concentrations.[162,163]

IV infusion of low doses of ANP (10 ng/kg/min) to women with preeclampsia has been shown to induce a mean uteroplacental blood flow increase of 28%.[164] An individual increase in placental blood flow correlates with increased cGMP synthesis and with a decrease in maternal blood pressure, indicating effective uteroplacental vasodilatation.[164]

Atrial Natriuretic Peptide in Fetal Life

Several studies indicate that ANP levels in fetal blood are not related to maternal ANP concentrations. In rat embryos, gene expression of ANP mRNA is detectable at 8.5 days of gestation.[165] Fetal ANP levels during pregnancy are higher than maternal levels, in murine and ovine experimental models.[166,167] Higher fetal ANP levels do not result from slower removal rates by developing kidneys or by transfer from maternal circulation.[168,169] In fact, ANP secretion is markedly increased in rats during midgestation, although the major site of synthesis is in the ventricles rather than the atria.[166,170] Similarly, at 17 to 19 weeks' gestation human fetuses, ANP expression is higher in the ventricles.[148] In ovine fetuses, on the other hand, ANP is mainly synthesized in the atria.[171] These differences may be relevant when translating animal data to humans because the mechanisms stimulating NP release may not be entirely comparable.

A number of experimental data, mostly obtained in murine and ovine fetal models, have shown that mid- and late-gestation animals can readily release NPs in response to various stimuli, including ATII infusion, AVP infusion, indomethacin treatment, acute fetal volume expansion, hypertonicity, and fetal hypoxia.[166,169,172,173] Nonetheless, NPs probably have little role in renal homeostasis and fluid balance during intrauterine life, which is chiefly ensured by the placenta. In general, ANP infusion at supraphysiologic doses in fetal animals decreases arterial blood pressure, has a moderate diuretic effect, but does not increase natriuresis significantly.[170,173]

Atrial Natriuretic Peptide in Newborns

At birth, loss of the placenta circulation produces dramatic hemodynamic changes that significantly modify the atria sizes and pressures and stimulates NP secretion. Increased perinatal secretion of ANP and BNP has been well established in both preterm and term newborns. This secretion starts at birth and peaks at days 1 to 2 of life and decreases thereafter, reaching a plateau after 1 to 2 weeks.[174] Because of their known natriuretic and diuretic action, it has been logically proposed that NPs play a predominant role in promoting the transition from fetal to postnatal circulation and stimulate the postnatal natriuretic phase that causes the contraction of the extracellular space.[175]

Plasma ANP levels and the onset of the postnatal diuretic phase in human newborns have been found, however, to be relatively poorly correlated, both in preterm and term infants.[176,177] This probably highlights the complexity of interactions between the cardiovascular and renal systems after birth, where NPs are only part of a complex hormonal and hemodynamic system that is activated after birth.

Several experimental data also indicate that the renal response to NPs is still largely immature at birth. ANP infusion, for example, induces a blunted natriuretic and diuretic response in newborn rabbits, which has been attributed to immaturity of ANP receptors and signal transduction pathways and to overriding interactions with other hormonal systems.[178] Similarly, the natriuretic and diuretic response to ANP in sheep has been shown to undergo a maturation phase that extends well into the first postnatal weeks.[168] In rats, expression of renal ANP receptors is low at birth and increases thereafter to reach adult levels only at the end of the fifth week of life.[178] This correlates with a parallel maturation of their signal transduction pathways, as demonstrated by a progressive increase in ANP-induced renal cGMP synthesis during the first weeks of life.[179]

In humans, a similar pattern of postnatal increase in cGMP urinary excretion has also been documented, although it is highly variable.[180]

In summary, these data indicate that the sensor and synthesis mechanisms leading to ANP and BNP secretion are mature at birth. The vasodilatory response to NPs is also satisfactory in utero, but the renal responses require a phase of postnatal maturation.[181] Increased ANP levels in neonates, therefore, indicate primarily a state of volume expansion or disturbances of the pulmonary circulation related to cardiovascular and respiratory diseases,[175,182] but do not necessarily anticipate a phase of negative fluid balance related to increased renal fluid losses.

Role of Atrial Natriuretic Peptide in Pathologic Conditions of Newborns

Fetal Distress

Levels of ANP have been found to be elevated during fetal distress and fetal hypoxia.[183-186] On these bases, it has been postulated that increased cord levels of NPs may predict the development of periventricular leukomalacia lesions. One study has prospectively addressed this hypothesis.[187] No significant association was found between brain lesions and cord ANP or BNP levels in four patients who later developed periventricular leukomalacia compared with control infants.[188]

Postnatal Diseases

After birth, ANP levels often remain elevated in infants with respiratory distress. Most likely, high ANP levels indicate increased atrial wall stretch secondary to volume expansion, pulmonary hypertension, mechanical ventilation, or patent ductus arteriosus (PDA). In the hypothesis that ANP or BNP levels (or levels of both) could be predictive of the clinical outcome or may anticipate a phase of increased diuresis coinciding with clinical improvement, several investigators have studied NPs in sick neonates. Increased interest in NPs has also been stimulated by the recent availability of whole-blood assays, allowing onsite BNP measurements within 10 minutes from as little as 250 mcl of blood samples.[188]

The available data, however, have generated controversial results. Discrepancies between studies are probably related to differences in the studied populations, particularly to the coexistence of a PDA, and to differences in policies for fluid and respiratory management among centers and may reflect changes over time in these policies. In addition, ANP secretion is often variable in infants within a 24-hour period. This may be related to sudden changes in atrial filling pressures, secondary, for example, to small fluid boluses, variations in PDA shunting, or in the mean airway pressure when infants are mechanically ventilated.

In this respect, the study by Modi et al[189] is very illustrative. These authors measured ANP levels every 4 hours in 18 preterm infants with respiratory distress. A clear period of respiratory improvement was observed in 15 babies, which was preceded by a peak in circulating ANP in eight babies and was concomitant with the same peak in seven babies, demonstrating a temporal relationship between circulating ANP and improvement in respiratory function.[189] The same study, however, has also documented in several infants peaks of ANP that were not followed by immediate respiratory improvement.[189] This observation illustrates the problem of assessing the clinical usefulness of NP dosage in neonates and probably explains a significant part of the large variance that has been reported by several authors when correlating NP levels with respiratory improvement.[182,190-194] A similar variability has also been reported when NP levels have been correlated with the timing of onset of the postnatal diuretic phase. Overall, a majority of studies report nonetheless a temporal relationship between increased ANP or BNP levels and a phase of negative sodium and water balance.[177,189,190,192,195,196]

The persistence of a PDA is probably the most confounding factor in neonatal ANP and BNP studies. In fact, left-to-right shunting resulting from a PDA, by its dramatic hemodynamic effects on atrial filling pressures, is one of the most potent triggers for ANP and BNP secretion in the neonatal period. Infants with PDA have high levels of circulating NPs.[188,197-199] A recent study by Choi et al[188] has shown very significant correlations between BNP levels and PDA. Nonsymptomatic infants with PDA had a fivefold increase in their BNP levels compared with control infants, and infants with symptomatic PDA had five times higher levels than infants with asymptomatic PDA. BNP levels returned to normal concentrations after duct closure with indomethacin.[188] Other authors have also reported similar results, although their data were considerably less significant.[197-201] Similarly, increased levels of BNP have also been documented in infants with persistent pulmonary hypertension of the newborn compared with healthy infants or with infants with respiratory disease but no evidence of pulmonary hypertension.[202]

Congestive Heart Failure and Congenital Heart Diseases

ANP and BNP levels are increased during congestive heart failure and in most congenital heart diseases, including septal and atrial defects, transposition of the great arteries, tetralogy of Fallot, pulmonary stenosis, tricuspid valve atresia, and mitral valve stenosis or regurgitation.[203-206] In general, reported data indicate higher NP levels in conditions with marked atrial distension, left ventricle overload, left-to-right shunt, and pulmonary hypertension. In patients with these conditions, cardiopulmonary bypass has been shown to cause a dramatic decrease in NP levels.[204]

Reference values for BNP and its pro-peptides (NT-ProBNP) in infants and children, as well as comprehensive reviews of available data, are now available.[207] As indicated previously, most studies report high levels of BNP and NT-proBNP immediately after birth, which decrease in the following weeks.[207]

In clinical practice, measurement of cardiac NPs may help in the decision-making process of specific conditions. Based on available data, Smith et al[208] have defined clinical situations in which dosage of cardiac NPs helps clinicians in deciding the most appropriate treatment. These include PDA of preterm neonates, pulmonary regurgitation and tetralogy of Fallot, heart transplantation, and allograft rejection; on the other hand, measurement of cardiac peptides is of little value in the management of atrial septal defects.[208]

References

1. Goodman BE. Transport of small molecules across cell membranes: water channels and urea transporters. *Adv Physiol Educ.* 2002;26:146.
2. Shaffer SG, Weisman DN. Fluid requirements in the preterm infant. *Clin Perinatol.* 1992;19:233.
3. Robertson GL, Berl T. Pathophysiology of water metabolism. In: Brenner BM, ed. *The Kidney.* 5th ed. Philadelphia, PA: Saunders; 1996:873-928.
4. Miyata S, Takamatsu H, Maekawa S, et al. Plasticity of neurohypophysial terminals with increased hormonal release during dehydration: ultrastructural and biochemical analyses. *J Comp Neurol.* 2001;434:413.
5. Hoffman GE, McDonald T, Figueroa JP, Nathanielsz PW. Neuropeptide cells and fibers in the hypothalamus and pituitary of the fetal sheep: comparison of oxytocin and arginine vasopressin. *Neuroendocrinology.* 1989;50:633.
6. Azizi M, Iturrioz X, Blanchard A, et al. Reciprocal regulation of plasma apelin and vasopressin by osmotic stimuli. *J Am Soc Nephrol.* 2008;19:1015-1024.
7. Roberts EM, Newson MJ, Pope GR, et al. Abnormal fluid homeostasis in apelin receptor knockout mice. *J Endocrinol.* 2009;202:453-462.
8. Hammer M, Olgaard K, Schapira A, et al. Hypovolemic stimuli and vasopressin secretion in man. *Acta Endocrinol.* 1988;118:465.
9. Engelmann M, Ludwig M. The activity of the hypothalamo-neurohypophysial system in response to acute stressor exposure: neuroendocrine and electrophysiological observations. *Stress.* 2004;7:91.
10. Brenner BM, Ballermann BJ, Gunning ME, Zeidel ML. Diverse biological actions of atrial natriuretic peptide. *Physiol Rev.* 1990;70:665.
11. Toto KH. Regulation of plasma osmolality: thirst and vasopressin. *Crit Care Nurs Clin North Am.* 1994;6:661.
12. Mannix ET, Farber MO, Aronoff GR, et al. Hemodynamic, renal, and hormonal responses to lower body positive pressure in human subjects. *J Lab Clin Med.* 1996;128:585.
13. Schrier RW, Berl T, Anderson RJ. Osmotic and nonosmotic control of vasopressin release. *Am J Physiol.* 1979;236:F321.
14. Czaplewski C, Kazmierkiewicz R, Ciarkowski J. Molecular modeling of the human vasopressin V2 receptor/agonist complex. *J Comput Aided Mol Des.* 1998;12:275.
15. Ruiz-Opazo N, Akimoto K, Herrera VL. Identification of a novel dual angiotensin II/vasopressin receptor on the basis of molecular recognition theory. *Nat Med.* 1995;1:1074.
16. Thibonnier M, Conarty DM, Preston JA, et al. Human vascular endothelial cells express oxytocin receptors. *Endocrinology.* 1999;140:1301.
17. Bankir L. Antidiuretic action of vasopressin: quantitative aspects and interaction between V1a and V2 receptor-mediated effects. *Cardiovasc Res.* 2001;51:372.
18. Son MC, Brinton RD. Vasopressin-induced calcium signaling in cultured cortical neurons. *Brain Res.* 1998;793:244.
19. Krismer AC, Wenzel V, Stadlbauer KH, et al. Vasopressin during cardiopulmonary resuscitation: a progress report. *Crit Care Med.* 2004;32:S432.
20. Hiroyama M, Wang S, Aoyagi T, et al. Vasopressin promotes cardiomyocyte hypertrophy via the vasopressin V1A receptor in neonatal mice: *Eur J Pharmacol.* 2007;559:89-97.
21. Valenti G, Procino G, Tamma G, et al. Minireview: aquaporin 2 trafficking. *Endocrinology.* 2005;146:5063.
22. Kuwahara M, Fushimi K, Terada Y, et al. cAMP-dependent phosphorylation stimulates water permeability of aquaporin-collecting duct water channel protein expressed in Xenopus oocytes. *J Biol Chem.* 1995;270:10384.
23. Itoh T, Rai T, Kuwahara M, et al. Identification of a novel aquaporin, AQP12, expressed in pancreatic acinar cells. *Biochem Biophys Res Commun.* 2005;330:832.
24. Harris HW, Zeidel ML. Cell biology of vasopressin. In: Brenner BM, ed. *The Kidney.* 5th ed. Philadelphia, PA: Saunders; 1996:516-531.
25. Ecelbarger CA, Nielsen S, Olson BR, et al. Role of renal aquaporins in escape from vasopressin-induced antidiuresis in rat. *J Clin Invest.* 1997;99:1852.

26. Tian Y, Sandberg K, Murase T, et al. Vasopressin V2 receptor binding is down-regulated during renal escape from vasopressin-induced antidiuresis. *Endocrinology*. 2000;141:307.

27. Hebert SC, Brown EM, Harris HW: Role of the Ca2+-sensing receptor in divalent mineral ion homeostasis. *J Exp Biol*. 1997;200:295.

28. Marples D, Frokiaer J, Dorup J, et al. Hypokalemia-induced downregulation of aquaporin-2 water channel expression in rat kidney medulla and cortex. *J Clin Invest*. 1996;97:1960.

29. Apostol E, Ecelbarger CA, Terris J, et al. Reduced renal medullary water channel expression in puromycin aminonucleoside-induced nephrotic syndrome. *J Am Soc Nephrol*. 1997;8:15.

30. Wilke C, Sheriff S, Soleimani M, Amlal H. Vasopressin-independent regulation of collecting duct aquaporin-2 in food deprivation. *Kidney Int*. 2005;67:201.

31. Stachenfeld NS, Taylor HS, Leone CA, Keefe DL. Estrogen effects on urine concentrating response in young women. *J Physiol*. 2003;552:869.

32. Ge Y, Stricklett PK, Hughes AK, et al. Collecting duct-specific knockout of the endothelin A receptor alters renal vasopressin responsiveness, but not sodium excretion or blood pressure. *Am J Physiol Renal Physiol*. 2005;289:F692.

33. Walker RJ, Weggery S, Bedford JJ, et al. Lithium-induced reduction in urinary concentrating ability and urinary aquaporin 2 (AQP2) excretion in healthy volunteers. *Kidney Int*. 2005;67:291.

34. Agnoli GC, Borgatti R, Cacciari M, et al. Low-dose desmopressin infusion: renal action in healthy women in moderate salt retention and depletion, and interactions with prostanoids. *Prostaglandins Leukot Essent Fatty Acids*. 2002;67:263.

35. Koukoulas I, Risvanis J, Douglas-Denton R, et al. Vasopressin receptor expression in the placenta. *Biol Reprod*. 2003;69:679.

36. Herin P, Kim JK, Schrier RW, et al. Ovine fetal response to water deprivation: aspects on the role of vasopressin. *Q J Exp Physiol*. 1988;73:931.

37. Irion GL, Mack CE, Clark KE. Fetal hemodynamic and fetoplacental vascular response to exogenous arginine vasopressin. *Am J Obstet Gynecol*. 1990;162:1115.

38. Towstoless MK, Congiu M, Coghlan JP, Wintour EM. Placental and renal control of plasma osmolality in chronically cannulated ovine fetus. *Am J Physiol*. 1987;253:R389.

39. Liu H, Koukoulas I, Ross MC, et al. Quantitative comparison of placental expression of three aquaporin genes. *Placenta*. 2004;25:475.

40. Wang S, Chen J, Beall M, et al. Expression of aquaporin 9 in human chorioamniotic membranes and placenta. *Am J Obstet Gynecol*. 2004;191:2160.

41. Ishibashi K, Morinaga T, Kuwahara M, et al. Cloning and identification of a new member of water channel (AQP10) as an aquaglyceroporin. *Biochim Biophys Acta*. 2002;1576:335.

42. Mobasheri A, Wray S, Marples D. Distribution of AQP2 and AQP3 water channels in human tissue microarrays. *J Mol Histol*. 2005;36:1.

43. Bell RJ, Laurence BM, Meehan PJ, et al. Regulation and function of arginine vasopressin in pregnant sheep. *Am J Physiol*. 1986;250:F777.

44. Buemi M, D'Anna R, Di Pasquale G, et al. Urinary excretion of aquaporin-2 water channel during pregnancy. *Cell Physiol Biochem*. 2001;11:203.

45. Stegner H, Leake RD, Palmer SM, Fisher DA. Permeability of the sheep placenta to 125I-arginine vasopressin. *Dev Pharmacol Ther*. 1984;7:140.

46. Desai M, Guerra C, Wang S, Ross MG. Programming of hypertonicity in neonatal lambs: resetting of the threshold for vasopressin secretion. *Endocrinology*. 2003;144:4332.

47. Oosterbaan HP, Swaab DF, Boer GJ. Oxytocin and vasopressin in the rat do not readily pass from the mother to the amniotic fluid in late pregnancy. *J Dev Physiol*. 1985;7:55.

48. Mastorakos G, Ilias I. Maternal and fetal hypothalamic-pituitary-adrenal axes during pregnancy and postpartum. *Ann N Y Acad Sci*. 2003;997:136.

49. Gilbert WM, Cheung CY, Brace RA. Rapid intramembranous absorption into the fetal circulation of arginine vasopressin injected intraamniotically. *Am J Obstet Gynecol*. 1991;164:1013.

50. Oosterbaan HP, Swaab DF. Amniotic oxytocin and vasopressin in relation to human fetal development and labour. *Early Hum Dev*. 1989;19:253.

51. Young SF, Smith JL, Figueroa JP, Rose JC. Ontogeny and effect of cortisol on vasopressin-1b receptor expression in anterior pituitaries of fetal sheep. *Am J Physiol Regul Integr Comp Physiol*. 2003;284:R51.

52. Zhu L, Mao C, Wu J, et al. Ovine fetal hormonal and hypothalamic neuroendocrine responses to maternal water deprivation at late gestation. *Int J Devl Neuroscience*. 2009;27:385-391.

53. Shi L, Mao C, Wu J, et al. Effects of i.c.v. losartan on the angiotensin II-mediated vasopressin release and hypothalamic fos expression in near-term ovine fetuses. *Peptides*. 2006;27:2230-2238.

54. Shi L, Guerra C, Yao J, Xu Z. Vasopressin mechanism-mediated pressor responses caused by central angiotensin II in the ovine fetus. *Pediatr Res*. 2004;56:756.

55. Bonilla-Felix M. Development of water transport in the collecting duct. *Am J Physiol Renal Physiol*. 2004;287:F1093.

56. Bajoria R, Ward S, Sooranna SR. Influence of vasopressin in the pathogenesis of oligohydramnios-polyhydramnios in monochorionic twins. *Eur J Obstet Gynecol Reprod Biol*. 2004;113:49.

57. Robillard JE, Weitzman RE. Developmental aspects of the fetal renal response to exogenous arginine vasopressin. *Am J Physiol*. 1980;238:F407.

58. Ramin SM, Porter JC, Gilstrap LC, Rosenfeld CR. Stress hormones and acid-base status of human fetuses at delivery. *J Clin Endocrinol Metab*. 1991;73:182.

59. Pochard JL, Lutz-Bucher B. Vasopressin and oxytocin levels in human neonates. Relationships with the evolution of labour and beta-endorphins. *Acta Paediatr Scand*. 1986;75:774.

11

60. Vuohelainen T, Ojala R, Virtanen A, et al. Predictors of AVP and TSH levels and the timing of first voiding in the newborn. *Pediatr Res.* 2007;62:106-110.
61. Zelenina M, Zelenin S, Aperia A. Water channels (aquaporins) and their role for postnatal adaptation. *Pediatr Res.* 2005;57:47R.
62. Polacek E, Vocel J, Neugebauerova L, et al. The osmotic concentrating ability in healthy infants and children. *Arch Dis Child.* 1965;40:291.
63. Svenningsen NW, Aronson AS. Postnatal development of renal concentration capacity as estimated by DDAVP-test in normal and asphyxiated neonates. *Biol Neonate.* 1974;25:230.
64. Winberg J. Renal function in water-losing syndrome due to lower urinary tract obstruction before and after treatment. *Acta Paediatr.* 1959;48:149.
65. Ammar A, Roseau S, Butlen D. Pharmacological characterization of V1a vasopressin receptors in the rat cortical collecting duct. *Am J Physiol.* 1992;262:F546.
66. Bonilla-Felix M, Vehaskari VM, Hamm LL. Water transport in the immature rabbit collecting duct. *Pediatr Nephrol.* 1999;13:103.
67. Gengler WR, Forte LR. Neonatal development of rat kidney adenyl cyclase and phosphodiesterase. *Biochim Biophys Acta.* 1972;279:367.
68. Quigley R, Chakravarty S, Baum M. Antidiuretic hormone resistance in the neonatal cortical collecting tubule is mediated in part by elevated phosphodiesterase activity. *Am J Physiol Renal Physiol.* 2004;286:F317.
69. Sulyok E. Renal response to vasopressin in premature infants: what is new? *Biol Neonate.* 1988;53:212.
70. Celsi G, Jakobsson B, Aperia A. Influence of age on compensatory renal growth in rats. *Pediatr Res.* 1986;20:347.
71. Tsukahara H, Hata I, Sekine K, et al. Renal water channel expression in newborns: measurement of urinary excretion of aquaporin-2. *Metabolism.* 1998;47:1344.
72. Devuyst O, Burrow CR, Smith BL, et al. Expression of aquaporins-1 and -2 during nephrogenesis and in autosomal dominant polycystic kidney disease. *Am J Physiol.* 1996;271:F169.
73. Nyul Z, Vajda Z, Vida G, Sulyok E, et al. Urinary aquaporin-2 excretion in preterm and full-term neonates. *Biol Neonate.* 2002;82:17.
74. Bonilla-Felix M, Jiang W. Aquaporin-2 in the immature rat: expression, regulation, and trafficking. *J Am Soc Nephrol.* 1997;8:1502.
75. Yasui M, Serlachius E, Lofgren M, et al. Perinatal changes in expression of aquaporin-4 and other water and ion transporters in rat lung. *J Physiol.* 1997;505:3.
76. Yamamoto T, Sasaki S, Fushimi K, et al. Expression of AQP family in rat kidneys during development and maturation. *Am J Physiol.* 1997;272:F198.
77. Rutishauser J, Boni-Schnetzler M, Boni J, et al. A novel point mutation in the translation initiation codon of the pre-pro-vasopressin-neurophysin II gene: cosegregation with morphological abnormalities and clinical symptoms in autosomal dominant neurohypophyseal diabetes insipidus. *J Clin Endocrinol Metab.* 1996;81:192.
78. Knoers NVAM, Monnens LAH. Nephrogenic diabetes insipidus. In: Avner ED, Harmon WE, Niaudet P, eds. Pediatric Nephrology. 5th ed. Philadelphia, PA: *Lippincott Williams and Wilkins*; 2004:777-787
79. Knoers NV, Deen PM. Molecular and cellular defects in nephrogenic diabetes insipidus. *Pediatr Nephrol.* 2001;16:1146.
80. Abernethy LJ, Qunibi MA, Smith CS. Normal MR appearances of the posterior pituitary in central diabetes insipidus associated with septo-optic dysplasia. *Pediatr Radiol.* 1997;27:45.
81. Garofeanu CG, Weir M, Rosas-Arellano MP, et al. Causes of reversible nephrogenic diabetes insipidus: a systematic review. *Am J Kidney Dis.* 2005;45:626.
82. Wang W, Li C, Summer SN, Falk S, et al. Molecular analysis of impaired urinary diluting capacity in glucocorticoid deficiency. *Am J Physiol Renal Physiol.* 2006;290:F1135–F1142.
83. Baylis PH. The syndrome of inappropriate antidiuretic hormone secretion. *Int J Biochem Cell Biol.* 2003;35:1495.
84. Price JF, Towbin JA, Denfield SW, et al. Arginine vasopressin levels are elevated and correlate with functional status in infants and children with congestive heart failure. *Circulation.* 2004;109:2550.
85. Rocha JL, Friedman E, Boson W, et al. Molecular analyses of the vasopressin type 2 receptor and aquaporin-2 genes in Brazilian kindreds with nephrogenic diabetes insipidus. *Hum Mutat.* 1999;14:233.
86. Kavvadia V, Greenough A, Dimitriou G, et al. A comparison of arginine vasopressin levels and fluid balance in the perinatal period in infants who did and did not develop chronic oxygen dependency. *Biol Neonate.* 2000;78:86.
87. Kobayashi R, Iguchi A, Nakajima M, et al. Hyponatremia and syndrome of inappropriate antidiuretic hormone secretion complicating stem cell transplantation. *Bone Marrow Transplant.* 2004;34:975.
88. Papadimitriou A, Kipourou K, Manta C, et al. Adipsic hypernatremia syndrome in infancy. *J Pediatr Endocrinol Metab.* 1997;10:547.
89. Kanda K, Nozu K, Kaito H, et al. The relationship between arginine vasopressin levels and hyponatremia following a percutaneous renal biopsy in children receiving hypotonic or isotonic intravenous fluids. *Pediatr Nephrol.* 2011;26:99-104.
90. Henry JP, Gauer OH, Sieker HO. The effect of moderate changes in blood volume on left and right atrial pressures. *Circ Res.* 1956;4:91.
91. de Bold AJ, Borenstein HB, Veress AT, Sonnenberg H. A rapid and potent natriuretic response to intravenous injection of atrial myocardial extract in rats. *Life Sci.* 1981;28:89.

92. Kangawa K, Matsuo H. Purification and complete amino acid sequence of alpha-human atrial natriuretic polypeptide (alpha-hANP). *Biochem Biophys Res Commun*. 1984;118:131.
93. Sudoh T, Kangawa K, Minamino N, Matsuo H. A new natriuretic peptide in porcine brain. *Nature*. 1988;332:78.
94. Sudoh T, Minamino N, Kangawa K, Matsuo H. C-type natriuretic peptide (CNP): a new member of natriuretic peptide family identified in porcine brain. *Biochem Biophys Res Commun*. 1990;168:863.
95. de Bold AJ, Ma KK, Zhang Y, et al. The physiological and pathophysiological modulation of the endocrine function of the heart. *Can J Physiol Pharmacol*. 2001;79:705.
96. Kuhn M. Cardiac and intestinal natriuretic peptides: insights from genetically modified mice. *Peptides*. 2005;26:1078.
97. Chusho H, Tamura N, Ogawa Y, et al. Dwarfism and early death in mice lacking C-type natriuretic peptide. *Proc Natl Acad Sci USA*. 2001;98:4016.
98. Vesely DL. Natriuretic peptides and acute renal failure. *Am J Physiol Renal Physiol*. 2003;285:F167.
99. Wu Q, Xu-Cai YO, Chen S, Wang W. Corin: new insights into the natriuretic peptide system. *Kidney Int*. 2009;75:142-146.
100. Levin ER, Gardner DG, Samson WK. Natriuretic peptides. *N Engl J Med*. 1998;339:321.
101. Manganaro R, Mamì C, Mancuso A, et al. Urodilatin excretion and its correlation with sodium excretion in healthy full-term newborn infants. *Early Hum Dev*. 2006;82:645-647.
102. Ruskoaho H. Atrial natriuretic peptide: synthesis, release, and metabolism. *Pharmacol Rev*. 1992;44:479.
103. McGrath MF, de Bold AJ. Determinants of natriuretic peptide gene expression. *Peptides*. 2005;26:933.
104. Joubert S, Jossart C, McNicoll N, De Lean A. Atrial natriuretic peptide-dependent photolabeling of a regulatory ATP-binding site on the natriuretic peptide receptor-A. *FEBS J*. 2005;272:5572.
105. Inoue T, Nonoguchi H, Tomita K. Physiological effects of vasopressin and atrial natriuretic peptide in the collecting duct. *Cardiovasc Res*. 2001;51:470.
106. Garbers DL, Lowe DG. Guanylyl cyclase receptors. *J Biol Chem*. 1994;269:30741.
107. Fuller F, Porter JG, Arfsten AE, et al. Atrial natriuretic peptide clearance receptor. Complete sequence and functional expression of cDNA clones. *J Biol Chem*. 1988;263:9395.
108. Matsukawa N, Grzesik WJ, Takahashi N, et al. The natriuretic peptide clearance receptor locally modulates the physiological effects of the natriuretic peptide system. *Proc Natl Acad Sci USA*. 1999;96:7403.
109. Nonoguchi H, Knepper MA, Manganiello VC. Effects of atrial natriuretic factor on cyclic guanosine monophosphate and cyclic adenosine monophosphate accumulation in microdissected nephron segments from rats. *J Clin Invest*. 1987;79:500.
110. Terada Y, Moriyama T, Martin BM, et al. RT-PCR microlocalization of mRNA for guanylyl cyclase-coupled ANF receptor in rat kidney. *Am J Physiol Renal Physiol*. 1991;261:1080.
111. Gunning ME, Brenner BM. Natriuretic peptides and the kidney: current concepts. *Kidney Int Suppl*. 1992;38:S127.
112. Lewko B. [Interaction between guanylate cyclases in the kidney glomerulus]. *Postepy Hig Med Dosw*. 1999;53:225.
113. Nonoguchi H, Sands JM, Knepper MA. ANF inhibits NaCl and fluid absorption in cortical collecting duct of rat kidney. *Am J Physiol*. 1989;256:F179.
114. Zeidel ML, Silva P, Brenner BM, Seifter JL. cGMP mediates effects of atrial peptides on medullary collecting duct cells. *Am J Physiol*. 1987;252:F551.
115. Zeidel ML, Kikeri D, Silva P, et al. Atrial natriuretic peptides inhibit conductive sodium uptake by rabbit inner medullary collecting duct cells. *J Clin Invest*. 1988;82:1067.
116. Sonnenberg H, Honrath U, Chong CK, Wilson DR. Atrial natriuretic factor inhibits sodium transport in medullary collecting duct. *Am J Physiol*. 1986;250:F963.
117. Harris PJ, Thomas D, Morgan TO. Atrial natriuretic peptide inhibits angiotensin-stimulated proximal tubular sodium and water reabsorption. *Nature*. 1987;326:697.
118. Nonoguchi H, Sands JM, Knepper MA. Atrial natriuretic factor inhibits vasopressin-stimulated osmotic water permeability in rat inner medullary collecting duct. *J Clin Invest*. 1988;82:1383.
119. Nonoguchi H, Tomita K, Marumo F. Effects of atrial natriuretic peptide and vasopressin on chloride transport in long- and short-looped medullary thick ascending limbs. *J Clin Invest*. 1992;90:349.
120. Baum M, Toto RD. Lack of a direct effect of atrial natriuretic factor in the rabbit proximal tubule. *Am J Physiol*. 1986;250:F66.
121. Capasso G, Rosati C, Giordano DR, De Santo NG. Atrial natriuretic peptide has no direct effect on proximal tubule sodium and water reabsorption. *Pflugers Arch*. 1989;415:336.
122. Kondo Y, Imai M, Kangawa K, Matsuo H. Lack of direct action of alpha-human atrial natriuretic polypeptide on the in vitro perfused segments of Henle's loop isolated from rabbit kidney. *Pflugers Arch*. 1986;406:273.
123. Herten M, Lenz W, Gerzer R, Drummer C. The renal natriuretic peptide urodilatin is present in human kidney. *Nephrol Dial Transplant*. 1998;13:2529.
124. Villarreal D, Freeman RH, Taraben A, Reams GP. Modulation of renin secretion by atrial natriuretic factor prohormone fragment 31-67. *Am J Med Sci*. 1999;318:330.
125. Burnett JC, Granger JP, Opgenorth TJ. Effects of synthetic atrial natriuretic factor on renal function and renin release. *Am J Physiol*. 1984;247:F863.
126. Aguilera G. Differential effects of atrial natriuretic factor on angiotensin II- and adrenocorticotropin-stimulated aldosterone secretion. *Endocrinology*. 1987;120:299.

11

127. Holtwick R, Gotthardt M, Skryabin B, et al. Smooth muscle-selective deletion of guanylyl cyclase-A prevents the acute but not chronic effects of ANP on blood pressure. *Proc Natl Acad Sci USA*. 2002;99:7142.

128. Nakayama T. The genetic contribution of the natriuretic peptide system to cardiovascular diseases. *Endocr J*. 2005;52:11.

129. Calderone A, Thaik CM, Takahashi N, et al. Nitric oxide, atrial natriuretic peptide, and cyclic GMP inhibit the growth-promoting effects of norepinephrine in cardiac myocytes and fibroblasts. *J Clin Invest*. 1998;101:812.

130. Cao L, Gardner DG. Natriuretic peptides inhibit DNA synthesis in cardiac fibroblasts. *Hypertension*. 1995;25:227.

131. Potter LR, Abbey-Hosch S, Dickey DM. Natriuretic peptides, their receptors, and cyclic guanosine monophosphate-dependent signaling functions. *Endocr Rev*. 2006;27:47-72.

132. Charloux A, Piquard F, Doutreleau S, et al. Mechanisms of renal hyporesponsiveness to ANP in heart failure. *Eur J Clin Invest*. 2003;33:769.

133. Stevens TL, Wei CM, Aahrus LL, et al. Modulation of exogenous and endogenous atrial natriuretic peptide by a receptor inhibitor. *Hypertension*. 1994;23:613.

134. Ledoux S, Dussaule JC, Chatziantoniou C, et al. Protein kinase A activity modulates natriuretic peptide-dependent cGMP accumulation in renal cells. *Am J Physiol*. 1997;272:C82.

135. Sasser JM, Ni XP, Humphreys MH, Baylis C. Increased renal phosphodiesterase-5 activity mediates the blunted natriuretic response to a nitric oxide donor in the pregnant rat. *Am J Physiol Renal Physiol*. 2010;299:F810-F814.

136. Aviv R, Gurbanov K, Hoffman A, et al. Urinary neutral endopeptidase 24.11 activity: modulation by chronic salt loading. *Kidney Int*. 1995;47:855.

137. Ebihara F, Di Marco GS, Juliano MA, Casarini DE. Neutral endopeptidase expression in mesangial cells. *J Renin Angiotensin Aldosterone Syst*. 2003;4:228.

138. Bianciotti LG, de Bold AJ. Modulation of cardiac natriuretic peptide gene expression following endothelin type A receptor blockade in renovascular hypertension. *Cardiovasc Res*. 2001;49:808.

139. Boric MP, Bravo JA, Corbalan M, et al. Interactions between bradykinin and ANP in rat kidney in vitro: inhibition of natriuresis and modulation of medullary cyclic GMP. *Biol Res*. 1998;31:281.

140. McDougall JG, Yates NA. Natriuresis and inhibition of Na+/K(+)-ATPase: modulation of response by physiological manipulation. *Clin Exp Pharmacol Physiol Suppl*. 1998;25:S57.

141. Yoshimura T, Yoshimura M, Yasue H, et al. Plasma concentration of atrial natriuretic peptide and brain natriuretic peptide during normal human pregnancy and the postpartum period. *J Endocrinol*. 1994;140:393.

142. Schrier RW, Briner VA. Peripheral arterial vasodilation hypothesis of sodium and water retention in pregnancy: implications for pathogenesis of preeclampsia-eclampsia. *Obstet Gynecol*. 1991;77:632-639.

143. Almeida FA, Pavan MV, Rodrigues CI. The haemodynamic, renal excretory and hormonal changes induced by resting in the left lateral position in normal pregnant women during late gestation. *BJOG*. 2009;116:1749-1754.

144. Mulay S, Varna DR. Placental barrier to atrial natriuretic peptide in rats. *Can J Physiol Pharmacol*. 1989;67:1.

145. Graham CH, Watson JD, Blumenfeld AJ, Pang SC. Expression of atrial natriuretic peptide by third-trimester placental cytotrophoblasts in women. *Biol Reprod*. 1996;54:834.

146. Cai WQ, Terenghi G, Bodin P, et al. In situ hybridization of atrial natriuretic peptide mRNA in the endothelial cells of human umbilical vessels. *Histochemistry*. 1993;100:277.

147. Itoh H, Sagawa N, Hasegawa M, et al. Transforming growth factor-beta stimulates, and glucocorticoids and epidermal growth factor inhibit brain natriuretic peptide secretion from cultured human amnion cells. *J Clin Endocrinol Metab*. 1994;79:176.

148. Cameron VA, Aitken GD, Ellmers LJ, et al. The sites of gene expression of atrial, brain, and C-type natriuretic peptides in mouse fetal development: temporal changes in embryos and placenta. *Endocrinology*. 1996;137:817.

149. Huang W, Lee D, Yang Z, et al. Evidence for atrial natriuretic peptide-(5-28) production by rat placental cytotrophoblasts. *Endocrinology*. 1992;131:919.

150. Inglis GC, Kingdom JC, Nelson DM, et al. Atrial natriuretic hormone: a paracrine or endocrine role within the human placenta? *J Clin Endocrinol Metab*. 1993;76:1014.

151. Hatjis CG, Grogan DM. Atrial natriuretic peptide receptors in normal human placentas. *Am J Obstet Gynecol*. 1988;159:587.

152. Zhang LC, Liang GD, Zhang YH, et al. Distribution and characteristics of placental ANP receptors in normal and hypertensive pregnancy. *Chin Med J*. 1992;105:39.

153. McQueen J, Kingdom JC, Whittle MJ, Connell JM. Characterization of atrial natriuretic peptide receptors in human fetoplacental vasculature. *Am J Physiol*. 1993;264:H798.

154. Itoh H, Zheng J, Bird IM, et al. Basic FGF decreases clearance receptor of natriuretic peptides in fetoplacental artery endothelium. *Am J Physiol*. 1999;277:R541.

155. Szukiewicz D, Szukiewicz A, Maslinska D, Markowski M. In vitro effect of bioactive natriuretic peptides on perfusion pressure in placentas from normal and pre-eclamptic pregnancies. *Arch Gynecol Obstet*. 1999;263:37.

156. Thomsen JK, Storm TL, Thamsborg G, et al. Atrial natriuretic peptide concentrations in pre-eclampsia. *Br Med J (Clin Res Ed)*. 1987;294:1508.

157. Fievet P, Fournier A, de Bold A, et al. Atrial natriuretic factor in pregnancy-induced hypertension and preeclampsia: increased plasma concentrations possibly explaining these hypovolemic states with paradoxical hyporeninism. *Am J Hypertens*. 1988;1:16.
158. Miyamoto S, Shimokawa H, Sumioki H, Nakano H. Physiologic role of endogenous human atrial natriuretic peptide in preeclamptic pregnancies. *Am J Obstet Gynecol*. 1989;160:155.
159. Hatjis CG, Greelish JP, Kofinas AD, et al. Atrial natriuretic factor maternal and fetal concentrations in severe preeclampsia. *Am J Obstet Gynecol*. 1989;161:1015.
160. Bond AL, August P, Druzin ML, et al. Atrial natriuretic factor in normal and hypertensive pregnancy. *Am J Obstet Gynecol*. 1989;160:1112.
161. McQueen J, Jardine A, Kingdom J, et al. Interaction of angiotensin II and atrial natriuretic peptide in the human fetoplacental unit. *Am J Hypertens*. 1990;3:641.
162. Holcberg G, Kossenjans W, Brewer A, et al. Selective vasodilator effects of atrial natriuretic peptide in the human placental vasculature. *J Soc Gynecol Investig*. 1995;2:1.
163. Stebbing PN, Gude NM, King RG, Brennecke SP. Alpha-atrial natriuretic peptide-induced attenuation of vasoconstriction in the fetal circulation of the human isolated perfused placenta. *J Perinat Med*. 1996;24:253.
164. Grunewald C, Nisell H, Jansson T, et al. Possible improvement in uteroplacental blood flow during atrial natriuretic peptide infusion in preeclampsia. *Obstet Gynecol*. 1994;84:235.
165. Zeller R, Bloch KD, Williams BS, et al. Localized expression of the atrial natriuretic factor gene during cardiac embryogenesis. *Genes Dev*. 1987;1:693.
166. Wei YF, Rodi CP, Day ML, et al. Developmental changes in the rat atriopeptin hormonal system. *J Clin Invest*. 1987;79:1325.
167. Cheung CY, Gibbs DM, Brace RA. Atrial natriuretic factor in maternal and fetal sheep. *Am J Physiol*. 1987;252:E279.
168. Robillard JE, Nakamura KT, Varille VA, et al. Ontogeny of the renal response to natriuretic peptide in sheep. *Am J Physiol*. 1988;254:F634.
169. Deloof S, Chatelain A. Effect of blood volume expansion on basal plasma atrial natriuretic factor and adrenocorticotropic hormone secretions in the fetal rat at term. *Biol Neonate*. 1994;65:390.
170. Cameron VA, Ellmers LJ. Minireview: natriuretic peptides during development of the fetal heart and circulation. *Endocrinology*. 2003;144:2191.
171. Cheung CY, Roberts VJ. Developmental changes in atrial natriuretic factor content and localization of its messenger ribonucleic acid in ovine fetal heart. *Am J Obstet Gynecol*. 1993;169:1345.
172. Rosenfeld CR, Samson WK, Roy TA, et al. Vasoconstrictor-induced secretion of ANP in fetal sheep. *Am J Physiol*. 1992;263:E526.
173. Cheung CY. Regulation of atrial natriuretic factor secretion and expression in the ovine fetus. *Neurosci Biobehav Rev*. 1995;19:159.
174. Mir TS, Laux R, Hellwege HH, et al. Plasma concentrations of aminoterminal pro atrial natriuretic peptide and aminoterminal pro brain natriuretic peptide in healthy neonates: marked and rapid increase after birth. *Pediatrics*. 2003;112:896.
175. Bierd TM, Kattwinkel J, Chevalier RL, et al. Interrelationship of atrial natriuretic peptide, atrial volume, and renal function in premature infants. *J Pediatr*. 1990;116:753.
176. Ekblad H, Kero P, Vuolteenaho O, et al. Atrial natriuretic peptide in the preterm infant. Lack of correlation with natriuresis and diuresis. *Acta Paediatr*. 1992;81:978.
177. Shaffer SG, Geer PG, Goetz KL. Elevated atrial natriuretic factor in neonates with respiratory distress syndrome. *J Pediatr*. 1986;109:1028.
178. Semmekrot B, Roseau S, Vassent G, Butlen D. Developmental patterns of renal atrial natriuretic peptide receptors: [125I]alpha-rat atrial natriuretic peptide binding in glomeruli and inner medullary collecting tubules microdissected from kidneys of young rats. *Mol Cell Endocrinol*. 1990;68:35.
179. Chevalier RL, Fern RJ, Garmey M, et al. Localization of cGMP after infusion of ANP or nitroprusside in the maturing rat. *Am J Physiol*. 1992;262:F417.
180. Midgley J, Modi N, Littleton P, et al. Atrial natriuretic peptide, cyclic guanosine monophosphate and sodium excretion during postnatal adaptation in male infants below 34 weeks gestation with severe respiratory distress syndrome. *Early Hum Dev*. 1992;28:145.
181. Norling LL, Vaughan CA, Chevalier RL. Maturation of cGMP response to ANP by isolated glomeruli. *Am J Physiol*. 1992;262:F138.
182. Stephenson TJ, Broughton Pipkin F, Hetmanski D, Yoxall B. Atrial natriuretic peptide in the preterm newborn. *Biol Neonate*. 1994;66:22.
183. Itoh H, Sagawa N, Hasegawa M, et al. Brain natriuretic peptide levels in the umbilical venous plasma are elevated in fetal distress. *Biol Neonate*. 1993;64:18.
184. Andersson S, Hallman M, Tikkanen I, Fyhrquist F. Birth stress increase fetal atrial natriuretic factor. *Am J Obstet Gynecol*. 1990;162:872.
185. Itoh H, Sagawa N, Hasegawa M, et al. Umbilical venous guanosine 3′,5′-cyclic phosphate (cGMP) concentration increases in asphyxiated newborns. *Reprod Fertil Dev*. 1995;7:1515.
186. Yamada J, Fujimori K, Ispida T, et al. Plasma endothelin-1 and atrial natriuretic peptide levels during prolonged (24-h) non-acidemic hypoxemia in fetal goats. *J Matern Fetal Med*. 2001;10:409.
187. Okumura A, Toyota N, Hayakawa F, et al. Cerebral hemodynamics during early neonatal period in preterm infants with periventricular leukomalacia. *Brain Dev*. 2002;24:693.
188. Choi BM, Lee KH, Eun BL, et al. Utility of rapid B-type natriuretic peptide assay for diagnosis of symptomatic patent ductus arteriosus in preterm infants. *Pediatrics*. 2005;115:e255.
189. Modi N, Betremieux P, Midgley J, Hartnoll G. Postnatal weight loss and contraction of the extracellular compartment is triggered by atrial natriuretic peptide. *Early Hum Dev*. 2000;59:201.

11

190. Rozycki HJ, Baumgart S. Atrial natriuretic factor and postnatal diuresis in respiratory distress syndrome. *Arch Dis Child*. 1991;66:43.
191. Bauer K, Buschkamp S, Marcinkowski M, et al. Postnatal changes of extracellular volume, atrial natriuretic factor, and diuresis in a randomized controlled trial of high-frequency oscillatory ventilation versus intermittent positive-pressure ventilation in premature infants <30 weeks gestation. *Crit Care Med*. 2000;28:2064.
192. Kojima T, Hirata Y, Fukuda Y, et al. Plasma atrial natriuretic peptide and spontaneous diuresis in sick neonates. *Arch Dis Child*. 1987;62:667.
193. Ronconi M, Fortunato A, Soffiati G, et al. Vasopressin, atrial natriuretic factor and renal water homeostasis in premature newborn infants with respiratory distress syndrome. *J Perinat Med*. 1995;23:307.
194. Onal EE, Dilmen U, Adam B, et al. Serum atrial natriuretic peptide levels in infants with transient tachypnea of the newborn. *J Matern Fetal Neonatal Med*. 2005;17:145.
195. Tulassay T, Rascher W, Seyberth HW, et al. Role of atrial natriuretic peptide in sodium homeostasis in premature infants. *J Pediatr*. 1986;109:1023.
196. Kojima T, Fukuda Y, Hirata Y, et al. Effects of aldosterone and atrial natriuretic peptide on water and electrolyte homeostasis of sick neonates. *Pediatr Res*. 1989;25:591.
197. Holmstrom H, Hall C, Thaulow E. Plasma levels of natriuretic peptides and hemodynamic assessment of patent ductus arteriosus in preterm infants. *Acta Paediatr*. 2001;90:184.
198. Holmstrom H, Omland T. Editorial Board: natriuretic peptides as markers of patent ductus arteriosus in preterm infants. *Clin Sci*. 2002;103:79.
199. Puddy VF, Amirmansour C, Williams AF, Singer DR. Plasma brain natriuretic peptide as a predictor of haemodynamically significant patent ductus arteriosus in preterm infants. *Clin Sci*. 2002;3:75.
200. Kaapa P, Seppanen M, Kero P, et al. Hemodynamic control of atrial natriuretic peptide plasma levels in neonatal respiratory distress syndrome. *Am J Perinatol*. 1995;12:235.
201. Pesonen E. Role of natriuretic hormones in the diagnosis of patent ductus arteriosus in newborn infants. *Acta Paediatr*. 2001;90:363.
202. Reynolds EW, Ellington JG, Vranicar M, Bada HS. Brain-type natriuretic peptide in the diagnosis and management of persistent pulmonary hypertension of the newborn. *Pediatrics*. 2004;114:1297.
203. Holmgren D, Westerlind A, Lundberg PA, Wahlander H. Increased plasma levels of natriuretic peptide type B and A in children with congenital heart defects with left compared with right ventricular volume overload or pressure overload. *Clin Physiol Funct Imaging*. 2005;25:263.
204. Costello JM, Backer CL, Checchia PA, et al. Alterations in the natriuretic hormone system related to cardiopulmonary bypass in infants with congestive heart failure. *Pediatr Cardiol*. 2004;25:347.
205. Ootaki Y, Yamaguchi M, Yoshimura N, et al. Secretion of A-type and B-type natriuretic peptides into the bloodstream and pericardial space in children with congenital heart disease. *J Thorac Cardiovasc Surg*. 2003;126:1411.
206. Oberhansli I, Mermillod B, Favre H, et al. Atrial natriuretic factor in patients with congenital heart disease: correlation with hemodynamic variables. *J Am Coll Cardiol*. 1990;15:1438.
207. Nir A, Lindinger A, Rauh M, et al. NT-Pro-B-type Natriuretic Peptide in infants and children: reference values based on combined data from four studies. *Pediatr Cardiol*. 2009;30:3-8.
208. Smith J, Goetze JP, Andersen CB et al. Practical application of natriuretic peptides in pediatric cardiology. *Cardiology in the Young*. 2010;20:353-363.

CHAPTER 12

Acute Problems of Prematurity: Balancing Fluid Volume and Electrolyte Replacements in Very Low Birth Weight and Extremely Low Birth Weight Neonates

Stephen Baumgart, MD

- Immature Epidermal Barrier Function and the Extremely Low Birth Weight Habitus
- Transcutaneous (Insensible) Water Loss
- Water Loss and Pathogenesis of Transcutaneous Dehydration
- Salt Restriction Prophylaxis
- Nonoliguric Hyperkalemia in Extremely Low Birth Weight Babies
- The Epidermal Barrier: Reducing Transcutaneous Evaporation
- Pulmonary Edema Formation
- Electrolyte Imbalances and Neurodevelopment
- Areas for Further Investigation
- Between a Rock and a Hard Place: Suggestions for Vigilant Fluid Balance Therapy in Extremely Low Birth Weight Babies

This chapter discusses three problem areas for achieving fluid and electrolyte balance in extremely low birth weight (ELBW) infants less than 1000 g at birth and for very low birth weight (VLBW) infants less than 1500 g at birth. The most recent clinical research on fluid and electrolyte therapy addresses these groups as separate; however, the principals for achieving fluid balance in each group represent the same physiology at different phases of fetal development.

The first of these problems is poor epidermal barrier function. Especially in ELBW babies, thin, gelatinous skin promotes rapid transcutaneous evaporation, producing severe electrolyte disturbances in the first few days of life, as well as presenting a poor barrier to the invasion of infections and is also subject to trauma from tape or adhesive injury and from routine contact with bedclothes and handling.

A second area of major concern is pulmonary edema formation. Increased lung water (pulmonary edema) has been suggested in the pathogenesis of several conditions (including patent ductus arteriosus [PDA], congestive heart failure, and bronchopulmonary dysplasia [BPD]), leading to the controversy of fluid restriction versus fluid replenishment in preventing chronic lung disease in both VLBW and ELBW babies. Also controversial is the routine use of diuretics and steroids for the treatment of pulmonary edema with acute respiratory distress syndrome (RDS) and with BPD and chronic lung disease.

Finally, a relatively new area of concern is the neurodevelopmental outcome of infants manifesting severe electrolyte imbalances early in life, particularly in those who develop hyponatremia, hypernatremia, or hyperosmolality in the first few weeks of life.

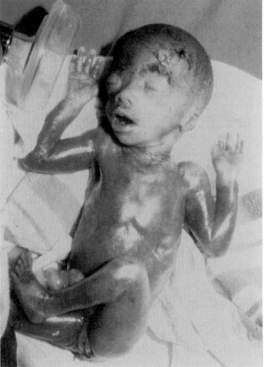

Figure 12-1 Photograph at birth of a 23-3/7 weeks gestation, 530 g extremely low birth weight infant born in 1980 showing that the extremely immature skin has little in the way of skin keratin content and appears translucent, gelatinous, and shiny as if moist with body water rapidly evaporating into the cool-dry delivery room air. Her eyelids are fused, and she is pink, well perfused, and making breathing efforts. She is moving all extremities with apparently good postural tone and spontaneous activity. She went on to survive relatively intact.

Immature Epidermal Barrier Function and the Extremely Low Birth Weight Habitus

ELBW infants experience large transepidermal water losses (TEWLs) immediately upon birth.[1,2] ELBW infants have little in the way of skin keratin content, and the skin appears translucent, gelatinous, and shiny (Fig. 12-1). In addition, these infants have a proportionally larger extracellular pool (with a nearly normal saline content in equilibrium with the plasma compartment)[3] from which to evaporate body water, leaving the sodium behind (Fig. 12-2).[4,5] During early fetal life, more than 85% of body mass may be composed of water, with two-thirds residing in the extracellular space and only one-third of this water residing in the intracellular space. In contrast,

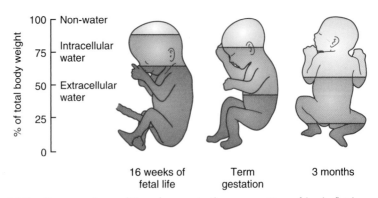

Figure 12-2 From previous edition changes in the composition of body fluids occurring during normal fetal and neonatal development. Note the sizeable extracellular water compartment (an extension of the amniotic fluid space) during fetal life shown at the left. (With permission W.B. Saunders Co. from Costarino AT, Baumgart S. Modern fluid and electrolyte management of the critically ill premature infant. *Pediatr Clin North Am.* 1986;33:153-178. Derived from a summary by Friis-Hansen B. Body water compartments in children. *Pediatrics.* 1961;28:169-181.)

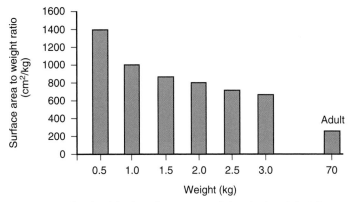

Figure 12-3   Compared with adult physiology, extremely low birth weight infants proportionally have more than six times the skin surface area exposed per kilogram of body weight, with at least three times the mass of water content vulnerable to evaporation. (Adapted with permission from Cambridge University Press, Cambridge, UK from Sridhar S, Baumgart S. Water and electrolyte balance in newborn infants. In: Hay WW, Thureen PJ, eds. *Neonatal Nutrition and Metabolism*, 2nd ed. Cambridge, UK, Cambridge University Press, 2006.)

by term gestation, the infant is composed of about 75% water, with approximately half in the extracellular space and half in the intracellular space. By 3 months postnatal age, only 60% of body mass is water, with two-thirds residing in the intracellular compartment and only one-third in the extracellular space. Finally, ELBW neonates have a geometrically larger skin surface area exposed for evaporation from the extracellular compartment than in more mature infants and adults (Fig. 12-3).[6] Compared with adult physiology, ELBW infants proportionally have more than six times the skin surface area exposed per kilogram of body weight, with at least three times the mass of water content vulnerable to evaporation.[5,6] A 500-g infant has as much as 1400 cm^2 skin exposed per kilogram compared with about 750 cm^2/kg in a term infant and 240 cm^2/kg in the adult. And remember, this exposed body mass is largely composed of extracellular, sodium-rich water exposed for evaporation.

Transcutaneous (Insensible) Water Loss

In 1981, we proposed a geometric model (Fig. 12-4) for estimating insensible water loss (IWL) in ELBW infants using a metabolic balance (Potter Baby Scale, Hartford, CN) for the continuous measurement of body weight loss over a 1- to 3-hour

Figure 12-4   From previous edition concept of a geometric model for estimating insensible water loss in extremely low birth weight infants using a metabolic balance for the continuous measurement of body weight loss over a 3-hour period. (With permission from JB Lippincott Co. from Baumgart S, Langman CB, Sosulski R, Fox WW, Polin RA. Fluid, electrolyte and glucose maintenance in the very low birthweight infant. *Clin Pediatr*. 1982;21:199-206.)

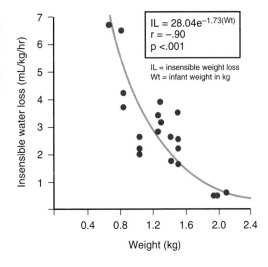

$$IL = 28.04e^{-1.73(Wt)}$$
$$r = -.90$$
$$p < .001$$

IL = insensible weight loss
Wt = infant weight in kg

D

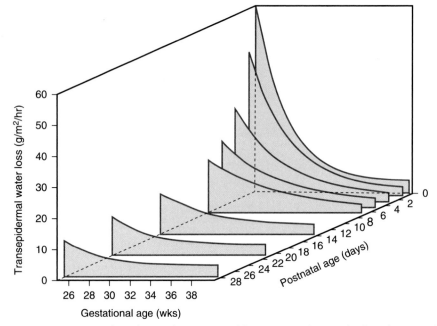

Figure 12-5 Transepidermal water loss measured for gestational age at birth and postnatal age. (Adapted with permission from Scandinavian University Press, Stockholm, Sweden from Hammarlund K, Sedin G. Transepidermal water loss in newborn infants. VIII. Relation to gestational age and post-natal age in appropriate and small for gestational age infants. *Acta Paediatr Scand*. 1983;72:721.)

period.[1,7] Although not widely accepted at the time (IWL estimates in ELBW babies ≤700 g were as high as 7.0 mL/kg/hr approaching 170 mL/day), these findings were exactly reproduced by Hammerlund and Sedin in 1983[2] using an entirely different method to measure water evaporation directly from the skin (transcutaneous water loss [TEWL]) by measuring vapor gradients (Transcutaneous Evaporimeter, Servomed, Stockholm) measured over the immature skin surface of ELBW and VLBW premature neonates during the first weeks of life. These investigators reported similar estimations of transcutaneous evaporation, yielding rates of 50 to 60 g/m²/hr or approximately 170 to 200 mL/kg/day in the first 1 to 3 days of life (Fig. 12-5).[2]

Water Loss and Pathogenesis of Transcutaneous Dehydration

Also in 1982, we reported a small series of ELBW infants who, despite fluid replenishment to as much as 250 mL/kg/day, nevertheless developed hypernatremic serum sodium concentrations by day 3 of life, with values averaging 155 mEq/L (Fig. 12-6),

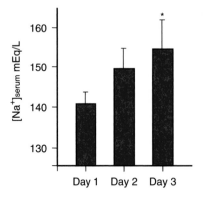

Figure 12-6 Extremely low birth weight babies are prone to developing hypernatremic serum sodium concentrations by day 3 of life, with values averaging 155 mEq/L and peaking in the smallest babies at a serum sodium of nearly 180 mEq/L (2 standard deviations). (With permission from JB Lippincott Co. from Baumgart S, Langman CB, Sosulski R, Fox WW, Polin RA. Fluid, electrolyte and glucose maintenance in the very low birthweight infant. *Clin Pediatr*. 1982;21:199-206.)

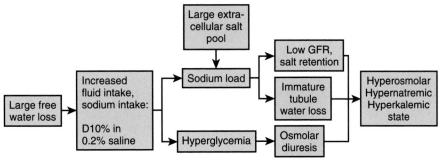

Figure 12-7   Large free water loss through transcutaneous evaporation is balanced by clinicians increasing the rates of fluid replacement, usually adding sodium on the second day of life to match anticipated urinary sodium losses. These influxes contribute to an immense sodium load presented to an immature kidney glomerular apparatus. Added to this exogenous sodium load, the large salt reservoir in the extracellular space is subjected to rapid transcutaneous dehydration, and the low glomerular filtration rate (GFR) of the fetal kidneys leads to salt retention. Immature renal tubules with poor concentrating ability tended to waste additional free water, and osmolar diuresis may also result from dextrose overload and hyperglycemia. The result is that by 48 to 72 hours of life, a hyperosmolar, hypernatremic state evolves, and hyperkalemia is likely to occur as well. (Adapted with permission from WB Saunders Co. from Baumgart S. Fluid and electrolyte therapy in the premature infant: Case management. In: Burg F, Polin RA, eds. *Workbook in Practical Neonatology*. Philadelphia, WB Saunders, 1983, pp. 25-39.)

and peaking in the smallest babies at a serum sodium of nearly 180 mEq/L.[1] These observations led to our first description of the pathogenesis of water depletion, with the development of hypernatremia, hyperglycemia, hyperosmolarity, and a hyperkalemic state peculiar to ELBW infants and developing in the first 72 hours of life (Fig. 12-7).[8] In Fig. 12-5, large free water loss through transcutaneous evaporation is balanced by clinicians increasing the rates of fluid replacement, usually adding sodium in the second day of life to match anticipated urinary sodium losses. These influxes contributed to an immense sodium load presented to an immature kidney glomerular apparatus. Added to this exogenous sodium load, the large salt reservoir in the extracellular space was subjected to rapid transcutaneous dehydration, and the low glomerular filtration rate (GFR) of fetal kidneys led to salt retention. Immature renal tubules with poor concentrating ability tended to waste additional free water, and an osmolar diuresis may also have resulted from dextrose overload and hyperglycemia. The result was that by 48 to 72 hours of life, a hyperosmolar, hypernatremic state evolved. This state contributed to the development of life-threatening hyperkalemia, as discussed later.

Salt Restriction Prophylaxis

To prevent this syndrome, Costarino and coworkers[9] in Philadelphia conducted a randomized, blinded control trial of sodium restriction versus maintenance sodium administration during the first 5 days of life in infants born weighing less than 1000 g and at less than 28 weeks' gestation. Infants were randomly assigned to either a low-sodium group who received no maintenance sodium additive with their parenteral nutrition or to a high sodium replenishment group who received 3 to 4 mEq/kg/day added to their daily maintenance fluids and administered beginning on day 2 of life.

A safety committee analyzed data at half-enrollment and stopped the study. Two of the nine infants in the sodium-restricted group became hyponatremic with serum sodium concentrations of 130 mEq/L or less by day 5 of life and were taken out of the study. Conversely, two of the eight infants in the sodium replenishment

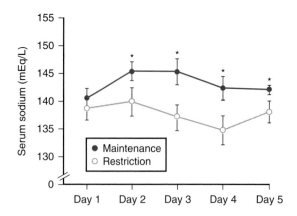

Figure 12-8 Infants randomly assigned to either a low-sodium group who received no maintenance sodium additive with their parenteral nutrition or to a high-sodium replenishment group who received 3 to 4 mEq/kg/day added to their daily maintenance fluids and administered beginning on day 2 of life. Daily assessments of serum sodium concentrations were significantly and consistently higher in the sodium supplemented infants after day 1 of life. (Adapted with permission from Elsevier, Inc. from Costarino AT, Gruskay JA, Corcoran L, et al. Sodium restriction vs. daily maintenance replacement in very low birthweight premature neonates, a randomized and blinded therapeutic trial. *J Pediatr.* 1992;120: 99-106.)

group became hypernatremic with a serum sodium of 150 mEq/L or greater by day 4, and they were also removed from the study. None of these occurrences was reversed. Daily assessments of serum sodium concentrations were significantly and consistently higher in the sodium-supplemented infants after day 1 of life (Fig. 12-8).[9]

By study design, sodium intake (seen in Fig. 12-9, *top graph*) ranged between 4 and 6 mEq/kg/day in the sodium-supplemented maintenance group (*solid shaded bars*).[9] Infants in the restricted group inadvertently received between 1 and 1.75 mEq/kg/day of sodium as additives (shown as *light shaded bars* in the graph) with medications containing sodium (sodium heparin, sodium ampicillin, and sodium citrate transfusions, and so on). It was impossible to eliminate sodium intake entirely because of these often unrecognized sources of exogenously applied salt. Sodium output in the urine (shown in Fig. 12-9, *middle graph*) remained the same for the first 3 days of the study, but began to increase after day 4 in infants in the sodium-supplemented group. And shown in the *bottom graph* (Fig. 12-9), calculated sodium balance was nearly zero in the sodium-supplemented group (*shaded bars*) when intake matched urinary sodium excretion, but remained markedly negative in the sodium-restricted group by as much as 6 mEq/kg/day net sodium loss (*light shaded bars*).

Fluid intakes, prescribed independent of the study by the physicians (who did not know the group assignment), were similar in both groups of babies, ranging between 90 and 130 mL/kg/day throughout the first 3 days of life (Fig. 12-10, *top graph*). However, after 3 days, fluid volume exceeded 130 mL/kg/day in the sodium-supplemented infants (indicated by *black circles*) and was significantly higher than in the salt-restricted babies, who only received approximately 90 mL/kg/day (shown by *open circles*). These results suggest that infants in the sodium-supplemented group were prescribed increasing amounts of fluid to compensate for their increasing serum sodium concentrations. Conversely, infants in the sodium-restricted group required relative fluid restrictions, probably in response decreasing falling serum sodium concentrations. Failure to restrict fluid intake volume after 5 days may result in clinically significant hyponatremia.

Of interest (as seen in the *bottom graph*, Fig. 12-10), urine output was fixed throughout the study in both groups at between 2 and 4 mL/kg/hr (or about 50–100 mL/kg/day) and was not dependent on either the volume of fluid administered or the amount of sodium intake.

Survival was similar in both groups at about two-thirds, and the comorbidities of intraventricular hemorrhage (IVH) and PDA were also similar. There was a trend, however, toward infants developing BPD in the high-sodium, high-fluid intake group (seven of seven infants vs. four of eight infants in the low-sodium, low-fluid intake group; *P* = .08). However, this safety analysis was underpowered to detect the impact of fluid volume administration on these comorbidities.

Figure 12-9 Sodium intake (*top*) ranged between 4 and 6 mEq/kg/day in the sodium-supplemented maintenance group (2–4 mEq/kg/day, *solid shaded bars*). Infants in the restricted group received between 1 and 1.75 mEq/kg/day of sodium as additives (*light shaded bars*) with medications containing sodium (see text). It was impossible to eliminate sodium intake entirely because of these often unrecognized sources of exogenously applied salt. In the *bottom graph*, calculated sodium balance was nearly zero in the sodium-supplemented group (*solid shaded bars*) in whom intake matched urinary sodium excretion, but remained markedly negative in the sodium restricted group by as much as 6 mEq/kg/day net sodium loss (2 standard deviations, *light shaded bars*). (Adapted with permission from Elsevier, Inc. from Costarino AT, Gruskay JA, Corcoran L, et al. Sodium restriction vs. daily maintenance replacement in very low birthweight premature neonates, a randomized and blinded therapeutic trial. *J Pediatr.* 1992;120:99-106.)

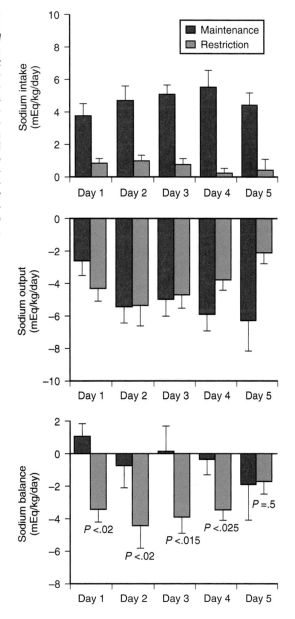

Nonoliguric Hyperkalemia in Extremely Low Birth Weight Babies

During these studies, we encountered an additional electrolyte disturbance that was further investigated by Gruskay et al,[10] who first reported nonoliguric hyperkalemia in ELBW babies in the absence of renal failure. These authors measured renal functions in a group of ELBW infants, some of whom developed serum potassium concentrations of 6.8 mEq/L or greater, a level first identified by Usher[11] that increases the risk for life-threatening cardiac arrhythmias in neonates. Gruskay et al[10] described eight ELBW infants in a hyperkalemic group with slightly lower birth weights and compared them with 10 comparable ELBW infants who remained normokalemic. Peak serum potassium concentrations averaged 8.0 + 0.3 mEq/L in

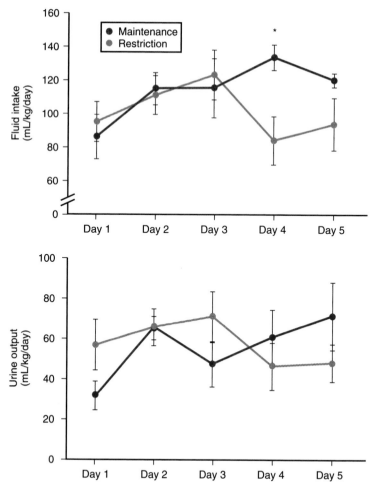

Figure 12-10 Fluid intakes prescribed by the physicians unaware of the sodium-supplemental group assignment were similar in both groups of babies, ranging between 90 and 130 mL/kg/day throughout the first 3 days of life (*top graph*). However, after 3 days, fluid volume exceeded 130 mL/kg/day in the sodium-supplemented infants (*solid red circles*) and was significantly higher than in the salt-restricted babies, who only received approximately 90 mL/kg/day (*light pink circles*). These results suggest that infants in the sodium-supplemented group were prescribed increasing amounts of fluid to compensate for their increasing serum sodium concentrations. Conversely, infants in the sodium-restricted group required relative fluid volume restriction, probably in response to decreasing serum sodium concentrations. Failure to restrict fluid intake volume after 5 days, however, may result in clinically significant hyponatremia. Urine output (*bottom graph*) was fixed throughout the study in both groups at between 2 and 4 mL/kg/hr (or about 50–100 mL/kg/day) and was not dependent on either the volume of fluid administered or the amount of sodium intake. (Adapted with permission from Elsevier, Inc. from Costarino AT, Gruskay JA, Corcoran L, et al. Sodium restriction vs. daily maintenance replacement in very low birthweight premature neonates, a randomized and blinded therapeutic trial. *J Pediatr.* 1992;120:99-106.)

the hyperkalemic babies, and *all* of these infants developed electrocardiographic abnormalities requiring treatment.

Renal functions for these two groups of babies demonstrated similar serum creatinine concentrations and GFRs (Fig. 12-11). In contrast, urine sodium excretion was markedly increased in hyperkalemic infants, with urine concentrations of sodium exceeding 140 mEq/L (Fig. 12-12) and fractional excretion of sodium nearly 15% in the hyperkalemic group compared with only 5% in the normokalemic infants. Both of these observations suggest a profoundly immature tubular conservation of filtered sodium. Moreover, potassium excess is normally *secreted* from the distal tubule. Hyperkalemic infants' urine revealed significantly less potassium

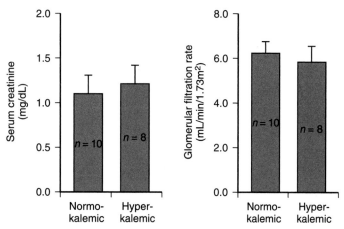

Figure 12-11 Eight hyperkalemic extremely low birth weight (ELBW) infants compared with 10 comparable ELBW infants who remained normokalemic. Renal functions for these two groups of babies demonstrated similar serum creatinine and glomerular filtration rates. (With permission from Elsevier, Inc. from Gruskay J, Costarino AT, Polin RA, Baumgart S. Non-oliguric hyperkalemia in the premature infant less than 1000 grams. *J Pediatr.* 1988;113:381-386.)

excretion than normal infants' urine (Fig. 12-13). These authors suggested an immaturity in renal tubular response to aldosterone, resulting in these electrolyte disturbances.

However, Stefano et al,[12] working independently in Philadelphia, reported a similar investigation of 12 ELBW infants developing nonoliguric hyperkalemia and compared them with 27 babies of similar gestation who remained normokalemic. In addition to urine and renal function studies, these authors reported erythrocyte Na^+, K^+-ATPase activity that was significantly higher in normokalemic infants, suggesting that the cellular maturation of this enzyme was markedly more immature in the hyperkalemic babies and contributed to the exudation of potassium from the intracellular compartment. Potassium leakage can be exacerbated by high serum sodium levels when sodium leaks into cells and competitively exceeds the Na^+, K^+-ATPase pump capacity to exclude sodium, further promoting intracellular potassium leak into the extracellular compartment. These authors concluded that hyperkalemia was attributable to an intracellular-to-extracellular potassium shift with diminished

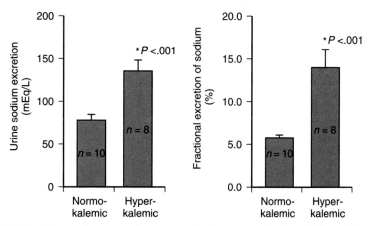

Figure 12-12 Urine sodium excretion was markedly increased in hyperkalemic infants, with urine concentrations of urine sodium sometimes exceeding 140 mEq/L (standard deviation), and mean fractional excretion of sodium was nearly 15% in the hyperkalemic group compared with only 5% in the normokalemic infants. Both of these observations suggest a profoundly immature tubular conservation of filtered sodium. (With permission from Elsevier, Inc. from Gruskay J, Costarino AT, Polin RA, Baumgart S. Non-oliguric hyperkalemia in the premature infant less than 1000 grams. *J Pediatr.* 1988;113:381-386.)

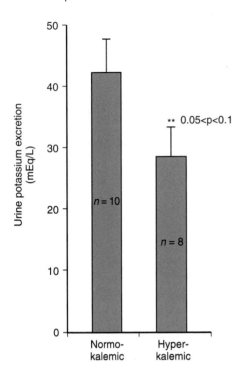

Figure 12-13 Potassium excess is normally *secreted* from the distal tubule. Hyperkalemic infants' urine had significantly less potassium excretion than the urine of normokalemic infants, suggesting an immaturity in renal tubular response to aldosterone resulting in these electrolyte disturbances. (With permission from Elsevier, Inc. from Gruskay J, Costarino AT, Polin RA, Baumgart S. Non-oliguric hyperkalemia in the premature infant less than 1000 grams. *J Pediatr.* 1988;113:381-386.)

Na^+, K^+-ATPase and that glomerular–tubular imbalance the kidneys did not completely explain why hyperkalemia was developing in these babies. Subsequent observational studies by Lorenz and Kleinman[13] and others have confirmed their findings.

The Epidermal Barrier: Reducing Transcutaneous Evaporation

Other than manipulating water and electrolyte administration to ELBW babies, an alternative strategy for preventing these disturbances is to reduce the large TEWL that creates an electrolyte imbalance in the first place. Several techniques have been proposed to accomplish this, including incubator humidification, "swamping" babies in mist either within incubators or within plastic body chambers under radiant warmers, application of petroleum-based ointments used on the skin as emollients, polyvinyl chloride plastic blankets or body bags, and nonocclusive semiadherent polyurethane artificial skins. Native transepidermal water evaporation gradually lessens because spontaneous keratinization of the epidermis develops over a 1- to 4-week period after birth in these babies, probably too late to prevent the acute dehydration syndrome just described.[14]

Environmental Humidification

Incubator humidification for premature babies is recommended by the American Academy of Pediatrics and the American College of Obstetricians' guidelines.[14] Levels suggested are between 40% to 50% percent relative humidity. Saturated environments for "swamping" babies at 80% to 100% relative humidity may lead to "rain-out" (a term used to describe "swamp-like" condensation of water on the interior surfaces of incubators or other plastic covers for tiny babies), and raises concern for water-borne infections.

Harpin and Rutter (1985)[15] used 80% to 90% humidified incubators for 33 VLBW infants and compared them with 29 historical control participants nurtured in dry incubators. All infants were born at less than 30 weeks' gestation and were studied for the first 2 weeks of life. Two infants developed *Pseudomonas* sepsis in the humidified group, and one died, and one developed *Pseudomonas* sepsis in the dry group and died. These authors concluded that saturated humidification was effective, but may be associated with water-borne nosocomial infection.

More recently, Gaylord et al (2001)[16] studied 70 infants in dry incubators, comparing them with 85 babies nursed in humidified incubators, again using historical control participants. Despite similar fluid balance, babies kept in dry incubators were significantly more likely to develop hypernatremia, hyperkalemia, azotemia, and oliguria and to receive more fluid volume replacements; babies in humidified incubators did not have these problems, but had more gram-negative isolates (62%) recovered from surface cultures.

Additionally, servo-regulated humidification is supplied within the closed-incubator condition (Giraffe OmniBed) and may set a determined *relative humidity* between 70% to 80%, which is optimal to avoid excessive IWL and electrolyte disturbances in ELBW premature neonates in the first week of life, which are often experienced when they are incubated dry. One recent report of a clinical series compared the use of initial stabilization of ELBW babies (<1000 g at birth) under a radiant warmer followed by conventional incubation, dry versus the use of humidity control in OmniBeds. The authors demonstrated that humidification improved care by decreasing fluid intake, with more stable electrolyte balance and growth velocity. (Boston AAP, Kim, *et al.* #7933.24, 2007) The authors did not address the risk-to-benefit issue of humidification and infection.

Therefore, humidity should be used cautiously. The author recommends not exceeding 80% relative humidity during incubator care. The author also suggests using the sophisticated humidification monitoring and control systems now incorporated into modern incubators. The author does not recommend "swamping" infants either within incubators or under radiant warmers. Any visible water (even mist) is condensation, which promotes bacterial and fungal growth.

The patented Giraffe Humidifier immerses a heating element in a reservoir of sterile water. Water temperature ranges from 52° to 58°C, which is bactericidal to most organisms thriving at temperatures of 20° to 45°C (human pathogens). As an added safety measure against reservoir contamination, water is boiled off the immersion element as the humidified air is passed inside the infant's compartment. Sterile humidity is created in a vapor state, with no airborne droplets. In an industry-sponsored study,[17] humidified OmniBeds (in vitro air control mode at 35°C and humidified to 65% relative humidity) were cultured (after investigator inoculation with reservoir contamination [four water-borne pathogens over a 4-week incubating period]. No infant environment culture revealed growth of any pathogen. The authors concluded that there is no concern for an increased risk of infection to an infant when the reservoir is filled daily with sterile distilled water and the bed is routinely cleaned according to their protocol.

Skin Emollients

Research on petroleum-based ointments to treat the skin of newborn babies began as early as 1981 when Rutter and Hull[18] first applied paraffin oil to premature infants every 4 to 6 hours, reducing TEWL, but not significantly altering fluid balance over the first several days of life. In 1996, Nopper et al[19] at Stanford University conducted a small randomized trial in 16 infants using Aquaphor, a preservative-free petroleum ointment to reduce TEWL, bacterial colonization, and sepsis. These authors claimed better skin integrity with this treatment, and many nurseries adopted this treatment as standard practice for ELBW babies. In 2000, however, Campbell et al[20] reported an increasing occurrence of candidiasis in their nurseries after the introduction of petroleum ointment use. The multicenter Vermont Oxford trial (2004) observed an increase in coagulase-negative staphylococcal sepsis occurring in babies who were treated with this petroleum preparation.[21] Because of these concerns for infection and the requirement for more frequent handling (it was necessary to repeatedly reapply ointment in ELBW babies to maintain an effective moisture barrier), the author no longer uses this technique in our nurseries.

Table 12-1   TRANSEPIDERMAL EVAPORATION (G/M²/HR) WITH AND WITHOUT A FLEXIBLE POLYURETHANE PLASTIC, NONOCCLUSIVE SKIN BARRIER*

	Day 1	Day 2	Day 3	Day 4	Day 5, Removal
Naked	27.5	31.3	21.4	18.8	20.8
Dressed	8.9†	9.5†	9.0†	10.6†	18.8

*OpSite, Smith Nephew Inc., Columbia, SC.[23] †Indicates significant reduction in TEE.

Plastic Shields, Bags, and Blankets

Alternatively, the author has reported the use of a single layer of Saran polyvinyl chloride to reduce IWL during the first few days of life by more than half in low birth weight (LBW) babies, and the author has advocated the use of this technique, especially for tiny infants under radiant warmers during the first 24 to 48 hours of life. To date, however, there have been no studies to evaluate the occurrence of infection or bacterial colonization with the use of these plastic "blankets."[22] Other investigators with our Philadelphia fluid study group, Knauth et al,[23] alternatively suggested the use of a flexible polyurethane plastic, nonocclusive skin barrier (the trade names of these barriers are familiar as Tegaderm and OpSite). Some of these barriers are treated with antimicrobial suppressants and are relatively infection neutral when used as total parenteral nutrition catheter site dressings. The author evaluated transcutaneous evaporation using these materials and produced a two-thirds reduction in TEWL (Table 12-1) during the first 4 days of life in a series of premature babies. However, as seen on the right side of Table 12-1, after removal on the fifth day, evaporation again increased,[24] either with reexposure of the immature skin or with the exfoliation of the developing keratin underneath this gently adhesive barrier. The Israelis have produced a membrane material for this application that is completely adhesive free to avoid such debridement.

Porot and Brodsky[25] recently published data on the use of polyurethane dressings completely covering LBW infants. They demonstrated significant reductions in hypernatremia, excessive fluid volume intake, weight loss, BPD, and mortality with the use of an artificial layer during the first few weeks of life.

Donahue et al[26] conducted a randomized trial of this technique in 61 babies, but did not reveal changes in fluid volume requirements, although improved skin integrity was suggested by these authors. For any of these strategies, a consistent effect in reducing electrolyte disturbances has not been demonstrated. Humidification and emollient ointments may increase the risk of infection. Some randomized data exist, none of which supports their use. Alternatively, standard incubation at moderate humidity between 40% to 70%, with or without a plastic barrier, remains the most popular practice in the author's nurseries.

Pulmonary Edema Formation

After the initial first week of life, the risk for dehydration diminishes as the skin barrier matures. Thereafter, and usually during the second or third week of life in ELBW babies, many authors have now described water overload in the pathogenesis of pulmonary edema, probably resulting from continuing overzealous fluid replenishment therapy continued past the first week when these babies were more subject to dehydration.

Suggested pathogenesis for water overload is depicted in Figure 12-14.[8] Fluid replenishment volume, when administered too aggressively, may result in increased lung water and may contribute to the pathogenesis of BPD.[27-29] Moreover, high fluid intakes have been associated with the development of clinically significant PDA and congestive heart failure,[30-32] also contributing to the pathogenesis of BPD.[33] Increased

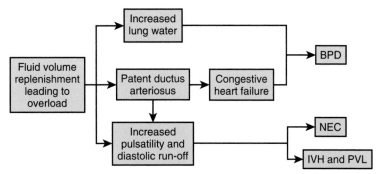

Figure 12-14 When administered too aggressively, fluid replenishment volume may result in increased lung water, and contribute to the pathogenesis of bronchopulmonary dysplasia (BPD).[27-29] Moreover, high fluid intakes have been associated with the development of clinically significant patent ductus arteriosus (PDA) and congestive heart failure,[30-32] also contributing to the pathogenesis of BPD.[33] Increased pulsatility and diastolic run-off with a clinically signifi-cant PDA may contribute to the development of necrotizing enterocolitis (NEC),[34] and intra-ventricular hemorrhage (IVH).[35] (Adapted with permission W.B. Saunders Co. from Baumgart S: Fluid and electrolyte therapy in the premature infant: Case management. In: *Workbook in Practical Neonatology.* Burg F, and Polin RA, eds. WB Saunders, Philadelphia, pp. 25-39, 1983.)

pulsatility and diastolic runoff with a clinically significant PDA may contribute to the development of necrotizing enterocolitis (NEC)[34] and IVH.[35]

Perhaps the root cause of this problem is premature infants' markedly immature renal development. At 25 weeks' gestation, the fetal kidneys have a lobulated appear-ance, with a thin cortex predominated by small, less well-developed juxtamedullary nephrons and entirely lacking the robust cortical nephron population. The result of diminutive anatomy is less glomerular surface available for filtration of any fluid volume or salt excess. We can only imagine even more immature nephrons and the severe functional limitations present in the tiny kidneys of ELBW infants between 500 to 1000 g in development.

Prevention of Iatrogenic Fluid Overload

In testing the prevention strategy of low versus high fluid volume administration for the development of fluid overload in premature infants, Bell and Acarregui[33] recently reviewed a meta-analysis of four randomized controlled trials (Table 12-2).[30-34] Of

Table 12-2 META ANALYSIS OF FOUR STUDIES EVALUATING HIGH-VERSUS LOW-FLUID VOLUME INTAKE STRATEGIES FOR MAINTENANCE THERAPY IN VERY LOW BIRTH WEIGHT INFANTS*

	Study Design	Weights and Gestational Age	High-/Low-Fluid Volume Limits	Outcomes
Bell et al[30]	170 sequential matched pairs, 30 days	1.41 kg 31 wk	122/169	PDA, CHF, NEC in high-fluid group
von Stackhauser and Struve[31]	56 random pairs, 3 days	1.9/2.0 kg 34.6/34.2 wk	60/150	No differences
Lorenz et al[32]	88 random matched pairs, 5 days	1.20 kg 29 wk	60–85/80–140	No differences
Tammela and Koivisto[33]	100 random pairs, 28 days	1.30 kg 31 wk	50–150/80–200	Death, BPD in high-fluid group

*PDA, congestive heart failure (CHF), and necrotizing enterocolitis (NEC) were significantly more common with high fluid volumes administered.
BPD, bronchopulmonary dysplasia.
Adapted from Bell, EF, Acarregui MJ. Restricted versus liberal water intake for preventing morbidity and mortality in preterm infants. Cochrane Database Syst Rev. 2001;3:CD000503.

the studies reported, fluid intakes ranged from as low as 50 mL/kg/day to as high as 200 mL/kg/day routinely, depending on the study designs used. All four were conducted primarily in VLBW (and not ELBW) populations, and only two of the studies demonstrated significant differences in the occurrences of PDA, congestive heart failure, BPD, NEC, or death in the high-fluid groups. The meta-analysis of all randomized data, however, favored low-fluid volume infusions, revealing that PDA with congestive heart failure and NEC were more frequently observed in the high-fluid group and that death was significantly higher as well. More recently, Kavvidia et al[36] reported the only randomized series including a number of ELBW infants, with gestational ages ranging between 23 and 33 weeks, and offered only modest differences in high- versus low-fluid volumes prescribed. No beneficial or adverse effects could be demonstrated.

Finally, Oh et al,[29] for the Neonatal Research Network, summarized a cohort of 1382 ELBW babies born at between 401 and 1000 g who were followed prospectively at Network centers to characterize their daily fluid volume intakes prescribed (both parenteral and enteral; net intake, mL/kg/day; Fig. 12-15) and percent of birth weight loss daily over the first 10 days of life and analyzed retrospectively for adverse outcomes of BPD and death. Multivariate logistic regression demonstrated that higher fluid intake volumes with weight retention over the first 10 days of life were significantly associated with higher risk of death or BPD. As in other studies, however, higher birth weight was associated with a lower risk for death or BPD, suggesting that even slightly more developmentally mature infants are less likely to require excessive fluid replenishment to maintain electrolyte balance described above in sections on epidermal barrier and renal organogenesis in ELBW babies. Wide ranges of daily fluid volume prescriptions (41–389 mL/kg/day) were observed in this study, with average group differences of as little as 7 to 24 mL/kg/day.

Even more recently, Stephens et al[37,38] reported on 204 surviving ELBW (<32 weeks and <1250 g at birth),ranked into low-, intermediate-, and high-fluid groups, concluding: "High fluid intake (>170 mL/kg/day) in the first days of life is associated with increased risk of PDA." These authors concluded that intakes less than 170 mL/

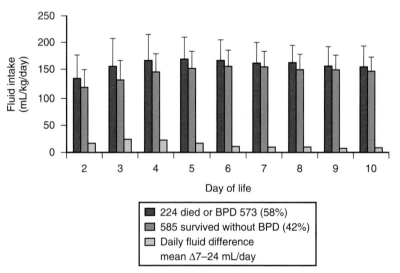

Figure 12-15   Multivariate logistic regression demonstrated that higher fluid intake volumes with weight retention over the first 10 days of life were significantly associated with higher risk of death or bronchopulmonary dysplasia (BPD) in 1382 extremely low birth weight infants followed prospectively from day 1 of life. Wide ranges of daily fluid volume prescriptions (41–389 mL/kg/day) were observed in this study, with average group differences of as little as 7 to 24 mL/kg/day. (Adapted with permission from Elsevier, Inc. from Oh W, Poindexter BB, Perritt R, et al for the Neonatal Research Network. Association between fluid intake and weight loss during the first ten days of life and risk of bronchopulmonary dysplasia in extremely low birth weight infants. J Pediatr 2005;147:786-790.)

kg/day could be provided at as little as less than 126 mL/kg/day during the first week with similar nutritional caloric intakes and is advisable.

Another recent report by Niwas et al[39] compared restricted 125 mL/kg/day versus more liberal fluid administration of 155 mL/kg/day in 113 ELBW infants (<900 g at birth), finding no association with any mortality or morbidities. This study may have been underpowered to detect such differences and did not combine death and BPD as an outcome as was done for the NETWORK analysis.

The author concludes from these published data that careful fluid volume restriction reduces death, PDA, and NEC in VLBW infants and may also be prudent for the ELBW population and that there is also a trend toward less chronic lung disease in infants from both categories. However, we cannot readily extrapolate a more restricted fluid strategy to the treatment of ELBW babies during the first 1 to 3 days of life because of the risk for dehydration with severe electrolyte disturbances already described. Randomized trials of either artificial epidermal barriers to circumvent hypernatremia or hyperkalemia, with or without free water restriction to avoid weight retention and to allow body water and sodium pool contraction over the first week after birth, are wanting and warranted.

Diuretic Therapy

Diuretic therapy to treat fluid overload and pulmonary edema after it occurs also remains controversial. In 2002, Brion et al[40] reported a meta-analysis of six randomized controlled trials for the combination of spironolactone and thiazide diuretics given for 3 weeks' duration or longer, with some success in the treatment of chronic lung disease. A year later, they conducted a second meta-analysis, describing six randomized controlled trials for the use of furosemide in treating lung edema in acute RDS.[41] Oxygenation was only transiently improved with furosemide. However, furosemide is also a vasodilator and was associated with the development of symptomatic PDA in RDS babies. Moreover, in some cases, significant hypovolemia developed, requiring excess fluid administration to recover blood pressure. Brion and Sol[41] concluded that furosemide should not be recommended for treating acute RDS. Of note, none of these studies was done in the era of prenatal prophylactic steroid therapy. Therefore, combinations of therapies effective for treating pulmonary edema and the development of BPD have not been adequately tested or reported in the present era.

Regarding lung edema, in a 1990 review, Bland[42] summarized perinatal animal models, describing lung water physiology. Prenatally, the pulmonary epithelium actively secretes chloride ion with water; but the postnatal lung changes to an active Na+/K+ exchange-mediated absorbing mechanism. This transitional change from a secretory organ to a dry organ may be disrupted by RDS or a clinically significant PDA with congestive heart failure, becoming involved in the pathogenesis of pulmonary edema, and BPD.

Corticosteroid Therapy

Helve et al[43] reported the use of postnatal steroids on the epithelial sodium channel and described mRNA expression as diminished in VLBW babies with RDS comparing them with normal term control infants. All five RDS subjects' mothers had received prenatal β-methasone therapy. Subsequently, when given dexamethasone for the treatment of BPD occurring after 1 month of age in four of these subjects, increased sodium channel mRNA expression was again observed, suggesting a potential role for postnatal steroids in resorbing lung edema and diminishing lung water.

In the only study of ELBW babies and steroids, Omar et al[44] in 1999 reported prenatal corticosteroid effects on development in ELBW infants ranging from 565 to 865 g. They noted higher urine output during the first 2 days of life in babies receiving prenatal steroids when compared with control participants. The authors speculated that natriuresis may be attributable to better mobilization of lung fluid through the augmentation of Na^+, K^+-ATPase in the pulmonary epithelium. These authors also commented on a lower calculated IWL during the first 4 days of life in these infants, speculating that prenatal steroids may also have improved epidermal barrier function. In the author's opinion, results of studies on corticosteroids and fluid balance remain highly speculative at this time, and unfortunately, no recommendations for routine therapy should be made.

Electrolyte Imbalances and Neurodevelopment

Hyponatremia

Finally, in examining the effects of fluid and electrolyte imbalances on later neurodevelopment, Bhatty et al[45] have given us a preliminary description of hyponatremia occurring in a group of ELBW infants less than 1000 g. These authors defined a serum sodium concentration of less than 125 mEq/L as clinically significant hyponatremia. Thirty-five babies developing hyponatremia during the first few weeks of life were compared retrospectively with 43 nonhyponatremic birth weight–matched control infants using multivariate regression analysis.

Although not statistically significant, hyponatremic babies in general seemed more critically ill: all of them subsequently developed BPD, had longer ventilator and oxygen courses, and had longer hospital stays. Moreover, more severe IVH (grades 3 and 4) were observed in 23% of the hyponatremic subjects and only 5% of the nonhyponatremic infants. Similarly, significant retinopathy (grades 3 and 4) was more prevalent in the hyponatremic subjects.

On follow-up through early infancy, Bhatty et al[45] observed a higher occurrence of spastic cerebral palsy in infants who had developed hyponatremia, more hypotonia, and an increased occurrence of sensorineural hearing loss, as well as behavioral problems reported by parents later in childhood. Using regression analysis, the authors suggested a specific association between recovery from hyponatremia and neurodevelopmental problems subsequently developing in the ELBW population.

When evaluating the degree of hyponatremia at onset, the degree of worst hyponatremia (lowest serum sodium concentration), and the duration of hyponatremia, they found no correlation to subsequent neurodevelopmental outcomes. In contrast, when looking at the speed of recovery from hyponatremia, the 11 infants with more rapid correction of serum sodium concentrations (by >10 mEq/L in 24 hours) experienced the worst neurodevelopmental outcomes later on. The authors concluded that rapid correction of hyponatremia, particularly within the first 24 hours of onset of serum sodium concentration below 125 mEq/L, may be associated with adverse neurodevelopmental sequelae and that the calculated sodium correction should provide a rate no more than 0.4 mEq/L/hr or at most 10 mEq/L/day. The author presently do not recommend any more rapid correction, and in most situations, we avoid entirely the use of 3% hypertonic saline acutely for correction of hyponatremia in ELBW and VLBW neonates.

Many other studies have suggested an association between hyponatremia and later neurodevelopmental problems (Table 12-3). In 1995, Leslie et al[46] matched case control participants revealing significant sensorineural hearing deficits in ELBW babies under 28 weeks of gestation and 1000 g at birth. Hyponatremia in this study

Table 12-3 PUBLISHED STUDIES SUGGESTING HYPONATREMIA IS ASSOCIATED WITH ADVERSE NEURODEVELOPMENTAL OUTCOMES[46-48]

	Study Design	Population	Developmental Deficits
Leslie et al[46]	Case controls	ELBW	Sensorineural hearing loss
Murphy et al[47]	Case controls	VLBW	Cerebral palsy
Ertl et al[48]	Multi-variate analysis, case controls	VLBW	Sensorineural hearing loss

ELBW, extremely low birth weight; VLBW, very low birth weight.

was also diagnosed at a sodium concentration below 125 mEq/L. In 1997, Murphy et al[47] reported 134 case controls for 59 VLBW babies developing cerebral palsy and associated cerebral palsy with hyponatremia. Ertl et al[48] matched 22 babies with sensorineural hearing loss to 25 case control participants for multivariate analysis and found an association between hearing impairment and hyponatremia specifically. None of these studies reported the course of development or treatment of hyponatremia nor made recommendations for therapy.

And in a fascinating long-term follow-up study, Al-Dahhana et al[49] reported that sodium-supplemented VLBW babies less than 32 weeks gestation given 4 to 5 mEq/kg/day in their diets and lasting from 4 to 14 days of life had better performance IQs, better motor and memory indices, and improved parental behavioral assessments at 10 years of age. This report suggests that routine sodium restriction in premature babies, although expedient to prevent hypernatremia, may not be beneficial with respect to long-term outcomes.

Hypernatremia

In contrast (and despite the frequent observation of hypernatremia in ELBW babies already described), the data associating hypernatremia with central nervous system disruptions have not been as closely examined. In 1974, Simmons et al[50] suggested restricting hypertonic sodium bicarbonate use, associating the resulting hypernatremia with significant IVHs. However, in 1990, Lupton et al[51] reevaluated serum sodium concentrations during the first 4 days of life in VLBW premature infants weighing less than 1500 g who had developed IVH in that time period and found no association with hypernatremia. Lupton et al's[51] study, however, defined hypernatremia at serum sodium levels greater than 145 mEq/L, which may not comprise a critical threshold for evaluating neurologic impairment. The author certainly have seen more severe hypernatremia in the ELBW population with serum sodium concentrations ranging from greater than 150 to as high as 180 mEq/L.[1]

None of these reports on hypernatremia directly addresses the occurrences of developmental delays with electrolyte imbalance in the ELBW population, and further investigation is needed. Existing developmental follow-up data for this population should probably be examined for routinely recorded serum sodium concentrations.

Areas for Further Investigation

There are many areas for further investigation. For ELBW infants, in whom virtually every therapy is experimental, protocols to standardize care should be developed in each provider's institution along with safety and outcome evaluations. Epidermal barrier augmentation seems to be a first, natural step in these investigations to avoid the disruption of fluid and electrolyte balance in the first place. Materials for promoting a temporary artificial skin barrier that is neutral to infection are more elusive than we might have imagined.

Manipulations of both sodium and free water volume intake are also warranted. Testing specified wet versus dry net volume intakes seems to me to be a dogmatic approach. Rather, a more strict and precise definition of fluid balance is needed. Right now, we depend on serial measurements of serum sodium concentration to evaluate whether ELBW babies need more or less water volume replenishment. The trouble with this approach is that the serum sodium concentration must be abnormal before fluid intake can be adjusted to offset changing losses. Further investigation of sodium channel development and the promotion of natural lung water resorption through endogenous means is a more complex area for basic science investigations. Clinical trials of diuretics and steroids should be performed *before* prescribing these therapies routinely.

In the area of neurodevelopmental outcomes, hyponatremia, water restriction, and sodium supplementation are hot topics for investigation given the numerous associations with sensorineural hearing loss and cerebral palsy reviewed previously.

Randomized controlled trials for routine sodium replacement versus restriction therapy may now be warranted. Regarding life-threatening hypernatremia and hyperkalemia, no investigative reports to date have described late adverse neurodevelopmental outcomes, and such investigations should at least include multivariate analysis of presently existing databases in this regard.

Between a Rock and a Hard Place: Suggestions for Vigilant Fluid Balance Therapy in Extremely Low Birth Weight Babies

Maintenance fluid therapy is at best a moving target that should be addressed by adjusting fluid volumes required frequently, at least two or three times daily, depending on a periodic clinical assessment of hydration and balance (intake and output). Practitioners should try to anticipate and to avoid both extremes of under- and overhydration in ELBW babies by anticipating their physiologic progress as demonstrated in a hypothetical 600-g patient shown in Figure 12-16.[52] On day 1 of life,

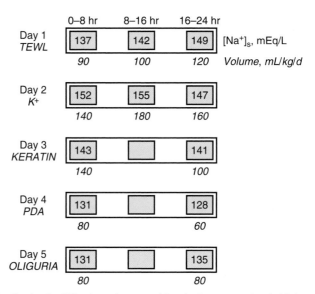

Figure 12-16   On day 1 of life, the primary problem is the tremendously high transepidermal water loss (TEWL). We recommend checking serum electrolytes every 8 hours during the first day or 2 of life and adjusting an electrolyte-free solution upward in 10- to 20-mL increments every 6 to 8 hours, depending on the rate of increase in the measured serum sodium concentration. The key to this strategy is checking serum or urine electrolytes more frequently because once the serum sodium rises, the practitioner is already behind. By day 2, the problem of hyperkalemia often emerges – volume replacement maximizes, as serum sodium concentration peaks, and sodium leaks into the cells displacing potassium outwards from the intracellular compartment. Then on day 3 TEWL begins to diminish as keratin deposition occurs, or in response to incubator care with additional humidification. At this juncture, the serum sodium concentration may suddenly decrease. We should anticipate this change by diminishing water volume *immediately* when we first see the serum sodium concentrations fall, thus anticipating fluid overload and the risk for promoting a hemodynamically significant PDA by day 4 of life, imaging the ductus prospectively may be of consequential benefit. The occurrence of iatrogenic hyponatremia is most often observed at this time and may be associated with patent ductus physiology, and is best addressed by aggressive water volume restriction to as little as 60 mL/kg/day, minimizing the *rate* of sodium correction and avoiding entirely the use of hypertonic salt infusions. Oliguria observed while treating for PDA and hyponatremia should not be addressed by liberalizing fluid volume administration, nor by the use of furosemide which may actually dilate the PDA. Rather, maintenance fluid restriction should be continued while the PDA is addressed definitively either with Indocin, or by surgical ligation. (Adapted with permission from Cambridge University Press, Cambridge, UK from Sridhar S, Baumgart S. Water and electrolyte balance in newborn infants. In: Hay WW, Thureen PJ, eds. *Neonatal Nutrition and Metabolism*, 2nd ed. Cambridge, UK, Cambridge University Press, 2006.)

the primary problem is the tremendously high TEWL; the author recommends checking serum electrolytes every 8 hours during the first day or two of life and adjusting an electrolyte-free solution upward in 10- to 20-mL increments every 6 to 8 hours, depending on the rate of increase in the measured serum sodium concentration. The key to this strategy is checking serum and urine electrolytes more frequently because when the serum sodium rises, the practitioner is already behind in water volume administration, as shown. By day 2, the problem of hyperkalemia often emerges—volume replacement maximizes as serum sodium concentration peaks, and sodium leaks into the cells, displacing potassium outward from the intracellular compartment. Then on day 3, TEWL begins to diminish as keratin deposition occurs or in response to incubator care with additional humidification. At this juncture, the serum sodium concentration may suddenly decrease. Practitioners should anticipate this change by diminishing water volume *immediately* when first seeing the serum sodium concentrations decrease, thus anticipating fluid overload and the risk for promoting a hemodynamically significant PDA by day 4 of life. Imaging the ductus prospectively may be of consequential benefit. The occurrence of iatrogenic hyponatremia is most often observed at this time and may be associated with ductal physiology[53] and is best addressed by aggressive water volume restriction to as little as 60 mL/kg/day, minimizing the *rate* of sodium correction *and* avoiding entirely the use of hypertonic salt infusions. Oliguria observed while treating for PDA, and hyponatremia should not be treated by liberalizing fluid volume administration, nor by the use of furosemide, which may actually dilate the PDA.[40] Rather, maintenance fluid restriction should be continued while the PDA is addressed definitively either with indomethacin or by surgical ligation.

A Parting Shot at Aggressive Patent Ductus Arteriosus Management

Much of this discussion regarding fluids and electrolyte imbalances in ELBW premature infants revolves around the prevention of a clinically significant PDA. In a recent and controversial opinion paper, Laughon et al[54] questioned the significance of a PDA and how it can and should be managed. These authors remind us of our assumption that a PDA is, per se, pathologic. Indeed, the ductus before birth is essential to maintain systemic circulation in fetuses delivering oxygenated blood to vital organs while bypassing the lungs. After birth at term, the ductus usually closes within 3 days. In LBW premature infants of 30 weeks gestation or later, the ductus usually closes within 5 days. In the ever troublesome VLBW premature newborn less than 30 weeks' gestation and certainly in the ELBW population less than 1000 g birth weight, at least two-thirds of infants have PDAs that do not close, and, incidentally, this is the group with serious pulmonary disease and high pulmonary vascular resistance to shunting left to right (resulting in lung congestion). The importance of diagnosis of a clinically significant PDA (i.e., pulmonary congestive) is raised by these authors. It seems that echocardiography invariably demonstrates an anatomically patent ductus in these critically ill babies with refractory respiratory distress; however, identifying the significance of this finding when screening for a ductus with echocardiography routinely on day 4 of life, as suggested above, requires examining the patient, not just for the presence of a systolic heart murmur (difficult to auscultate while on an oscillatory ventilator), nor just for echogenic evidence of an otherwise normal structure but for bounding pulses, a hyperactive precordium, and a widened pulse pressure (systolic value more than double the diastolic). Doppler evidence of a significant left-to-right ductal shunt is often vaguely represented as "bidirectional" on an echocardiogram, and deleterious effects of diastolic run-off flow velocities seem exaggerated. Failure to improve oxygenation despite prenatal corticosteroid and postnatal surfactant therapies often leads to frustration when asking, "What stone can be left unturned?" Therefore, treating the PDA aggressively seems prudent even though a markedly premature lung morphology and fluid physiology (secretory vs. dry organogenesis) may remain the true culprits of premature lung disease. Surgical ligation is the gold standard for premature ductal closure. Although 40% of murmurs observed remain asymptomatic, the majority of symptomatic murmurs become asymptomatic with fluid restriction alone (a strong recommendation for a "dry" approach to parenteral fluid prescription during the first week of life in ELBW infants).[55] And surgery is not without risks for a hemodynamically unstable patient: bleeding, pneumothorax, vocal cord paralysis, grades 3 to 4 retinopathy, and infection have all been associated with PDA surgical ligation.

Then there is indomethacin medical therapy to avoid surgery in patients not responding to fluid restriction within 48 hours. In the landmark multicenter collaborative trial authored by Gersony et al[55] (1983), more than 3500 infants with significant PDAs failing fluid restriction received indomethacin for one or two courses by 2 weeks postnatal age (with 79% closure) before surgery was offered (35%). There were no differences in mortality or duration of mechanical ventilation, hospital stay, IVH, or NEC in the medical versus the surgical treatment groups. At the end of the study, however, all PDAs were closed. Other landmark studies of indomethacin therapy have followed (e.g., prophylactic treatment for all vulnerable premature infants to prevent PDA and IVHs or only for those with asymptomatic PDAs having echocardiographic evidence of PDA on screening), but amelioration of final adverse outcomes remains wanting (neurodevelopmental delays persist, as does chronic lung disease at $\geq$36 weeks postconceptional age).[56,57]

Conclusion

If judicious fluid and electrolyte balance is achievable in ELBW babies, neither indomethacin nor surgery may be required.[58]

References

1. Baumgart S, Langman CB, Sosulski R, et al. Fluid, electrolyte and glucose maintenance in the very low birthweight infant. *Clin Pediatr.* 1982;21:199-206.
2. Hammarlund K, Sedin G. Transepidermal water loss in newborn infants. VIII. Relation to gestational age and post-natal age in appropriate and small for gestational age infants. *Acta Paediatr Scand.* 1983;72:721.
3. Michel CC. Fluid movements through capillary walls. Chapter 9. In: Renkin EM, Michel CC, eds. *Handbook of Physiology, Section II Vol II.* Bethesda, MD: American Physiologic Society; 1984.
4. Costarino AT, Baumgart S. Modern fluid and electrolyte management of the critically ill premature infant. *Ped Clin No Amer.* 1986;33:153-178.
5. Friis-Hansen B. Body water compartments in children. *Pediatrics.* 1961;28:169-181.
6. Haycock GB, Schwartz GJ, Wisotsky DH. Geometric method for measuring body surface areas: A height-weight formula validated in infants, children and adults. *J Pediatr.* 1978;93:62-66.
7. Baumgart S, Engle WD, Fox WW, et al. Radiant warmer power and body size as determinants of insensible water loss in the critically ill neonate. *Pediatr Res.* 1981;15:1495-1499.
8. Baumgart S. Fluid and electrolyte therapy in the premature infant: Case management. In: Burg F, Polin RA, eds. *Workbook in Practical Neonatology.* Philadelphia: WB Saunders; 1983:25-39.
9. Costarino AT, Gruskay JA, Corcoran L, et al. Sodium restriction vs. daily maintenance replacement in very low birthweight premature neonates, a randomized and blinded therapeutic trial. *J Pediatr.* 1992;120:99-106.
10. Gruskay J, Costarino AT, Polin RA, Baumgart S. Non-oliguric hyperkalemia in the premature infant less than 1000 grams. *J Pediatr.* 1988;113:381-386.
11. Usher RH. The respiratory distress syndrome of prematurity. I. Change in potassium in the serum and the electrocardiogram and effects of therapy. *Pediatrics.* 1959;24:562.
12. Stefano JL, Norman ME, Morales MC, et al. Decreased erythrocyte Na+, K+ ATPase activity associated with cellular potassium loss in extremely low birth weight infants with nonoliguric hyperkalemia. *J Pediatr.* 1993;122:276-284.
13. Lorenz, JM, Kleinman LI. Nonoliguric hyperkalemia in preterm neonates (Letter). *J Pediatr.* 1989; 114:507.
14. *Guidelines for perinatal care.* 2nd ed. Elk Grove Village, IL: American Academy of Pediatrics and American College of Obstetricians and Gynecologists; 1988:278.
15. Harpin VA, Rutter N. Humidification of incubators. *Arch Dis Child.* 1985;60:219.
16. Gaylord MS, Wright K, Lorch K, et al. Improved fluid management utilizing humidified incubators in extremely low birth weight infants. *J Perinatol.* 2001;21:438-443.
17. Lynam L, Biagotti L. Testing for bacterial colonization in a Giraffe humidification system. *Neonatal Intensive Care.* 2002;15(2).
18. Rutter N, Hull D. Reduction of skin water loss in the newborn. I. Effect of applying topical agents. *Arch Dis Child.* 1981;56:669.
19. Nopper AJ, Horii KA, Sookdeo-Drost S, et al. Topical ointment therapy benefits premature infants. *J Pediatr.* 1996;128:660.

20. Campbell JR, Zaccaria E, Baker CJ. Systemic candidiasis in extremely low birth weight infants receiving topical petrolatum ointment for skin care: a case-control study. *Pediatrics* 2000;105:1041-1045.
21. Edwards WH, Conner JM, Soll RF/Vermont Oxford Network Neonatal Skin Care Study Group. The effect of prophylactic ointment therapy on nosocomial sepsis rates and skin integrity in infants with birth weights of 501-1000 g. *Pediatrics.* 2004;113:1195-1203.
22. Baumgart S. Reduction of oxygen consumption, insensible water loss and radiant heat demand with use of a plastic blanket for low birthweight infants under radiant warmers. *Pediatrics.* 1984;74: 1022-1028.
23. Knauth A, Gordin M, McNelis W, Baumgart S. A semipermeable polyurethane membrane as an artificial skin in the premature neonate. *Pediatrics.* 1989;83:945-950.
24. Kalia Yn, Nonato LB, Lund CH, Guy RH. Development of skin barrier function in premature infants. *J Investig Derm.* 1998;111:320-326.
25. Porat R, Brodsky N. Effect of Tegederm use on outcome of extremely low birth weight (ELBW) infants. *Pediatr Res.* 1993;33:231(A).
26. Donahue ML, Phelps DL, Richter SE, Davis JM. A semipermeable skin dressing for extremely low birth weight infants. *Journal of Perinatology.* 1996;16(1):20-26.
27. Palta M, Babbert D, Weinstein MR, Peters ME. Multivariate assessment of traditional risk factors for chronic lung disease in very low birth weight neonates. *J Pediatr.* 1991;119:285-292.
28. Van Marter LJ, Pagano M, Allred EN, et al. Rate of bronchopulmonary dysplasia as a function of neonatal intensive care practices. *J Pediatr.* 1992;120:938-946.
29. Oh W, Poindexter BB, Perritt R, et al. for the Neonatal Research Network: Association between fluid intake and weight loss during the first ten days of life and risk of bronchopulmonary dysplasia in extremely low birth weight infants. *J Pediatr.* 2005;147:786-790.
30. Bell, EF, Warburton D, Stonestreet BS, Oh W. Effect of fluid administration on the development of symptomatic patent ductus arteriosus and congestive heart failure in premature infants. *N Engl J Med.* 1980;302:598-604.
31. von Stockhausen HB, Struve M. Die Auswirkungen einer stark unterschiedlichen parenteral en Flussigkeitszufuhr bei Fruh- und Neugeborenen in den ersten drei Lebenstagen. *Klin Padiatr.* 1980;192: 539-546.
32. Lorenz JM, Kleinman LI, Kotagal UR, Reller MD. Water balance in very low-birth weight infants: relationship to water and sodium intake and effect on outcome. *J Pediatr.* 1982;101:423-432.
33. Tammella OKT, Koivisto ME. Fluid restricton for preventing bronchopulmonary dysplasia? Reduced fluid intake during the first weeks of life improves the outcome of low-birth-weight infants. *Acta Paediatr.* 1992;81:207-212.
34. Bell EF, Acarregui MJ. Restricted versus liberal water intake for preventing morbidity and mortality in preterm infants. *Cochrane Database Syst Rev.* 2001;3:CD000503.
35. Perlman JM, McMenamin JB, Volpe JJ. Fluctuating cerebral blood flow velocity in respiratory distress syndrome: Relationship to the development of intraventricular hemorrhage. *N Engl J Med.* 1983;309:209-213.
36. Kavvidia V, Greenough A, Dimitriou G, Forsling ML. Randomized trial of two levels of fluid input in the perinatal period – effect on fluid balance, electrolyte and metabolic disturbances in ventilated VLBW infants. *Acta Paediatr.* 2000;89:237-241.
37. Stephens BE, Gargus FA, Walden RV, et al. Fluid regimens in the first week of life may increase risk of patent ductus arteriosus in extremely low birth weight infants. *J Perinatol.* 2007;28:123-128.
38. Stephens BE, Vohr BR. Fluid regimens and risk of patent ductus arteriosus in extremely low birth weight infants. *J Perinatol.* 2008;28:653.
39. Niwas R, Baumgart S, DeCristofaro JD. Fluid intake in the first week of life: effect on morbidity and mortality in extremely low birth weight infants (less than 900 grams). *J of Med And Med Sciences.* 2010;1(5):156-161.
40. Brion LP, Primhak RA, Ambrosio-Perez I. Diuretics acting on the distal renal tubule for preterm infants with (or developing) chronic lung disease. *Cochrane Database Syst Rev.* 2000;3:CD001817; PMID:10908511:156-161.
41. Brion LP, Sol RF. Diuretics for respiratory distress syndrome in preterm infants. *Cochrane Database Syst Rev.* 2000;2:CD001454;PMID:10796265.
42. Bland RD. Lung epithelial ion transport and fluid movement during the perinatal period. *Am J Physiol* 1990;259:L30-L37.
43. Helve O, Pitkanen OM, Andersson S, et al. Low expression of human epithelial sodium channel in airway epithelium of preterm infants with respiratory distress. *Pediatrics.* 2004;113:1267-1272.
44. Omar SA, Decristofaro JD, Agarwal BI, La Gamma E, et al. Effects of prenatal steroids on water and sodium homeostasis in extremely low birth weight Neonates. *Pediatrics.* 1999;104:482-488.
45. Bhatty SB, Tsirka A, Quinn PB, et al. Rapid correction of hyponatremia in extremely low birth weight (ELBW) premature neonates is associated with long term developmental delay. *Pediatr Res.* 1997;41:140A and Privileged Communication, Dr. DeCristofaro, Stony Brook University Hospital, Stony Brook, New York.
46. Leslie GI, Kalaw MB, Bowen JR, Arnold JD. Risk factors for sensorineural hearing loss in extremely premature infants. *J Paediatr Child Health.* 1995;312-316.
47. Murphy DJ, Hope PL, Johnson A. Neonatal risk factors for cerebral palsy in very preterm babies: case-control study. *BMJ.* 1997;314:404-408.
48. Ertl T, Hadzsiev K, Vincze O, et al. Hyponatremia and sensorineural hearing loss in preterm infants. *Biology of the Neonate.* 2001;79:109-112.

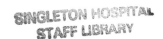

49. Al-Dahhana J, Jannoun L, Haycock G. Developmental risks and protective factors for influencing cognitive outcome at 5-1/2 years of age in very low birthweight children. *Dev Med Child Neurol.* 2002;44:508-516.

50. Simmons MA, Adcock EW III, Bard H, Battaglia FC. Hypernatremia and intracranial hemorrhage in neonates. *New Engl J Med.* 1974;291:6-10.

51. Lupton BA, Roland EH, Whitfield MF, Hill A. Serum sodium concentration and intraventricular hemorrhage in premature infants*Am J Dis Child.* 1990;144:1019-1021.

52. Baumgart S. Water and electrolyte balance in low birth weight infants. In: Burg FD, Inglefinger JR, Polin RA, Gershon AA, eds. *Current Pediatric Therapy.* 18th ed. USA, Philadelphia, PA: Elsevier Science; 2005:85-88, in press.

53. Gupta J, Sridhar S, Baumgart S, DeCristofaro JD. Hyponatremia in extremely low birth weight (ELBW) infants may precede the development of a significant patent ductus arteriosus (PDA) in the first week of life. *Pediatric Res.* 2002;51:387A.

54. Laughon MM, Simmons MA, Bose CL. Patency of the ductus arteriosus in the premature infant: is it pathologic? Should it be treated? *Curr Opin Pediatr.* 2004;16:146-151.

55. Gersony WM, Peckham GJ, Ellison RC, et al. Effects of indomethacin in premature infants with patent ductus arteriosus: Results of a national collaborative study. *J Pediatr.* 1983;102:895-906.

56. Fowlie P, Davis PG. Prophylactic intravenous indomethacin for preventing mortality and morbidity in preterm infants. *Cochrane Database Syst Rev.* 2002;(3):CD000174.

57. Cooke L, Steer P, Woodgate P. Indomethacin for asymptomatic patent ductus arteriosus in preterm infants. *Cochrane Database Syst Rev.* 2003;(2):CD003745.

58. Benitz WE. Treatment of persistent patent ductus arteriosus in preterm infants: time to accept the null hypothesis? *J Perinat.* 2010;30:241-252.

CHAPTER 13

Lung Fluid Balance in Developing Lungs and Its Role in Neonatal Transition

Sarah D. Keene, MD, Richard D. Bland, MD, Lucky Jain, MD, MBA

Often signaled by a loud cry, the birth of a neonate marks a remarkable transition from its dependence for gas exchange on the placenta to an independent state of air breathing and gas exchange in the lungs. Clearing the fluid filled lungs is a significant component of this transition. Scientists have long known that fetal lungs are full of fluid, initially presumed to be an extension of the amniotic fluid pool. However, studies have confirmed[1,2] that fetal lungs themselves, rather than the amniotic sac, are the source of the chemically distinct liquid that fills the lungs during development. Through an active process involving chloride secretion by the respiratory epithelium, this liquid forms a slowly expanding structural template that prevents collapse and is essential for growth of fetal lungs.[3,4]

For effective gas exchange to occur, rapid clearance of liquid from potential alveolar airspaces during and soon after birth is essential for establishing the timely switch from placental to pulmonary gas exchange. It is clear now that traditional explanations that relied on mechanical factors and Starling forces can only account for a small fraction of the fluid absorbed[5,6] and that the normal transition from liquid to air inflation is considerably more complex than the characteristic "vaginal squeeze" theory suggests. Physiologic events beginning days before spontaneous delivery are accompanied by changes in the hormonal milieu of the fetus that pave the way for a smooth neonatal transition, including clearance of the large body of lung fluid. Respiratory morbidity resulting from failure to clear the lung fluid is common and can be particularly problematic in some infants delivered prematurely or when delivery occurs operatively before the onset of spontaneous labor. The same pathways are involved in the development of pulmonary edema in acute respiratory distress syndrome (ARDS) that develops in response to infections such as respiratory syncytial virus.[7] This chapter considers some of the experimental work that provides the basis for our current understanding of lung liquid dynamics before, during, and after birth, focusing on the various pathways and mechanisms by which this process occurs.

Fetal Lung Liquid and Its Physiologic Significance

As stated, the lung is a secretory organ during development, displaying breathing-like movements, but without any contribution to respiratory gas exchange. The small fraction of the combined ventricular output of blood from the heart that circulates through the pulmonary circulation[8] allows the delivery to the lung epithelium of the substrates needed to make surfactant and secretion of up to 5 mL/kg/hr lung fluid at term gestation.[9,10] Several studies have shown that the presence of an appropriate

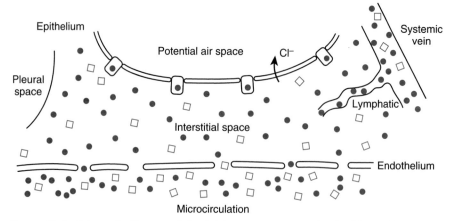

Figure 13-1   Schematic diagram of the fluid compartments in the fetal lung, showing the tight epithelial barrier to protein and the more permeable vascular endothelium, which restricts the passage of globulins (□) more than it restricts albumin (•). In the fetal mammalian lung, chloride secretion in the respiratory epithelium is responsible for liquid production within potential air spaces. (After Bland RD: *Adv Pediatr.* 34:175–222, 1989.)

volume of secreted liquid within the fetal respiratory tract is essential for normal lung growth and development before birth.[1,2,11] Conditions that interfere with normal production of lung liquid, such as pulmonary artery occlusion,[12] diaphragmatic hernia with displacement of abdominal contents into the chest,[13] and uterine compression of the fetal thorax from chronic leak of amniotic fluid,[14] also inhibit lung growth. Conversely, excessive accumulation of lung fluid, such as that after tracheal occlusion, leads to excessive but abnormal lung growth.[1]

Figure 13-1 is a schematic diagram showing the fluid compartments of the fetal lung. Potential air spaces are filled with liquid that is rich in chloride ($\approx$150 mEq/L) and almost free of protein (< 0.03 mg/mL).[15] Whereas the lung epithelium has tight intercellular junctions that provide an effective barrier to macromolecules, including albumin, the vascular endothelium has wider openings that allow passage of large plasma proteins, including globulins and fibrinogen.[16-18] Consequently, liquid in the interstitial space, which was sampled in fetal sheep by collecting lung lymph, has a protein concentration that is about 100 times greater than the protein concentration of liquid contained in the lung lumen.[19] Despite the large transepithelial difference in protein osmotic pressure, which tends to inhibit fluid flow out of the interstitium, active transport of chloride (Cl^-) ions across the fetal lung epithelium generates an electrical potential difference that averages about −5 mV, luminal side negative.[4]

The osmotic force created by this secretory process overcomes that of the protein gradient, pulling liquid from the pulmonary microcirculation through the interstitium into potential air spaces.

In vitro experiments using cultured explants of lung tissue and monolayers of epithelial cells harvested from human fetal lung have indicated that cation-dependent chloride transport, driven by epithelial cell Na^+, K^+-ATPase, is the mechanism responsible for liquid secretion into the lumen of the mammalian lung during fetal life.[20-22] In fetal sheep and lambs, lung epithelial Cl^- transport is inhibited by diuretics that block Na^+, K^+, $2Cl^-$, co-transport.[23-25] This finding supports the concept that the driving force for transepithelial Cl^- movement in the fetal lung is similar to the mechanism described for Cl^- transport across other epithelia, although the specific anion channels responsible have not yet been definitively identified.[26] Accordingly, Cl^- enters the epithelial cell across its basal membrane linked to sodium (Na^+) and potassium (K^+) (Fig. 13-2). Na^+ enters the cell down its electrochemical gradient and is subsequently extruded in exchange for K^+ (three Na^+ ions exchanged for two K^+ ions) by the action of Na^+, K^+-ATPase located on the basolateral surface of the cell. This energy-dependent process increases the concentration of Cl^- within the

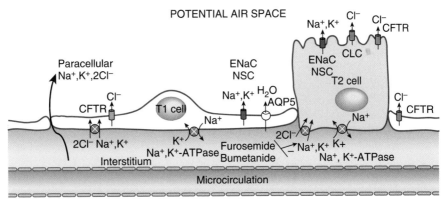

Figure 13-2 Schematic drawing of the fluid compartments of the fetal lung, highlighting the lung epithelium, consisting of type I cells that occupy most of the surface area of the lung lumen and type II cells that manufacture and secrete surfactant. These cells also secrete Cl by a process that involves Na^+, K^+, $2Cl^-$ co-transport and Na^+, K^+-ATPase (Na pump) activity. This energy-dependent process, which can be blocked by loop diuretics, furosemide, and bumetanide, increases the concentration of Cl within the cell so that it exceeds its electrochemical equilibrium, with resultant extrusion of Cl through anion-selective channels on the apical membrane surface (cystic fibrosis transmembrane conductance regulator [CFTR] or chloride channels [CLCs]). Sodium (Na) and water follow the movement of Cl into the lung lumen. AQP, aquaporin; ENaC, epithelial sodium channel; NSC, nonselective channel.

cell so that it exceeds its electrochemical equilibrium. Cl^- then passively exits the epithelial cell through anion-selective channels that are located on the apical membrane surface. Na^+ traverses the epithelium via paracellular pathways or via nonselective cation channels that have been identified in fetal distal airway epithelium; water can flow either between epithelial cells or through water channels, one of which (aquaporin 5) is abundantly expressed in alveolar type I (AT-I) lung epithelial cells.[27,28]

Although the Cl^- concentration of liquid withdrawn from the lung lumen of fetal sheep is about 50% greater than that of plasma, the Na^+ concentration is virtually identical to that of plasma.[3,16] The concentration of bicarbonate in lung liquid of fetal sheep is less than 3 mEq/L, yielding a pH of approximately 6.3 and indicating that that the lung epithelium may actively transport bicarbonate out of the lung lumen. The demonstration that acetazolamide, a carbonic anhydrase inhibitor, blocks secretion of lung liquid in fetal sheep supports this view. Both physiologic and immunohistochemical studies have shown that H^+-ATPases are present on the respiratory epithelium of fetal sheep, where they likely provide an important mechanism for acidification of liquid within the lung lumen during development. In vitro electrophysiologic studies using fetal rat lung epithelial cells provided evidence that exposure to an acid pH might activate Cl^- channels and thereby contribute to the production of fetal lung liquid.[29] In fetal dogs and monkeys, however, the bicarbonate concentration of lung luminal liquid is not significantly different from that of fetal plasma.[30] Thus, the importance of lung liquid pH and acidification mechanisms during human lung development in utero remains unclear.

The volume of liquid within the lung lumen of fetal sheep increases from 4 mL/kg to 6 mL/kg at midgestation[25] to more than 20 mL/kg near term.[18,19] The hourly flow rate of lung liquid increases from approximately 2 mL/kg body weight at midgestation to approximately 5 mL/kg body weight at term.[9,10,31] Increased production of luminal liquid during development reflects a rapidly expanding pulmonary microvascular and epithelial surface area that occurs with proliferation and growth of lung capillaries and respiratory units.[25,32] The observation that unilateral pulmonary artery occlusion decreases lung liquid production in fetal sheep by at least 50%[33] shows that the pulmonary circulation, rather than the bronchial circulation, is the major source of fetal lung liquid. Intravenous infusion of isotonic saline at a rate sufficient to increase lung microvascular pressure and lung lymph flow in fetal lambs

Table 13-1 FACTORS THAT CAN DELAY CLEARANCE OF FETAL LUNG FLUID

Failure of antenatal decrease in fetal lung fluid	• Delivery without labor • Prematurity
Excessive production of fluid	• Elevated transvascular pressure (e.g., cardiogenic edema) • Increased vascular permeability
Decreased epithelial transport of sodium and water	• Decreased number or function of type I and II cells • Decreased sodium-channel expression and activity • Loss of function mutations of ENaC • Decreased Na^+, K^+-ATPase function

ENaC, epithelial sodium channel.

had no effect on liquid flow across the pulmonary epithelium.[34] Thus, transepithelial Cl^- secretion appears to be the major driving force responsible for the production of liquid in the fetal lung lumen. In vitro studies of epithelial ion transport across the fetal airways indicate that the epithelium of the upper respiratory tract also secretes Cl^-, thereby contributing to lung liquid production.[35-37] However, most of this liquid forms in the distal portions of the fetal lung, where total surface area is many times greater than it is in the conducting airways.

How Is the Fetal Lung Fluid Cleared?

Several studies have demonstrated that both the rate of lung liquid production and the volume of liquid within the lumen of the fetal lung normally decrease before birth, most notably during labor.[19,31,38-40] Thus, lung water content is about 25% greater after premature delivery than it is at term, and newborn animals that are delivered by cesarean section without prior labor have considerably more liquid in their lungs than do animals that are delivered either vaginally or operatively after the onset of labor (Table 13-1).[41,42] In studies with fetal sheep, extravascular lung water was 45% less in mature fetuses that were in the midst of labor than in fetuses that did not experience labor, and there was a further 38% decrease in extravascular lung water measured in term lambs that were studied 6 hours after a normal vaginal birth.[19]

To achieve this, the lung epithelium is believed to switch from a predominantly Cl^--secreting membrane at birth to a predominantly Na^+-absorbing membrane after birth. Work performed over the past 2 decades to understand the mechanism(s) responsible for fetal lung fluid clearance have shown that active Na^+ transport across the pulmonary epithelium drives liquid from lung lumen to the interstitium, with subsequent absorption into the vasculature.[43-46] In the lung, Na^+ reabsorption is a two-step process (Fig. 13-3).[47] The first step is passive movement of Na^+ from the lumen across the apical membrane into the cell through Na^+ permeable ion channels. The second step is active extrusion of Na^+ from the cell across the basolateral membrane into the serosal space. Several investigators have demonstrated that the initial entry step primarily involves sodium-specific apical channels (epithelial sodium channels [ENaC]) that are particularly sensitive to amiloride, a diuretic. Indeed, cDNAs that encode amiloride-sensitive Na^+ channels in other Na^+ transporting epithelia have also been cloned from airway epithelial cells.[48-50] This is consistent with studies by O'Brodovich et al,[51] who have shown that intraluminal instillation of amiloride in fetal guinea pigs delays lung fluid clearance.

More recent studies using the patch-clamp technique have confirmed the role of ENaC channels in AT-I and AT-II cells in the vectorial transport of Na^+ from the apical surface.[48,52,53] Increased production of the mRNA for amiloride-sensitive epithelial Na^+ channels (ENaC) in the developing lung[54] has been correlated with the transition from a secretory to absorptive state. Much of this information has come from studies using AT-II cells. Recent studies have shown that AT-I cells also express functional Na^+ channels and other transporters capable of salt and fluid transport.[55-57]

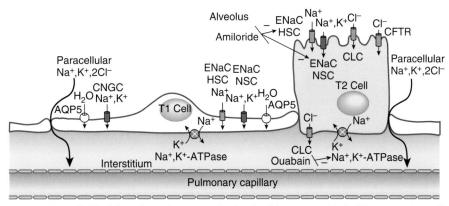

Figure 13-3 Epithelial sodium absorption in the fetal lung near birth. Na enters the cell through the apical surface of both alveolar type I (AT-I) and AT-II cells via amiloride-sensitive epithelial sodium channels (ENaCs), both highly selective channels (HSCs) and nonselective channels (NSCs), and via cyclic nucleotide gated channels (seen only in AT-I cells). Electroneutrality is conserved with chloride movement through the cystic fibrosis transmembrane conductance regulator (CFTR) or through chloride channels (CLCs) in AT-I and AT-II cells or paracellularly through tight junctions. The increase in cell Na stimulates Na^+, K^+-ATPase activity on the basolateral aspect of the cell membrane, which drives out three Na ions in exchange for two K ions, a process that can be blocked by the cardiac glycoside ouabain. If the net ion movement is from the apical surface to the interstitium, an osmotic gradient would be created, which would in turn direct water transport in the same direction, either through aquaporins (AQPs) or by diffusion.

Based on work in animals and humans, ENaC channels are thought to be responsible for 40% to 70% of sodium transport.[58] Nonspecific cation channels and cyclic nucleotide gated channels are also present in alveolar cells and contribute to the amiloride-insensitive sodium and fluid uptake.

Sodium Channel Pathology in the Lung

ENaC channels are primarily composed of three subunit types, α, β, and γ, each with a role in sodium transport but with varied relative importance in mammalian species. A fourth subunit, δ, first identified in the brain and since shown to be coexpressed with the other subunits in lung tissue, is of uncertain significance.[59,60] Hummler et al[61] have shown that inactivating the α-ENaC (a-subunit of the epithelial Na^+ channel) leads to defective lung liquid clearance and premature death in mice. Inactivating β- and γ-ENaC subunits also leads to early death in newborn mice, albeit because of fluid and electrolyte imbalances, suggesting that α-ENaC expression is critical for fetal lung fluid absorption. In later work, Hummler et al[62] showed that a mouse model of increased α-ENaC activity demonstrated increased alveolar fluid clearance after induction of pulmonary edema. This is direct evidence that in vivo ENaC constitutes the rate-limiting step for Na^+ absorption in epithelial cells of the lung, and thus in the adaptation of newborn lungs to air breathing. It also supports the hypothesis that in many newborns who have difficulty in the transition to air breathing, Na^+ channel activity may be diminished, albeit transiently.

Studies in human neonates have shown that immaturity of Na^+ transport mechanisms contributes to the development of transient tachypnea of the newborn (TTN) and respiratory distress syndrome (RDS) (Table 13-2).[63,64] Gowen et al[64] were the first to show that human neonates with TTN had an immaturity of the lung epithelial transport, measured as an amiloride induced drop in the potential difference between the nasal epithelium and subcutaneous space. Nasal potential difference is a good measure of the net electrogenic transport of Na^+ and Cl^- (dominant ion) across the epithelial layer (PD = Resistance × Current) and has been shown to mirror image ion transport occurring in the lower respiratory tract. The potential

Table 13-2 PATHOLOGIC STATES ASSOCIATED WITH ABNORMAL LUNG
ION TRANSPORT

Decreased sodium and water transport	• Respiratory distress syndrome • Transient tachypnea of the newborn • Pulmonary edema
Excessive sodium and water transport	• Cystic fibrosis

difference was reduced in infants with TTN (suggesting a defect in Na^+ transport), and recovery from TTN in 1 to 3 days was associated with an increase in potential difference to normal level.

Similar studies have now been conducted in premature newborns with RDS, and the results are consistent with impaired Na^+ transport in these infants.[63] Barker et al[63] measured nasal transepithelial potential difference in premature infants less than 30 weeks' gestation. Authors found that maximal nasal epithelial potential difference increased with birth weight and was lower in infants with RDS. Premature infants without RDS had a nasal potential difference similar to normal full-term infants. Furthermore, the ability of amiloride to affect the potential difference was lower in preterm infants with RDS on day 1 of life, reflecting lower amiloride-sensitive Na transport. Helve et al[65,66] studied ENaC RNA levels in full-term and preterm infants with and without RDS. Lower α- and β-ENaC levels were noted in preterm infants, correlated with decreasing gestational age. Interestingly, full-term infants born via cesarean section did not demonstrate a decrease in ENaC levels at 22 hours of life, although those born by vaginal delivery did show a decrease. These studies provide important evidence for the role of Na channel activity in the pathogenesis of RDS and TTN.

Additional evidence indicates that the ability of various agents to increase lung fluid absorption in fetal lambs is gestational age dependent.[38,67-72] The mechanism for poor response of immature lungs to agents that stimulate Na^+ transport is not known. Deficiencies could exist in one or more of several steps, including β-receptor, GTP-binding proteins, adenyl cyclase, protein kinase A, or the Na^+ channel and its regulatory proteins. Studies have shown that the expression of α-subunit of ENaC is developmentally regulated in rats[54] and in humans.[70] However, several questions remain to be answered. For example, pseudohypoaldosteronism type I (a renal salt-wasting disease) has been reported to be associated with mutations involving the α-subunit of ENaC.[72] One would have expected these patients to have trouble clearing fluid from their spaces considering that the α-subunit is so critical for ENaC function. However, the incidence of RDS or TTN is not increased in infants who have this syndrome.

A complex and yet incompletely defined relationship exists between Na^+ and Cl^- channels. Cystic fibrosis (CF) is a genetic disease caused by mutations of the CF transmembrane conductance regulator (CFTR), which has been identified as a cyclic AMP (cAMP)-dependent Cl channel.[73] In the lungs of CF patients, amiloride-sensitive Na^+ absorption is increased, and aerosolized amiloride has been used to reverse this imbalance.[61,74,75] However, despite the absence of functional CFTR activity in fetuses who will go on to develop CF, fetal lung fluid production during gestation is unaffected, and the lungs are normally developed at birth. These findings are in contrast to recent studies on infants with congenital diaphragmatic hernia (CDH), who do not have a specific deficiency in ENaC or other channels. However, these infants do have respiratory distress at birth and may have this compounded by decreased alveolar fluid clearance. Animal models of term equivalent CDH rats show net lung fluid secretion rather than the absorption seen in control subjects.[76] Animal and human studies have also shown decreased levels of various ENaC subunits (α- and β-subunits in rats; β- and γ-subunits in humans) in term infants with CDH, the cause of which is unknown.[77]

Therefore, examining the molecular mechanisms and the cellular regulation of Na^+ reabsorption is important in understanding both normal lung development and physiology, but also abnormalities in lung Na and water balance in both fetal and adult lungs.

What Causes the Neonatal Lung Epithelium to Switch to an Absorptive Mode?

Developmental changes in transepithelial ion and fluid movement in the lung can be viewed as occurring in three distinct stages.[78] In the first (fetal) stage, the lung epithelium remains in a secretory mode, relying on active Cl^- secretion via Cl^- channels and relatively low reabsorption activity of Na^+ channels. The second (transitional) stage involves a reversal in the direction of ion and water movement. A multitude of factors may be involved in this transition, including exposure of epithelial cells to high concentrations of steroids and cyclic nucleotides and to an air interface. This stage involves not only increased expression of Na^+ channels in the lung epithelia but possibly a switch from nonselective cation channels to highly selective Na^+ channels. The net increase in Na^+ movement into the cell can also cause a change in resting membrane potential, leading to a slowing and eventually a reversal of the direction of Cl^- movement through Cl^- channels. The third and final (adult) stage represents lung epithelia with predominantly Na^+ reabsorption through Na^+ channels and possibly Cl^- reabsorption through Cl^- channels, with a fine balance between the activity of ion channels and tight junctions. Such an arrangement can help ensure adequate humidification of alveolar surface while preventing excessive buildup of fluid. There is also recent evidence to show that fetal lung fluid clearance is facilitated by ciliary function[79] and that term neonates with genetic defects of cilia structure or function (primary ciliary dyskinesia) have a high prevalence of neonatal respiratory disease.[79]

A considerable amount of research effort in this area has focused on physiologic changes that trigger the change in lung epithelia from a Cl^- secretory to a Na^+ reabsorption mode.[23,45,52,78,80-82] Although several endogenous mediators (Table 13-3), including catecholamines, vasopressin, and prolactin, have been proposed to increase lung fluid absorption, none explains this switch convincingly.[71,83,84] Mechanical factors, such as stretch and exposure of the epithelial cells to air interface, are other probable candidates that have not been well studied. Jain et al[52] have shown that alveolar expression of highly selective Na^+ channels in the lung epithelia is regulated by the lung microenvironment, especially the presence of glucocorticoids, air interface, and oxygen concentration.[85] Furthermore, regulation of Na^+ channels is mediated through these factors in a tissue-specific manner.[86,87] For example, aldosterone is a major factor in the kidneys and colon, but probably not in the lungs.[88] In the kidneys, it works by activating transcription of genes for ENaC subunits.[88] Of the several factors that have been proposed to have a lung-specific effect on Na^+

Table 13-3 ENDOGENOUS FACTORS THAT CAN ENHANCE LUNG FLUID CLEARANCE

β-Adrenergics and catecholamines
Dopamine
Arginine vasopressin
Prostaglandin E_2
Prolactin
Surfactant
Oxygen
Tumor necrosis factor α
Epidermal growth factor
Steroids
Alveolar expansion (stretch)

D

reabsorption, some have been investigated, including glucocorticoids, oxygen, β-adrenergics, and surfactant.[81,83,89]

High doses of glucocorticoids, acting through serum and glucocorticoid regulated kinase,[26] have been shown to stimulate transcription of ENaC in several Na^+-transporting epithelia as well as in the lung.[70] In the alveolar epithelia, glucocorticoids were found to induce lung Na^+ reabsorption in the late gestation fetal lung.[71] In addition to increasing transcription of Na^+ channel subunits, steroids increase the number of available channels by decreasing the rate at which membrane associated channels are degraded and increase the activity of existing channels. Glucocorticoids have also been shown to enhance the responsiveness of lungs to β-adrenergic agents and thyroid hormones.[90] The enhanced Na^+ reabsorption induced by glucocorticoids can be blocked by amiloride, suggesting a role for ENaC. This effect was not observed with triiodothyronine (T_3) or with cAMP. Glucocorticoid induction was found to be receptor mediated and primarily transcriptional. This observation is important because it provides an additional explanation for the beneficial effect of antenatal steroids on the lung.

In the rat fetal lung, O'Brodovich et al[51,54] have previously shown that the expression of α-ENaC is markedly increased at about 20 days' gestation (corresponding to the saccular stage of lung development) and can be accelerated by exposure to dexamethasone and increased levels of thyroid hormone. Such an effect would translate into accelerated fetal lung fluid reabsorption at birth. Jain et al[52] have shown that steroids are highly effective in enhancing the expression of highly selective Na^+ channels in lung epithelial cells. Under conditions of steroid deprivation, alveolar cells express predominantly a nonselective cation channel that is unlikely to transport the large load of Na^+ and alveolar fluid clearance imposed at birth. However, when these steroid-deprived (both fetal and adult) cells are exposed to dexamethasone, there is a rapid transition to highly selective Na^+ channels, which are readily seen in other Na^+ and fluid transporting systems such as the kidneys and colon.[52] In addition, steroids have been shown to have beneficial effects on the surfactant system as well as pulmonary mechanics.[90-95]

Considerable evidence shows that high levels of endogenous catecholamines at birth may be important for accelerating alveolar fluid clearance.[96-98] It would be logical to conclude that in the absence of an endogenous surge in fetal catecholamines, exogenous catecholamines would be effective in initiating fetal lung fluid clearance. However, recent studies show that exogenous addition of epinephrine in guinea pigs failed to stimulate fluid clearance in the newborn lungs.[98] There are several possible explanations for this finding. First, catecholamines work on the fetal Na^+ channel (mostly nonselective) by increasing its activity, not by increasing the gene transcription or translation of the proteins required to assemble the channel.[78,83] Thus, if the developmentally regulated ENaC channels are not available in adequate numbers at birth, no amount of extra catecholamines will make a difference. Steroids, on the other hand, increase the transcription of the ENaC genes and, through another mechanism involving proteosomal degradation, increase the total number of ENaC channels available at birth; however, a longer duration (4–24 hr) of exposure is required for such an effect. Indeed, if these in vitro findings were to hold true in vivo, then neonates exposed to antenatal steroids would be more responsive to other exogenous agents that enhance Na^+ channel activity (i.e., catecholamines). Helms et al[55,99] have recently shown that dopamine can greatly enhance Na^+ channel activity working via a non–cAMP-dependent posttranslational mechanism. However, because a significant ($\cong$40%) reduction in fetal lung fluid occurs before spontaneous delivery and rapid clearance of the remaining fluid has to occur within hours after birth, it is doubtful if postnatal steroid treatment initiated after the infant has become symptomatic would be a successful alternate strategy. In adult ARDS, clinical trials of β-agonist and steroid therapy have shown improvement in lung fluid clearance or ventilator-free days but not definitively in mortality.[100] It remains to be seen if this is applicable to neonates.

Summary

The transition from placental gas exchange to air breathing is a complex process that requires adequate removal of fetal lung fluid and a concomitant increase in perfusion of the newly ventilated alveoli. In neonates who are unable to make this transition, varying degrees of respiratory distress and impairment of gas exchange are common. Therapeutic approaches that can facilitate fetal lung fluid clearance are likely to reduce pulmonary morbidity in the neonatal period and help in designing therapies to combat lung edema formation in postnatal life.

References

1. Alcorn D, Adamson TM, Lambert TF, et al. Morphological effects of chronic tracheal ligation and drainage in the fetal lamb lung. *J Anat.* 1977;123:649–660.
2. Moessinger AC, Singh M, Donnelly DF, et al. The effect of prolonged oligohydramnios on fetal lung development, maturation and ventilatory patterns in the newborn guinea pig. *J Dev Physiol.* 1987;9:419–427.
3. Adams FH, Fujiwara T, Rowshan G. The nature and origin of the fluid in the fetal lamb lung. *J Pediatr.* 1963;63:881–888.
4. Olver RE, Strang LB. Ion fluxes across the pulmonary epithelium and the secretion of lung liquid in the foetal lamb. *J Physiol.* 1974;241:327–357.
5. Karlberg P, Adams FH, Geubelle F, Wallgren G. Alteration of the infant's thorax during vaginal delivery. *Acta Obstet Gynecol Scand.* 1962;41:223–229.
6. Olver RE, Walters DV, Wilson SM. Developmental regulation of lung liquid transport. *Annu Rev Physiol.* 2004;66:77–101.
7. Song W, Wei S, Matalon S. Inhibition of epithelia sodium channels by respiratory syncytial virus in vitro and in vivo. *Ann N Y Acad Sci.* 2010;1203:79-84.
8. Rudolph AM, Heymann MA. Circulatory changes during growth in the fetal lamb. *Circ Res.* 1970;26:289–299.
9. Adamson TM, Brodecky V, Lambert TF, et al. Lung liquid production and composition in the 'in utero' foetal lamb. *Aust J Exp Biol Med Sci.* 1975;53:65–75.
10. Mescher EJ, Platzker AC, Ballard PL, et al. Ontogeny of tracheal fluid, pulmonary surfactant, and plasma corticoids in the fetal lamb. *J Appl Physiol.* 1975;39:1017–1021.
11. Harding R, Hooper SB. Regulation of lung expansion and lung growth before birth. *J Appl Physiol.* 1996;81:209–224.
12. Wallen LD, Kulisz E, Maloney JE. Main pulmonary artery ligation reduces lung fluid production in fetal sheep. *J Dev Physiol.* 1991;16:173–179.
13. Harrison MR, Bressack MA, Churg AM, de Lorimier AA. Correction of congenital diaphragmatic hernia in utero. II. Simulated correction permits fetal lung growth with survival at birth. *Surgery.* 1980;88:260–268.
14. Walters DV, Ramsden CA, Olver RE. Dibutyryl cAMP induces a gestation-dependent absorption of fetal lung liquid. *J Appl Physiol.* 1990;68:2054–2059.
15. Adamson TM, Boyd RD, Platt HS, Strang LB. Composition of alveolar liquid in the foetal lamb. *J Physiol.* 1969;204:159–168.
16. Body RD, Hill JR, Humphreys PW, et al. Permeability of lung capillaries to macromolecules in foetal and new-born lambs and sheep. *J Physiol.* 1969;201:567–588.
17. Normand IC, Olver RE, Reynolds EO, Strang LB. Permeability of lung capillaries and alveoli to non-electrolytes in the foetal lamb. *J Physiol.* 1971;219:303–330.
18. Normand IC, Reynolds EO, Strang LB. Passage of macromolecules between alveolar and interstitial spaces in foetal and newly ventilated lungs of the lamb. *J Physiol.* 1970;210:151–164.
19. Bland RD, Hansen TN, Haberkern CM, et al. Lung fluid balance in lambs before and after birth. *J Appl Physiol.* 1982;53:992–1004.
20. Barker PM, Boucher RC, Yankaskas JR. Bioelectric properties of cultured monolayers from epithelium of distal human fetal lung. *Am J Physiol.* 1995;268:L270–L277.
21. McCray PB, Bettencourt JD, Bastacky J. Developing bronchopulmonary epithelium of the human fetus secretes fluid. *Am J Physiol.* 1992;262:L270–L279.
22. McCray PB, Bettencourt JD, Bastacky J. Secretion of lung fluid by the developing fetal rat alveolar epithelium in organ culture. *Am J Respir Cell Mol Biol.* 1992;6:609–616.
23. Carlton DP, Cummings JJ, Chapman DL, Poulain FR, Bland RD: Ion transport regulation of lung liquid secretion in foetal lambs. *J Dev Physiol.* 1992;17:99–107.
24. Cassin S, Gause G, Perks AM. The effects of bumetanide and furosemide on lung liquid secretion in fetal sheep. *Proc Soc Exp Biol Med.* 1986;181:427–431.
25. Olver RE, Schneeberger EE, Walters DV. Epithelial solute permeability, ion transport and tight junction morphology in the developing lung of the fetal lamb. *J Physiol.* 1981;315:395–412.
26. Wilson SM, Olver RE, Walters DV. Developmental regulation of lumenal lung fluid and electrolyte transport. *Respir Physiol Neurobiol.* 2007;159:247-255.
27. Borok Z, Lubman RL, Danto SI, et al. Keratinocyte growth factor modulates alveolar epithelial cell phenotype in vitro: expression of aquaporin 5. *Am J Respir Cell Mol Biol.* 1998;18:554–561.

13

28. Dobbs LG, Gonzalez R, Matthay MA, et al. Highly water-permeable type I alveolar epithelial cells confer high water permeability between the airspace and vasculature in rat lung. *Proc Natl Acad Sci USA.* 1998;95:2991–2996.

29. Blaisdell CJ, Edmonds RD, Wang XT, et al. pH-regulated chloride secretion in fetal lung epithelia. *Am J Physiol Lung Cell Mol Physiol.* 2000;278:L1248–L1255.

30. O'Brodovich H, Merritt TA. Bicarbonate concentration in rhesus monkey and guinea pig fetal lung liquid. *Am Rev Respir Dis.* 1992;146:1613–1614.

31. Kitterman JA, Ballard PL, Clements JA, et al. Tracheal fluid in fetal lambs: spontaneous decrease prior to birth. *J Appl Physiol.* 1979;47:985–989.

32. Schneeberger EE. Plasmalemmal vesicles in pulmonary capillary endothelium of developing fetal lamb lungs. *Microvasc Res.* 1983;25:40–55.

33. Shermeta DW, Oesch I. Characteristics of fetal lung fluid production. *J Pediatr Surg.* 1981;16: 943–946.

34. Carlton DP, Cummings JJ, Poulain FR, Bland RD: Increased pulmonary vascular filtration pressure does not alter lung liquid secretion in fetal sheep. *J Appl Physiol.* 1992;72:650–655.

35. Cotton CU, Lawson EE, Boucher RC, Gatzy JT. Bioelectric properties and ion transport of airways excised from adult and fetal sheep. *J Appl Physiol.* 1983;55:1542–1549.

36. Krochmal EM, Ballard ST, Yankaskas JR, et al. Volume and ion transport by fetal rat alveolar and tracheal epithelia in submersion culture. *Am J Physiol.* 1989;256:F397–F407.

37. Zeitlin PL, Loughlin GM, Guggino WB. Ion transport in cultured fetal and adult rabbit tracheal epithelia. *Am J Physiol.* 1988;254:C691–C698.

38. Brown MJ, Olver RE, Ramsden CA, et al. Effects of adrenaline and of spontaneous labour on the secretion and absorption of lung liquid in the fetal lamb. *J Physiol.* 1983;344:137–152.

39. Chapman DL, Carlton DP, Nielson DW, et al. Changes in lung lipid during spontaneous labor in fetal sheep. *J Appl Physiol.* 1994;76:523–530.

40. Dickson KA, Maloney JE, Berger PJ. Decline in lung liquid volume before labor in fetal lambs. *J Appl Physiol.* 1986;61:2266–2272.

41. Bland RD. Dynamics of pulmonary water before and after birth. *Acta Paediatr Scand Suppl.* 1983;305: 12–20.

42. Bland RD, Bressack MA, McMillan DD. Labor decreases the lung water content of newborn rabbits. *Am J Obstet Gynecol.* 1979;135:364–367.

43. Bland RD. Loss of liquid from the lung lumen in labor: more than a simple 'squeeze'. *Am J Physiol Lung Cell Mol Physiol.* 2001;280:L602–L605.

44. Guidot DM, Folkesson HG, Jain L, et al. Integrating acute lung injury and regulation of alveolar fluid clearance. *Am J Physiol Lung Cell Mol Physiol* 2006;291:L301–L306.

45. Jain L, Eaton DC. Alveolar fluid transport: a changing paradigm. *Am J Physiol Lung Cell Mol Physiol.* 2006;290:L646–L648.

46. Uchiyama M, Konno N. Hormonal regulation of ion and water transport in anuran amphibians. *Gen Comp Endocrinol.* 2006;147:54–61.

47. Matthay MA, Folkesson HG, Verkman AS. Salt and water transport across alveolar and distal airway epithelia in the adult lung. *Am J Physiol.* 1996;270:L487–L503.

48. Voilley N, Lingueglia E, Champigny G, et al. The lung amiloride-sensitive Na^+ channel: biophysical properties, pharmacology, ontogenesis, and molecular cloning. *Proc Natl Acad Sci USA.* 1994;91: 247–251.

49. Canessa CM, Horisberger JD, Rossier BC. Epithelial sodium channel related to proteins involved in neurodegeneration [see comments]. *Nature.* 1993;361:467–470.

50. Canessa CM, Schild L, Buell G, et al. Amiloride-sensitive epithelial Na^+ channel is made of three homologous subunits. *Nature.* 1994;367:463–467.

51. O'Brodovich H, Hannam V, Seear M, Mullen JB. Amiloride impairs lung water clearance in newborn guinea pigs. *J Appl Physiol.* 1990;68:1758–1762.

52. Jain L, Chen XJ, Ramosevac S, et al. Expression of highly selective sodium channels in alveolar type II cells is determined by culture conditions. *Am J Physiol Lung Cell Mol Physiol.* 2001;280: L646–L658.

53. O'Brodovich H. Epithelial ion transport in the fetal and perinatal lung. *Am J Physiol.* 1991;261: C555–C564.

54. O'Brodovich H, Canessa C, Ueda J, et al. Expression of the epithelial Na^+ channel in the developing rat lung. *Am J Physiol.* 1993;265:C491–C496.

55. Helms MN, Self J, Bao HF, et al. Dopamine activates amiloride-sensitive sodium channels in alveolar type 1 cells in a lung slice preparation. *Am J Physiol Lung Cell Mol Physiol* 2006; 291:L610–L618.

56. Johnson MD, Bao HF, Helms MN, et al. Functional ion channels in pulmonary alveolar type I cells support a role for type I cells in lung ion transport. *Proc Natl Acad Sci USA.* 2006;103: 4964–4969.

57. Johnson MD, Widdicombe JH, Allen L, et al. Alveolar epithelial type I cells contain transport proteins and transport sodium, supporting an active role for type I cells in regulation of lung liquid homeostasis. *Proc Natl Acad Sci USA.* 2002;99:1966–1971.

58. Matthay MA, Folkesson HG, Clerici C. Lung epithelial fluid transport and the resolution of pulmonary edema. *Physiol Rev.* 2002;82:569-600.

59. Ji HL, Su XF, Kedar S, Li J, et al. Delta-subunit confers novel biophysical features to alpha beta gamma-human epithelial sodium channel (ENaC) via a physical interaction. *J Biol Chem.* 2006;281: 8233-8241.

60. Bangel-Ruland N, Sobczak K, Christmann T, et al. Characterization of the epithelial sodium channel delta-subunit in human nasal epithelium. *Am J Respir Cell Mol Biol.* 2010;42: 498-505.

61. Hummler E, Barker P, Gatzy J, et al. Early death due to defective neonatal lung liquid clearance in alpha-ENaC-deficient mice. *Nat Genet.* 1996;12:325–328.

62. Hummler E, Planès C. Importance of ENaC-mediated sodium transport in alveolar fluid clearance using genetically-engineered mice. *Cell Physiol Biochem.* 2010;25:63-70.

63. Barker PM, Gowen CW, Lawson EE, Knowles MR. Decreased sodium ion absorption across nasal epithelium of very premature infants with respiratory distress syndrome [see comments]. *J Pediatr.* 1997;130:373–377.

64. Gowen CW, Lawson EE, Gingras J, et al. Electrical potential difference and ion transport across nasal epithelium of term neonates: correlation with mode of delivery, transient tachypnea of the newborn, and respiratory rate. *J Pediatr.* 1988;113:121–127.

65. Helve O, Pitkänen O, Janér C, Andersson S. Pulmonary fluid balance in the human newborn infant. *Neonatology* 2009;95:347-352.

66. Helve O, Janér C, Pitkänen O, Andersson S. Expression of the epithelial sodium channel in airway epithelium of newborn infants depends on gestational age. *Pediatrics.* 2007;120:1311-1316.

67. Barker PM, Brown MJ, Ramsden CA, et al. The effect of thyroidectomy in the fetal sheep on lung liquid reabsorption induced by adrenaline or cyclic AMP. *J Physiol.* 1988;407:373–383.

68. Barker PM, Gowen CW, Lawson EE, Knowles MR. Decreased sodium ion absorption across nasal epithelium of very premature infants with respiratory distress syndrome. *J Pediatr.* 1997;130: 373–377.

69. Perks AM, Cassin S. The effects of arginine vasopressin and epinephrine on lung liquid production in fetal goats. *Can J Physiol Pharmacol.* 1989;67:491–498.

70. Venkatesh VC, Katzberg HD. Glucocorticoid regulation of epithelial sodium channel genes in human fetal lung. *Am J Physiol.* 1997;273:L227–L233.

71. Wallace MJ, Hooper SB, Harding R. Regulation of lung liquid secretion by arginine vasopressin in fetal sheep. *Am J Physiol.* 1990;258:R104–R111.

72. Chang SS, Grunder S, Hanukoglu A, et al. Mutations in subunits of the epithelial sodium channel cause salt wasting with hyperkalaemic acidosis, pseudohypoaldosteronism type 1. *Nat Genet.* 1996;12:248–253.

73. Liedtke CM. Electrolyte transport in the epithelium of pulmonary segments of normal and cystic fibrosis lung. *Faseb J.* 1992;6:3076–3084.

74. Knowles MR, Olivier K, Noone P, Boucher RC. Pharmacologic modulation of salt and water in the airway epithelium in cystic fibrosis. *Am J Respir Crit Care Med.* 1995;151:S65–S69.

75. Mall M, Grubb BR, Harkema JR, et al. Increased airway epithelial Na$^+$ absorption produces cystic fibrosis-like lung disease in mice. *Nat Med.* 2004;10:487–493.

76. Folkesson HG, Chapin CJ, Beard LL, et al. Congenital diaphragmatic hernia prevents absorption of distal air space fluid in late-gestation rat fetuses. *Am J Physiol Lung Cell Mol Physiol.* 2006;290: L478–L484.

77. Ringman Uggla A, von Schewelov K, Zelenina M, et al. Low Pulmonary Expression of Epithelial Na Channel and Na(+), K(+)-ATPase in Newborn Infants with Congenital Diaphragmatic Hernia. *Neonatology.* 2010;99:14–22.

78. Jain L, Eaton DC. Physiology of fetal lung fluid clearance and the effect of labor. *Semin Perinatol.* 2006;30:34–43.

79. Noone PG, Leigh MW, Sannuti A, et al. Primary ciliary dyskinesia: diagnostic and phenotypic features. *Am J Respir Crit Care Med.* 2004;169:459–467.

80. Jain L. Alveolar fluid clearance in developing lungs and its role in neonatal transition. *Clin Perinatol.* 1999;26:585–599.

81. Jain L, Chen XJ, Brown LA, Eaton DC. Nitric oxide inhibits lung sodium transport through a cGMP-mediated inhibition of epithelial cation channels. *Am J Physiol.* 1998;274: L475–L484.

82. Jain L, Chen XJ, Malik B, et al. Antisense oligonucleotides against the alpha-subunit of ENaC decrease lung epithelial cation-channel activity. *Am J Physiol.* 1999;276:L1046–L1051.

83. Chen XJ, Eaton DC, Jain L. Beta-adrenergic regulation of amiloride-sensitive lung sodium channels. *Am J Physiol Lung Cell Mol Physiol.* 2002;282:L609–L620.

84. Cummings JJ, Carlton DP, Poulain FR, et al. Vasopressin effects on lung liquid volume in fetal sheep. *Pediatr Res.* 1995;38:30–35.

85. Bouvry D, Planes C, Malbert-Colas L, et al. Hypoxia-induced cytoskeleton disruption in alveolar epithelial cells. *Am J Respir Cell Mol Biol.* 2006;35:519–527.

86. Anantharam A, Tian Y, Palmer LG. Open probability of the epithelial sodium channel is regulated by intracellular sodium. *J Physiol.* 2006;574:333–347.

87. Renard S, Voilley N, Bassilana F, et al. Localization and regulation by steroids of the alpha, beta and gamma subunits of the amiloride-sensitive Na$^+$ channel in colon, lung and kidney. *Pflugers Arch.* 1995;430:299–307.

88. Eaton D, Ohara A, Ling BN. Cellular regulation of amiloride blockable Na$^+$ channels. *Biomed Res.* 1991;12:31–35.

89. Guidot DM, Modelska K, Lois M, et al. Ethanol ingestion via glutathione depletion impairs alveolar epithelial barrier function in rats. *Am J Physiol Lung Cell Mol Physiol.* 2000;279: L127–L135.

90. Jobe AH, Ikegami M, Padbury J, et al. Combined effects of fetal beta agonist stimulation and glucocorticoids on lung function of preterm lambs. *Biol Neonate.* 1997;72:305–313.

91. Ervin MG, Berry LM, Ikegami M, et al. Single dose fetal betamethasone administration stabilizes postnatal glomerular filtration rate and alters endocrine function in premature lambs. *Pediatr Res.* 1996;40:645–651.

92. Pillow JJ, Hall GL, Willet KE, et al. Effects of gestation and antenatal steroid on airway and tissue mechanics in newborn lambs. *Am J Respir Crit Care Med.* 2001;163:1158–1163.

93. Smith LM, Ervin MG, Wada N, et al. Antenatal glucocorticoids alter postnatal preterm lamb renal and cardiovascular responses to intravascular volume expansion. *Pediatr Res.* 2000;47:622–627.

94. Willet KE, Jobe AH, Ikegami M, et al. Lung morphometry after repetitive antenatal glucocorticoid treatment in preterm sheep. *Am J Respir Crit Care Med.* 2001;163:1437–1443.

95. Willet KE, Jobe AH, Ikegami M, et al. Antenatal endotoxin and glucocorticoid effects on lung morphometry in preterm lambs. *Pediatr Res.* 2000;48:782–788.

96. Baines DL, Folkesson HG, Norlin A, et al. The influence of mode of delivery, hormonal status and postnatal O_2 environment on epithelial sodium channel (ENaC) expression in perinatal guinea-pig lung. *J Physiol.* 2000;522(Pt 1):147–157.

97. Berthiaume Y, Staub NC, Matthay MA. Beta-adrenergic agonists increase lung liquid clearance in anesthetized sheep. *J Clin Invest.* 1987;79:335–343.

98. Finley N, Norlin A, Baines DL, Folkesson HG. Alveolar epithelial fluid clearance is mediated by endogenous catecholamines at birth in guinea pigs. *J Clin Invest.* 1998;101:972–981.

99. Helms MN, Chen XJ, Ramosevac S, et al. Dopamine regulation of amiloride-sensitive sodium channels in lung cells. *Am J Physiol Lung Cell Mol Physiol.* 2006;290:L710–L722.

100. Morty RE, Eickelberg O, Seeger W. Alveolar fluid clearance in acute lung injury: what have we learned from animal models and clinical studies? *Intensive Care Med.* 2007;33:1229–1240.

D

CHAPTER 14

Use of Diuretics in the Newborn

Jean-Pierre Guignard, MD

Diuretics are pharmacologic agents that increase the excretion of water and electrolytes. They are primarily used in states of inappropriate salt and water retention. Such states can be the consequence of congestive heart failure (CHF), renal diseases, and liver disease. Diuretics are also used in various conditions not evidently associated with salt retention. Such conditions include oliguric states, respiratory disorders, electrolyte disorders, and nephrogenic diabetes insipidus. Diuretics can also be valuable tools in the laboratory differential diagnosis of congenital tubulopathies.

The rationale use of diuretics in newborn infants requires a clear understanding of the physiology and physiopathology of immature kidneys.[1,2]

Body Fluid Homeostasis

The kidney is responsible for maintaining the extracellular fluid (ECF) volume and osmolality constant despite larges variations in salt and water intake.

Extracellular Fluid Volume

NaCl, the major osmotically active solute in ECF, determines its volume. The overall balance between sodium intake and its urinary excretion thus regulates ECF volume and consequently cardiac output and blood pressure. Volume receptors are distributed in the low-pressure capacitance vessels (great veins and atria) as well as in the high-pressure resistance vessels (arterial vascular tree). Arterial sensors perceive the adequacy of blood flow in the arterial circuit, a parameter coined as *effective arterial circulating volume*. This volume is also monitored by baroreceptors located in the juxtaglomerular apparatus of the kidney. When sensed by these receptors, a decrease in renal perfusion pressure leads to the activation of the renin–angiotensin–aldosterone system (RAAS). Aldosterone stimulates sodium reabsorption and potassium excretion. Although aldosterone is the main hormone regulating long-term changes in sodium excretion, other hormones and paracrine factors, including angiotensin II, the prostaglandins, dopamine, the catecholamines, and atrial natriuretic peptide (ANP), also modulate sodium renal handling. The release of the latter, a potent vasodilator and natriuretic agent, is modulated by sensors (the stretch receptors) that sense the atrial filling volume.[3]

Plasma Osmolality

The plasma osmolality is maintained within narrow limits.[3] Small 2% to 3% changes in plasma osmolality are sensed by osmoreceptors located in the hypothalamus, which by stimulating or inhibiting the release of vasopressin, lead to increases or decreases in the excretion of free water. By acting on the baroreceptors, the effective circulating volume also influence the release of vasopressin. Dilution of urine depends on sodium delivery to the distal nephron diluting site, and the concentration of urine, modulated by vasopressin, requires the presence of a hypertonic renal medullary interstitium.[3]

Clinical Use of Diuretics

Sodium-Retaining States

Sodium retention is the primary target of diuretics. Salt and water retention with or without edema formation can occur as a primary event or as a consequence of reduced effective circulating volume with secondary hyperaldosteronism. CHF is the main neonatal condition associated with sodium retention.[4] The increased pressure in the venous circulation and capillaries favors the movement of fluid into the interstitium and leads to the formation of edema. Failure of the heart to provide normal tissue perfusion is sensed as a decrease in effective circulating volume by the kidney, which retains sodium and water. Treatment of the condition consists in restoring normal cardiac output. By mobilizing the edematous fluid, diuretics improve the symptoms of CHF. The pulmonary edema secondary to left heart failure requires the urgent use of diuretics to reduce the life-threatening pulmonary congestion.[5,6] The use of diuretics can be lifesaving when the ECF volume is expanded.

Diuretics may on the contrary further compromise the patient's condition when sodium retention occurs in response to homeostatic mechanisms mobilized to defend the circulating volume. The same reasoning applies to states of nephrotic or liver cirrhosis edemas.[7,8] The use of diuretics (loop diuretics, thiazides, and potassium-sparing diuretics) in these conditions requires a clear understanding of the patient's underlying pathophysiologic condition and careful monitoring of the hemodynamic state.[5,6]

Oliguric States

Loop diuretics are often administered to patients with oliguric renal insufficiency in the hope of promoting diuresis and improving renal perfusion and glomerular filtration rate (GFR). When present, the diuretic response may actually worsen the renal hypoperfusion.[9,10]

Respiratory Disorders

Interstitial and alveolar edema is present in idiopathic respiratory distress syndrome (RDS) of preterm babies as well as in transient tachypnea of term neonates. Inadequate fetal lung fluid clearance is partly responsible for the edema. Administration of diuretics (loop diuretics) could accelerate the reabsorption of lung fluid and ameliorate pulmonary recovery in these patients with lung edema.[11]

Central Nervous System Disorders

Large hemorrhages into the brain ventricles may result in fluid retention and dilatation of the fluid-producing brain cavities. Diuretics (acetazolamide, furosemide) are sometimes used to prevent or reduce the accumulation of fluid in the ventricles.[12]

Electrolyte Disorders

Diuretics can be used in various situations associated with dyselectrolytemia. They can increase potassium excretion in hyperkalemic states (loop diuretics, thiazides), increase calcium excretion in hypercalcemia (loop diuretics), or decrease the rate of calcium excretion in hypercalciuric states (thiazides). Increased bicarbonate excretion can be achieved by acetazolamide, and increased excretion of hydrogen ions can be stimulated by loop diuretics.[5,13,14]

Nephrogenic Diabetes Insipidus

Diuretics (thiazides) can paradoxically decrease urine output in nephrogenic diabetes insipidus.[15]

Arterial Hypertension

Arterial hypertension may be a consequence of or aggravated by sodium retention and consecutive expansion of the ECF volume. This type of hypertension responds to diuretic-induced natriuresis.[16]

Differential Diagnosis of Congenital Tubulopathies

Diuretics such as acetazolamide, furosemide, and hydrochlorothiazide can be used to test distal tubular acidification or distal sodium reabsorption defects in patients with congenital tubulopathies.

Classification of Diuretics According to the Site of Action

Diuretics can be classified according to their site and mode of action (Fig. 14-1 and Table 14-1). They all increase sodium and water excretion and variably modify the excretion of other electrolytes (Table 14-2). *Filtration diuretics* increase salt and water excretion by primarily increasing GFR. *Osmotic diuretics* depress salt and electrolyte reabsorption in the proximal tubule and in Henle loop. *Carbonic anhydrase inhibitors* act primarily on the proximal tubule. *Loop diuretics*, the most potent diuretics, inhibit Na^+ reabsorption in the ascending limb of Henle loop. *The thiazide and thiazide-like diuretics* act in the distal convoluted tubule and *potassium-sparing diuretics* in the late distal tubule and collecting duct.[13,14] New diuretics with different modes of action (*adenosine antagonists, natriuretic peptides, vasopressin antagonists*) are being developed and tested. All diuretics share adverse effects that are actually extensions of their primary effects on electrolyte excretion (Table 14-3), as well as non-electrolyte adverse effects (Table 14-4).

Although diuretics are very widely used in intensive care neonatal units, the extent of and expectations for diuretic therapy by neonatologists caring for low birth weight neonates may, as stated in a recent survey,[17] exceed evidence for efficacy (Table 14-5). The dosages of diuretics commonly used in neonates are given in Table 14-6.

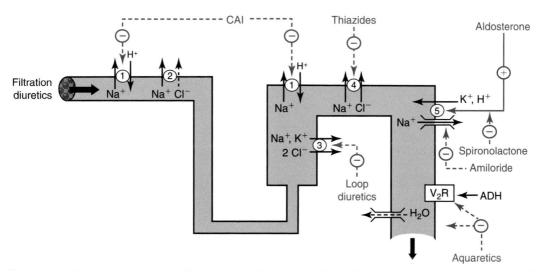

Figure 14-1   Sites 1 to 5: sites of sodium transport along the nephron. Numbers 1 to 5 represent the sites and mechanisms of Na^+ transport. The group of diuretics acting at the different sites is indicated in brackets. *1*, Na^+ / H^+ exchanger NHE1. *2*, Na^+glucose cotransporter SLGT2. *3*, Na^+, K^+, $2Cl^-$ cotransporter (furosemide receptor): NKCC2 (loop diuretics). *4*, Na^+, Cl^- cotransporter (thiazide receptor): NCC (thiazides). *5*, H^+, K^+ ATPase and epithelial sodium channel (amiloride receptor): ENaC (potassium-sparing diuretics). The aquaretics act on the collecting duct V_2R arginine vasopressin receptor. CAI, carbonic anhydrase inhibitor; ENaC, sodium epithelium channel.

Table 14-1 CLINICAL USE OF DIURETICS IN NEONATES

Filtration diuretics

- Oliguric prerenal failure

Osmotic diuretics

- Oliguric prerenal failure
- Elevated intracranial pressure

Carbonic anhydrase inhibitors

- Production of alkaline diuresis
- Posthemorrhagic ventricular dilatation
- Assessment of distal urinary acidification

Loop diuretics

- Edematous states (congestive heart failure, renal and liver diseases)
- Respiratory disorders (transient tachypnea, respiratory distress syndrome,
- chronic lung disease in preterm neonates, compromised lung mechanics)
- Prerenal failure (asphyxia)
- Transient tachypnea of the term neonate
- Chronic lung disease in preterm neonates
- Compromised lung mechanics
- Posthemorrhagic ventricular dilatation
- Indomethacin-induced oliguria
- Electrolyte disorders (hyperkalemia, hypercalcemia, severe hyponatremia)
- Assessment of distal urinary acidification

Thiazides

- Edematous states (congestive heart failure, renal and liver diseases)
- Respiratory disorders (chronic lung diseases in preterm neonates
- Hypercalciuria
- Proximal renal tubular acidosis
- Nephrogenic diabetes insipidus
- Diagnosis of renal tubular hypokalemic disorders

Potassium-sparing diuretics

- Adjunctive therapy with loop or thiazide diuretics
- Prevention of hypokalemia
- Nephrogenic diabetes insipidus
- Cystic fibrosis

Table 14-2 ACUTE EFFECTS OF DIURETICS ON ELECTROLYTE EXCRETION*

	Na^+	K^+	Ca^{++}	Mg^{++}	H^+	Cl^-	HCO_3^-	$H_2PO_4^-$
Carbonic anhydrase inhibitors	↑	↑↑	=	~	↓	(↑)	↑↑	↑↑
Loop diuretics	↑↑	↑↑	↑↑	↑↑	↑	↑↑	↑	↑
Thiazide diuretics	↑	↑↑	~	(↑)	↑	↑	↑	↑
K+-sparing diuretics	↑	↓	↓	↓	↓	↑	(↑)	=

*In the absence of significant volume depletion, which would trigger complex adjustments.
(↑), slight increase; ↑, moderate increase; ↑↑, marked increase; ↓, decrease; =, no change; ~, variable effects.

Filtration Diuretics

Agents that increase diuresis by increasing GFR are called *filtration diuretics*. These agents include the glucocorticoids; theophylline; and inotropic agents such as iso-proterenol, dopamine, and dobutamine. By increasing GFR, these drugs only moderately increase Na^+ excretion. Dopamine and theophylline are sometimes used in neonates in the hope of improving renal perfusion and GFR rather than for their natriuretic and diuretic effect. They are discussed in Chapter 5.

Table 14-3 ELECTROLYTE DISTURBANCES INDUCED BY DIURETICS COMMONLY USED IN NEONATES

	Loop	Thiazides	K⁺-Sparing
Hypovolemia	+++	+	+
Hyponatremia	++	+++	-
Hypokalemia	+++	++	-
Hyperkalemia	-	-	++
Hypercalciuria	++	-	-
Hypercalcemia	-	+	-
Hypomagnesemia	+	+	-
Hypophosphatemia	+	+	-
Hyperuricemia	++	++	-
Metabolic acidosis	-	-	+
Metabolic alkalosis	++	++	-

+++, marked increase in electrolyte disturbances; ++, moderate increase in electrolyte disturbances; +, mild increase in electrolyte disturbances. A . indicates no effects.
Adapted from ref 13.

Table 14-4 GENERAL NON-ELECTROLYTE SIDE EFFECTS OF DIURETICS

Diuretic		Non-electrolyte Side Effects
Carbonic anhydrase inhibitors		CNS depression, paresthesia, calculus formation
Loop diuretics		Ototoxicity (usually reversible), nephrocalcinosis in neonates, PDA in neonates, hyperuricemia, hyperglycemia, hyperlipidemia, hypersensitivity
Thiazides		Hyperglycemia, insulin resistance, hyperlipidemia, hypersensitivity (fever, rash, purpura, anaphylaxis, interstitial nephritis), hyperuricemia
K+-sparing	Amiloride	Diarrhea, headache
	Triamterene	Glucose intolerance, interstitial nephritis, blood dyscrasias
	Spironolactone	Gynecomastia, hirsutism, peptic ulcers, ataxia, headache

CNS, central nervous system; PDA, patent ductus arteriosus.

Table 14-5 SPECIFIC INDICATIONS WITH QUESTIONABLE BENEFITS IN CLINICAL TRIALS

Condition	Diuretic(s)	Reference
Oliguric prerenal failure	Mannitol Furosemide	Better et al,[18] Rigden et al[19] Kellum,[9] Dubourg et al[40]
Respiratory distress syndrome	Furosemide	Jain and Eaton[41]
Transient tachypnea of the newborn	Furosemide	Wiswell et al,[43] Lewis and Whitelaw[44]
Chronic lung disease	Furosemide Thiazides Thiazides + spironolactone Furosemide + thiazides Furosemide + metolazone Intratracheal furosemide	Brio and Primhak,[45] Brion et al[46] Brion et al[70] Brion et al[70] Brion et al[70] Segar et al[47] Aufricht et al[56]
Posthemorrhagic ventricular dilatation	Furosemide + acetazolamide	International PHVD Drug Trial Group,[21] Kennedy et al,[22] International PHVD Drug Trial Group,[49] Whitelaw et al[50]

Continued

Table 14-5 SPECIFIC INDICATIONS WITH QUESTIONABLE BENEFITS IN CLINICAL TRIALS—cont'd

Condition	Diuretic(s)	Reference
Indomethacin-induced oliguria	Furosemide Dopamine	Eades and Christensen,[24] Brion et al,[51] Andriessen et al,[52] Lee et al[53] Barrington and Brion[55]
Furosemide-induced nephrocalcinosis	Thiazides	Campfield et al[61]
Nephrocalcinosis secondary to the use of vitamin D in hypophosphatemic rickets	Thiazides	Seikaly and Baum[66]
Compromised lung mechanics after cardiac surgery	Intratracheal furosemide	Aufricht et al[56]
Cystic fibrosis	Aerolized amiloride	Pons et al,[75] Ratjen and Bush[76]
Asthma	Intratracheal furosemide	Aufricht et al[56]

Table 14-6 DOSAGES OF DIURETICS COMMONLY USED IN NEONATES

Drug	Route/Interval (qh)	Dosage (mg/kg/day)	Half-life (h)	Comments
Furosemide	PO: 12–24 IV: 12–24 CIVI	1–2 0.5–1.5 100–200 µg/kg/h	≈1.5 idem	Effective at GFR <10 Doses may be increased up to 5 mg/kg in CRF Hypokalemia; Mg, Ca depletion Ototoxicity; metabolic alkalosis
Torasemide	PO	0.5–1	≈3.5	Longer half-life and larger duration than furosemide Effective at GFR <10 Idem furosemide
Ethacrynic acid	PO: 12–24	1–2	≈1	Effective at GFR <10 Idem furosemide
Bumetanide	PO: 12–24 IV: 12–24 CIVI	0.01–0.10 0.01–0.05 5–10 µg/kg/h	≈1 idem	Effective at GFR <10 Idem furosemide
Hydrochlorothiazide	PO: 12–24	1–3	≈2.5	Not effective at GFR <20 Hypokalemia metabolic alkalosis
Chlorthalidone	PO: 24–48	0.5–2.0	45	Not effective at GFR <20 Hypokalemia metabolic alkalosis
Metolazone	PO: 12–24	0.2–0.4	8–10	Effective at GFR <20 Hypokalemia
Spironolactone	PO: 6–12	1–3	≈1.6	Delayed effect. Cave CRF or K suppl. Hyperkalemia, acidosis
Canrenoate-K	IV: 24	4–10	≈16	Single IV dose Hyperkalemia, acidosis
Triamterene	PO: 12–24	2–4	≈4.2	Cave RF or K suppl. Hyperkalemia, acidosis
Amiloride	PO: 24	0.5	≈21	Cave RF or K suppl. Hyperkalemia, acidosis

CIVI, constant IV infusion; CRF: chronic renal failure; GFR: glomerular filtration rate (mL/min/1.73 m^2); IV, intravenous; PO, oral.
Adapted from Guignard JP. Diuretics. In: Yaffe S and Aranda J, eds. *Neonatal and Pediatric Pharmacology – Therapeutic Principles in Practice.* 4th ed. Philadelphia: Lippincott Williams & Wilkins, Wolters Kluwer, 2011:629-645.

Osmotic Diuretics

Osmotic diuretics are agents that inhibit the reabsorption of solute and water by altering osmotic driving forces along the nephron.

Chemistry

Mannitol, a hexahydric alcohol related to mannose with a molecular weight of 182 d, is the main representative of this class of agents.[18]

Mechanisms and Sites of Action

Freely filtered and (mostly) not reabsorbed, osmotic diuretics increase the tubular fluid osmolality, thus impairing the diffusion of water out of the tubular lumen, as well as that of NaCl by a solvent drag effect. The osmotic diuretics act in the proximal tubule and in the loop of Henle. By attracting water from the intracellular compartment, osmotic diuretics increase ECF volume and renal blood flow. Increased medullary blood flow washes out the hypertonic medulla, thus impairing the concentrating mechanism. By inhibiting NaCl reabsorption out of the water-impermeable thick ascending limb, osmotic diuretics also impair the dilution of urine. Osmotic diuretics increase nonspecifically the excretion of all electrolytes. The natriuresis induced by osmotic diuretics is only about 10% of the filtered load.

Efficacy and Therapeutic Uses

Osmotic diuretics increase the excretion of Na^+, K^+, Cl^-, Mg^{++}, Ca^{++}, Cl^-, and HCO_3^-. They improve renal perfusion without significantly affecting GFR. Mannitol has been used to increase urine flow rate in patients with prerenal failure,[18,19] promote the excretion of toxic substances by forced diuresis, and reduce elevated intracranial and intraocular pressures.

Adverse Effects: Interactions

Circulatory overload, acute renal tubular necrosis, intracranial hemorrhage, and CHF have been described in patients given intravenous (IV) mannitol. Mannitol is presently not recommended in neonates.

Carbonic Anhydrase Inhibitors

Agents in this group act by inhibiting the carbonic anhydrase in renal tubular cells and in the brush border of proximal tubular cells.

Chemistry

Acetazolamide, a sulfonamide derivative, is the main inhibitor of carbonic anhydrase used in humans.

Mechanisms and Sites of Action

Inhibition of carbonic anhydrase results in depressed cellular formation and subsequent secretion of H^+. As a consequence, the HCO_3^- ions that are normally reabsorbed by combining to H^+ in the tubular lumen are excreted in the urine. Acetazolamide is a weak diuretic agent, at best producing the excretion of 5% of the Na^+ and water filtered load.

Pharmacokinetic Properties

Acetazolamide is readily absorbed and is eliminated in the urine. It crosses the placental barrier and is secreted in breast milk.

Efficacy and Therapeutic Uses

Acetazolamide increases the urinary excretion of HCO_3^-, Na^+, and K^+, promoting alkaline diuresis with consequent systemic metabolic acidosis. Acetazolamide may be useful to alkalinize the urine when necessary, such as when chemotherapy is given. Acetazolamide can also be used to assess reliably the distal acidification ability by measuring the urine minus blood PCO_2 in alkaline urine.[20]

14

Specific Indications with Questionable Benefits (Table 14-5)

Posthemorrhagic Ventricular Dilatation. Acetazolamide has been used alone or in association with furosemide in the treatment of posthemorrhagic ventricular dilatation (PHVD) in the hope of avoiding the need for surgical management. Randomized controlled studies have led to the conclusion that this treatment was ineffective in decreasing the rate shunt placement and that it was associated with increased neurologic morbidity. The use of diuretics in PHVD is thus not recommended.[21,22]

Adverse Effects: Interactions

The occurrence of metabolic acidosis is common if the urinary losses of HCO_3^- are not substituted. Side effects include paresthesias, drowsiness, rash, fever, and the formation of renal calculi. Blood dyscrasias and hepatic failure are occasionally seen.

Loop Diuretics: Inhibition of Na$^+$, K$^+$, 2Cl$^-$ Cotransport

Loop diuretics induce natriuresis by inhibiting the active reabsorption of NaCl in Henle loop.

Chemistry

Loop diuretics form a group of diuretics with diverse chemical structures.[23,24] Furosemide and bumetanide are sulfonamide derivatives, torsemide is a sulfonylurea, and ethacrynic acid is a phenoxyacetic acid derivative.

Mechanisms and Sites of Action

Loop diuretics block the Na$^+$, K$^+$, 2Cl$^-$ cotransporter in the thick ascending limb of Henle loop, where 25% of NaCl filtered load are usually reabsorbed. They are consequently highly efficacious because only a small proportion of the filtered Na$^+$ that escapes reabsorption in the loop can be reabsorbed downstream. Loop diuretics act from within the tubular lumen where they are actively secreted by the organic acid pump. The effect of loop diuretics is more closely related to their urinary excretion rate than to their plasma concentration. By inhibiting NaCl reabsorption in Henle loop, loop diuretics abolish the lumen-positive voltage and thus the driving force for Ca^{++} and Mg^{++} reabsorption. They consequently increase Ca^{++} and Mg^{++} excretion. Inhibition of NaCl transport upstream of the distal tubule results in increased Na$^+$ delivery to the late portion of the distal tubule and cortical collecting duct. This part of the nephron responds by increasing the tubular secretion of K$^+$ and H$^+$, thus decreasing urine pH and increasing the urinary excretion of K$^+$. This secretion is also stimulated by the state of secondary hyperaldosteronism usually present as a consequence of diuretic-induced decrease in ECF volume.[3] By inhibiting NaCl reabsorption in the water-impermeable thick ascending limb of Henle loop, loop diuretics interfere with both the diluting and the concentrating mechanism.

Pharmacokinetic Properties

Furosemide is rapidly reabsorbed from the gastrointestinal (GI) tract and is mainly excreted unchanged in the urine. It is 99% bound to plasma albumin and has a bioavailability close to 60% to 70%. Furosemide and ethacrynic acid displace bilirubin from albumin-binding sites.[13] Loop diuretics cross the placental barrier and are secreted in breast milk. The diuretic response to loop diuretics appears within a few minutes after IV administration and within 30 to 60 minutes after oral administration. The effect does not last over 2 hours after IV injection and 6 hours after oral administration. Compared with furosemide, torsemide's release and half-life are prolonged.[25-27] The nonrenal clearance of loop diuretics is increased in patients with chronic renal failure. The half-life is prolonged in patients with renal and liver insufficiency and in premature and term neonates in whom half-lives as long as 45 hours have been observed.[28] Although the pharmacology of furosemide has been well studied in children[29] and neonates,[28] that of other loop diuretics is not as well defined. The pharmacokinetics and pharmacodynamics of bumetanide have been studied in critically ill children[30] and infants.[31]

Efficacy and Therapeutic Uses

Loop diuretics are the most potent natriuretic agents, also markedly increasing Cl^-, K^+, Ca^{++}, and Mg^{++} excretion.[23] They have steep dose-response curves. They remain active in patients with advanced renal failure. Loop diuretics are the most frequently used diuretics in neonates, infants, and children.[32]

Continuous Intravenous Infusion of Loop Diuretics

Clinical trials in infants indicate that continuous infusion therapy can produce more efficient and better-controlled diuresis with less fluid shifts and greater hemodynamic stability.[33] Administration of a small loading dose of the diuretic before starting the continuous infusion accelerates the diuretic response.[24] Alternatively, starting with a relatively high continuous infusion dose (0.2 mg/kg/h) of furosemide has been claimed to be optimal.[34] In hemodynamically stable postoperative cardiac patients, intermittent furosemide has been shown to be more efficacious than continuous infusion of furosemide.[35]

Indications

Edematous States. CHF is the most common indication to the use of loop diuretics in neonates and infants. In infants with severe CHF, the diuretic effect of furosemide is inversely related to the serum aldosterone level. The concomitant administration of a K^+-sparing diuretic improves the response to loop diuretics.[36] Furosemide increases the peripheral venous capacitance and can thus be useful independently from its diuretic effect. In adults, torsemide has been shown to be at least as effective as furosemide in reducing salt and water retention,[37] to have a longer duration of action, and to reduce the overall treatment costs of CHF compared with furosemide.[38]

Nephrotic Syndrome. In hypovolemic infants with massive nephrotic edema, IV furosemide can be used to promote sodium and water excretion. Furosemide (1–2 mg/kg) should only be given after careful expansion of the extracellular space with IV albumin (5 mL/kg of 20% albumin in 60 min). The dose can be repeated. The effect is transient but may be useful in patients with severe ascites or pulmonary edema. The therapy may be associated with potentially serious complications such as CHF or RDS.[39]

Specific Indications with Questionable Benefits (Table 14-5)

Oliguric States. Furosemide is frequently used in oliguric states secondary to prerenal or renal failure in the hope of promoting diuresis and improving renal function. Although furosemide may increase urine output and facilitate the clinical management of the patient, it is unlikely to improve GFR. By inducing diuresis and possibly hypovolemia, loop diuretics carry the risk of further stressing the oliguric kidney. There is as yet no clinical or experimental evidence that loop diuretics can prevent acute renal failure or improve the outcome of patients with acute renal failure.[9,40]

Respiratory Distress Syndrome. Furosemide administration has produced conflicting results in preterm neonates with RDS. Although furosemide usually acutely induces diuresis and a transient improvement in pulmonary function, a recent critical review of the literature failed to find evidence for long-term benefits of routine administration of furosemide (or any diuretic) in preterm infants with RDS.[41] The review also concluded that elective administration of furosemide should be weighed against the risk of precipitating hypovolemia or of developing a symptomatic patent ductus arteriosus (PDA) by stimulating prostaglandin synthesis.

Transient Tachypnea of the Newborn. Transient tachypnea of the newborn (TTN), sometimes called wet lungs, is a common self-limited disease of term newborns that results from delayed lung fluid clearance.[42] This deficit is probably secondary to immature sodium epithelium channel (ENaC). Furosemide has been proposed to hasten fluid lung clearance and thus improve the pulmonary condition. In a randomized study, the oral administration of 2 mg/kg followed by 1 mg/kg 12 hors later increased weight loss but did not improve the severity or duration of symptoms.[43] A Cochrane analysis of the study concluded that oral furosemide could not be recommended as treatment of TTN.[44] Whether infants with TTN could benefit from IV furosemide remains to be demonstrated.

Preterm Infants with or Developing Chronic Lung Disease. Loop diuretics have been given to preterm infants with chronic lung disease (CLD) in the hope of decreasing the need for oxygen or ventilatory support. A critical review of the available literature has concluded that (1) furosemide has very inconstant effects in preterm infants younger than 3 weeks of age developing CLD and (2) in infants older than 3 weeks of age with CLD, the acute IV administration of furosemide (1 mg/kg) improved lung compliance and airway resistance for only 1 hour. The chronic administration of furosemide improved both oxygenation and lung compliance.[45] The overall conclusion of the authors of the Cochrane review was that the routine use of loop diuretics in infants with or developing CLD, whether administered IV or enterally, cannot be recommended until randomized trials assessing their effects on survival, duration of oxygen administration and ventilatory support, and long-term outcome are available.[45]

A similar conclusion was drawn by the thorough analysis of studies on the effect of aerosolized furosemide in preterm infants with CLD.[46] Although data in preterm infants older than 3 weeks of age with CLD showed that a single dose of aerosolized furosemide improved pulmonary mechanisms, the data in premature infants younger than 3 weeks of age were too scarce to confirm this effect. Based on current available evidence, the routine or sustained use of IV or aerolized furosemide cannot be recommended.[45,46] The suggestion that adding metolazone to furosemide would overcome tolerance to the latter awaits confirmation.[47]

Posthemorrhagic Ventricular Dilatation. PHVD is a common complication of intraventricular hemorrhage in preterm infants. It carries a high risk of long-term disability. Combined furosemide–acetazolamide treatment has been used in the hope of avoiding the need of placing a ventriculoperitoneal shunt. A large trial in 177 infants showed that acetazolamide and furosemide treatment resulted in a borderline increase in the risk for motor impairment at 1 year and in an increased risk for nephrocalcinosis without evidently decreasing the risk for disability, chronic motor impairment, or death.[48] A critical review of the three available randomized trials in newborn infants with PHVD concluded that combined furosemide–acetazolamide therapy is neither effective nor safe in treating preterm infants with PHVD.[49,50]

Indomethacin-Induced Oliguria. Oliguria occurs frequently after administration of indomethacin to close a PDA. Inhibition of prostaglandin synthesis by indomethacin is responsible for the oliguria. Because furosemide increases the production of prostaglandins, it could potentially help prevent the indomethacin-related toxicity while at the same time decreasing the ductal response to indomethacin. A Cochrane analysis of studies available in 2001 demonstrated that furosemide increased urine output in all patients, leading to a 5% weight loss during a three-dose course. This diuretic response was considered as being risky in dehydrated neonates.[51] The review concluded that there was as yet not enough evidence to support the administration of furosemide to preterm infants with PDA treated with indomethacin.[51] This conclusion has been confirmed by more recent studies showing that (1) furosemide given before each indomethacin dose resulted in a significant increase in serum creatinine and worsening of hyponatremia without increasing urine output[52] and (2) furosemide increased the incidence of acute renal failure without, however, affecting the PDA closure rate.[53] A delay in ductus arteriosus closure has recently been demonstrated in neonatal rats given furosemide.[54] Noteworthy is also the conclusion that there is as yet no evidence from randomized trials to support the use of dopamine to prevent renal dysfunction in indomethacin-treated preterm infants.[55] The same conclusion probably applies to the premature infants presenting with ibuprofen-induced oliguria.

Hypercalcemic States. Loop diuretics can promote calcium excretion and decrease hypercalcemia. Isotonic saline must be infused concomitantly to prevent volume depletion.

Severe Hyponatremia. Severe hyponatremia can be treated by loop diuretics and the concomitant isovolumetric infusion of hypertonic saline.

Asthma and Compromised Lung Mechanics. Direct intratracheal administration of furosemide has been claimed to produce beneficial effects in patients with asthma, in infants with bronchopulmonary dysplasia, and in toddlers with compromised lung mechanics after cardiac surgery. In the latter study, a systemic effect was observed within 15 minutes after intratracheal instillation of the agent.[56] This technique has not yet been validated.

Laboratory Investigation: Assessment of Distal Tubular Acidification. The simultaneous administration of furosemide and fludrocortisone has been shown to be an easy, effective, and well-tolerated alternative to standard ammonium chloride loading to assess distal tubular urine acidification and confirm the diagnosis of distal renal tubular acidosis.[57]

Drug Dosage

See Table 14-6.

Adverse Effects: Interactions

Adverse effects, including volume depletion, postural hypotension, dizziness and syncope, hyponatremia, and hypokalemia, are commonly observed when using loop diuretics. These effects are dose dependent and often occur after overzealous use of large doses of diuretics or chronic administration.

Hypochloremic Metabolic Alkalosis

This occurs frequently as a consequence of direct stimulation by loop diuretics of H^+ secretion in the collecting tubule.

Hypercalciuria and Nephrocalcinosis

Elevated Ca^{++} urinary losses after chronic furosemide administration may lead to *nephrocalcinosis* in term[58] and premature infants[59] secondary hyperparathyroidism, bone resorption, and rickets. When prolonged, hypercalciuria may lead to renal impairment.[60] Although thiazide diuretics decrease calcium and oxalate excretion, adding thiazides to loop diuretics does not appear beneficial.[61]

Patent Ductus Arteriosus

The beneficial renal effect of combining furosemide and indomethacin is still controversial.[24] The suggestion that stimulating prostaglandin synthesis furosemide could promote PDA has not been confirmed (see earlier discussion).

Ototoxicity

The use of furosemide has been identified as an independent risk factor for sensorineural hearing loss in preterm infants.[62] Hearing loss may be transient or permanent. It is usually associated with elevated blood concentrations of loop diuretics. The coadministration of loop diuretics and aminoglycosides increases the risk of ototoxicity. By avoiding elevated peak concentrations of furosemide, the continuous infusion may decreases the risk of ototoxicity.[24]

Miscellaneous

Pancreatitis, jaundice, impaired glucose tolerance, thrombocytopenia, and serious skin disorders are occasionally observed. The majority of adverse effects occur with the use of high doses of the diuretics.

Interactions

Drug interactions may occur with the coadministration of nephrotoxic antibiotics, nonsteroidal antiinflammatory drugs, anticoagulants, and cisplatin.

Distal Convoluted Tubule: Inhibitors of Na⁺Cl⁻ Cotransport

The thiazides inhibit NaCl reabsorption in the distal convoluted tubule.

Chemistry

The benzothiadiazide derivatives are sulfonamides. They are weak diuretics that inhibit the reabsorption of NaCl at the diluting site in the early distal tubule. The main thiazides include chlorothiazide and hydrochlorothiazide. Thiazide-like agents such as chlorthalidone and metolazone belong to this group.

Mechanisms and Sites of Action

The thiazide diuretics are organic anions. They gain access to the tubular lumen by filtration and by secretion in the proximal tubule. They decrease NaCl reabsorption in the distal convoluted tubule by inhibiting the Na^+-Cl^- apical cotransporter. This cotransporter, sometimes called "thiazide-sensitive sodium chloride cotransporter (TSC)" is predominantly expressed in the epithelial cells of the distal convoluted tubule. Its expression is upregulated by aldosterone.[3] To reach their site of action on the luminal side of the tubular cells, the thiazides must be secreted by the anionic organic acid pathway in the proximal tubule. Approximately 4% to 5% of the Na^+ filtered load being reabsorbed in the distal tubule, inhibition of Na^+ reabsorption at this site can only modestly increase NaCl excretion. Some of the thiazides also slightly increase the excretion of HCO_3^- by weakly inhibiting the carbonic anhydrase. By increasing Na^+ delivery to the late distal tubule, the thiazides lead to increased reabsorption of Na^+ at this site in exchange for K^+ and H^+ which are then excreted in the urine.[13,14] By inhibiting NaCl reabsorption in the early distal tubule, the thiazides blunt the ability to dilute the urine. They do not interfere with the concentrating mechanism. The thiazides stimulate Ca^{++} reabsorption in the distal tubule, probably by opening the apical membrane Ca^{++} channels. The thiazides (but not metolazone) are ineffective at GFRs below 30 mL/min/1.73 m².

Pharmacokinetic Properties

The thiazides are rapidly absorbed after oral administration. They variably bind to plasma proteins. They are eliminated unchanged, exclusively (chlorothiazide, hydrochlorothiazide, chlorthalidone) or in great part (~80%) (metolazone) in the urine. Administration of thiazides initiates diuresis in 2 hours, an effect that lasts for 12 hours. The response to metolazone is somewhat more rapid (1 hour) and lasts longer (12–24 hours). The thiazides cross the placental barrier and are secreted in breast milk.

Efficacy and Therapeutic Uses

Thiazide diuretics moderately increase the excretion of Na^+, Cl^-, and water. All thiazides (chlorothiazide, hydrochlorothiazide) and thiazide-like diuretics have overall similar effects when used in maximal doses. When administered chronically, they decrease the excretion of Ca^{++}, as well as that of uric acid, probably as a consequence of increased proximal reabsorption because of volume depletion. The excretion of Mg^{++} is somewhat increased, as is the excretion of K^+ and fixed acids. The prophylactic coadministration of K^+-sparing diuretics can prevent the occurrence of severe hypokalemia. Alternatively, potassium and magnesium supplementation may be useful in patients at risk of symptomatic hypokalemia. The thiazides (but not metolazone) increase the excretion of HCO_3^-. In the absence of significant volume depletion, the thiazides do not normally influence renal hemodynamics and GFR. In contrast with the thiazides and chlorthalidone, metolazone remains effective at GFRs below 30 mL/min/1.73 m^2.

Indications

The main indications for the administration of thiazide diuretics include edematous states, hypertension, and a few specific indications.

Specific Indications with Questionable Benefits (Table 14-5)

Hypercalciuria

The thiazides decrease calcium excretion and this effect may be useful in states of idiopathic hypercalciuria, as well as to prevent calcium losses in patients receiving glucocorticoids.[63] They have been associated to loop diuretics in the hope of decreasing the risk of hypercalciuria and nephrocalcinosis in very low birth weight infants; disappointing results have been observed.[61] In young rats with established furosemide-induced nephrocalcinosis, thiazides failed to improve the calcinosis.[64] The use of thiazides has been associated with an increase in total serum cholesterol and in the ratio of low-density lipoprotein (LDL) to high-density lipoprotein (HDL).[65] In children with X-linked hypophosphatemia on renal phosphate and vitamin D therapy, hydrochlorothiazide decreased the urinary excretion of calcium but did not reverse the nephrocalcinosis.[66]

Proximal Renal Tubular Acidosis

The thiazides have been used to raise the plasma bicarbonate concentration in proximal renal tubular acidosis. This effect on bicarbonate reabsorption is the consequence of the chronic volume contraction induced by the thiazides, a condition that is deleterious for body growth.[67]

Nephrogenic Diabetes Insipidus

The thiazides have been successfully used in children with nephrogenic diabetes insipidus. By inducing volume contraction, they enhance the proximal tubular reabsorption of water and electrolytes, thus significantly decreasing urine output. Although usefully decreasing urine output, volume contraction may inhibit growth in young children with nephrogenic diabetes insipidus. The concomitant use of hydrochlorothiazide and amiloride obviates the need for the K$^+$ supplementation and has been shown as useful as the standard treatment with hydrochlorothiazide and indomethacin in reducing urine output.[68,69]

Chronic Lung Disease

The thiazide and thiazide-like diuretics have been used in the hope of improving pulmonary mechanisms and clinical outcome in preterm infants with CLD. A critical analysis of available well-planned studies led to the conclusion that in preterm infants older than 8 weeks of age with CLD, a 4-week treatment with thiazides and spironolactone reduced the need for furosemide, improved lung compliance, decreased the risk of death, and tended to decrease the risk for lack of extubation after 8 weeks in intubated infants without access to corticosteroids, bronchodilators, or aminophylline.[70] There was little evidence to support any benefit on the need for ventilatory support, length of hospital stay, or long-term outcome in infants receiving current therapy. There was also no evidence to support the hypothesis that adding spironolactone to thiazides or metolazone to furosemide improved the outcome of preterm infants.[70] The addition of K$^+$-sparing diuretics to thiazide did, however, decrease the risk of hypokalemia.

Laboratory Investigation: Diagnosis of Renal Hypokalemic Tubulopathies

Assessment of the maximal diuretic response induced by the administration of hydrochlorothiazide (1 mg/kg) orally allows to differentiate Bartter from Gitelman syndrome, the former presenting with a blunted response to the diuretic agent.[71]

Drug Dosage

See Table 14-6.

Adverse Effects: Interactions

The thiazides may adversely affect water balance and induce electrolyte imbalances (See Table 14-3). They induce an increase in total serum cholesterol and in the LDL-to-HDL ratio.[65] Other side effects include GI disturbances, hypersensitivity reactions, cholestatic jaundice, pancreatitis, thrombocytopenia, and hyperglycemia in diabetic and susceptible patients and hyperlipidemia. Precipitation of hepatic encephalopathy has been observed in patients with hepatic cirrhosis. The thiazides displace bilirubin from albumin and should be cautiously administered to patients with jaundice.

Cortical Collecting Duct: K$^+$-Sparing Drugs

Diuretics that inhibit Na$^+$ reabsorption in the cortical collecting duct decrease the urinary excretion of K$^+$ and H$^+$ and can produce hypokalemia and metabolic acidosis.[14]

Chemistry

Two types of diuretics form the group of K$^+$-sparing diuretics: the inhibitors of a renal epithelial Na$^+$ channels (ENaC) and the antagonists of mineralocorticoid receptors. The overall effects of these two groups of diuretics differ only in their mode of action.

Mechanisms and Sites of Action

The antagonists of the action of aldosterone on the principal cells of the collecting duct increase Na$^+$ excretion and decrease K$^+$ and H$^+$ secretion. Spironolactone, the main agent in this group, competitively inhibits the binding of aldosterone to the mineralocorticoid receptor, thus decreasing the synthesis of aldosterone-induced proteins. The aldosterone antagonists have greater effects in situations of hyperaldosteronism. They do not modify the renal hemodynamics. Highly selective antagonists of the mineralocorticoid receptor are currently under investigation.[72]

The K$^+$-sparing diuretics amiloride and triamterene block the entry of Na$^+$ into the cell through the ENaC Na$^+$ in the apical membrane. Because of changes in electrical profile across the apical membrane, the diffusion of both H$^+$ and K$^+$ from cells into tubular fluid decreases. Activation of the RAAS by the diuretics also impairs the excretion of K$^+$, H$^+$, Ca^{++}, and Mg^{++}. The ENaC blockers do not affect renal hemodynamics.

Pharmacokinetic Properties

Spironolactone is rapidly absorbed from the GI tract with a bioavailability close to 90%. It is 90% bound to plasma proteins and is excreted mainly in the urine and to a lesser extent in the feces. Spironolactone has a slow onset of action, requiring 2 to 3 days for maximum effect.[73] Canrenoate potassium has actions similar to those of spironolactone. It is available for IV administration.

Amiloride is incompletely absorbed from the GI tract with a bioavailability of only 50%. It is not bound to plasma proteins and is excreted unchanged in the urine. Its half-life is 6 to 9 hours. It is prolonged in patients with hepatic or renal failure. Triamterene is unreliably absorbed. It is metabolized by hepatic conjugation. One-fifth of the dose is excreted unchanged in the urine. Its half-life is 1 to 3 hours.

All K$^+$-sparing diuretics cross the placental barrier and are secreted in breast milk.

Efficacy and Therapeutic Uses

The overall effects on electrolyte excretion are similar for spironolactone, amiloride, and triamterene. They are weak natriuretic agents that reduce the excretion of potassium and hydrogen ions. K$^+$-sparing diuretics are mainly used in Na$^+$-retaining states in association with loop or thiazide diuretics. They enhance the natriuretic effect while at the same time limiting K⁺ losses. Refractory edema secondary to CHF, cirrhosis of the liver, and the nephrotic syndrome represent the most common indications for the use of K-sparing diuretics. In these conditions associated with secondary hyperaldosteronism, spironolactone is the first choice agent provided renal function is not impaired. Because they induce K⁺ retention, K⁺-sparing diuretics should not be used in patients with impaired renal function or in those receiving K⁺ supplementation. They should also be avoided in patients prone to developing metabolic acidosis. Amiloride has been successfully used in association with hydrochlorothiazide in patients with nephrogenic diabetes insipidus, obviating the need for using indomethacin.[68]

Specific Indications with Questionable Benefits (Table 14-5)

K⁺-sparing diuretics are often used in association with thiazide diuretics in the management of preterm infants with CLD. Although they certainly decrease the risk of hypokalemia and facilitate the clinical management of the infants, there is as yet no definite proof that their association to thiazide improve the long-term outcome of preterm infants with CLD.[70]

The respiratory function of patients with cystic fibrosis has been improved by the inhalation of amiloride,[74] possibly by the blocking effect of ENaC in pulmonary tissue. Such a beneficial effect has not been confirmed in placebo-controlled trials.[75,76]

Drug Dosage

See Table 14-6.

Adverse Effects: Interactions

The main adverse effects of K⁺-sparing diuretics is to increase the K⁺ plasma concentration to harmful levels. Close monitoring of K⁺ concentration is thus mandatory. GI disturbances, dizziness, photosensitivity, and blood dyscrasias have been reported after the use of triamterene.

Significant adverse effects have been observed with spironolactone; gynecomastia, hirsutism, impotence and menstrual irregularities can occur. Gynecomastia in men is related to both the dose and duration of treatment. Breast enlargement and tenderness occur in women. The pathogenesis of the adverse effects of spironolactone on the endocrine system is probably related to an antiadrenergic action and to reduced 17 hydroxylase activity.

Interactions

K⁺-sparing diuretics should not be used in patients receiving angiotensin-converting enzyme inhibitors because the association can worsen the risk of hyperkalemia.

New Developments in Diuretic Therapy

Three categories of diuretics are under investigation: the adenosine A_1 receptor antagonists, the natriuretic peptides, and the arginine-vasopressin antagonists.[77]

Adenosine A_1 Receptor Antagonists

Theophylline, an A_1 adenosine nonspecific receptor antagonist, presents with natriuretic and diuretic properties. It has been shown, both in experimental studies and clinical trials, to protect newborn kidneys in conditions of asphyxia and RDS. The effect and the use of theophylline are described in Chapter 5.

Natriuretic Peptides

ANP and B-type natriuretic peptide (BNP) are two peptides with natriuretic and diuretic properties.[77] Both are released by cardiac cells in the atria in response to increased blood volume. ANP (28 amino acids) and BNP (32 amino acids) act via the natriuretic peptide receptor A (NPR-A). In addition to increasing the excretion of Na⁺, both peptides inhibit the sympathetic system and the RAAS. They also relax vascular smooth muscle. ANP and BNP are degraded by the metalloproteinase neutral endopeptidase 24.11 (NEP). Urodilatin is a noncirculating natriuretic peptide

(32 amino acids) secreted by distal tubular cells that is not degraded by the NEP located in the proximal tubular cells.[78] ANP favors filtration by relaxing the afferent artery and the mesangial cells.[79] The NPs inhibit Na^+ proximal reabsorption and decrease distal Na^+ reabsorption indirectly by blunting angiotensin II and aldosterone synthesis and directly by inhibiting the thiazide-sensitive Na^+ channel. ANP increases diuresis by inhibiting the V2 receptor-mediated action of arginine vasopressin (AVP) on water permeability.

The natriuretic peptides have not yet been used as diuretic agents in neonates but may have interesting properties in patients presenting with inappropriate salt and water retention.

Arginine Vasopressin Antagonists

AVP acts on three type of receptors: (1) the V_{1A} receptors mediating vasoconstriction, (2) the V_{1B} mediating the release of ACTH, and (3) the V_2 receptors mediating free water reabsorption in the collecting duct. AVP also stimulates Na^+, K^+, $2Cl^-$ cotranspoort in the ascending limb of Henle loop via V_2 receptors. By selectively increasing the excretion of free water, the AVP antagonists may prove useful in the treatment of severe hyponatremic states.[77,80,81]

References

1. Guignard JP, John EG. Renal function in the tiny, premature infant. *Clin Perinatol*. 1986;13: 377-401.
2. Guignard JP. Renal morphogenesis and development of renal function. In: Taeusch HW, Ballard RA, Gleason CA, eds. *Avery's diseases of the newborn*. 8th ed. Philadelphia, PA: WB Saunders Co; 2005:1257-1266.
3. Giebisch G, Windhager E. The urinary system. Part VI. In: Boron WF, Boulpaep EL, eds. *Medical Physiology*. Philadelphia, PA: Saunders, 2003:735-876.
4. Guignard JP, Gouyon JB. Body fluid homeostasis in the newborn infant with congestive heart failure: effects of diuretics. *Clin Perinatol*. 1988;15:447-466.
5. Lowrie L. Diuretic therapy of heart failure in infants and children. *Prog Pediatr Cardiol*. 2000;12: 45-55.
6. Morrison RT. Edema and principles of diuretic use. *Med Clin North Am*. 1997;81:689-704.
7. Schrier RW, Fassett RG. A critique of the overfill hypothesis of sodium and water retention in the nephrotic syndrome. *Kidney Int*. 1998;53:1111-1111.
8. Vande Walle JG, Donckerwolcke RA. Pathogenesis of edema formation in the nephrotic syndrome. *Pediatr Nephrol*. 2001;16:283-293.
9. Kellum JA. Use of diuretics in the acute care setting. *Kidney Int Suppl*. 1998;66:S67-S70.
10. Gouyon JB, Guignard JP. Drugs and acute renal insufficiency in the neonate. *Biol Neonate*. 1986;50: 177-181.
11. Brion LP, Yong SC, Perez IA, et al. Diuretics and chronic lung disease of prematurity. *J Perinatol*. 2001;21:269-271.
12. Whitelaw A, Aquilina K. Management of posthaemorrhagic ventricular dilatation. *Arch Dis Child Fetal Neonatal Ed*. 2011 Feb 2. (Epub ahead of print).
13. Chemtob S, Kaplan BS, Sherbotie JR, et al. Pharmacology of diuretics in the newborn. *Pediatr Clin North Am*. 1989;36:1231-1250.
14. Wells TG. The pharmacology and therapeutics of diuretics in the pediatric patient. *Pediatr Clin North Am*. 1990;37:463-504.
15. Knoers N, Monnens LA. Amiloride-hydrochlorothiazide versus indomethacin-hydrochlorothiazide in the treatment of nephrogenic diabetes insipidus. *J Pediatr*. 1990;117:499-502.
16. Ong WH, Guignard JP, Sharma A, et al. Pharmacological approach to the management of neonatal hypertension. *Seminars in Neonatology*. 1998;3:149-163.
17. Hagadorn JL, Sanders MR, Staves C, et al. Diuretics for very low birth weight infants in the first 28 days: a survey of the US neonatologists. *J Perinatol*. 2011, in press.
18. Better OS, Rubinstein I, Winaver JM, et al. Mannitol therapy revisited (1940–1997). *Kidney Int*. 1997; 52:886-894.
19. Rigden SP, Dillon MJ, Kind PR, et al. The beneficial effect of mannitol on post-operative renal function in children undergoing cardiopulmonary bypass surgery. *Clin Nephrol*. 1984;21:148-151.
20. Alon U, Hellerstein S, Warady BA. Oral acetazolamide in the assessment of (urine-blood) PCO2. *Pediatr Nephrol*. 1991;5:307-311.
21. International PHVD Drug Trial Group. International randomized controlled trial of acetazolamide and furosemide in posthaemorrhagic ventricular dilatation in infancy. *Lancet*. 1998;352:433-440.
22. Kennedy CR, Ayers S, Campbell MJ, et al. Randomized, controlled trial of acetazolamide and furosemide in posthemorrhagic ventricular dilatation in infancy: follow-up at 1 year. *Pediatrics*. 2001;198: 597-607.
23. Brater DC. Diuretic therapy. *N Engl J Med*. 1998;339:387-395.

24. Eades SK, Christensen ML. The clinical pharmacology of loop diuretics in the pediatric patient. *Pediatr Nephrol*. 1998;12:603-616.

25. Dubourg L, Mosig D, Drukker A, et al. Torasemide is an effective diuretic in the newborn rabbit. *Pediatr Nephrol*. 2000;14:476-479.

26. Wargo KA. A comprehensive review of the loop diuretics. *Ann Pharmacother*. 2009;43:1836-1847.

27. Lyseng-Williamson KA. Torasemide prolonged release. *Drugs*. 2009:1363-1372.

28. Mirochnick MH, Miceli JJ, Kramer PA, et al. Furosemide pharmacokinetics in very low birth weight infants. *J Pediatr*. 1988;112:653-657.

29. Prandota J. Clinical pharmacology of furosemide in children: a supplement. *Am J Ther*. 2001;8: 275-289.

30. Marshall JD, Wells TG, Letzig L, et al. Pharmacokinetics and pharmacodynamics of bumetanide in critically ill pediatric patients. *J Clin Pharmacol*. 1998;38:994-1002.

31. Sullivan JE, Witte MK, Yamashita TS, et al. Pharmacokinetics of bumetanide in critically ill infants. *Clin Pharmacol Ther*. 1996;60:405-413.

32. Hagadorn JL, Sanders MR, Staves C, et al. Diuretics for very low birth weight infants in the first 28 days: a survey of the US neonatologists. *J Perinatol*. 2011; in press.

33. Luciani GB, Nichani S, Chang AC, et al. Continuous versus intermittent furosemide infusion in critically ill infants after open heart operations. *Ann Thorac Surg*. 1997;64:1133-1139.

34. van der Vorst MM, Ruys-Dudok van Heel I, Kist-van Holthe JE, et al. Continuous intravenous furosemide in haemodynamically unstable children after cardiac surgery. *Intensive Care Med*. 2001;27: 711-715.

35. Klinge JM, Scharf J, Hofbeck M, et al. Intermittent administration of furosemide versus continuous infusion in the postoperative management of children following open heart surgery. *Intensive Care Med*. 1997;23:693-697.

36. Baylen BG, Johnson G, Tsang R, et al. The occurrence of hyperaldosteronism in infants with congestive heart failure. *Am J Cardiol*. 1980;45:305-310.

37. Knauf H, Mutschler E. Clinical pharmacokinetics and pharmacodynamics of torasemide. *Clin Pharmacokinet*. 1998;34:1-24.

38. Young M, Plosker GL. Torasemide: a pharmacoeconomic review of its use in chronic heart failure. *Pharmacoeconomics*. 2001;19:679-703.

39. Haws RM, Baum M. Efficacy of albumin and diuretic therapy in children with nephrotic syndrome. *Pediatrics*. 1993;91:1142-1146.

40. Dubourg L, Drukker A, Guignard J-P. Failure of the loop diuretic torasemide to improve renal function of hypoxemic vasomotor nephropathy in the newborn rabbit. *Pediatr Res*. 2000;47:504-508.

41. Brion LP, Soll RF. Diuretics for respiratory distress syndrome in preterm infants. *Cochrane Database Syst Rev* 2008; (1):CD001454.

42. Jain L, Eaton DC. Physiology of fetal lung fluid clearance and the effect of labor. *Semin Perinatol*. 2006;30:34-43.

43. Wiswell MC, Rawings JS, Smith FR, et al. Effect of furosemide on the clinical course of transient tachypnea of the newborn. *Pediatrics*. 1985;75:908-910.

44. Lewis V, Whitelaw A. Furosemide for transient tachypnea of the newborn. *Cochrane Database Syst Rev*. 2002;(1):CD003064.

45. Brion LP, Primhak RA. Intravenous or enteral loop diuretics for preterm infants with (or developing) chronic lung disease: *Cochrane Database Syst Rev* 2002;(1):CD001453.

46. Brion LP, Primhak RA, Yong W. Aerosolized diuretics for preterm infants with (or developing) chronic lung disease. *Cochrane Database Syst Rev* 2006;(3):CD001694.

47. Segar JL, Robillad JE, Jonason KJ, et al. Addition of metolazone to overcome tolerance to furosemide in infants with bronchopulmonary dysplasia. *J Pediatr*. 1992;120:966-973.

48. Kennedy CR, Ayers S, Campbell MJ, et al. Randomized, controlled trial of acetazolamide and furosemide in posthemorrhagic ventricular dilatation in infancy: follow-up at 1 year. *Pediatrics*. 2001;198: 597-607.

49. International PHVD Drug Trial Group. International randomized controlled trial of acetazolamide and furosemide in posthaemorrhagic ventricular dilatation in infancy. *Lancet*. 1998;352:433-440.

50. Whitelaw A, Kennedy CR, Brion LP. Diuretic therapy for newborn infants with posthemorrhagic ventricular dilatation. *Cochrane Database Syst Rev* 2001;(2):CD 002270.

51. Brion LP, Campbell DE. Furosemide for symptomatic patent ductus arteriosus in indomethacin-treated infants. *Cochrane Database Syst Rev* 2001;(3):CD 001148.

52. Andriessen P, Struis NC, Niemarkt H, et al. Furosemide in preterm infants treated with indomethacin for patent ductus arteriosus. *Acta Paediatr*. 2009;98:797-803.

53. Lee BS, Byun SY, Chung ML, et al. Effect of furosemide on ductal closure and renal function in indomethacin-treated preterm infants during the early neonatal period. *Neonatology*. 2010;98: 191-199.

54. Toyoshima K, Momma K, Nakanishi T. In vivo dilatation of the ductus arteriosus induced by furosemide in the rat. *Pediatr Res*. 2010;67:173-176.

55. Barrington K, Brion LP. Dopamine versus no treatment to prevent renal dysfunction in indomethacin-treated preterm newborn infants. *Cochrane Database Syst Rev* 2002;(3):CD 003213.

56. Aufricht C, Votava F, Marx M, et al. Intratracheal furosemide in infants after cardiac surgery: its effects on lung mechanics and urinary output, and its levels in plasma and tracheal aspirate. *Intensive Care Med*. 1997;23:992-997.

57. Walsh SB, Shirley DG, Wrong OM, et al. Urinary acidification assessed by simultaneous furosemide and fludrocortisone treatment: an alternative to ammonium chloride. *Kidney Int*. 2007;71:1310-1316.

14

58. Saarela T, Laning P, Koivisto M, et al. Nephrocalcinosis in full-term infants receiving furosemide treatment for congestive heart failure: a study of the incidence and 2-year follow up. *Eur J Pediatr.* 1999;158:668-672.

59. Gimpel C, Krause A, Franck P, et al. Exposure to furosemide as the strongest risk factor for nephrocalcinosis in preterm infants. *Pediatr Int.* 2010;52:51-56.

60. Downing GJ, Egelhoff JC, Daily DK, et al. Kidney function in very low birth weight infants with furosemide-related renal calcifications at ages 1 to 2 years. *J Pediatr.* 1992;120:599-604.

61. Campfield T, Braden G, Flynn-Valone P, et al. Effect of diuretics on urinary oxalate, calcium, and sodium excretion in very low birth weight infants. *Pediatrics.* 1997;99:814-818.

62. Borradori C, Fawer CL, Buclin T, et al. Risk factors of sensorineural hearing loss in preterm infants. *Biol Neonate.* 1997;71:1-10.

63. Lukert BP, Raisz LG. Glucocorticoid-induced osteoporosis: pathogenesis and management. *Ann Intern Med.* 1990;112:352-364.

64. Knoll S, Alon US. Effect of thiazide on established furosemide-induced nephrocalcinosis in the young rat. *Pediatr Nephrol.* 2000;14:32-35.

65. Reusz GS, Dobos M, Tulassay T. Hydrochlorothiazide treatment of children with hypercalciuria: effects and side effects. *Pediatr Nephrol.* 1993;7:699-702.

66. Seikaly MG, Baum M. Thiazide diuretics arrest the progression of nephrocalcinosis in children with X-linked hypophosphatemia. *Pediatrics.* 2001;108:E6.

67. Kahlhoff H, Manz F. Nutrition, acid-base status and growth in early childhood. *Eur J Nutr.* 2001;40: 221-230.

68. Kirchlechner V, Koller DY, Seidl R, et al. Treatment of nephrogenic diabetes insipidus with hydrochlorothiazide and amiloride. *Arch Dis Child.* 1999;80:548-552.

69. Knoers N, Monnens LA. Amiloride-hydrochlorothiazide versus indomethacin-hydrochlorothiazide in the treatment of nephrogenic diabetes insipidus. *J Pediatr.* 1990;117:499-502.

70. Brion LP, Primhak RA, Ambrosio-Perez I. Diuretics acting on the distal renal tubule for preterm infants with (or developing) chronic lung disease. *Cochrane Database Syst Rev* 2002;(1):CD 001817.

71. Colussi G, Bettinelli A, Tedeschi S, et al. A thiazide test for the diagnosis of renal tubular hypokalemic disorders. *Clin J Am Soc Nephrol.* 2007;2:454-460.

72. Delyani JA. Mineralocorticoid receptor antagonists: the evolution of utility and pharmacology. *Kidney Int.* 2000;57:1408-1411.

73. Buck ML. Clinical experience with spironolactone in pediatrics. *Ann Pharmacother.* 2005;39:823-828.

74. Hofmann T, Senier I, Bittner P, et al. Aerosolized amiloride: dose effect on nasal bioelectric properties, pharmacokinetics, and effect on sputum expectoration in patients with cystic fibrosis. *J Aerosol Med.* 1997;10:147-158.

75. Pons G, Marchand MC, d'Athis P, et al. French multicenter randomized double-blind placebo-controlled trial on nebulized amiloride in cystic fibrosis patients. The amiloride-AFLM Collaborative Study Group. *Pediatr Pulmonol.* 2000;30:25-31.

76. Ratjen F, Bush A. Amiloride: still a viable treatment option in cystic fibrosis? *Am J Respir Crit Care Med.* 2008;178;1191-1192.

77. Costello-Boerrigter LC, Boerrigter G, Burnett JC Jr. Revisiting salt and water retention: new diuretics, aquaretics, and natriuretics. *Med Clin North Am.* 2003;87:475-491.

78. Forssmann W, Meyer M, Forssmann K. The renal urodilatin system: clinical implications. *Cardiovasc Res.* 2001;51:450-462.

79. Semmekrot B, Guignard J-P. Atrial natriuretic peptide during early human development. *Biol Neonate.* 1991;60:341-349.

80. Costello-Boerrigter LC, Boerrigter G, Burnett JC. Pharmacology of vasopressin antagonists. *Heart Fail Rev.* 2009;14:75-82.

81. Kumar S, Berl T. Vasopressin antagonists in the treatment of water-retaining disorders. *Semin Nephrol.* 2008;28:279-288.

CHAPTER 15

Neonatal Hypertension: Diagnosis and Management

Joseph T. Flynn, MD, MS

There has been increased awareness of neonatal hypertension over the past several decades since its first description in the 1970s.[1,2] Despite this, there is still uncertainty over which neonates require treatment for hypertension, primarily because of conflicting data on normative blood pressure (BP) values in neonates. This chapter reviews the existing data on normal neonatal BP and presents a reasonable approach to evaluation and management based on likely causes and pathophysiology. Finally, research needs, especially those related to late-onset hypertension and long-term outcome, are reviewed.

Normative Values for Neonatal Blood Pressure

There are many complexities to the changing patterns of BP in the newborn period, and consideration of gestational age at birth, postnatal and postconceptual age, and appropriateness of size for gestational age, are all contributory factors. As in older children, BP values in neonates may vary according to the method of BP assessment (e.g. intraarterial, Doppler, oscillometric) and according to the infant's state (e.g. sleeping, crying, feeding). All of these factors need to be taken into account when reviewing the literature on BP standards as well as in clinical practice. Even though neonatal BPs have been measured for decades, we are still in the early phase of identifying the normal patterns of infant BPs, and many physiologic changes still need further investigation.

Data on BP on the first day of life was published in 1995 by Zubrow et al.[3] From data on 329 infants on day 1 of life, they were able to define the mean plus upper and lower 95% confidence limits for BP; their data clearly demonstrated increases in BP with increasing gestational age and birth weight (Fig. 15-1). A more recent study by Pejovic et al,[4] limiting their analysis to hemodynamically stable premature and term infants admitted to the neonatal intensive care unit (NICU), also showed that BPs on day 1 of life correlated with gestational age and birth weight. Healthy term infants do not seem to demonstrate this same pattern.[5]

After the first day of life, it appears that BPs in premature newborns increase more rapidly over the first week or 2 of life followed by a slowing of the rate of increase. The previously mentioned Philadelphia study categorized more than 600 infants in the NICU into gestational age groups and showed a similar rate of BP

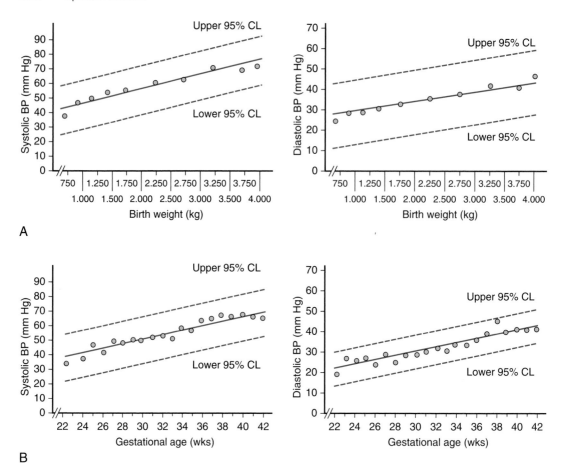

Figure 15-1 Linear regression of systolic and diastolic blood pressure (BP) by birth weight (A) and gestational age (B), with 95% CL (confidence limits); *upper* and *lower dashed lines.* (Reproduced from Zubrow AB, Hulman S, Kushner H, et al. Determinants of blood pressure in infants admitted to neonatal intensive care units: a prospective multicenter study. *J Perinatol.* 1995;15:470-479 with permission from Nature Publishing Group.)

increase over the first 5 days of life, regardless of gestational age.[3] The more recent study by Pejovic and colleagues[4] on stable NICU infants showed a similar pattern with BPs in each gestational age category of premature infants increasing at a faster rate over the first week of life with subsequent slowing.[4] In these infants, they determined that the rate of rise was more rapid in the preterm than full-term infants (Fig. 15-2). As premature neonates mature, it appears that the strongest predictor of BP is postconceptual age. Illustrated in Figure 15-3 from Zubrow et al[3] are the regression lines between postconceptual age and systolic and diastolic BP along with the upper and lower 95th confidence limits for systolic and diastolic BP for each week of postconceptual age.

In term infants, appropriateness for gestational age seems to be an important influence on BP. In the Australian study of healthy term infants,[5] BPs were higher on day 2 of life compared to day 1, but not thereafter. A Spanish study demonstrated that small for gestational age infants had the lowest BPs at birth, but subsequently the fastest rate of rise, so that by 1 month of age, all term infants had similar BPs.[6]

Normal BPs in infants older than 1 month of age have not been extensively studied recently. The percentile curves reported by the Second Task Force of the National High Blood Pressure Education Program (NHBPEP)[7] (Fig. 15-4) remain the most widely available reference values. These curves allow BP to be characterized as normal or elevated not only by age and gender, but also by length (provided in the legend below the curves). Unfortunately, these BP values were determined by a single

Figure 15-2 Increase in systolic (A), diastolic (B), and mean (C) blood pressure (BP) during the first month of life in infants classified by estimated gestational age: A, 28 weeks or younger; B, 29 to 32 weeks; C, 33 to 36 weeks; and D, 37 weeks or older. (Reproduced from Zubrow AB, Hulman S, Kushner H, et al. Determinants of blood pressure in infants admitted to neonatal intensive care units: a prospective multicenter study. *J Perinatol.* 1995;15:470-479 with permission from Nature Publishing Group.)

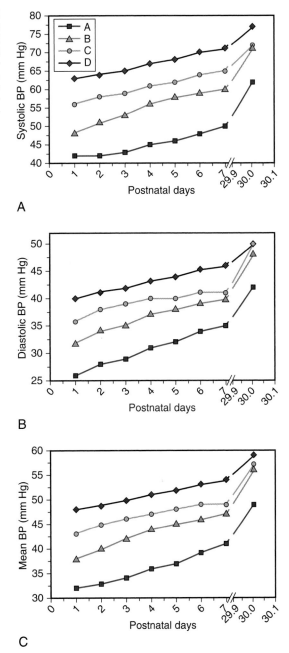

15

measurement on awake infants by the Doppler method, which reduced the number of diastolic BP readings by more than half. Comparison with the more recently published values for 1 year-old infants in the Fourth Report from the NHBPEP[8] reveals significant differences that further call into question the validity of the 1987 curves. Additionally, a recent study of 406 healthy term infants with BPs measured by the oscillometric method on day 2 of life and then at 6 and 12 months of age demonstrated BPs that are slightly higher than the Task Force values.[9] Although there is clearly a pressing need for new normative BP data on infants during the first year of life, at present, the Task Force values should be used in most circumstances.

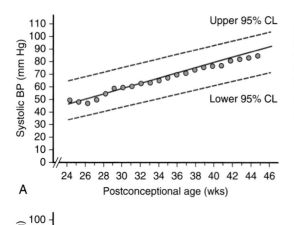

Figure 15-3 Linear regression of mean systolic (A) and diastolic (B) blood pressure (BP) by postconceptual age in weeks, with 95% confidence limits (CLs; *upper* and *lower dashed lines*). (Reproduced from Zubrow AB, Hulman S, Kushner H, et al. Determinants of blood pressure in infants admitted to neonatal intensive care units: a prospective multicenter study. *J Perinatol.* 1995;15:470-479 with permission from Nature Publishing Group.)

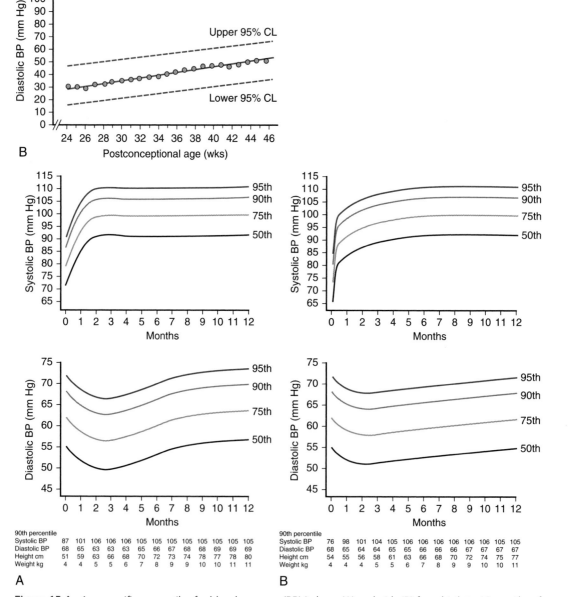

Figure 15-4 Age-specific percentiles for blood pressure (BP) in boys (A) and girls (B) from birth to 12 months of age. (Reprinted from Task Force on Blood Pressure Control in Children. Report of the Second Task Force on Blood Pressure Control in Children—1987. National Heart, Lung and Blood Institute, National Institutes of Health, Bethesda, MD, January 1987.)

What Level of Blood Pressure Should Be Considered Hypertensive?

In older children, the definition of hypertension is persistent systolic or diastolic BP equal to or greater than the 95th percentile for age, gender, and height.[8] As can be deduced from the preceding discussion, there is considerable variation in neonatal BP, and no generally agreed upon reference values are available. For term infants and infants between 1 and 12 months of age, the best available reference data are those from the Second Task Force Report[7] (Fig. 15-4). In this age group, one could diagnose hypertension if the infant's BP was repeatedly greater than or equal to the 95th percentile for an infant of comparable age (also note that weight and height are given below the curves and could also be used to help determine if an infant's BP is normal or elevated).

The major unresolved question is how to diagnose hypertension in preterm infants. From the limited published data, it is possible to derive systolic and diastolic BP percentiles, as well as mean arterial pressure percentiles, according to postconceptual age (Table 15-1).[3-6,9,10] Although not derived from a large-scale study (which is sorely needed), these values may be useful clinically. Specifically, infants with BP values persistently at or above the 99th percentile clearly would warrant investigation and possibly initiation of antihypertensive drug therapy. Whatever reference data are used, clinical circumstances and personal experience need to be brought to bear in interpreting an individual infant's BP and entertaining a possible diagnosis of hypertension.

Incidence and Differential Diagnosis

Most reports indicate that the incidence of hypertension in neonates is low, ranging from 0.2% to 3%.[1,2,11,12] It is so unusual in otherwise healthy term infants that routine BP determination is not advocated for this group.[13] For preterm and otherwise high-risk newborns admitted to modern NICUs, however, the picture can be quite different. In a recent Australian study of approximately 2500 infants followed for more than 4 years, the prevalence of hypertension was 1.3%.[14] Antenatal steroids, maternal hypertension, umbilical arterial catheter placement, postnatal acute renal failure, and chronic lung disease were among the most common concurrent conditions in babies with elevated BP.

Hypertension may also be detected long after discharge from the NICU. In a retrospective review of more than 650 infants seen in follow-up after discharge from a tertiary level NICU, Friedman and Hustead[15] found an incidence of hypertension (defined as a systolic BP of >113 mm Hg on three consecutive visits over 6 weeks) of 2.6%. Hypertension in this study was detected at a mean age of approximately 2 months postterm when corrected for prematurity. Infants in this study who developed hypertension tended to have lower initial Apgar scores and slightly longer NICU stays than infants who remained normotensive, indicating a somewhat greater likelihood of developing hypertension in sicker babies. Unfortunately, this study has not been replicated, so the current prevalence of hypertension in high-risk infants remains unclear. However, these data do support routine BP monitoring after NICU discharge, as advocated by the NHBPEP.[8]

As in older infants and children, the causes of hypertension in neonates are numerous (Table 15-2), with the largest number of cases probably accounted for by umbilical artery catheter-associated thromboembolism affecting the aorta, the renal arteries, or both. This was first demonstrated in the early 1970s by Neal and colleagues[16] and later confirmed by other investigators. Hypertension was reported to develop in infants who had undergone umbilical arterial catheterization even when thrombi were unable to be demonstrated in the renal arteries. Reported rates of thrombus formation have generally been about 25%.[17]

Although several studies have examined duration of line placement and line position as factors involved in thrombus formation, these data have not been conclusive.[18] Longer duration of umbilical catheter placement has been associated with

Table 15-1   NEONATAL BLOOD PRESSURE PERCENTILES*

Postconceptual Age	50th Percentile	95th Percentile	99th Percentile
44 Weeks			
SBP	88	105	110
DBP	50	68	73
MAP	63	80	85
42 Weeks			
SBP	85	98	102
DBP	50	65	70
MAP	62	76	81
40 Weeks			
SBP	80	95	100
DBP	50	65	70
MAP	60	75	80
38 Weeks			
SBP	77	92	97
DBP	50	65	70
MAP	59	74	79
36 Weeks			
SBP	72	87	92
DBP	50	65	70
MAP	57	72	77
34 Weeks			
SBP	70	85	90
DBP	40	55	60
MAP	50	65	70
32 Weeks			
SBP	68	83	88
DBP	40	55	60
MAP	49	64	69
30 Weeks			
SBP	65	80	85
DBP	40	55	60
MAP	48	63	68
28 Weeks			
SBP	60	75	80
DBP	38	50	54
MAP	45	58	63
26 Weeks			
SBP	55	72	77
DBP	30	50	56
MAP	38	57	63

*Derived from data in references Zubrow et al,[3] Pejovic et al,[4] Kent et al,[5] Lurbe et al,[6] Kent et al,[9] and Kent et al.[10]
DBP, diastolic blood pressure; MAP, mean arterial pressure; SBP, systolic blood pressure.

Table 15-2 CAUSES OF NEONATAL HYPERTENSION

Renovascular
- Thromboembolism
- Renal artery stenosis
- Mid-aortic coarctation
- Renal venous thrombosis
- Compression of renal artery
- Idiopathic arterial calcification
- Congenital rubella syndrome

Renal parenchymal disease
- Congenital
  - Polycystic kidney disease
  - Multicystic-dysplastic kidney disease
  - Tuberous sclerosis
  - Ureteropelvic junction obstruction
  - Unilateral renal hypoplasia
  - Congenital nephrotic syndrome
  - Renal tubular dysgensis
- Acquired
  - Acute tubular necrosis
  - Cortical necrosis
  - Interstitial nephritis
  - Hemolytic-uremic syndrome
  - Obstruction (stones, tumors)

Pulmonary
- Bronchopulmonary dysplasia
- Pneumothorax

Cardiac
- Thoracic aortic coarctation

Endocrine
- Congenital adrenal hyperplasia
- Hyperaldosteronism
- Hyperthyroidism
- Pseudohypoaldosteronism type II

Medications and intoxications
- Infant
  - Dexamethasone
  - Adrenergic agents
  - Vitamin D intoxication
  - Theophylline
  - Caffeine
  - Pancuronium
  - Phenylephrine
- Maternal
  - Cocaine
  - Heroin

Neoplasia
- Wilms tumor
- Mesoblastic nephroma
- Neuroblastoma
- Pheochromocytoma

Neurologic
- Pain
- Intracranial hypertension
- Seizures
- Familial dysautonomia
- Subdural hematoma

Miscellaneous
- Total parenteral nutrition
- Closure of abdominal wall defect
- Adrenal hemorrhage
- Hypercalcemia
- Traction
- Extracorporeal membrane oxygenation
- Birth asphyxia

15

higher rates of thrombus formation.[19] A recent Cochrane review comparing "low" versus "high" umbilical artery catheters determined that the "high" catheter placement was associated with fewer ischemic events such as necrotizing enterocolitis, but that hypertension occurred at equal frequency with either position.[20] Thus, it is assumed that catheter-related hypertension is related to thrombus formation at the time of line placement because of disruption of the vascular endothelium of the umbilical artery, particularly in preterm infants.

Fibromuscular dysplasia leading to renal arterial stenosis is an extremely important cause of renovascular hypertension in neonates. Many of these infants may have main renal arteries that appear normal on angiography, but demonstrate significant branch vessel disease that can cause severe hypertension.[21] In addition, renal arterial stenosis may also be accompanied by mid-aortic coarctation and cerebral vascular stenoses.[21,22] Several other vascular problems may also lead to neonatal hypertension, including renal venous thrombosis, idiopathic arterial calcification, and compression of the renal arteries by tumors.

After renovascular causes, the next largest group of infants with hypertension are those with congenital renal abnormalities. While both autosomal dominant and autosomal recessive polycystic kidney disease (PKD) may present in the newborn period with severe nephromegaly and hypertension,[23,24] recessive PKD more commonly leads to hypertension early, sometimes in the first month of life. Hypertension has also been reported in infants with unilateral multicystic dysplastic kidneys,[25] possibly because of another coexisting urologic abnormality such as parenchymal scarring. Renal obstruction may be accompanied by hypertension, for example, in infants with congenital ureteropelvic junction obstruction, and sometimes may persist after surgical correction of the obstruction.[26] The importance of congenital urologic malformations as a cause of neonatal hypertension was recently highlighted in a referral series from Brazil[27] in which 13 of 15 hypertensive infants had urologic causes. The median age at diagnosis of hypertension was 20 days (range, 5–70 days), emphasizing the need for regular BP measurement in infants with urologic malformations to detect hypertension.

The other important group of hypertensive neonates are those with bronchopulmonary dysplasia (BPD). BPD-associated hypertension was first described in the mid-1980s by Abman and colleagues,[28] who found the incidence of hypertension in infants with BPD was 43% versus an incidence of 4.5% in infants without BPD. More than half of the infants with BPD who developed hypertension did not display it until after discharge from the NICU, again highlighting the need for measurement of BP in NICU "graduates."

Other studies have subsequently confirmed that hypertension occurs more commonly in infants with BPD compared with infants of similar gestational age or birthweight without BPD. Factors such as hypoxemia and increased severity of BPD appear to correlate with the development of hypertension.[29] Because many of these infants will have had an umbilical line placed, it is also possible that BPD is a comorbidity for line-associated thromboembolic disease (see above). Although updated studies are needed, these observations reinforce the impression that infants with severe BPD are clearly at increased risk and need close monitoring for the development of hypertension. This is especially true in infants who require ongoing treatment with theophylline preparations, diuretics, or corticosteroids.

Hypertension may also be secondary to disorders of several other organ systems or may develop as a consequence of treatment with various pharmacologic agents (Table 15-2). Interested readers are encouraged to consult more comprehensive reviews for a full discussion of these causes.[30,31]

Diagnostic Evaluation

Except in critically ill infants with severely elevated BP, in many infants, elevated BP is detected on routine monitoring of vital signs, making it difficult to identify infants with true hypertension that warrants further evaluation or treatment. This is primarily a consequence of the changing nature of BP in neonates and the difficulty in knowing what BP level should be considered elevated (see preceding sections). However, some classic presentations of neonatal hypertension have been described, including congestive heart failure and cardiogenic shock.[32] In less acutely ill infants, feeding difficulties, unexplained tachypnea, apnea, lethargy, irritability, or seizures may constitute symptoms of unsuspected hypertension. In older infants who have been discharged from the NICU, unexplained irritability or failure to thrive may be the only manifestations of hypertension.

Accurate BP measurement is crucial so that hypertension will be correctly identified. The gold standard for BP measurement in neonates remains direct intra-arterial measurement. There is reasonable correlation between umbilical artery and peripheral artery catheter BPs in neonates,[33] so no specific site is preferred. Indirect methods of measuring BP such as palpation and auscultation are not practical in neonates, especially in the NICU setting, and ultrasonic Doppler assessment has largely been replaced by oscillometric devices.[34]

Oscillometric devices are easy to use and provide the ability to follow BP trends over time. Studies have shown reasonably good correlation between oscillometric and umbilical or radial artery BP in neonates and young children.[35,36] They are especially useful for infants who require BP monitoring after discharge from the NICU.[37] However, not all oscillometric devices are equal. A few studies have compared different oscillometric BP monitors with direct arterial measurements in neonates and have shown that accuracy varied depending on the size of the infant[38] with a higher likelihood of oscillometric methods to overread BP compared with direct measurement.[39] Given this, consistent technique becomes of paramount importance in obtaining accurate BP values. A standard protocol as suggested by

Nwankwo and colleagues[40] may result in decreased variability of BP readings, ensuring that accurate BP values will be available to guide clinical decision making.

Diagnosing the cause of the elevated BP should be fairly straightforward. A relatively focused history should be obtained, paying attention to determining whether there were any pertinent prenatal exposures, as well as to the details of the infant's clinical course and any concurrent conditions. The procedures that the infant has undergone (e.g., umbilical catheter placement) should be reviewed, and his or her current medication list should be reviewed for substances that can elevate BP.

The physical examination should focus on obtaining information to assist in narrowing the differential diagnosis. BP readings should be obtained in all four extremities at least once to rule out coarctation of the aorta.[41] The general appearance of the infant should be assessed, with particular attention paid to the presence of any dysmorphic features that may indicate an obvious diagnosis such as congenital adrenal hyperplasia.[42] Careful cardiac and abdominal examination should be performed. The presence of a flank mass or of an epigastric bruit may point the clinician toward diagnosis of either ureteropelvic junction obstruction or renal artery stenosis, respectively.

Because the correct diagnosis is usually suggested by the history and physical examination and there is typically ample prior laboratory data available for review, few additional studies are needed in most instances. It is important to assess renal function and to examine a specimen of the urine to ascertain the presence of renal parenchymal disease. Chest radiography may be useful in infants with signs of congestive heart failure and in those with a murmur on physical examination. Other diagnostic studies, such as cortisol, aldosterone, or thyroxine levels, should be obtained when there is pertinent history (Table 15-3). Plasma renin activity is typically quite high in infancy, particularly in premature infants,[43-45] making renin values difficult to interpret. Given this, assessment of plasma renin activity in the initial evaluation of hypertension in infants may be deferred. An exception to this is infants with electrolyte abnormalities such as hypokalemia that suggest a genetic disorder in tubular sodium handling.[46]

The role of imaging in the evaluation of neonates with hypertension has been reviewed extensively elsewhere,[47] so only a few comments are made here. Renal ultrasonography with Doppler should be obtained in all infants with hypertension because it can help uncover potentially correctable causes of hypertension such as renal venous thrombosis,[48] may detect aortic or renal arterial thrombi,[17] and can identify anatomic renal abnormalities and other congenital renal diseases. Although nuclear scanning has been shown in some studies to demonstrate abnormalities of renal perfusion caused by thromboembolic phenomenon,[47] in the author's experience, it has had little role in the assessment of infants with hypertension, primarily because of the difficulties in obtaining accurate, interpretable results in this age

Table 15-3 DIAGNOSTIC TESTING IN NEONATAL HYPERTENSION

Generally Useful	Useful in Selected Infants
Urinalysis (± culture)	Thyroid studies
CBC and platelet count	Urine VMA and HVA
Electrolytes	Plasma renin activity
BUN, creatinine	Aldosterone
Calcium	Cortisol
Chest radiography	Echocardiography
Renal ultrasonography with Doppler	Abdominal and pelvic ultrasonography
	VCUG
	Aortography
	Renal angiography
	Nuclear scan (DTPA/Mag-3)

BUN, blood urea nitrogen; CBC, complete blood count; DTPA, diethylene-triamine-penta-acetic acid; HVA, homovanillic acid; Mag-3, mercapto acetyl triglycine; VCUG, voiding cystourethrography; VMA, vanillylmandelic acid.

group. Other studies, including echocardiograms and voiding cystourethrograms, should be obtained as indicated.

For infants with extremely severe BP elevation, angiography may be necessary. In the author's experience, a formal arteriogram using the traditional femoral approach offers the only accurate method of diagnosing renal artery stenosis, particularly given the high incidence of branch vessel disease in children with fibromuscular dysplasia.[21] Although theoretically possible in infants, size is obviously a limiting factor. Computed tomography and magnetic resonance angiography will not detect branch stenosis in neonates and should not be ordered. Given these considerations, it may be necessary to defer angiography, managing the hypertension medically until the baby is large enough for an arteriogram to be performed safely.

Treatment

The first step in treatment should be correction of any iatrogenic causes of hypertension, such as excessive or unnecessary inotrope administration, dexamethasone or other corticosteroids, hypercalcemia, volume overload, and pain. Hypoxemia should be treated in infants with BPD, and appropriate hormonal replacement should be initiated in those with endocrine disorders.

Surgery is indicated for treatment of neonatal hypertension in a limited set of circumstances, most notably in infants with ureteral obstruction or aortic coarctation.[49] For infants with renal artery stenosis, it may be necessary to manage the infant medically until he or she has grown sufficiently to undergo definitive repair of the vascular abnormalities.[50] However, unilateral nephrectomy may be needed in rare cases. Infants with hypertension secondary to Wilms tumor or neuroblastoma require surgical tumor removal, possibly after chemotherapy. A case has also been made by some authors for removal of multicystic-dysplastic kidneys because of the risk of development of hypertension,[24,51] although this is controversial. Infants with malignant hypertension secondary to recessive PKD may require bilateral nephrectomy. Fortunately, such severely affected infants are rare.

At some point, a decision will need to be made as to whether antihypertensive medications are indicated. Except in severely hypertensive infants with obvious end-organ manifestations (e.g., congestive heart failure or seizures), this can be a difficult decision. No data exist on the adverse effects of chronic BP elevation in infancy, and few, if any, antihypertensive medications have ever been studied in neonates. Additionally, as noted earlier, determining what BP threshold at which to consider treatment can be difficult because of the lack of robust normative BP data. Therefore, clinical expertise and expert opinion must be relied upon to guide decision making.

Oral antihypertensive agents (Table 15-4) are best reserved for infants with less severe hypertension and infants whose acute hypertension has been controlled with intravenous (IV) infusions and who are ready to be transitioned to chronic therapy. The author typically starts with the calcium channel blocker isradipine[52,53] because it can be compounded into a stable 1-mg/mL suspension,[54] facilitating dosing in small infants. Amlodipine may also be used, but its slow onset of action and prolonged duration of effect may be problematic in the acute setting. "Sublingual" nifedipine should be avoided for several reasons, including the lack of an appropriate oral formulation and unpredictable magnitude of antihypertensive effect.[55] Other potentially useful vasodilators include hydralazine and minoxidil. β-Blockers may need to be avoided in infants with chronic lung disease. In such infants, diuretics may have a beneficial effect not only in controlling BP but also in improving pulmonary function.[56] On the other hand, it should be noted that propranolol is available commercially as a suspension, which makes it convenient to use when β-blockade is not contraindicated.

Use of angiotensin-converting enzyme (ACE) inhibitors in neonates is controversial. Captopril is one of the only antihypertensive agents that has actually been shown to be effective in infants,[57] but it is well known to cause an exaggerated decrease in BP in premature infants.[58] This effect is related to the activation of the renin–angiotensin system in neonates mentioned previously, which in turn is a

Table 15-4 RECOMMENDED DOSES FOR SELECTED ANTIHYPERTENSIVE AGENTS FOR TREATMENT OF HYPERTENSION IN INFANTS

Class	Drug	Route	Dose	Interval	Comments
*ACE inhibitors	Captopril	PO	<3 months: 0.01-0.5 mg/kg/dose Maximum, 2 mg/kg/day >3 months: 0.15–0.3 mg/kg/dose Maximum, 6 mg/kg/day	TID	First dose may cause a rapid decrease in BP, especially if receiving diuretics Monitor serum creatinine and K+ IV enalaprilat not recommended; see text
	Enalapril	PO	0.08–0.6 mg/kg/day	QD–BID	
	Lisinopril	PO	0.07-0.6 mg/kg/day	QD	
α- and β-Antagonists	Labetalol	Oral	0.5–1.0 mg/kg/dose Maximum, 10 mg/kg/day	BID-TID	Heart failure, BPD relative contraindications
		IV	0.20–1.0 mg/kg/dose 0.25–3.0 mg/kg/hr	Q4–6hr Infusion	
	Carvedilol	PO	0.1 mg/kg/dose, ≤0.5 mg/kg/dose	BID	May be useful in heart failure
β-Antagonists	Esmolol	IV	100–500 µg/kg/min	Infusion	Very short acting; constant infusion necessary
	Propranolol	PO	0.5–1.0 mg/kg/dose Maximum, 8–10 mg/kg/day	TID	Monitor heart rate; avoid in BPD
Calcium channel blockers	Amlodipine	PO	0.05–0.3 mg/kg/dose Maximum, 0.6 mg/kg/day	QD	All may cause mild reflex tachycardia
	Isradipine	PO	0.05–0.15 mg/kg/dose Maximum, 0.8 mg/kg/day	QID	
	Nicardipine	IV	1–4 µg/kg/min	Infusion	
Central α-agonist	Clonidine	PO	5–10 µg/kg/day Maximum, 25 µg/kg/day	TID	May cause mild sedation
Diuretics	Chlorothiazide	PO	5–15 mg/kg/dose	BID	Monitor electrolytes
	Hydrochlorothiazide	PO	1–3 mg/kg/dose	QD	
	Spironolactone	PO	0.5–1.5 mg/kg/dose	BID	
Vasodilators	Hydralazine	PO	0.25–1.0 mg/kg/dose Maximum, 7.5 mg/kg/day	TID–QID	Tachycardia and fluid retention are common side effects
		IV	0.15– 0.6 mg/kg/dose	Q4hr	
	Minoxidil	PO	0.1–0.2 mg/kg/dose	BID–TID	Tachycardia and fluid retention are common side effects; prolonged use causes hypertrichosis
	Sodium Nitroprusside	IV	0.5–10 µg/kg/min	Infusion	Thiocyanate toxicity can occur with prolonged (>72 hr) use or in renal failure.

*ACE, angiotensin-converting enzyme; BID, twice daily; BPD, bronchopulmonary dysplasia; IV, intravenous; QD, once daily; QID, four times daily; PO, oral; TID, three times daily.

15

reflection of the importance of the renin–angiotensin system in nephron development.[59] Although few data exist on this topic, the concern over use of ACE inhibitors in infants is that they may impair the final stages of renal maturation. Based on this concern, the author typically avoids use of captopril (and other ACE inhibitors) until the preterm infant has reached a corrected postconceptual age of 44 weeks.

Intermittently administered IV agents have a role in therapy in selected infants with hypertension. Hydralazine and labetalol in particular may be useful in infants with mild to moderate hypertension who are not yet candidates for oral therapy because of necrotizing enterocolitis or other forms of gastrointestinal dysfunction. Enalaprilat, the IV ACE inhibitor, has also been used in the treatment of neonatal renovascular hypertension.[60,61] However, in the author's experience, this agent should be used with great caution. Even doses at the lower end of published ranges may lead to significant, prolonged hypotension and oliguric acute renal failure. It should also be noted that all available doses for enalaprilat are based on the previously mentioned uncontrolled case series. For these reasons, the author does not recommend its use in neonates with hypertension.

In infants with acute severe hypertension, continuous IV infusions of antihypertensive agents should be used.[62] The advantages of IV infusions are numerous, most importantly including the ability to quickly titrate the infusion rate to achieve the desired level of BP control. As in patients of any age with malignant hypertension, care should be taken to avoid too rapid a reduction in BP[62,63] to avoid cerebral ischemia and hemorrhage, problems that premature infants, in particular, are already at increased risk of because of the immaturity of their periventricular circulation. Here again, continuous infusions of IV antihypertensive agents offer a distinct advantage. Published experience[64,65] suggests that the calcium channel blocker nicardipine may be particularly useful in infants with acute severe hypertension. Other drugs that have been successfully used in neonates include esmolol,[66] labetalol,[67] and nitroprusside.[68] Oral agents in general are probably not appropriate given their variable onset and duration of effect and unpredictable antihypertensive response.[52] Whatever agent is used, BP should be monitored continuously via an indwelling arterial catheter or by frequently repeated (every 10–15 min) BP cuff readings with an oscillometric device so the dosage can be titrated to achieve the desired degree of BP control.

Outcome

For most infants with hypertension, the long-term prognosis should be good, depending on the underlying etiology of the hypertension. For infants with hypertension related to an umbilical artery catheter, available information suggests that the hypertension will usually resolve over time.[14,69,70] These infants may require increases in their antihypertensive medications over the first several months after discharge from the NICU as they undergo rapid growth. After this, it is usually possible to wean their antihypertensive agents by making no further dose increases as the infant continues to grow. Because home BP monitoring is crucially important for following these infants, home BP equipment, usually an oscillometric device, should be obtained for all infants discharged from the NICU on antihypertensive medications.

Some forms of neonatal hypertension may persist beyond infancy, usually hypertension related to PKD and other forms of renal parenchymal disease.[22,23,26,71] Infants with renal venous thrombosis may also remain hypertensive,[72] and some of these children will ultimately benefit from removal of the affected kidney. Persistent or late hypertension may also be seen in children who have undergone repair of renal artery stenosis or thoracic aortic coarctation.[73] Reappearance of hypertension in these situations should prompt a search for restenosis by the appropriate imaging studies.

Better long-term outcome studies of infants with neonatal hypertension are needed. Because many of these infants are delivered before the completion of nephron development, it is possible that they may not develop the full complement of glomeruli normally seen in term infants. Reduced nephron mass is hypothesized to be a risk factor for the development of adult hypertension.[74,75] Thus, it may be possible that hypertensive neonates (and possibly also normotensive premature neonates) are at increased risk compared with term infants for the development of hypertension in late adolescence or early adulthood.[76] Because we are now entering an era in which the first significantly premature NICU "graduates" are reaching their second and third decades of life, it is possible that appropriate studies can be conducted to address this question.

Conclusion

Although better data are needed in many areas, particularly with respect to pathophysiology, diagnostic thresholds, and antihypertensive medications, much has been learned about neonatal hypertension over the past decades. Normal BP in neonates depends on a variety of factors, including gestational age, postnatal age, and birth weight. Hypertension is more often seen in infants with concurrent conditions such as BPD and in those who have undergone umbilical arterial catheterization. A careful diagnostic evaluation should lead to determination of the underlying cause of hypertension in most infants. Treatment decisions should be tailored to the severity of the hypertension and may include IV or oral therapy (or both). Most infants will resolve their hypertension over time, although a small number may have persistent BP elevation throughout childhood.

Acknowledgements
The author would like to thank Dr. Carolyn Abitbol for her permission to use Table 15-1 in this chapter.

References
1. Adelman RD. Neonatal hypertension. *Pediatr Clin North Am.* 1978;25:99-110.
2. Watkinson M. Hypertension in the newborn baby. *Arch Dis Child Fetal Neonatal Ed.* 2002;86: F78-F88.
3. Zubrow AB, Hulman S, Kushner H, et al. Determinants of blood pressure in infants admitted to neonatal intensive care units: A prospective multicenter study. *J Perinatol.* 1995;15:470-479.
4. Pejovic B, Peco-Antic A, Marinkovic-Eric J. Blood pressure in non-critically ill preterm and full-term neonates. *Pediatr Nephrol.* 2007;22:249-257.
5. Kent A, Kecskes Z, Shadbolt B, et al. Normative blood pressure data in the early neonatal period. *Pediatr Nephrol.* 2007;22:1335-1341.
6. Lurbe E, Garcia-Vicent C, Torro I, et al. First-year blood pressure increase steepest in low birthweight newborns. *J Hypertens.* 2007;25:81-86.
7. Task Force on Blood Pressure Control in Children. Report of the Second Task Force on Blood Pressure Control in Children – 1987. National Heart, Lung and Blood Institute, National Institutes of Health, Bethesda, MD, January 1987.
8. National High Blood Pressure Education Program Working Group on High Blood Pressure in Children and Adolescents. The fourth report on the diagnosis, evaluation, and treatment of high blood pressure in children and adolescents. *Pediatrics.* 2004;114(2 Suppl 4th Report):555-576.
9. Kent A, Kecskes Z, Shadbolt B, et al. Blood pressure in the first year of life in healthy infants born at term. *Pediatr Nephrol.* 2007;22:1743-1749.
10. Kent A, Meskell S, Falk M, et al. Normative blood pressure data in non-ventilated premature neonates from 28-36 weeks gestation. *Pediatr Nephrol.* 2009;24:141-146.
11. Buchi KF, Siegler RL. Hypertension in the first month of life. *J Hypertens.* 1986;4:525-528.
12. Singh HP, Hurley RM, Myers TF. Neonatal hypertension: incidence and risk factors. *Am J Hypertens.* 1992;5:51-55.
13. American Academy of Pediatrics Committee on Fetus and Newborn. Routine evaluation of blood pressure, hematocrit and glucose in newborns. *Pediatrics.* 1993;92:474-476.
14. Seliem WA, Falk MC, Shadbolt B, et al. Antenatal and postnatal risk factors for neonatal hypertension and infant follow-up. *Pediatr Nephrol.* 2007;22:2081-2087.
15. Friedman AL, Hustead VA. Hypertension in babies following discharge from a neonatal intensive care unit. *Pediatr Nephrol.* 1987;1:30-34.
16. Neal WA, Reynolds JW, Jarvis CW, et al. Umbilical artery catheterization: demonstration of arterial thrombosis by aortography. *Pediatrics.* 1972;50:6-13.
17. Seibert JJ, Taylor BJ, Williamson SL, et al. Sonographic detection of neonatal umbilical-artery thrombosis: clinical correlation. *Am J Radiol.* 1987;148:965-968.
18. Wesström G, Finnström O, Stenport G. Umbilical artery catheterization in newborns. I. Thrombosis in relation to catheter type and position. *Acta Paediatr Scand.* 1979;68:575-581.
19. Boo NY, Wong NC, Zulkifli SS, et al. Risk factors associated with umbilical vascular catheter-associated thrombosis in newborn infants. *J Paediatr Child Health.* 1999;35:460-465.

15

20. Barrington KJ. Umbilical artery catheters in the newborn: effects of position of the catheter tip. Cochrane Database of Systematic Reviews, 2009. Issue 1, Art. No.: CD000505. DOI: 10.1002/14651858.CD000505.
21. Tullus K, Brennan E, Hamilton G, et al. Renovascular hypertension in children. *Lancet*. 2008; 371:1453-1663.
22. Das BB, Recto M, Shoemaker L, et al. Midaortic syndrome presenting as neonatal hypertension. *Pediatr Cardiol*. 2008;29:1000-1001.
23. Fick GM, Johnson AM, Strain JD, et al. Characteristics of very early onset autosomal dominant polycystic kidney disease. *J Am Soc Nephrol*. 1993;3:1863-1870.
24. Guay-Woodford LM, Desmond RA. Autosomal recessive polycystic kidney disease: the clinical experience in North America. *Pediatrics*. 2003;111(5 Pt 1):1072-1080.
25. Angermeier KW, Kay R, Levin H. Hypertension as a complication of multicystic dysplastic kidney. *Urology*. 1992;39:55-58
26. Gilboa N, Urizar RE. Severe hypertension in newborn after pyeloplasty of hydronephrotic kidney. *Urology*. 1983;22:179-182.
27. Lanzarini VV, Furusawa EA, Sadeck L, et al. Neonatal arterial hypertension in nephro-urological malformations in a tertiary care hospital. *J Hum Hypertens*. 2006;20:679-683.
28. Abman SH, Warady BA, Lum GM, et al. Systemic hypertension in infants with bronchopulmonary dysplasia. *J Pediatr*. 1984;104:929-931.
29. Anderson AH, Warady BA, Daily DK, et al. Systemic hypertension in infants with severe bronchopulmonary dysplasia: associated clinical factors. *Am J Perinatol*. 1993;10:190-193
30. Nafday SM, Brion LP, Benchimol C, et al. Renal Disease. In: MacDonald MG, Seshia MMK, Mullett MD, eds. *Avery's Neonatology: Pathophysiology and Management of the Newborn*, 6th ed. Philadelphia, PA: Lippincott-Williams and Wilkins; 2005:981-1065.
31. Flynn JT. Neonatal Hypertension. In: Flynn JT, Ingelfinger J, Portman R, eds. *Pediatric Hypertension*, 2nd ed. New York, NY: Humana Press; 2011, pp. 375-396.
32. Hawkins KC, Watson AR, Rutter N. Neonatal hypertension and cardiac failure. *Eur J Pediatr*. 1995; 154:148-149.
33. Butt W, Whyte H. Blood pressure monitoring in neonates: comparison of umbilical and peripheral artery catheter measurements. *J Pediatr*. 1984;105:630-632.
34. Low JA, Panagiotopoulos C, Smith JT, et al. Validity of newborn oscillometric blood pressure. *Clin Invest Med*. 1995;18:163-167.
35. Kimble K, Darnall R, Yelderman M, et al An automated oscillometric technique for estimating mean arterial pressure in critically ill newborns. *Anesthesiology*. 1981;54:423-425.
36. Park M, Menard S. Accuracy of blood pressure measurement by the Dinamap monitor in infants and children. *Pediatrics*. 1987;79:907-914.
37. Park MK, Menard SM. Normative oscillometric blood pressure values in the first 5 years of life in an office setting. *Am J Dis Child*. 1989;143:860-864.
38. Dannevig I, Dale H, Liestol K, et al. Blood pressure in the neonate: three non-invasive oscillometric pressure monitors compared with invasively measure blood pressure. *Acta Pediatrica*. 2005; 94:191-196.
39. O'Shea J, Dempsey E. A comparison of blood pressure measurements in newborns. *Am J Perinatol*. 2009;26:113-116.
40. Nwankwo M, Lorenz J, Gardiner J. A standard protocol for blood pressure measurement in the newborn. *Pediatrics*. 1997;99:E10.
41. Rao PS, Jureidini SB, Balfour IC, et al. Severe aortic coarctation in infants less than 3 months: successful palliation by balloon angioplasty. *J Invasive Cardiol*. 2003;15:202-208.
42. Speiser PW, White PC. Congenital Adrenal Hyperplasia. *New Engl J Med*. 2003;349:776-788.
43. Tannenbaum J, Hulman S, Falkner B. Relationship between plasma renin concentration and atrial natriuretic peptide in the human newborn. *Am J Perinatol*. 1990;7:174-177.
44. Krüger C, Rauh M, Dörr HG. Immunoreactive renin concentration in healthy children from birth to adolescence. *Clinica Chimica Acta*. 1998;274:15-27.
45. Richer C, Hornych H, Amiel-Tison C, et al. Plasma renin activity and its postnatal development in preterm infants. Preliminary report. *Biol Neonate*. 1977;31:301-304.
46. Vehaskari VM. Heritable forms of hypertension. *Pediatr Nephrol*. 2009;24:1929-1937.
47. Roth CG, Spottswood SE, Chan JC, et al. Evaluation of the hypertensive infant: a rational approach to diagnosis. *Radiol Clin North Am*. 2003;41:931-944.
48. Elsaify WM. Neonatal renal vein thrombosis: grey-scale and Doppler ultrasonic features. *Abdom Imaging*. 2009;34:413-418.
49. Rajpoot DK, Duel B, Thayer K, Shanberg A. Medically resistant neonatal hypertension: revisiting the surgical causes. *J Perinatol*. 1999;19(8 Pt 1):582-583.
50. Bendel-Stenzel M, Najarian JS, Sinaiko AR. Renal artery stenosis: long-term medical management before surgery. *Pediatr Nephrol*. 1995;10:147-151.
51. Webb NJA, Lewis MA, Bruce J, et al. Unilateral multicystic dysplastic kidney: the case for nephrectomy. *Arch Dis Child*. 1997;76:31-34.
52. Flynn JT, Warnick SJ. Isradipine treatment of hypertension in children: a single-center experience. *Pediatr Nephrol*. 2002;17:748-753.
53. Miyashita Y, Peterson D, Rees JM, et al. Isradipine treatment of acute hypertension in hospitalized children and adolescents. *J Clin Hypertens (Greenwich)*. 2010;12:850-855.
54. MacDonald JL, Johnson CE, Jacobson P. Stability of isradipine in an extemporaneously compounded oral liquid. *Am J Hosp Pharm*. 1994;51:2409-2411.

55. Flynn JT. Safety of short-acting nifedipine in children with severe hypertension. *Expert Opin Drug Saf*. 2003;2:133-139.
56. Kao LC, Durand DJ, McCrea RC, et al. Randomized trial of long-term diuretic therapy for infants with oxygen-dependent bronchopulmonary dysplasia. *J Pediatr*. 1994;124(5 Pt 1):772-781.
57. O'Dea RF, Mirkin BL, Alward CT, et al. Treatment of neonatal hypertension with captopril. *J Pediatr*. 1988;113:403-406.
58. Tack ED, Perlman JM. Renal failure in sick hypertensive premature infants receiving captopril therapy. *J Pediatr*. 1988;112:805-810.
59. Guron G, Friberg P. An intact renin-angiotensin system is a prerequisite for normal renal development. *J Hypertens*. 2000;18:123-137.
60. Wells TG, Bunchman TE, Kearns GL. Treatment of neonatal hypertension with enalaprilat. *J Pediatr*. 1990;117:664-667.
61. Mason T, Polak MJ, Pyles L, et al. Treatment of neonatal renovascular hypertension with intravenous enalapril. *Am J Perinatol*. 1992;9:254-257.
62. Flynn JT, Tullus, K. Severe hypertension in children and adolescents: pathophysiology and treatment. *Pediatr Nephrol*. 2009;24:1101-1112.
63. Adelman RD, Coppo R, Dillon MJ. The emergency management of severe hypertension. *Pediatr Nephrol*. 2000;14:422-427.
64. Flynn JT, Mottes TA, Brophy PB, et al. Intravenous nicardipine for treatment of severe hypertension in children. *J Pediatr*. 2001;139:38-43.
65. Gouyon JB, Geneste B, Semama DS, et al. Intravenous nicardipine in hypertensive preterm infants. *Arch Dis Child Fetal Neonatal Ed*. 1997;76:F126-F127.
66. Wiest DB, Garner SS, Uber WE, et al. Esmolol for the management of pediatric hypertension after cardiac operations. *J Thorac Cardiovasc Surg*. 1998;115:890-897.
67. Thomas CA, Moffett BS, Wagner JL, et al. Safety and efficacy of intravenous labetalol for hypertensive crisis in infants and small children. *Pediatr Crit Care Med*. 2011;12:28-32.
68. Benitz WE, Malachowski N, Cohen RS, et al. Use of sodium nitroprusside in neonates: efficacy and safety. *J Pediatr*. 1985;106:102-110.
69. Adelman RD. Long-term follow-up of neonatal renovascular hypertension. *Pediatr Nephrol*. 1987;1:35-41.
70. Caplan MS, Cohn RA, Langman CB, et al. Favorable outcome of neonatal aortic thrombosis and renovascular hypertension. *J Pediatr*. 1989;115:291-295.
71. Roy S, Dillon MJ, Trompeter RS, Barratt TM. Autosomal recessive polycystic kidney disease: long-term outcome of neonatal survivors. *Pediatr Nephrol*. 1997;11:302-306.
72. Mocan H, Beattie TJ, Murphy AV. Renal venous thrombosis in infancy: long-term follow-up. *Pediatr Nephrol*. 1991;5:45-49.
73. O'Sullivan JJ, Derrick G, Darnell R. Prevalence of hypertension in children after early repair of coarctation of the aorta: a cohort study using casual and 24 hour blood pressure measurement. *Heart*. 2002;88:163-166.
74. Mackenzie HS, Lawler EV, Brenner BM. Congenital olionephropathy: the fetal flaw in essential hypertension? *Kidney Int*. 2006;55:S30-S34.
75. Keller G, Zimmer G, Mall G, et al. Nephron number in patients with primary hypertension. *N Engl J Med*. 2003;348:101-108.
76. Shankaran S, Das A, Bauer CR, et al. Fetal origin of childhood disease: intrauterine growth restriction in term infants and risk for hypertension at 6 years of age. *Arch Pediatr Adolesc Med*. 2006;160:977-981.

15

CHAPTER 16

Edema

Yosef Levenbrown, DO, Andrew T. Costarino, MD

Several systems act in concert to regulate total body water (TBW), allowing homeostasis of the circulating intravascular volume and maintenance of cellular and extracellular electrolytes in the appropriate concentrations. Edema, defined here as an abnormal accumulation of extracellular water (ECW), can result from malfunction of these fluid regulatory systems. This chapter provides an overview of the water regulatory mechanisms and then examines how the dysfunction of these mechanisms can lead to a state of edema. Lastly, the chapter examines some common clinical scenarios of the neonatal population that are associated with edema.

The Basics: Body Water Compartments

The volume and distribution of body water changes significantly during gestation and infancy. TBW is 78% of body weight at birth, but by 1 year of age, the percent of TBW declines to approximately 60%. There is a parallel decline in the ECW volume, which demonstrates a decrease from 45% of the TBW to 27% during the first postnatal year. As a result of the loss of ECW, the percentage of body weight that is intracellular water (ICW) increases during the first 3 months of age from 34% to 43%. This transient increase in ICW volume is followed by a decrease to around 35% at 1 year of age. At around 3 months of age, the ICW overtakes the ECW as the major contributor to TBW. This trend continues until, eventually, the ICW volume doubles that of the ECW.[1]

Between 1 and 3 years of age, a slight increase is found in all three body water components, after which TBW and ECW decrease slightly until around puberty, at which point the adult values are reached. This decline in TBW and ECW that occurs between age 3 years and puberty is likely a result of the increase in both the quantity and size of cells in the major organ systems, especially the cells of the musculoskeletal system, the skin, and central nervous system (CNS). These three organ systems tend to retain more water in the intracellular compartment, leading to the decrease in both TBW and the proportion of ECW. TBW also is inversely proportional to the amount of body fat because of the low content of water in fat cells. During the first year of life, there is a very rapid increase in the amount of body fat. This is followed by a decrease during the preschool years and finally by a slight increase in amount of body fat during the prepubescent years. These changes in body fat composition correlate well with the above-mentioned changes in TBW. Overall, ICW appears to remain relatively constant, likely because the composition of the intracellular content remains constant.[1]

Starling Forces

Water movement across an idealized capillary wall was described qualitatively by Starling[2] in 1896 and can be defined by the following equation:

$$J_v = K_{fc}[(P_c - P_t) - \sigma_d(\pi_p - \pi_t)]$$

where J_v is the volume flow of fluid across the capillary wall, K_{fc} is the filtration coefficient of the capillary wall (volume flow/unit time per 100 g of tissue per unit pressure), P_c is the capillary hydrostatic pressure, P_t is the interstitial fluid or tissue hydrostatic pressure, σ_d is the osmotic reflection coefficient of all plasma proteins, π_p is the colloid osmotic pressure (COP) of the plasma, and π_t is the COP of the tissue fluids. To best understand how the interplay of these forces affects overall fluid balance, it is best to analyze them individually.

Hydrostatic Forces

The hydrostatic pressure in the intravascular space (P_c) is the principle force driving water and electrolytes out of the capillary into the interstitial space. The filtration force of the capillary hydrostatic pressure is opposed by the tissue pressure surrounding the capillaries (P_t). Thus, the net difference between capillary and tissue hydrostatic pressure ($P_c - P_t$) is the driving force promoting filtration or absorption of fluid out of or into the capillary lumen.

Under physiologic conditions, the average capillary hydrostatic pressure is estimated to be about 17 mm Hg.[3] An increase in small artery, arteriolar, or venous pressure will increase the capillary hydrostatic pressure favoring filtration. A reduction of these pressures will have the opposite effect. Whereas an increased arteriolar resistance or closure of arteries reduces the downstream capillary hydrostatic pressure, an increase in the venous resistance results in increased upstream capillary hydrostatic pressure. In general, changes in the venous resistance result in a greater effect on the capillary pressure than changes in arteriolar resistance.[4]

In the nonedematous state, P_t in loose tissues is close to zero or even negative (−1 to −4 mm Hg). Negative interstitial pressure often occurs under physiologic conditions when the lymphatic system is pumped from muscle contraction while there is minimal leakage of fluid from the intravascular space.[3] Tissue pressure can change significantly if fluid moves into tissue space.[5]

Osmotic Forces

The plasma COP (π_p) is the primary counterbalancing force to capillary hydrostatic pressure that promotes fluid retention in intravascular space. In his landmark publication, Starling[2] demonstrated that this force is generated from the osmotic pressure associated with the plasma proteins. Total osmotic pressure of plasma approximates 6000 mm Hg, but most of this pressure is generated by the electrolytes, which are present in almost equal concentrations in both the intravascular and extravascular compartments of the ECW. In contrast, the plasma proteins are minimally present in the tissue surrounding the capillary.[2] Therefore, the direct and indirect effect of the charged plasma proteins generates the difference in osmotic pressure, the plasma oncotic pressure. Normally, the plasma oncotic pressure averages 28 mm Hg.[3,4]

Albumin is the primary plasma protein that is responsible for approximately 80% of the total COP. The other 20% is generated by globulins. It is the number of particles rather than the mass of a solute that determines its osmotic pressure. Thus, while albumin compromises only 50% of total plasma protein concentration, it has the greatest number of molecules present in the plasma and therefore makes the greatest contribution to the plasma oncotic pressure[6].

Another characteristic of albumin plays an important role through its effect on osmotic pressure. The albumin molecule has a net negative charge as the protein binds chloride anions. The charged albumin, and its bound chloride, attract cations (mainly Na+). The excess cations within the intravascular space due to the albumin binding increases the osmotic pressure within the plasma significantly more than the albumin particles alone would generate. This is known as the Gibbs-Donnan effect. On average, the normal human COP is 28 mm Hg. Whereas 19 mm Hg is attributable to dissolved proteins, 9 mm Hg is generated by the imbalance of cations associated with the Gibbs-Donnan effect.[3,4]

The interstitial fluid COP (π_t) is generated from smaller size proteins and the minimal amount of albumin that manages to leak out of the pores in the capillary walls. In healthy adults, the percentage of albumin that leaks into the interstitial space each hour is approximately 4% to 5%. This leakage of albumin is known as the transcapillary escape rate (TER), and it varies with capillary permeability, capillary recruitment, and hydrostatic pressure.[6] The concentration of these proteins in the interstitial fluid is approximately 40% of the protein concentration in the plasma. Thus, the average colloid osmotic interstitial pressure is about 8 mm Hg, favoring the movement of fluid into the intravascular compartment.

The Osmotic Reflection Coefficient

The reflection coefficient is the relative impediment to the passage of a substance through the capillary wall. The reflection coefficient of water across a capillary wall (fully permeable) is zero, and that of albumin (fully impermeable) is 1. Thus, all solutes that can be filtered across a capillary wall will have a reflection coefficient between 0 and 1. The reflection coefficient of a substance depends both on the nature of the solute and the characteristics of the endothelial wall being crossed.

The reflection coefficient is a key component of the COP. True COP (π) is determined by the following equation:

$$\pi = \sigma RT(C_i - C_o)$$

where σ is the reflection coefficient, R is the gas constant, T is the absolute temperature (in degrees Kelvin), C_i is the albumin concentration inside the capillary, and C_o is the albumin concentration outside the capillary.[4,5]

The Filtration Coefficient

The filtration coefficient is an expression that quantifies the ability of a given fluid to cross the capillary wall. The filtration coefficient is proportional to the surface area of the capillaries, to the number of pores per centimeter squared, and to the radius of the pores raised to the fourth power. It is inversely proportional to the thickness of the capillary wall and to the viscosity of the fluid being filtered. Not only does K_{fc} differ among the various organs, it may even increase or decrease within the same organ because of the closure or opening of more capillaries with similar conductance characteristics within a given organ.

Alterations in permeability of fluid or osmotic particles (either K_{fc} or σ_d) may lead to edema formation without changes in either hydrostatic or osmotic pressure.[6]

The Starling Hypothesis

The Starling hypothesis includes the factors previously described to relate direction movement across a capillary membrane. It is expressed mathematically as follows:

$$Q_f = k[(P_c + \pi_i) - (P_i + \pi_p)]$$

where Q_f is the fluid movement across the capillary wall, k is the filtration constant for the capillary membrane, P_c is the capillary hydrostatic pressure, π_i is the interstitial fluid oncotic pressure, P_i is the interstitial fluid hydrostatic pressure, and π_p

is the plasma oncotic pressure. When Q_f yields a positive value, it indicates that the sum flow of fluid will be out of the capillaries into the vascular space (filtration). A negative value for Q_f indicates net flow of fluid into the vascular space (absorption). During normal tissue hydration, the values of the elements of this relationship result in a near zero balance across the capillary wall. Some fluid ($\approx 0.5\%$ of the plasma volume) is filtered out of the capillary at the arterial end of the capillary, where the average capillary pressure tends to be 15 to 25 mm Hg greater than at the venous side. Most of this fluid is subsequently reabsorbed at the venous end of the capillaries where the capillary pressure is lower.[3] Over the entire length of the capillary, the small net amount of fluid filtered out and not subsequently reabsorbed is cleared by the lymphatic system, through which it makes its way back into the blood circulation.

Under physiologic conditions, arterial pressure, venous pressure, postcapillary resistance, interstitial fluid hydrostatic and oncotic pressures, and plasma oncotic pressure all remain relatively constant. Therefore, the primary variable that determines net fluid movement across a capillary wall under physiologic conditions is change in the precapillary resistance, which influences the capillary hydrostatic pressure.[4]

The Role of Aquaporins in Regulating Fluid Balance

The Importance of Aquaporins in Maintaining Water Homeostasis

Four pathways appear to be responsible for water transport in mammalian tissues. They include (1) passive diffusion of water across the cell membrane lipid bilayer; (2) movement of water through cotransporter channels, such as the Na–glutamate or the Na–glucose cotransporter; (3) paracellular water transport through tight junctions between cells; and (4) water transport via a family of transmembrane proteins called the aquaporins (AQPs).[7] Predicted to exist in the 1950s, these molecules were characterized in the 1990s as facilitators of water movement across the plasma membrane down osmotic gradients. More than 10 isoforms of these aquaporins (AQPs) have been identified, with specific ones isolated in different organ systems (e.g., AQP1 through AQP4, as well as APQ6 and APQ7 are highly expressed in the kidneys). Most of these proteins have a common molecular structure, with six transmembrane domains and intracellular NH_2^- and COOH-terminal. Although all the AQPs facilitate the transport of water, a subclass of AQPs, the aquaglyceroporins, transport both water and small nonpolar molecules such as glycerol and urea.[8]

The AQPs serve to allow water movement to occur much faster than passive diffusion across the lipid bilayer, and they are more efficient than cotransporter-associated water transport. Paracellular transport of water plays a minimal role in water transport within healthy tissues. Thus, the AQPs appear to be responsible for the high water permeability and water transport regulation in various tissues, including the erythrocytes and the nephron tubules. Conversely, dysfunction or lack of expression of AQPs likely plays a role in the pathogenesis in diseases such as nephrogenic diabetes insipidus, cataracts, Sjögren syndrome, congestive heart failure, syndrome of inappropriate antidiuretic hormone secretion (SIADH), and traumatic CNS edema.

The Role of Aquaporins in the Kidneys

The majority of water reabsorption that occurs in the nephron is facilitated by the AQPs. Most of the fluid that is filtered at the glomerulus is then reabsorbed in the proximal tubule and the descending limb of the loop of Henle. AQP1, which is expressed in the apical and basolateral segment of the renal tubular epithelial cell plasma membrane, is primarily responsible for this water transport.[8] Additionally, in the outer medullary descending vasa recta, which is rich in AQP1 channels, water resorption occurs despite the existence of hydrostatic forces that favor influx. This observation suggests that in this portion of the vasa recta, water transport involves the water only AQP1 pathway, facilitated by transtubular sodium and urea concentration gradients creating the osmotic driving force for water movement.[9]

In the distal tubule and collecting duct, other AQPs serve to regulate water resorption with a dominant role played by AQP2 and its interaction with arginine vasopressin (AVP). Although only 15% of the filtrate reaches the distal nephron, regulation of water resorption in this segment allows the kidneys to "fine tune" water balance to accommodate the needs of the body. The osmotic driving force for the water movement through the collecting duct epithelia is the hypertonic milieu of the medullary portion of the kidneys created by active transport of sodium and urea from the lumen of the thick ascending loop of Henle into the interstitial space surrounding the collecting ducts. AVP secretion by the pituitary gland, in response to central volume and osmoreceptors, upregulates AQP2 expression to match the fluid needs of the body. This occurs when AVP binds to the V2 receptor in the collecting duct of the nephron, increasing intracellular cyclic adenosine monophosphate (cAMP) production. The cAMP in turn stimulates protein kinase A–dependent phosphorylation of the AQP2 protein. Vesicles carrying the phosphorylated AQP, then fuse with the nephron epithelial cells, implanting the AQP in the wall of the apical plasma membrane. This results in dramatically increased water permeability of the collecting duct epithelial cell. After entering the duct cell from the collecting duct lumen through the AQP2 channels, the water exits the cell through the AQP3 and AQP4 channels located in the cell basolateral membrane, causing the water to enter the interstitial space of the nephron. AVP is also responsible for upregulating the AQP4 channels, but not the AQP3 channels.[8,10]

The Role of Aquaporins in the Lungs

Both the presence of AQPs in lung tissue, as well as physiologic studies of lung water permeability, indicate a role of these proteins in lung water homeostasis. AQPs 1, 3, 4, and 5 have been isolated in human lungs. AQP1 is expressed in the plasma membrane of the endothelial cells lining the pulmonary capillaries and in some pneumocytes. AQP4 has been isolated in the basolateral membrane of the airway epithelium of the trachea as well as in the large airways, and AQP5 has been identified in the apical membrane of type I alveolar epithelial cells.[11-13] The observation that different AQPs are concentrated in different regions of lung tissue suggests that the different AQPs play different roles within the pulmonary system.[8,14]

The flow of water through a membrane down its osmotic gradient can be quantified as the coefficient of osmotic water permeability (P_f). Studies on whole-lung preparations of sheep and mouse lung tissue have demonstrated a relatively high P_f across the alveolar to epithelial barriers. In other words, water freely flows across the alveolar epithelium. Such high values for P_f are similar to the P_f values in the renal tubular epithelium, suggesting the presence of lung AQPs.[14]

Studies of knockout mice provide further insight into the role of AQPs in the lung. Bai et al[11] demonstrated that water permeability of lung epithelium was decreased more than 10-fold in AQP1 knockout mice. Ma et al[12] observed that a similar decrement in osmotic water movement occurs in AQP5 null mice, but a 30% decrease was present in AQP1/AQP5 double knockout mice. In this study, Ma et al[12] demonstrated that without the benefit of AQP5, the P_f of the type I alveoli epithelia were similar to the water permeability of cells that did not contain water channels at all.[15] The AQPs are likely also critical in the osmotic flow of water in the lung microvasculature because water movement in the pulmonary capillary is greatly decreased by AQP1 deletion.[11,15]

Lung water homeostasis changes dramatically as an infant moves from the intrauterine to the extrauterine environment. By term, human fetal lungs are producing approximately 500 mL of fluid each day. At birth, a volume of water approximately 30 mL/Kg body weight must be emptied or resorbed, and the lung epithelium must abruptly switch from net secretion to net absorption of lung water. Most of the lung fluid is emptied mechanically during delivery and as the baby takes its first breath. However, a significant amount of fluid remains to be absorbed during the first postnatal days. Understanding the operative factors in the transition in lung

16

water homeostasis at birth is clinically important because premature infants and critically ill term infants appear to have an impaired this ability for the lung to reabsorb water that is associated with the occurrence of acute respiratory distress syndrome (RDS) and chronic bronchopulmonary dysplasia (BPD).

The evidence indicating an important role of AQPs in lung water homeostasis during usual conditions makes these proteins a natural object of study for understanding the sudden birth-associated changes in lung water. However, although the switch from net water secretion to absorption in newborn lungs involves an increased expression of the epithelial membrane sodium channels and of the sodium pump, current evidence for the role of AQPs is conflicting. Yasui et al[16] observed a transient increase in AQP4 mRNA in rat lungs that occurs just after birth. This increase in AQP4 coincides with the time period when lung water content decreases from prenatal to neonatal values. The increased AQP4 mRNA was specific to the lung and was not found in other organs that express AQP4. Moreover, it was shown by immunocytochemistry that this induction of AQP4 occurred specifically in the bronchial epithelium of newborn rats, the area in the lungs identified as the primary location of postnatal lung liquid absorption.[16] Also, fetal lung AQP4 mRNA was induced by maternal administration of β-agonists and glucocorticoids. This finding is consistent with the observation that both substances have been shown to accelerate the clearance of lung water at birth.[16] These observations led Yasui and colleagues[16] to believe that AQP4 contributes to lung fluid transition shortly after birth.

In contrast, several investigators studying AQP1, AQP4, and APQ5 knockout mice have failed to observe an effect on neonatal alveolar fluid clearance in the absence of these AQPs. The apparent benign nature of these knockout conditions was present even when fluid production was maximally stimulated with β-agonists and upregulation of type II alveoli cells. Furthermore these findings were consistent whether the alveolar fluid was simply fluid that was not removed postnatally or whether it was fluid that was a result of alveolar injury.[11-13] Conversely, these studies did show that alveolar fluid clearance was significantly impaired by the transport inhibitors of the membrane Na channels and Na/K pumps (amiloride and ouabain, respectively). These studies seem to suggest that alveolar fluid clearance during the neonatal transition occurs through an active process driven by osmolar gradients that are generated by Na channels and Na/K pumps.[11,12]

Factors That Combat the Development of Edema

The Lymphatic System

The lymphatic system plays an important role in preventing accumulation of fluid in the interstitial space. In most organ systems, when the capillary pressure is increased enough to increase fluid filtration into the interstitial space, lymph flow subsequently increases in a linear fashion. The ability of lymph flow to prevent the accumulation of fluid in the interstitial space depends not on the absolute quantity of lymph flow, but on the amount of lymph flow relative to the filtration coefficient (K_{fc}) of a given tissue. Tissues that do not have adequate lymphatic flow to drain the fluid that naturally filters out of the capillaries are often equipped with secondary overflow systems that directly drain this excess fluid. Without a secondary overflow system, the inadequate flow of lymph would lead to edema in these tissues. Examples of such overflow systems include the arachnoid granulations in the brain and the canal of Schlemm in the eye. In the lung and the liver, capillary filtration overflow causes pulmonary edema and ascites. Although these are generally considered pathologic processes, they protect these vital organs from the harmful effects that fluid engorgement would have on the actual parenchyma of these organs.[5]

The lymphatic system also plays an important role in preventing accumulation of proteins that have been filtered out of the capillaries. Removal of these proteins prevents an increase in the tissue oncotic pressure that would tend to draw more fluid into the interstitial space.[5]

Alterations in Starling Forces

The filtration of fluids from the intravascular compartment in response to an eleva-tion of the capillary pressure causes an increase in the surrounding tissue pressure in response to this accumulation of fluid. At first, when fluid begins to accumulate, there is a large increase in the interstitial pressure for a small increase in fluid volume (i.e., low tissue compliance). This increased interstitial pressure further opposes fluid filtration. However, as fluid continues to leak into the interstitial space, the tissue compliance eventually increases, thereby decreasing the effectiveness of this protec-tive mechanism.

Filtration of fluid into the interstitial space causes a decline in the tissue COP by diluting the interstitial proteins. This buffers further fluid filtration by decreasing the tissue COP (π_t), which increases the second term in the Starling relationship ($\sigma_d(\pi_p - \pi_t)$). The ability of these forces to change as needed to protect the tissues from further fluid accumulation, as well as the ability of the lymph flow to increase in response to increased filtration, provides an "edema safety factor" that is able to prevent further translocation of fluids into the interstitial space.[5]

Various tissues within the body have different methods of compensating for changes in interstitial fluid. In the liver, where the sinusoids are extremely porous and permeable to plasma proteins, alteration in the oncotic pressure ($\pi_p - \pi_t$) is not an effective method to prevent increased capillary filtration. Therefore, acceleration of lymph flow and ascites formation (the overflow system) along with elevations in interstitial pressure provides the forces to counteract the increased capillary filtra-tion. Functionally, when fluid leaks from the circulation into the liver stroma, venting fluid from the parenchyma into the peritoneal space is more effective and less harmful to the organ function than if excess fluid were to accumulate in the liver parenchyma. As fluid accumulates in the peritoneal space, the peritoneal pressure increases. This impedes the further accumulation of ascites by reducing the pressure gradient driving surface transudation and by increasing the rate of reabsorption by the peritoneal capillaries and lymphatics.[17]

The lung combats increased capillary filtration by increasing lymphatic flow and by decreasing the colloid osmotic gradient. Erdmann et al[18] demonstrated that every increase in left atrial pressure caused an elevation in lung lymph flow to a new steady state within 1 to 2 hours. This increase in lymph flow was approximately linear in relation to the increase in microvascular hydrostatic pressure. The lym-phatic system of the lungs is extremely efficient in preventing lung water accumula-tion. The microvascular hydrostatic pressure had to increase to 50 cmH$_2$0 before lung water accumulation rose 25%, with an increase in lung water of 50% to 100% being the typical threshold for developing pulmonary edema.[5,18]

Factors That Promote the Development of Edema

At the most basic level, edema results from any pathologic state that causes an imbal-ance in the Starling forces. The following discussion reviews the most common categories of conditions that can cause these Starling force disruptions.

The Porous Nature of the Capillary Wall

The first factor that may promote the development of edema is related to the capil-lary wall itself. With the exception of the capillaries in the brain, which do not contain open junctions, the walls of most capillary beds contain many different openings through which fluid can move from the lumen into the surrounding tissues.[5] Capillaries within organs, such as the intestinal tract, the bronchial system, and the kidney glomeruli, are fenestrated, with thick diaphragms interspaced between the endothelial cells. The capillaries in the liver and spleen contain walls that are described as discontinuous, containing very large openings. Thus, in these capillary beds, fluid has the ability to cross the capillary walls either through junc-tions between endothelial cells or through larger openings in the microvessel wall.[5]

In addition to the paracellular route, substances can cross the endothelial barrier through caveoli, which are specialized plasmalemmal vesicles containing a

16

protein known as caveolin-1. This mode of molecular transport is the method by which larger molecules such as proteins cross the capillary wall. The cell surface docking protein gp60 binds to plasma proteins greater than 3 nm. After binding to the plasma protein, gp60 interacts with caveolin-1 as well as various signaling intermediaries, including a G protein and an Src family tyrosine kinase. This cascade results in the formation and subsequent release of plasma protein containing caveolae from the apical side of the cell membrane. These vesicles are transported to the basal membrane and release their contents through exocytosis. In addition, caveolae like vesiculo-vacuolar organelles similar to caveolae can interconnect to form secondary structures that function as transmembrane channels for molecular trafficking across a cell. Receptors of endogenous permeability-enhancing agents have been indentified on the surface of these channels, leaving open the possibility that they play a role in endothelial permeability.[19]

Loss of the "Edema Safety Factor"

Under normal circumstances, when fluid is filtered out of the capillary space into the interstitium, there is both an increase in the tissue hydrostatic pressure and a simultaneous decline in the tissue COP. These changes, which occur in response to fluid accumulation in the tissues, impede further filtration of fluid out of the capillaries. Lymph flow also has the ability to greatly increase in response to enhanced capillary filtration. If fluid continues to accumulate, these protective forces can become overwhelmed and will be unable to counteract additional fluid filtration. At that point, even small changes in capillary pressure will lead to translocation of large amounts of fluid into the interstitial space.

Chen et al[20] demonstrated, in a study using the hind paw of a dog, that with the protective alterations in tissue Starling forces and increases in lymphatic flow, fluid accumulation in the interstitium was prevented with an increases in capillary hydrostatic pressure up to 12 mm Hg. Although no visible edema was noted at this pressure threshold, there was a 10% increase in interstitial fluid volume. When the capillary pressure was elevated further to 37.9 mm Hg, gross edema developed as the protective system was overwhelmed.[5,20]

Any condition that increases the permeability of the capillary endothelial wall also impairs the protective efforts of the edema safety factor because proteins leak into the interstitial space, raising the tissue COP. The effect of the increased osmotic pressure ($\sigma_d(\pi_p - \pi_t)$) that occurs with the increase in the tissue COP is magnified by the decrease in σ_d that occurs as the capillaries become "leakier." The overall result of these changes is to decrease fluid reabsorption ($\sigma_d(\pi_p - \pi_t)$), which leads to increased accumulation of fluids in the tissues.[5] Drake et al[21] were able to define the capillary pressure in the dog lung, above which the lung will gain weight because of accumulation of filtered fluid. They termed this the *critical capillary pressure*, and it represents the limits of the total edema safety factor of the lung. Predictably, when the lung capillaries become leaky to plasma proteins, the critical capillary pressure decreases.[21]

As long as there is an appropriate compensatory increase in the flow rate of the lymphatics in response to changes in the Starling forces, edema will not occur. Initially, there is a linear increase in lymph flow in response to increased filtration, but eventually, with continued filtration, lymph flow plateaus. If there is lymphatic dysfunction, as is often present in critically ill patients,[6] edema will develop even at normal capillary filtration flow rates. A seemingly paradoxical decrease in lymphatic flow occurs in the lung and intestine when edema accumulates. This occurs in these two organs because the high fluid states promote translocation of fluid into the alveoli or into the peritoneum (the overflow systems), decreasing the filling pressure of the lymphatics.[5]

Factors That Increase Permeability of the Vascular Endothelium

Under physiologic conditions, the vascular endothelium cells in most blood vessels are linked with tight junctions that are relatively impermeable to proteins and larger molecules. However, under certain conditions, the permeability of these blood vessels to these larger molecules is increased. The vascular reactivity to the mediators of the systemic inflammatory response in sepsis is one model of endothelial dysfunction. In this model, the vascular endothelium response reacts in a highly coordinated loss of junctional integrity that allows recoil, or active retraction, of cell borders, resulting in an increased width of the endothelial clefts. These changes allow increased junctional leakage of solute.[22] When this occurs, tissue COP increases, promoting fluid accumulation in the extravascular space. The changes in response to the vascular mediators is represented mathematically by a smaller σ_d that lowers the absolute value of the forces that promote absorption ($\sigma_d(\pi_p - \pi_t)$).

Paracellular flux of plasma fluid and proteins at endothelial cell–cell junctions contributes significantly to endothelial dysfunction in inflammation. Under physiologic conditions, adherens junctions maintain the state of vascular integrity in nearly all vascular beds. Its molecular structure is based on vascular endothelial (VE) cadherin, a transmembrane receptor whose extracellular domain binds to the extracellular domain of another VE cadherin molecule from an adjacent cell. The intracellular domain of the VE cadherin is anchored to the cell cytoskeleton via a family of actin-binding proteins called *catenins*. The stability of this complex is able to withstand fluid shear stress and is essential in maintaining endothelial barrier integrity. During inflammation, the humoral proinflammatory mediators disrupt this assembly, leading to endothelial dysfunction and hyperpermeability[19] (Fig. 16-1).

The loss of endothelial integrity that occurs during inflammatory states typically occurs in three stages. In the first stage, inflammatory agents induce transient vascular leakage through the formation of minute gaps between endothelial cells. During the second stage, activated leukocytes prolong the hyperpermeability. Finally, the microvasculature undergoes remodeling under the influence of angiogenic factors that affect the integrity of the cell junctions.[22]

Recently, vascular endothelial growth factor (VEGF) has been identified as a major angiogenic factor that induces the hyperpermeable state, particularly in the microvasculature of the lungs. Within the lung, the mesenchymal cells, alveolar macrophages, and epithelial cells are the primary cells that express VEGF. Therefore, although VEGF is constantly present in the fluid lining the lung epithelium, VEGF overexpression leads to increased permeability to macromolecules within the pulmonary vasculature and subsequently to pulmonary edema.[22,23] It has been demonstrated that patients with acute RDS, as well as patients at risk for developing this syndrome, have elevated levels of VEGF compared with control subjects.[24] This finding suggests a significant role for VEGF in the high-permeability model of pulmonary edema and in ARDS. The exact mechanism by which VEGF increases endothelial permeability is unclear. Current evidence indicates its action results in fusion of intracellular vesicles, which then form transcellular pathways through vesiculovacuolar organelles, resulting in fenestrations and ultimately transcellular gaps.[22]

The Role of Hypoalbuminemia

Hypoalbuminemia is a common finding in critically ill patients of all ages, and is often proportional to the severity of illness. When hypoalbuminemia occurs, it commonly is the result of an altered distribution of albumin between the intravascular and extravascular compartments. This is most often the result of the capillary leak associated with cytokine release in combination with decreased lymphatic flow.[6] Direct measurements of albumin permeability have demonstrated a threefold increase in TER in patients experiencing sepsis. In the presence of increased TER, infusion of exogenous albumin will distribute the protein to both the extravascular as well as the intravascular space. Thus, in conditions associated with increased capillary permeability, albumin supplementation may lead to increased albumin leakage across the capillary membrane and worsening edema without any improvement in outcome.[6,25]

After surgery, it is common for patients to develop hypoalbuminemia. Postoperative hypoalbuminemia is often the result of a redistribution of albumin between the intravascular and extravascular spaces after surgical trauma. Studies in this

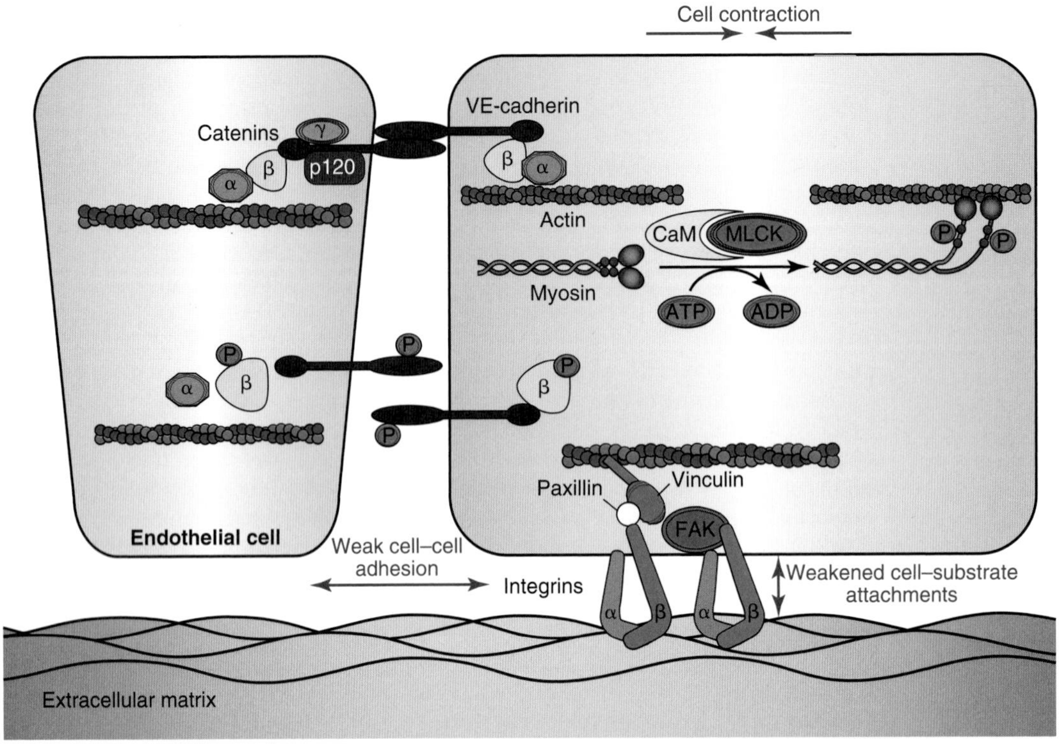

Figure 16-1 Schematic diagram of microvascular endothelial barrier structure. The barrier is formed by endothelial cells that connect to each other through the junctional adhesive molecule vascular endothelial (VE)–cadherin, which binds to another VE–cadherin molecule from an adjacent cell and connects to the actin cytoskeleton via a family of catenins (a, b, g, and p120). This endothelial lining is tethered to the extracellular matrix through focal adhesions mediated by transmembrane integrins composed of a and b subunits, focal adhesion kinase (FAK), and cytoskeleton-linking proteins including paxillin and vinculin. The integrity of this barrier is maintained by VE-cadherin–mediated cell–cell adhesions and focal adhesion-supported cell matrix attachment. A dynamic interaction among these structural elements controls the opening and closing of the paracellular pathways for fluid, proteins, and cells to move across the endothelium. In particular, the Ca2þ/calmodulin (CaM)–dependent myosin light chain kinase (MLCK) catalyses phosphorylation of myosin light chains (*small red circles*), triggering binding of the myosin heavy chain motor domains to actin and their cross-bridge movement. This reaction promotes cytoskeleton contraction and cell retraction. In parallel, phosphorylation of VE-cadherin, catenins, or both may cause the junction complex to dissociate from its cytoskeletal anchor, leading to weakened cell–cell adhesion. The cytoskeletal and junctional responses act in concert, causing paracellular hyperpermeability. (Reprinted with permission from Kumar P, Shen Q, Pivetti CD, Lee ES, Wu MH, Yuan SY. Molecular mechanisms of endothelial hyperpermeability: implications in inflammation. *Expert Rev Mol Med.* 2009; 11:1-20.)

patient population indicate that although albumin supplementation can result in a higher serum albumin concentration, morbidity, mortality and glomerular filtration rate (used as a marker of intravascular fluid volume) remain unchanged whether or not supplemental albumin is given.[26,27]

In healthy people, albumin is the main determinant of COP. However, in critically ill patients, there is a low correlation between serum albumin concentration and COP. Instead, in critically ill patients, there is a stronger relationship between COP and total protein concentration. This difference in the relative contribution of albumin to COP may be attributable to elevations in acute-phase reactant proteins or immunoglobulins during states of acute illness. Therefore, in critically ill patients, hypoalbuminemia does not necessarily correlate with edema formation[6,28] and may explain why the use of albumin supplementation is ineffective in changing the course of the critically ill state of edema, as well as outcome. Typically, as the acute disease process improves and endothelial dysfunction recovers, patients improve with or without administration of supplemental albumin.[6,29] In fact, in the Cochrane meta-analysis, the subgroup of critically ill patients who received exogenous albumin in states of sepsis, burns, and hypoalbuminemia suggested an increase in mortality in these groups of patients with the use of exogenous albumin. The exceptions to this finding were in clinical settings in which the low albumin was not attributable to redistribution, but occurred after acute blood loss or loss of other protein-rich fluid during surgery.[29]

Unique Features of Water Homeostasis in the Neonatal Population

Changes in Body Water Composition in the Neonate

Neonates must make a transition from the fluid-filled fetal environment to the relatively dry extrauterine world. Remarkably, the majority of this transition occurs over a few minutes in the immediate postnatal life. As a result, there are several challenges to fluid regulation unique to this time of life.

As noted above, a full-term newborn is 75% TBW with 40% of the TBW contained in the extracellular fluid (ECF) compartment. This proportion is significantly different than in adults, in whom the TBW concentration is reduced to 60% of total body weight and water in the ECF compartment is only 20% of total body weight. The difference between a preterm infant and an adult is even more dramatic. In babies born between 26 and 31 weeks' gestational age, the TBW is approximately 80% to 85% of total body weight, with 65% of body weight from water in the extracellular compartment.

Immediately after birth, the body water mass rapidly declines, mainly because of a decrease in ECF volume as it changes from its postnatal value of 45% of TBW to 30% by 3 months of age. This initial rapid decline in ECF volume is followed by a more gradual decline until age 10 years, when the adult ECF value of 20% total body weight is achieved.[8,30]

In healthy babies, there is a fairly rapid loss of extracellular isotonic fluid. This fluid loss is mainly from the intestinal compartment, and it is evidenced by the expected postnatal weight loss over the first few weeks of life. Infants who do not have an early negative fluid balance often demonstrate RDS. Contraction of the extracellular compartment is facilitated partly by secretion of atrial natriuretic peptide, which is produced by the cells of the myocardium in response to atrial stretch.[31] This occurs in the immediate postnatal period secondary to the dramatic decrease in pulmonary vascular resistance that occurs as the lung is inflated and alveolar gas tensions change. The pulmonary vasculature for the first time accepts the entire cardiac output, delivering it to and stretching the left atria.

Solute Balance in Healthy Neonates

Healthy neonates have an intact ability to excrete sodium. This allows them to maintain an isotonic loss of fluid with the postnatal contraction of the ECF compartment. In addition, neonates have the ability to increase their excretion of sodium in response to the administration of a sodium load. When the contraction of the extracellular compartment is complete, a state of positive sodium balance is reached. This allows neonates to retain the sodium necessary for appropriate growth.[30]

A relatively low albumin concentration in both term and preterm infants is a normal finding in the newborn period, and it does not appear to be associated with the formation of edema.[6,32] Mean values of albumin concentration at birth increases from 1.9 g/dL in infants of gestational ages less than 30 weeks to 3.1 g/dL at term. There is a postnatal increase in serum albumin concentration of approximately 15% in the first 3 weeks of life regardless of the gestational age of the infant. Greenough et al[33] administered albumen to premature neonates (24–34 weeks' gestational age) at 7 days of age in an attempt to increase serum albumin concentration and promote a diuresis. The investigators' hypothesis was that this therapy would improve pulmonary function by decreasing lung fluid. They observed that compared with the placebo control infants, the albumin-treated infants demonstrated higher serum albumin concentrations, a negative water balance, and weight loss. However, no differences between groups were noted in the amount of ventilator support required.[33] In another study examining the effect of albumin supplementation of parenteral nutrition in preterm infants with RDS, the treatment group demonstrated improved weight gain and blood pressure, but failed to show any benefit in the duration of mechanical ventilation, time of requirement for supplemental oxygen, or time to full enteral feeding. There was also no difference in the incidence of necrotizing enterocolitis or intraventricular hemorrhage between the two groups.[34]

Resistance to the Effect of Arginine Vasopressin in Neonates

Neonatal kidneys demonstrate resistance to the effect of AVP, impairing the ability of this patient population to concentrate urine in response to even very high levels of exogenous vasopressin.[35] The observation of increased urinary excretion of AQP2 (a marker of AQP activity) during the first 2 to 3 postnatal weeks suggested that a deficiency of AQP2 was associated with the impaired ability to concentrate urine during the first few weeks of postnatal life. Subsequent studies, however, have demonstrated that both dehydration and DDAVP (desmopressin) administration appropriately stimulate production of AQP2 in infants' kidneys even during the first 2 to 3 weeks of life.[10]

Current evidence indicates that the inability of immature kidneys to maximally concentrate urine is attributable to multiple deficiencies in several steps in the AVP transduction pathway, including:

- Prostaglandin E_2 (PGE_2) induced upregulation of a Gi (inhibitory) protein, which results in inhibitory feedback decreasing the production of cAMP. Because cAMP production is a necessary step for AVP-stimulated production of AQP2, enhanced PGE_2 stimulation of inhibiting G proteins will decrease the responsiveness of the kidneys to the effects of the AVP.
- High levels of phosphodiesterase in the cells of the infant collecting duct, which lead to rapid degradation of cAMP
- Low concentration of urea and sodium in the infant medullary interstitium limit the osmotic gradient available for water reabsorption. This reduced gradient in infants is likely a result of low dietary protein, low expression of urea transporters, and low rates of sodium absorption from the ascending loop of Henle.[10]

The limited ability to concentrate urine in the immediate postnatal period may serve to benefit neonates in making the transition to extrauterine life because it promotes the rapid clearing of the excess extracellular pulmonary fluid.

It is important to note that neonates have intact pituitary production of AVP and only a diminished, not absent, renal response to this hormone. Therefore, even in the neonatal period, an underfilled intravascular compartment is associated with high circulating AVP. This high-AVP state may place hospitalized neonates at risk for water retention. If these patients receive hypotonic intravenous or hypotonic enteral fluids as is typical in this age group, hyponatremia can occur.

True syndrome of inappropriate anti-diuretic hormone (SIADH), although possible in the neonatal population, is uncommon. A low serum sodium concentration during stress states, as in the postoperative period, is often the result of unrecognized intravascular volume depletion with appropriate AVP water retention and hypotonic fluid administration rather than SIADH. These aspects of neonatal water and solute management can be challenging to clinicians because it is difficult to recognize inadequate intravascular volume in this age group. In investigations of acutely ill infants and children, as few as one third of subjects demonstrated overt signs of dehydration.[30]

Increase in Vascular Endothelial Growth Factor Expression

Vascular endothelial growth factor (VEGR) may be associated with the tendency of neonates to retain water.[32] Newborns and young infants are more likely to retain fluid in response to stimuli such as cardiopulmonary bypass compared with older children and adults. Similarly, the lungs of neonates are more susceptible to alveolar edema in response to infectious and chemical injury. In the first month of life, full-term neonates have higher plasma levels of VEGF, which gradually decrease to the normal values within the first few months after birth.[34,36] The increased baseline serum level of VEGF has been implicated as part of the cause of the edema in neonates after cardiopulmonary bypass.[37] Further studies are necessary to delineate the role of VEGF in neonatal edema.

Special Circumstances in the Neonatal Population

Preterm Neonates

Newborn preterm neonates have a limited ability to excrete sodium. Although they can increase sodium excretion in response to a sodium load, they still have a tendency toward a positive sodium balance. Even with "maintenance" sodium intake (1–3 mEq/kg/day), preterm neonates are often in a state of positive sodium balance. When water losses exceed intake, their relative inability to excrete sodium will result in hypernatremia. If water intake is liberalized, the serum osmolality will be maintained at the expense of expansion of the ECF compartment. Expansion of the ECF compartment superimposed on a preexisting state of impaired diuresis may be the reason that in the immediate postnatal period, sodium supplementation of preterm neonates is associated with a worse respiratory outcome with an increased incidence of BPD.[31,38] Early fluid management of these patients should allow isotonic contraction of the extracellular compartment, with a brief period of negative sodium and water balance.

Edema After Indomethacin Closure of Patent Ductus Arteriosus

The use of indomethacin to close patent ductus arteriosus (PDA) has become common in the neonatal population. After indomethacin treatment, infants often go through a state of fluid retention. The mechanism of this effect relates to AQP2 metabolism and its regulation by PGE_2. As discussed previously, the insertion of AQP2 into the apical membrane of the collecting duct within the kidney occurs through a cAMP second messenger system. The absorptive effect of the AVP-stimulated increase in AQP2 insertion into the apical membrane of the collecting duct is regulated and counterbalanced by the effect of PGE_2. PGE_2 binding to the EP3 receptor activates the inhibitory G_i protein, which decreases cyclic adenosine monophosphate (cAMP) generation, thereby decreasing the cAMP-dependent insertion of AQP2 into the collecting duct. This results in an increase excretion of water in the urine. Indomethacin and the other nonsteroidal antiinflammatory drugs decrease PGE production and there-fore cause a loss of the counterbalancing inhibitory effect of the PGE_2. This leads to an unopposed upregulation of the AQP2 channels with enhanced fluid reabsorption.[8,10]

Pulmonary Edema in Neonates

Compromised lung water clearance is a prominent feature of neonatal RDS and BPD. The pulmonary edema can lead to respiratory failure by impairing respiratory mechanics and causing ventilation–perfusion mismatching.

Similar to all capillary beds, the mechanism of edema formation in the pulmonary vasculature is the result of either increased permeability of the pulmonary vasculature or an increase in the capillary hydrostatic pressure. Clinicians therefore often classify patients based on the primary mechanism associated with the disease. Often, however, it is difficult to make a clear assignment to one of these two categories because each primary mechanism has features of the other.

Of the two primary types, high-permeability edema is frequently more difficult to manage. A breakdown in capillary endothelial tight junctions and the alveolar epithelial barrier leads to the development of protein-rich alveolar edema. High-permeability edema often occurs as the result of an inflammatory insult, and it is typically seen in acute lung injury. Inflammation, the most likely cause of the breakdown in the endothelial–epithelial barrier, very often causes myocardial dysfunction as well.[39]

Cardiogenic pulmonary edema is a result of acute or chronic myocardial or valvular dysfunction, causing increased left ventricular end-diastolic volume and pressure, which then leads to increased pulmonary venous and capillary hydrostatic pressures.[22] Studies of adults have shown that the respiratory gas exchange abnormalities present in the setting of cardiogenic pulmonary edema is worse than predicted simply by the perturbations in the Starling capillary fluid relationship. West and Mathieu-Costello[40] have demonstrated that in the presence of conditions that can increase the pulmonary capillary pressure, the pulmonary capillary walls undergo structural changes. These structural changes result in endothelial and alveolar epithelial disruption as well as increased capillary permeability known as *capillary stress fracture*. The end result of this process is the development of high-permeability pulmonary edema,[40] causing the endothelial permeability to increase. Similar capillary stress fractures can also occur as a result of pulmonary arterial hypertension and in response to elevated alveolar pressures that can sometimes occur during mechanical ventilation. VEGF levels are increased in patients with cardiogenic pulmonary edema and may play a role in its production.[22,41]

Several developmental changes may place neonates at risk for pulmonary edema. For example, in fetuses, the pulmonary endothelial intracellular junctions are fenestrated. By comparison, in adults, the endothelial cells are more tightly joined, creating an intact barrier. The higher endothelial permeability observed in fetuses is likely attributable to the combined actions of lower blood oxygen tensions, as well as a high level of circulating endothelin-1, VEGF, and angiotensin II. Each of these factors creates a tendency to increase vascular permeability. Additionally, nitric oxide (NO), which has been shown to prevent endothelial leakage in the lung, is produced in lower amounts in premature neonates. NO production in the pulmonary vasculature increases as fetuses approach term, subsequently reaching a maximum concentration at age 2 to 3 days.[42,43] Finally, various scaffolding proteins in the pulmonary endothelium, important for endothelial barrier function, change at birth, contributing to the perinatal changes in vascular permeability.[42]

The pulmonary endothelial cells contain microdomains of anionic charge and glycoconjugate specificity located on cell organelles that are responsible for the transport of water, small solutes, and other macromolecules. Mills and Haworth[44] demonstrated that alterations within these domains, rather than the intercellular junctions, have the biggest impact on the change in pulmonary capillary endothelial permeability during the first week of life. Transport of water and small solutes are associated primarily with areas of anionic charge. They demonstrated that in newborn pigs, a greater proportion of the endothelial plasmalemma and its vesicles had anionic charge, suggesting greater transport of fluid into the interstitium. By 1 week of life, the composition of the pulmonary capillary endothelium had altered and was similar to that seen in adults.[44] Neonates are susceptible to pulmonary edema until the maturational changes in these factors that regulate endothelial permeability are complete.

This tendency for neonates to develop pulmonary edema is even greater in preterm neonates. As stated previously, the switch in prenatal ion transport in the fetal airway epithelium from Cl^- secretion to Na^+ absorption plays a significant role in the transition from lung liquid secretion to lung liquid reabsorption. The Na^+ absorption is facilitated primarily from the amiloride-sensitive sodium channels (ENaCs). This transition is necessary for postnatal adaption to air breathing. Compared with neonates born at gestational ages greater than 30 weeks, the stable maximal baseline nasal potential difference, a surrogate marker for ENaC activity, was lower in infants born at gestational ages less than 30 weeks. Thus, although preterm infants do demonstrate the same transition from Cl- secretion to Na^+ absorption as full-term infants do, the ENaC activity, which is necessary to facilitate lung fluid clearance, is reduced in preterm neonates compared with term neonates.[45]

Respiratory Distress Syndrome and Bronchopulmonary Dysplasia

Inadequate lung water clearance may cause lung edema in both neonatal RDS and in BPD. At birth, the pulmonary epithelium, which was secreting water into the airway during fetal life, must rapidly begin water absorption. This functional change involves an upregulation of the AQPs, specifically AQP4, and an upregulation of epithelial cell membrane sodium–potassium ATPase and sodium channels. The later epithelial membrane compounds establish the osmotic gradients needed to drive the water movement through the AQPs. In most healthy infants, the majority of the lung water present before birth is cleared mechanically in the first minutes of life as the baby fills the alveolar sacs with air. The rest of the water remains in the lungs to be cleared over the first several postnatal days. Premature infants often seem to lack the ability to clear this excess fluid from the lungs, which contributes to the pathogenesis RDS and BPD in this patient population. A long-noted clinical observation is that diuresis precedes the improvement in respiratory function from acute RDS, and therapeutic diuretics improve outcome in chronic BPD.[10,16,30]

Several investigators have speculated that impaired clearance of pulmonary fluid in premature infants is attributable to a unique feature of the AQP3 water channel. AQP3, which has been localized to the type II pneumocyte, is pH sensitive. Acidification of the ECF decreases the water permeability of these channels. Thus, acidosis caused by impaired oxygen delivery or poor ventilation in a premature infant with RDS leads to an impaired ability to clear the alveolar fluid through AQP3.[8,14]

In addition to the AQPs, other channels play important roles in the clearance of lung fluid in the perinatal period. In fetuses, active secretion of chloride ions (Cl^-) across the pulmonary epithelium generates the osmotic force that causes water to move from the lung microcirculation into the future airspaces of the lungs. Several days before birth, the Cl^- secretion decreases, and Na^+ uptake by the lung epithelium increases. Lung fluid follows the sodium, causing the fluid from the lung lumen to move into the interstitial space and then into the bloodstream or lymphatic system.[46]

Because the transition within the lungs from the state of secretion to that of absorption takes place a few days before birth, preterm delivery as well as operative delivery without labor are both associated with increased fluid in the pulmonary airspaces. This hypothesis is supported in a rabbit animal model investigation demonstrating that lung water content is 25% greater after preterm delivery compared with term delivery. In addition, the term rabbits born after the onset of labor had less water in their lungs than did rabbits that were delivered operatively without prior onset of labor.[46]

Recent studies have identified amiloride sensitive sodium channels (ENaCs) on the apical surface of the airway epithelium, which appear to be critical in the process of lung fluid clearance. In human fetal lungs, these ENaC subunits are present in the earliest stages of lung development but at a lower concentrations than observed in mature fetuses. In preterm infants, there is a significant decrease in the β subunit of the ENaC during the first day of life. The resultant impairment of neonatal lung fluid clearance that results from this decrease in the β subunit may contribute to respiratory distress often seen in these infants.[47] The observation that both term neonates with transient tachypnea of the newborn and older infants with BPD have decreased levels of amiloride-sensitive N-PD (nasal potential difference, a correlate for ENaC activity) support the relationship between ENaC activity and lung fluid clearance.[45,48] Additionally, glucocorticoids, which when given antenatally decrease the incidence of RDS, cause an upregulation of all three ENaC subunits.

Although surfactant deficiency has been implicated as the primary pathology of RDS, it is also likely that the factors that impair fluid clearance from the lung outlined above play a prominent role in the pathogenesis of this condition.[47,49] Fluid management in newborn infants with acute respiratory failure should be undertaken, keeping in mind that these infants are at great risk for expansion of the ECW. Therefore, routine sodium supplementation and excessive parenteral fluid administration should be carefully managed in infants with respiratory distress until postnatal diuresis and naturesis are observed.[30]

Fluid Retention After Cardiopulmonary Bypass

Cardiopulmonary bypass in infants and children is associated with a generalized disturbance of vascular permeability with significant edema formation as well as effusions. This can lead to a state of extravascular fluid accumulation with severe edema, secondary intravascular volume depletion, and significant organ dysfunction. The basis of this syndrome is thought to be a systemic inflammatory response caused by a mixture of stimuli, including cardiopulmonary bypass circuit–induced complement activation, circulatory shock, and endotoxemia.[37,50] Symptoms of multiple-organ dysfunction such as delayed myocardial recovery, a need for respiratory support, and renal and hepatic abnormalities, are more pronounced in patients with higher degrees of postbypass fluid retention. A longer length of stay postoperatively in the intensive care unit is also associated with a higher fluid retention rate.[51]

In contrast to the generalized edema caused by inflammatory states from other etiologies such as sepsis, the microvascular permeability that occurs after cardiopulmonary bypass may begin to resolve within hours after the surgery.[51] The rapid reversibility of this state suggests that bradykinin, which rapidly and reversibly increases vascular permeability by receptor-mediated endothelial cell contraction and intercellular gap formation, is the primary mediator responsible for this state. In fact, one study demonstrated approximately three times higher plasma concentrations of bradykinin in neonates, infants, and children with higher fluid retention rates after cardiopulmonary bypass. In this context, contact activation of Hageman factor with subsequent formation of prekallikrein and kallikrein, as well as the direct release of bradykinin from kininogens present in mast cells through the activity of proteases such as tryptase can be implicated as a major cause of the increased bradykinin level. Additionally, bypassing the pulmonary circulation decreases the exposure of the blood to angiotensin-converting enzyme located on the pulmonary endothelium, which typically inactivates bradykinin. The end result is that cardiopulmonary bypass is associated with both an increase in bradykinin production and a decrease in its degradation.[51] In another study, it was found that there was a strong correlation between post–cardiopulmonary bypass fluid retention and preoperative elevated levels of VEGF. Although an underlying reason for this elevation in VEGF in this patient population was not identified, the positive correlation with increased fluid retention has been noted.[37]

Although both these studies implicate different mediators as the underlying cause of the increased state of fluid retention, both studies demonstrated a significant association between younger age and greater degrees of postbypass fluid retention. In both studies, almost all patients operated on in the neonatal period demonstrated greater degrees of postbypass fluid retention. Although the underlying cause for this difference based on age is unclear, it is important for clinicians treating neonates after cardiopulmonary bypass to be aware of this increased incidence of postbypass fluid retention and therefore to expect a more complicated postoperative course with these patients.

Conclusion

Edema in the neonatal population is similar to edema in older children and adults in that it is caused by an imbalance in Starling capillary forces. A number of factors make neonates more prone to these perturbations. Importantly, their vasculature is more permeable compared with older patients, newborns have very high levels of total body fluid, and the high pulmonary vascular resistance renders them vulnerable to developing lung edema. The acute and chronic respiratory disease such as RDS and BPD may be partly attributable to an inability to adequately rid the prenatally acquired fluid. Clinicians treating infants in this population should be aware of these factors that render neonates more prone to edema and to adjust fluid management carefully.

References

1. Friis-Hansen B. Body water compartments in children: changes during growth and related changes in body composition. *Pediatrics*. 1961;28:169-181.
2. Starling EH. On the Absorption of Fluids from the Connective Tissue Spaces. *J Physiol*. 1896;19: 312-326.
3. Guyton AC, Hall JE. Textbook of Medical Physiology. Philadelphia: W.B. Saunders Company; 2000.
4. Berne RM, Levy MN. *Cardiovascular Physiology*. St. Louis: Mosby, Inc; 2001.

5. Taylor AE. Capillary fluid filtration. Starling forces and lymph flow. *Circ Res*. 1981;49:557-575.
6. Uhing MR. The albumin controversy. *Clin Perinatol*. 2004;31:475-488.
7. Verkman AS. Aquaporin water channels and endothelial cell function. *J Anat*. 2002;200:617-627.
8. Zelenina M, Zelenin S, Aperia A. Water channels (aquaporins) and their role for postnatal adaptation. *Pediatr Res*. 2005;57:47R-53R.
9. Edwards A, Silldforff EP, Pallone TL. The renal medullary microcirculation. *Front Biosci*. 2000;5: E36-E52.
10. Bonilla-Felix M. Development of water transport in the collecting duct. *Am J Physiol Renal Physiol*. 2004;287:F1093-F1101.
11. Bai C, Fukuda N, Song Y, et al. Lung fluid transport in aquaporin-1 and aquaporin-4 knockout mice. *J Clin Invest*. 1999;103:555-561.
12. Ma T, Fukuda N, Song Y, et al. Lung fluid transport in aquaporin-5 knockout mice. *J Clin Invest*. 2000;105:93-100.
13. Song Y, Fukuda N, Bai C, et al. Role of aquaporins in alveolar fluid clearance in neonatal and adult lung, and in oedema formation following acute lung injury: studies in transgenic aquaporin null mice. *J Physiol*. 2000;525(Pt 3):771-779.
14. Kreda SM, Gynn MC, Fenstermacher DA, et al. Expression and localization of epithelial aquaporins in the adult human lung. *Am J Respir Cell Mol Biol*. 2001;24:224-234.
15. Borok Z, Verkman AS. Lung edema clearance: 20 years of progress: invited review: role of aquaporin water channels in fluid transport in lung and airways. *J Appl Physiol*. 2002;93:2199-2206.
16. Yasui M, Serlachius E, Lofgren M, et al. Perinatal changes in expression of aquaporin-4 and other water and ion transporters in rat lung. *J Physiol*. 1997;505(Pt 1):3-11.
17. Laine GA, Hall JT, Laine SH, Granger J. Transsinusoidal fluid dynamics in canine liver during venous hypertension. *Circ Res*. 1979;45:317-323.
18. Erdmann AJ 3rd, Vaughan TR Jr, Brigham KL, et al. Effect of increased vascular pressure on lung fluid balance in unanesthetized sheep. *Circ Res*. 1975;37:271-284.
19. Kumar P, Shen Q, Pivetti CD, et al. Molecular mechanisms of endothelial hyperpermeability: implications in inflammation. *Expert Rev Mol Med*. 2009;11:1-20.
20. Chen HI, Granger HJ, Taylor AE. Interaction of capillary, interstitial, and lymphatic forces in the canine hindpaw. *Circ Res*. 1976;39:245-254.
21. Drake RE, Smith JH, Gabel JC. Estimation of the filtration coefficient in intact dog lungs. *Am J Physiol*. 1980;238:H430-H438.
22. Kosmidou I, Karmpaliotis D, Kirtane AJ, et al. Vascular endothelial growth factors in pulmonary edema: an update. *J Thromb Thrombolysis*. 2008;25:259-264.
23. Kaner RJ, Ladetto JV, Singh R, et al. Lung overexpression of the vascular endothelial growth factor gene induces pulmonary edema. *Am J Respir Cell Mol Biol*. 2000;22:657-664.
24. Thickett DR, Armstrong L, Christie SJ, Millar AB. Vascular endothelial growth factor may contribute to increased vascular permeability in acute respiratory distress syndrome. *Am J Respir Crit Care Med*. 2001;164:1601-1605.
25. Fleck A, Raines G, Hawker F, et al. Increased vascular permeability: a major cause of hypoalbuminaemia in disease and injury. *Lancet*. 1985;1:781-784.
26. Nielsen OM, Engell HC. Effects of maintaining normal plasma colloid osmotic pressure on renal function and excretion of sodium and water after major surgery. A randomized study. *Dan Med Bull*. 1985;32:182-185.
27. Zetterstrom H, Hedstrand U. Albumin treatment following major surgery. I. Effects on plasma oncotic pressure, renal function and peripheral oedema. *Acta Anaesthesiol Scand*. 1981;25:125-132.
28. Barclay SA, Bennett D. The direct measurement of plasma colloid osmotic pressure is superior to colloid osmotic pressure derived from albumin or total protein. *Intensive Care Med*. 1987;13: 114-118.
29. Cochrane Injuries Group Albumin Reviewers. Human albumin administration in critically ill patients: systematic review of randomised controlled trials. *BMJ*. 1998;317:235-240.
30. Modi N. Clinical implications of postnatal alterations in body water distribution. *Semin Neonatol*. 2003;8:301-306.
31. Betremieux P, Modi N, Hartnoll G, Midgley J. Longitudinal changes in extracellular fluid volume, sodium excretion and atrial natriuretic peptide, in preterm neonates with hyaline membrane disease. *Early Hum Dev*. 1995;41:221-233.
32. Cartlidge PH, Rutter N. Serum albumin concentrations and oedema in the newborn. *Arch Dis Child*. 1986;61:657-660.
33. Greenough A, Emery E, Hird MF, Gamsu HR. Randomised controlled trial of albumin infusion in ill preterm infants. *Eur J Pediatr*. 1993;152:157-159.
34. Kanarek KS, Williams PR, Blair C. Concurrent administration of albumin with total parenteral nutrition in sick newborn infants. *JPEN J Parenter Enteral Nutr*. 1992;16:49-53.
35. Heller H. The renal function of newborn infants. *J Physiol*. 1944;102:429-440.
36. Himeno W, Akagi T, Furui J, et al. Increased angiogenic growth factor in cyanotic congenital heart disease. *Pediatr Cardiol*. 2003;24:127-132.
37. Abrahamov D, Erez E, Tamariz M, et al. Plasma vascular endothelial growth factor level is a predictor of the severity of postoperative capillary leak syndrome in neonates undergoing cardiopulmonary bypass. *Pediatr Surg Int*. 2002;18:54-59.
38. Costarino AT Jr, Gruskay JA, Corcoran L, et al. Sodium restriction versus daily maintenance replacement in very low birth weight premature neonates: a randomized, blind therapeutic trial. *J Pediatr*. 1992;120:99-106.

16

39. Merx MW, Weber C. Sepsis and the heart. *Circulation*. 2007;116:793-802.
40. West JB, Mathieu-Costello O. Vulnerability of pulmonary capillaries in heart disease. *Circulation*. 1995;92:622-631.
41. Chin BS, Chung NA, Gibbs CR, et al. Vascular endothelial growth factor and soluble P-selectin in acute and chronic congestive heart failure. *Am J Cardiol*. 2002;90:1258-1260.
42. Haworth SG. Pulmonary endothelium in the perinatal period. *Pharmacol Rep*. 2006;58(Suppl): 153-164.
43. Schutte H, Mayer K, Burger H, et al. Endogenous nitric oxide synthesis and vascular leakage in ischemic-reperfused rabbit lungs. *Am J Respir Crit Care Med*. 2001;164:412-418.
44. Mills AN, Haworth SG. Greater permeability of the neonatal lung. Postnatal changes in surface charge and biochemistry of porcine pulmonary capillary endothelium. *J Thorac Cardiovasc Surg*. 1991;101:909-916.
45. Gaillard EA, Shaw NJ, Wallace HL, et al. Electrical potential difference across the nasal epithelium is reduced in premature infants with chronic lung disease but is not associated with lower airway inflammation. *Pediatr Res*. 2007;61:77-82.
46. Bland RD. Lung epithelial ion transport and fluid movement during the perinatal period. *Am J Physiol*. 1990;259:L30-37.
47. Helve O, Pitkanen O, Janer C, Andersson S. Pulmonary fluid balance in the human newborn infant. *Neonatology*. 2009;95:347-352.
48. Gowen CW Jr, Lawson EE, Gingras J, et al. Electrical potential difference and ion transport across nasal epithelium of term neonates: correlation with mode of delivery, transient tachypnea of the newborn, and respiratory rate. *J Pediatr*. 1988;113:121-127.
49. Venkatesh VC, Katzberg HD. Glucocorticoid regulation of epithelial sodium channel genes in human fetal lung. *Am J Physiol*. 1997;273:L227-233.
50. Nilsson L, Kulander L, Nystrom SO, Eriksson O. Endotoxins in cardiopulmonary bypass. *J Thorac Cardiovasc Surg*. 1990;100:777-780.
51. Neuhof C, Walter O, Dapper F, et al. Bradykinin and histamine generation with generalized enhancement of microvascular permeability in neonates, infants, and children undergoing cardiopulmonary bypass surgery. *Pediatr Crit Care Med*. 2003;4:299-304.

D

CHAPTER 17

Kidney Injury in the Neonate

Sharon P. Andreoli, MD

Acute kidney injury (AKI; previously known as acute renal failure) and chronic kidney disease (CKD; previously known as chronic renal failure) in neonates is a very common problem, and there are many different causes of kidney injury in newborns (Table 17-1). Although many cases of AKI can resolve with return of kidney function to normal, some causes of AKI result in permanent kidney injury that is apparent immediately. Others may result in kidney disease years after the initial insult. It is well known that kidney diseases such as kidney dysplasia, obstructive uropathy, and cortical necrosis can lead to CKD. In contrast, it has been thought in the past that AKI caused by hypoxic ischemic and nephrotoxic insults was reversible with return of kidney function to normal. However, recent studies have demonstrated that hypoxic and ischemic insults can result in physiologic and morphologic alterations in the kidney that can lead to kidney disease at a later time.[1,2] Thus, as will be discussed in more detail later, AKI in neonates from any cause is a risk factor for later development of CKD.[1-3]

AKI is classified as prerenal, intrinsic kidney disease including vascular insults and obstructive uropathy. In newborns, kidney injury may have a prenatal onset in congenital diseases such as kidney dysplasia with or without obstructive uropathy and in genetic diseases such as autosomal recessive polycystic kidney disease. Newborns with congenital and genetic kidney diseases that have a prenatal onset may have stigmata of Potter syndrome caused by in utero oliguria with resultant oligohydramnios. Newborns with Potter syndrome may have life-threatening pulmonary insufficiency, a flattened nasal bridge, low-set ears, joint contractures, and other orthopedic anomalies caused by fetal constraint as a result of the oligohydramnios.

AKI and CKD may also result from the in utero exposure of the developing kidneys to agents that may interfere with nephrogenesis such as angiotensin-converting enzyme (ACE) inhibitors, angiotensin II receptor blockers (ARBs), and perhaps cyclooxygenase (COX) inhibitors.[4-7] Exposure of a developing fetus to ACE inhibitors and ARBs have each been associated with kidney dysfunction that is acute and chronic, fetal death, and undermineralization of the calvarial bones.[4,5] Exposure to ACE inhibitors or ARBs is most detrimental for kidney development when the fetus is exposed in the second and third trimesters, but it has recently been shown that exposure during the first trimester is also associated with congenital defects.[6]

Table 17-1   ETIOLOGY OF ACUTE KIDNEY INJURY IN NEONATES

Prerenal injury
• Decreased true intravascular volume
  • Dehydration
  • Gastrointestinal losses
  • Salt-wasting kidney or adrenal disease
  • Central or nephrogenic diabetes insipidus
  • Third-space losses (sepsis, traumatized tissue)
• Decreased effective intravascular blood volume
  • Congestive heart failure
  • Pericarditis, cardiac tamponade

Intrinsic kidney disease
• Acute tubular necrosis
  • Ischemic/hypoxic insults
  • Drug induced: aminoglycosides, intravascular contrast, NSAIDs
  • Toxin mediated: endogenous toxins, rhabdomyolysis, hemoglobinuria
• Interstitial nephritis
  • Drug induced: antibiotics, anticonvulsants
  • Idiopathic
• Vascular lesions
  • Cortical necrosis
  • Renal artery thrombosis
  • Renal venous thrombosis
• Infectious causes
  • Sepsis
  • Pyelonephritis

Obstructive uropathy
• Obstruction in a solitary kidney
• Bilateral ureteral obstruction
• Urethral obstruction

Congenital kidney diseases
• Dysplasia or hypoplasia
• Cystic kidney diseases
  • Autosomal recessive polycystic kidney disease
  • Autosomal dominant polycystic kidney disease
  • Cystic dysplasia
  • In utero exposure to ACE inhibitors or ARBs

ACE, angiotensin-converting enzyme; ARB, angiotensin II receptor blockers, NSAID, nonsteroidal antiinflammatory drug.

AKI in newborns is also commonly acquired in the postnatal period because of hypoxic ischemic injury and toxic insults. As in older children, hospital-acquired AKI in newborns is frequently multifactorial in origin.[3,8-14] Because nephrogenesis proceeds through approximately 34 weeks of gestation, ischemic or hypoxic and toxic insults in the developing kidney in a premature newborn can result not only in AKI, but also in long-term complications associated with potential interrupted nephrogenesis. Whether kidney disease is congenital or acquired, it is important to appropriately manage the fluid and electrolyte imbalances and other side effects of kidney injury in newborns.

Definition

Currently, there is no uniform definition of AKI in pediatric or neonatal patients, and AKI is defined in multiple ways, but the majority of definitions of AKI currently in use involve a change in the serum creatinine level; in neonates, AKI is frequently defined by a change in the serum creatinine according to gestational age. AKI is characterized by an increase in the blood concentration of creatinine and nitrogenous waste products, a decrease in the glomerular filtration rate (GFR), and the inability of the kidney to appropriately regulate fluid and electrolyte homeostasis. After birth, the serum creatinine in the newborn is a reflection of maternal kidney function and cannot be used as a measure of kidney function in the newborn shortly after birth.[15,16] In full-term healthy newborns, the GFR rapidly increases, and the serum creatinine declines to about 0.4 to 0.6 mg/dL (35.4–53.0 µmol/L) at about 2 weeks of age; the serum creatinine declines at a slower rate in premature infants.[14-16] Thus, use of serum creatinine as a determinate of kidney insufficiency requires that the gestational age at time of birth and the postnatal age, as well as maternal factors, be taken into account.

It is clear that a change in the serum creatinine is a rough measure of changes in kidney function and that better determinates of real-time kidney renal function are needed. Recent exciting studies have investigated the use of early biomarkers of AKI so that AKI can be diagnosed before changes in the serum creatinine are detected.[17-21] Biomarkers under investigation include changes in plasma neutrophil gelatinase-associated lipocalin (NGAL) and cystatin C levels and urinary changes in NGAL, interleukin-18 (IL-18) and kidney injury molecule-1 (KIM-1).[17,18] NGAL has shown promise in children undergoing cardiac surgery as an early marker of AKI.[17] Studies in premature and term infants document that urine NGAL is detectable and correlates with birth weight and gestational age; however, levels were increased in neonates with normal renal function.[19-21] Additional studies to determine the utility of biomarkers in neonates with AKI are warranted. The development, testing, and successful implementation of therapeutic strategies in AKI will require the development of sensitive biomarkers so that therapy can be initiated in a timely manner.

The definition of AKI in pediatric patients has been quite variable. A new classification system called the RIFLE criteria (risk for renal dysfunction, injury to the kidney, failure of kidney function, loss of kidney function, and end-stage kidney disease) has been proposed as a standardized classification of AKI in adults[22] and has been adapted for pediatric patients.[23] The pediatric RIFLE (pRIFLE) was found to better classify pediatric AKI and to reflect the course of AKI in children admitted to intensive care units (ICUs).[23] The pRIFLE criteria appear quite promising for better characterization of AKI and have been validated in children; additional studies need to be done to further validate this classification.[23] Further validation and utilization of the pRIFLE criteria would allow for intercenter comparisons of AKI in children. In a study of pediatric patients of whom 36% were neonates, AKI as classified by pRIFLE criteria was shown to correlate with mechanical ventilation, metabolic acidosis, and hypoxia in the neonate.[24]

Although a decrease in urine output is a common clinical manifestation of AKI, many forms of AKI are associated with normal urine output.[1,3] Whereas newborns with prerenal injury, AKI caused by hypoxic/ischemic insults, or cortical necrosis are more likely to have oligo/anuria (urine output <1.0 mL/kg/h), newborns with nephrotoxic kidney insults, including aminoglycoside nephrotoxicity and contrast nephropathy, are more likely to have AKI with normal urine output. The morbidity and mortality of nonoliguric AKI is substantially less than for oliguric AKI.[9-14]

This chapter reviews the epidemiology of kidney injury in newborns, the common causes of AKI and CKD in newborns with a focus on hypoxic ischemic and nephrotoxic insults, management of AKI and CKD in newborns, and long-term follow-up of neonates who have had AKI.

Epidemiology and Incidence of Kidney injury in Neonates

AKI in neonates is fairly common and is a major contributor to morbidity and mortality.[25] Although the precise incidence and prevalence of kidney disease in newborns is unknown, several studies have demonstrated that kidney injury is common in neonatal ICUs (NICUs) and pediatric ICUs (PICUs).[8-31] The incidence of kidney disease ranged from 6% to 24% of newborns in NICUs, and in at least one study, AKI was particularly common in neonates who had undergone cardiac surgery.[9,11,14-16] Neonates with severe asphyxia had a high incidence of AKI; AKI is less common in neonates with moderate asphyxia, and the AKI was nonoliguric, oliguric, and anuric in 60%, 25%, and 15%, respectively.[12]

Other studies have demonstrated that very low birth weight (VLBW; <1500 g), a low Apgar score, a patent ductus arteriosus (PDA), and maternal administration of antibiotics and nonsteroidal antiinflammatory drugs (NSAIDs) was associated with the development of AKI.[28] Other studies have also shown that low Apgar score and maternal ingestion of NSAIDs is associated with decreased kidney function in preterm infants.[29,30] A recent study demonstrated that AKI was diagnosed in 56% of infants with perinatal asphyxia.[31] The incidence of AKI in newborns in a developing country was 3.9 in 1000 live births and 34.5 in 1000 newborns admitted to the NICU.[32]

Several very interesting studies have demonstrated that some newborns may have genetic risk factors for AKI. Polymorphism of the ACE gene or the angiotensin receptor gene with resultant alterations in activity of the renin–angiotensin system might play a role in the development of AKI.[33] In studies in newborns, polymorphisms of tumor necrosis factor α (TNF-α), IL-1b, IL-6, and IL-10 genes were investigated in newborns to determine if polymorphisms of these genes would lead to a more intense inflammatory response and predispose newborns to AKI.[34] The allelic frequency of the individual genes did not differ between newborns with AKI and those without AKI, but the TNF-α/IL-6 AG/GC haplotypes were present in 26% of newborns who developed AKI compared with 6% of newborns who did not. The investigators suggested that the combination of these polymorphisms might lead to a greater inflammatory response and the development of AKI in neonates with infection.[34] As described below, future therapies for AKI might involve strategies to interrupt the inflammatory response. In other studies, the incidence of ACE I/D allele genotypes or the variants of the angiotensin I receptor gene did not differ in neonates with AKI compared with neonates without AKI, but they may be associated with PDA and heart failure and indirectly contribute to CKD.[33,35] AKI occurred more commonly in VLBW neonates carrying the heat shock protein 72 (1267) GG genetic variation, which is associated with low inductability of heat shock protein 72.[36] Given the important role of heat shock proteins in ischemic kidney injury, these findings suggest that some neonates are more susceptible to ischemic injury.[37] Future studies of the genetic background of children at risk for AKI because of medication exposure, toxin exposure, ischemic hypoxic insults, or other insults will likely impact the management of children at risk for AKI and the management of AKI.

Etiology of Kidney Injury in Newborns

There are many different etiologies of AKI and CKD in neonates (Table 17-1), and the most common are related to prerenal mechanisms, including hypotension, hypovolemia, hypoxemia, perinatal and postnatal asphyxia, sepsis, and obstructive uropathy.[38,39]

Prerenal Injury

In prerenal injury, kidney function is decreased because of decreased kidney perfusion, but the kidney is intrinsically normal. Restoration of normal kidney perfusion results in a return of kidney function to normal; acute tubular necrosis (ATN) implies that the kidney has experienced intrinsic damage. However, the evolution of prerenal injury to intrinsic kidney injury is not sudden, and a number of compensatory mechanisms work together to maintain kidney perfusion when kidney perfusion is compromised.[40,41] When kidney perfusion is decreased, the afferent arteriole relaxes its vascular tone to decrease kidney vascular resistance and maintain kidney blood flow. Decreased kidney perfusion results in increased catecholamine secretion, activation of the renin–angiotensin system, and generation of prostaglandins. During kidney hypoperfusion, the intrarenal generation of vasodilatory prostaglandins, including prostacyclin, mediates vasodilatation of the kidney microvasculature to maintain kidney perfusion.[40,41] Administration of aspirin or NSAIDs can inhibit this compensatory mechanism and precipitate acute kidney insufficiency during kidney hypoperfusion. As discussed later, administration of indomethacin for closure of the PDA in premature newborns is associated with a substantial risk of kidney injury.[42-46] It was originally thought that selective COX-2 inhibitors would be kidney sparing, but it has been recognized that the selective COX-2 inhibitors can adversely affect kidney hemodynamics similar to the effects of nonselective COX inhibitors.[47,48] In addition, clinical use of selective COX-2 inhibitors has been associated with AKI in adult patients.[48] Similarly, when kidney perfusion pressure is low as in renal artery stenosis, the intraglomerular pressure necessary to drive filtration is partly mediated by increased intrarenal generation of angiotensin II to increase efferent arteriolar resistance.[40,49,50] Administration of ACE inhibitors in these conditions can eliminate the pressure gradient needed to drive filtration and precipitate AKI.[49,50] Thus, administration of medications that can interfere with compensatory mechanisms to maintain kidney perfusion can precipitate AKI in certain clinical circumstances.

Prerenal injury results from kidney hypoperfusion caused by true volume contraction or from a decreased effective blood volume.[40] Volume contraction results from hemorrhage, dehydration caused by gastrointestinal losses, salt-wasting kidney or adrenal diseases, central or nephrogenic diabetes insipidus, increased insensible losses, and in disease states associated with third-spaces losses such as sepsis, traumatized tissue, and capillary leak syndrome; decreased effective blood volume occurs when the true blood volume is normal or increased, but kidney perfusion is decreased because of diseases such as congestive heart failure and cardiac tamponade.[40] Whether prerenal injury is caused by true volume depletion or decreased effective blood volume, correction of the underlying disturbance will return kidney function to normal.

The urine osmolality, urine sodium concentration, fractional excretion of sodium (FENa), and renal failure index have all been proposed to be used to help differentiate prerenal injury from vasomotor nephropathy or ATN. This differentiation is based on the premise that the tubules are working appropriately in prerenal injury and are, therefore, able to conserve salt and water appropriately, but in vasomotor nephropathy, the tubules have progressed to irreversible injury and are unable to appropriately conserve sodium.[16] During prerenal injury, the tubules are able to respond to decreased kidney perfusion by appropriately conserving sodium and water such that the urine osmolality is greater than 400 to 500 mOsm/kg H_2O, the urine sodium is less than 10 to 20 mEq/L, and the FENa is less than 1% in children. Because the renal tubules in newborns and premature infants are relatively immature compared with those of older infants and children, the corresponding values suggestive of kidney hypoperfusion are urine osmolality greater than 350 mOsm/kg H_2O, urine sodium less than 20 to 30 mEq/L, and FENa of less than 2.5%.[3,16] When the renal tubules have sustained injury as occurs in ATN, they cannot appropriately conserve sodium and water such that the urine osmolality is less than 350 mOsm/kg H_2O, the urine sodium is greater than 30 to 40 mEq/L, and the FENa is greater than 2.5%. However, the use of these numbers to differentiate prerenal injury from ATN requires that the patient has normal tubular function initially. Although this may be the case in some pediatric patients, newborns, particularly premature newborns whose tubules are immature, may have kidney injury with urinary indices suggestive of ATN. Therefore, it is important to consider the state of the function of the tubules before the potential onset that might precipitate vasomotor nephropathy or ATN.

Acute Ischemic Kidney Injury and Nephrotoxic Kidney Injury

Acute Ischemic Kidney Injury

Ischemic AKI (also known as ATN) can evolve from prerenal injury if the insult is severe and sufficient enough to result in vasoconstriction and ATN. Recent studies suggest that the vasculature of the kidney may play a role in acute injury and chronic injury as well, and the endothelial cell has been identified as a target of injury. Peritubular capillary blood flow has been shown to be abnormal during reperfusion, and there is also a loss of normal endothelial cell function in association with distorted peritubular pericapillary morphology and function.[51,52] The mechanism of cellular injury in hypoxic/ischemic AKI is not known, but alterations in endothelin (ET) or nitric oxide (NO) regulation of vascular tone, adenosine triphosphate (ATP) depletion and alterations in the cytoskeleton, changes in heat shock proteins, initiation of the inflammatory response, and the generation of reactive oxygen and nitrogen molecules may each play a role in cell injury.[51-68]

NO is a vasodilator produced from endothelial NO synthase (eNOS), and NO helps regulate vascular tone and blood flow in the kidneys.[57,58] Recent studies suggest that loss of normal eNOS function occurs after ischemic/hypoxic injury, which could precipitate vasoconstriction.[57] In contrast, inducible NO synthase (iNOS) activity increases after hypoxic/ischemic injury, and iNOS can participate in the generation of reactive oxygen and nitrogen molecules. Inducible NO synthase with the generation of toxic NO metabolites, including peroxynitrate, has been shown to mediate tubular injury in animal models of AKI.[58,59] ET peptides are potent vasoconstrictors that have also been shown to play a role in the pathogenesis of AKI in animal models.[60] In animal models of AKI in rats, circulating levels of ET-1 and tissue expression of ET-1protein levels was substantially increased, and ET(A) and ET(B) receptor gene expression was also increased after ischemic injury.[61] ET receptor agonist for the A receptor have been shown to decrease AKI in animal models.[62] Thus, alterations in the balance of vasoconstrictive and vasostimulatory stimuli are likely to be involved in the pathogenesis of hypoxic/ischemic AKI.

An initial response to hypoxic/ischemic AKI is ATP depletion, which leads to a number of detrimental biochemical and physiologic responses, including disruption of the normal cytoskeletal organization with loss of the apical brush border and loss of polarity with Na^+, K^+-ATPase localized to the apical as well as the basolateral membrane.[63] This has been shown in several animal models of AKI and it has also been shown in human kidney allografts that loss of polarity with mislocation of Na^+, K^+-ATPase to apical membrane contributes to kidney dysfunction in transplanted kidneys.[64] Reactive oxygen molecules are also generated during reperfusion and can contribute to tissue injury.[54] Although tubular cells and endothelial cells are susceptible to injury by reactive oxygen molecules, studies have shown that endothelial cells are more sensitive to oxidant injury than tubular epithelial cells.[55] Other studies have shown an important role for heat shock protein in modifying the kidney response to ischemic injury as well as playing a role in promoting recovery of the cytoskeleton after AKI.[65]

In children and neonates with multiorgan failure, the systemic inflammatory response is thought to contribute to AKI as well as other organ dysfunction by the activation of the inflammatory response, including increased production of cytokines and reactive oxygen molecules, activation of polymorphonuclear leukocytes (PMNs), and increased expression of leukocyte adhesion molecules.[66] Reactive oxygen molecules can be generated by several mechanisms, including activated PMNs, which may cause injury by the generation of reactive oxygen molecules, including superoxide anion, hydrogen peroxide, hydroxyl radical, hypochlorous acid, peroxynitrite or by the release of proteolytic enzymes. Myeloperoxidase from activated PMNs converts hydrogen peroxide to hypochlorous acid, which may react with amine groups to form chloramines; each of these can oxidize proteins, DNA, and lipids, resulting in substantial tissue injury.[54,67] Leukocyte endothelial cell adhesion molecules have been shown to be upregulated in ATN, and administration of antiadhesion molecules can substantially decrease kidney injury in animal models of ATN.[56] As described later, several animal models have shown future therapies for hypoxic/ischemic AKI may involve manipulation of the inflammatory response. Studies in humans with AKI have demonstrated an increased evidence of oxidation of proteins, reflecting oxidant stress.[68]

In established ATN, the urinalysis may be unremarkable or demonstrate low-grade proteinuria and granular casts, and urine indices of tubular function demonstrate an inability to conserve sodium and water as described above. The creatinine

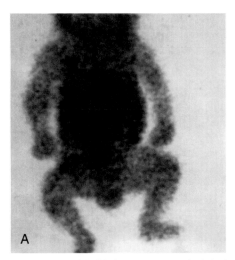 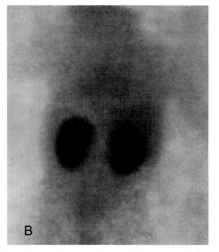

Figure 17-1 MAG3 (mercapto acetyl triglycine) renal scan in a newborn with acute tubular necrosis **B** and in a newborn with cortical necrosis (**A**). Each scan is at 4 hours after injection of isotope. **B** shows delayed uptake of isotope with parenchymal accumulation of isotope with little to no excretion of isotope into the collecting system. In contrast, **A** demonstrates no kidney parenchymal uptake of isotope in a neonate with cortical necrosis.

typically increases by about 0.5 to 1.0 mg/dL (44.2–88.4 µmol/L) per day. Radiographic studies demonstrate kidneys of normal size with loss of corticomedullary differentiation, but a radionucleotide kidney scan with technetium–99-MAG3 (mercapto acetyl triglycine) or technetium–99-DTPA (diethylene-triamine-penta-acetic acid) will demonstrate normal or slightly decreased kidney blood flow with poor function and delayed accumulation of the radioisotope in the kidney parenchyma without excretion of the isotope in the collecting system (Fig. 17-1B).

In the past, it was thought that the prognosis of ischemic AKI was good except in cases in which the insult was of sufficient severity to lead to vasculature injury and microthrombi formation with the subsequent development of cortical necrosis. However, recent studies demonstrate that chronic changes can occur and that such patients are at risk for later complications.[1,2] As discussed later, AKI before nephrogenesis is complete may also result in disrupted nephrogenesis and reduced nephron number.[69-73]

The recovery of the neonate and the recovery of kidney function depend on the underlying events that precipitated the ischemic/hypoxic insults. Recent studies also indicate that AKI contributes directly to the morbidity and mortality of neonates and children in the NICUs and PICUs.[25,26] In children who recover from ATN, the kidney function returns to normal, but the length of time before recovery is quite variable. Some children begin to recover kidney function within days of the onset of kidney injury, but recovery may not occur for several weeks in other children. Return of kidney function may be accompanied by a diuretic phase with excessive urine output at a time when the tubules have begun to recover from the insult but have not recovered sufficiently to appropriately reabsorb solute and water. When the diuretic phase occurs during recovery, close attention to fluid and electrolyte balance is very important to ensure adequate fluid management to promote recovery from ATN and prevent additional kidney injury. As described below, long-term follow-up of newborns with AKI is warranted to evaluate for late complications.

Nephrotoxic Acute Kidney Injury

Many different drugs and agents may result in nephrotoxic AKI. Nephrotoxic AKI may result from the administration of a number of different medications as well as from indigenous compounds such as hemoglobinuria and myoglobinuria.

Nephrotoxic AKI in newborns is commonly associated with aminoglycoside antibiotics, NSAIDs, intravascular contrast media, and amphotericin B; other medications have been implicated less commonly. Aminoglycoside nephrotoxicity usually presents with nonoliguric AKI with a urinalysis showing minimal urinary abnormalities. The incidence of aminoglycoside antibiotic nephrotoxicity is related to the dose and duration of the antibiotic therapy as well as the level of kidney function before the initiation of aminoglycoside therapy. The etiology of aminoglycoside nephrotoxicity is thought to be related to the lysosomal dysfunction of proximal tubules and is reversible after the aminoglycoside antibiotics have been discontinued. However, after the aminoglycoside is discontinued, the serum creatinine may continue to increase for several days because of ongoing tubular injury from continued high parenchymal levels of the aminoglycoside. AKI may also occur after administration of ACE inhibitors, probably by alteration in intrarenal hemodynamics.[49,50]

NSAIDs may also precipitate AKI by their effect on intrarenal hemodynamics.[40-48] Indomethacin therapy to promote closure of PDAs in premature neonates is associated with kidney dysfunction, including a 56% reduction in urinary flow rate, a 27% reduction in GFR, and a 66% reduction in free water clearance.[42,43] Other physiologic alterations after administration of indomethacin and ibuprofen include a decrease in urinary ET-1 and arginine vasopressin along with a reduction in urinary sodium excretion and FENa.[44] Alterations in kidney function occur in approximately 40% of premature newborns who have received indomethacin, and such alterations are usually reversible.[45] In a large study of more than 2500 premature newborns treated with indomethacin to promote closure of the PDA, infants with preexisting kidney and electrolyte abnormalities and infants whose mothers had received indomethacin tocolysis or who had chorioamnionitis were at significantly increased risk for the development of kidney impairment.[46]

Vascular Injury

Renal artery thrombosis and renal vein thrombosis will result in AKI if bilateral or if either occurs in a solitary kidney. Renal artery thrombosis is strongly associated with an umbilical artery line and a PDA.[74,75] In addition to AKI, children may demonstrate hypertension, gross or microscopic hematuria, thrombocytopenia, and oliguria. In renal artery thrombosis, the initial ultrasound scan may appear normal or demonstrate minor abnormalities, but a renal scan will demonstrate little to no blood flow. In renal vein thrombosis, the ultrasound scan demonstrates an enlarged, swollen kidney, but the renal scan typically demonstrates decreased blood flow and function. Therapy should be aimed at limiting extension of the clot by removal of the umbilical arterial catheter, and anticoagulate or fibrinolytic therapy can be considered, particularly if the clot is large.[74,75]

Cortical necrosis is associated with hypoxic/ischemic insults caused by perinatal anoxia, placenta abruption, and twin–twin or twin–maternal transfusions with resultant activation of the coagulation cascade.[76,77] Interestingly, intrauterine laser treatment in 18 sets of twins with twin–twin transfusion resulted in no long-term kidney impairment despite severe alterations of kidney function, including anuria and polyuria before the laser treatment.[78] Newborns with cortical necrosis usually have gross or microscopic hematuria and oliguria and may have hypertension as well. In addition to laboratory features of an elevated blood urea nitrogen (BUN) and creatinine, thrombocytopenia may also be present because of the microvascular injury. Radiographic features include a normal kidney ultrasound scan in the early phase, but ultrasound scans in the later phases may show that the kidney has undergone atrophy and has substantially decreased in size. A radionucleotide renal scan will show decreased to no perfusion with delayed or no function (Fig. 17-1A) in contrast to delayed uptake of the radioisotope, which is observed in ATN (see Fig. 17-1B). The prognosis of cortical necrosis is worse than that of ATN. Children with cortical necrosis may have partial recovery or no recovery at all. Typically, children with cortical necrosis need short- or long-term dialysis therapy, but children who do recover sufficient renal function are at risk for the late development of CKD as described below.

Obstructive Uropathy

Obstruction of the urinary tract can cause AKI if the obstruction occurs in a solitary kidney, if it involves the ureters bilaterally, or if there is urethral obstruction. Obstruction can result from congenital malformations such as posterior urethral valves, bilateral ureteropelvic junction obstruction, or bilateral obstructive ureteroceles. Acquired urinary tract obstruction can result from passage of kidney stones or rarely tumors. It is important to evaluate for obstruction because the management is to promptly relieve the obstruction.

Medical Management of Acute Kidney Injury in Neonates

Preventive Measures

It is thought that prenal injury is the most common cause of AKI in neonates in a resource-poor setting, and because dialytic resources are scarce in such settings, the mortality rate was high from prerenal failure.[79] Thus, on a global scale, the prevention of AKI in neonates with adequate hydration is likely to have a larger impact on mortality than other measures.

Intravenous (IV) infusion of theophylline in severely asphyxiated neonates given within the first hour after birth was associated with improved fluid balance, improved creatinine clearance, and reduced serum creatinine levels with no effects on neurologic and respiratory complications.[80] Other studies in asphyxiated neonates also demonstrated improved kidney function and decreased excretion of β-2 microglobulin in the neonates given theophylline within 1 hour of birth.[81,82] However, the clinical significance of the improved kidney function was not clear, and the incidence of persistent pulmonary hypertension was higher in the neonates who had received theophylline group. The beneficial effects of theophylline are likely to be mediated by its adenosine antagonistic properties.[83] Additional studies are needed to determine the significance of these findings and the potential side effects of theophylline.

Diuretic and Dopamine Receptor Agonist

After intrinsic kidney injury has become established, management of the metabolic complications of AKI involves appropriate monitoring of fluid balance, electrolyte status, acid–base balance, nutrition, and the initiation of renal replacement therapy when appropriate. Diuretic therapy to stimulate urine output eases management of AKI, but the conversion of oliguric to nonoliguric AKI has not been shown to alter the course of AKI.[84] Diuretic therapy has potential theoretical mechanisms to prevent, limit, or improve kidney function. Mannitol (0.5–1.0 g/kg over several minutes) may increase intratubular urine flow to limit tubular obstruction and may limit cell damage by prevention of swelling or by acting as a scavenger of free radicals or reactive oxygen molecules. Furosemide (1–5 mg/kg/dose) also increases urine flow rate to decrease intratubular obstruction and inhibit Na^+, K^+-ATPase, which limits oxygen consumption in already damaged tubules with a low oxygen supply. When using mannitol in children or neonates with AKI, a lack of response to therapy can precipitate congestive heart failure, particularly if the child's intravascular volume is expanded before mannitol infusion; caution should be used when considering mannitol therapy. In addition, lack of excretion of mannitol may also result in substantial hyperosmolality. Similarly, administration of high doses of furosemide in kidney injury has been associated with ototoxicity.[84] When using diuretic therapy in children with AKI, potential risks and benefits need to be considered. When the neonate is unresponsive to therapy, administering continued high doses of diuretics is not justified and is unlikely to be beneficial to the neonate. In neonates who do respond to therapy, continuous infusions may be more effective and may be associated with less toxicity than bolus administration.

The use of "renal"-dose dopamine (0.5–3-5 μg/kg/min) to improve kidney perfusion after an ischemic insult has become common in NICUs and PICUs.

Although dopamine increases kidney blood flow by promoting vasodilatation and may improve urine output by promoting natriuresis, no definitive studies have demonstrated that low-dose dopamine is effective in decreasing the need for dialysis or improving survival in patients with AKI.[85-90] In fact, a placebo-controlled randomized study of low-dose dopamine in adult patients demonstrated that low-dose dopamine was not beneficial and did not confer clinically significant protection from kidney dysfunction.[87] Other studies have demonstrated that renal-dose dopamine is not effective in the therapy of AKI, and one study demonstrated that low-dose dopamine worsened kidney perfusion and kidney function.[90]

Fenoldopam is a potent short-acting selective dopamine-1 receptor agonist that decreases vascular resistance while increasing kidney blood flow.[91] A recent meta-analysis of 16 trials of fenoldopam in adults concluded that therapy with fenoldopam decreased the incidence of AKI, decreased the need for renal replacement therapy, decreased length of ICU stay, and decreased death from any cause.[92] Fenoldopam has been used in a few children with AKI, including two children receiving therapy with a ventricular assist device as a bridge to cardiac transplantation; therapy with fenoldopam was thought to avoid the need for renal replacement therapy in one child.[93] Additional studies using fenoldopam need to be performed in children and neonates with AKI.

Electrolyte Management

Mild hyponatremia is very common in AKI and may be attributable to hyponatremia dehydration, but fluid overload with dilutional hyponatremia is much more common. If the serum sodium is greater than 120 mEq/L, fluid restriction or water removal by dialytic therapy will correct the serum sodium. However, if the serum sodium is less than 120 mEq/L, the neonate is at higher risk for seizures from hyponatremia, and correction to a sodium level of approximately 125 mEq/L with hypertonic saline should be considered. Because the kidney tightly regulates potassium balance and excretes approximately 90% of dietary potassium intake, hyperkalemia is a common and potentially life-threatening electrolyte abnormality in AKI in neonates.[94] The serum potassium level may be falsely elevated if the technique of the blood drawing is traumatic or if the specimen is hemolyzed. Hyperkalemia results in disturbances of cardiac rhythm by its depolarizing effect on the cardiac conduction pathways. The concentration of serum potassium that results in arrhythmia depends on the acid–base balance and the other serum electrolytes. Hypocalcemia, which is common in kidney injury, exacerbates the adverse effects of the serum potassium on cardiac conduction pathways. Tall peaked T waves are the first manifestation of cardiotoxicity, and prolongation of the PR interval, flattening of P waves, and widening of QRS complexes are later abnormalities. Severe hyperkalemia will eventually lead to ventricular tachycardia and fibrillation and requires prompt therapy with sodium bicarbonate, IV glucose and insulin, IV calcium gluconate, and albuterol.[95,96] Albuterol infusions of 400 μg given every 2 hours as needed have been shown to rapidly lower serum potassium levels.[96] All of these therapies are temporizing measures and do not remove potassium from the body. Kayexalate Na given orally per nasogastric tube, or per rectum will exchange sodium for potassium in the gastrointestinal tract and result in potassium removal.[94,97] Complications of Kayexalate Na therapy include possible hypernatremia, sodium retention, and constipation. In addition, Kayexalate therapy has been associated with colonic necrosis.[98] Depending on the degree of hyperkalemia and the need for correction of other metabolic derangements in AKI, hyperkalemia frequently requires the initiation of dialysis or hemofiltration.

Because the kidney excretes net acids generated by diet and intermediary metabolism, acidosis is very common in AKI. Severe acidosis can be treated with IV or oral sodium bicarbonate, oral sodium citrate solutions, or dialysis therapy. When considering treatment of acidosis, it is important to consider the serum ionized calcium level. Under normal circumstances, approximately half the total calcium is protein bound, and the other half is free and in the ionized form, which is what determines the transmembrane potential and electrochemical gradient. Hypocalcemia is common in AKI, and acidosis increases the fraction of total calcium to the ionized form. Treatment of acidosis can then shift the ionized calcium to the more normal ratio, decreasing the amount of ionized calcium and precipitating tetany or seizures.

Because the kidney excretes a large amount of ingested phosphorus, hyperphosphatemia is a very common electrolyte abnormality noted during AKI. Hyperphosphatemia should be treated with dietary phosphorus restriction and with oral calcium carbonate or other calcium compounds to bind phosphorus and prevent gastrointestinal absorption of phosphorus.[99] Because most neonates with AKI have hypocalcemia, use of calcium-containing phosphate binders provides a source of calcium as well as phosphate-binding capacity.

In many instances, AKI is associated with marked catabolism, and malnutrition can develop rapidly, leading to delayed recovery from AKI. Prompt and proper nutrition is essential in the management of newborns with AKI. If the gastrointestinal tract is intact and functional, enteral feedings with formula (PM 60/40) should be instituted as soon as possible. If the newborn is oligo/anuric and sufficient calories cannot be achieved while maintaining appropriate fluid balance, the earlier initiation of dialysis should be instituted.

Therapies to Decrease Injury and Promote Recovery

Although there is not a current specific therapy to prevent kidney injury or promote recovery in human ATN, several potential therapies are being studied, and future management of AKI may also include antioxidant, antiadhesion molecule therapy, the administration of vascular mediators, or mesenchymal stem cells (MSCs) to prevent injury or promote recovery.[100-107] Several different therapies have been shown to prevent, decrease, or promote recovery in animal models of AKI. Melanocyte-stimulating hormone has antiinflammatory activity and has been shown to protect renal tubules from injury.[100] Scavengers of free radicals and reactive oxygen and nitrogen molecules, as well as antiadhesion molecules, have been shown to decrease the degree of injury in animal models of AKI.[102] Recently, very interesting studies have also demonstrated that multipotent MSCs may play a role in promoting recovery from AKI in animal models.[103]

Despite the promise of animal models of intervention in AKI, clinical studies in humans have been largely disappointing, including studies using anaritide (atrial natriuretic peptide) and insulin-like growth factor 1.[104,105] Because therapy in these studies was initiated when kidney injury was well established, it is likely that the opportunity to intervene and impact the recovery from AKI had been missed.[106,107] As mentioned previously, the development and testing of interventions for AKI will require the development of early biomarkers of injury that are much more sensitive than serum creatinine.

Acute and Chronic Renal Replacement Therapy

Renal replacement therapy is provided to remove endogenous and exogenous toxins and to maintain fluid, electrolyte, and acid–base balance until kidney function returns or to maintain the neonate until kidney transplantation is possible. Renal replacement therapy may be provided by peritoneal dialysis, intermittent hemodialysis, and hemofiltration with or without a dialysis circuit. Whereas peritoneal dialysis and hemodialysis are options for long-term dialysis in infants whose kidney function does not improve, hemofiltration is used for AKI. Each mode of renal replacement therapy has specific advantages and disadvantages (Table 17-2). For AKI, the preferential use of hemofiltration by pediatric nephrologists is increasing, and the use of peritoneal dialysis is decreasing except for in neonates and small infants.[108]

No studies in newborns have compared the outcome of AKI or CKD when different renal replacement therapies are used in the treatment of AKI or CKD. Many factors, including the age and size of the child, the cause of kidney injury, the degree of metabolic derangements, blood pressure, and nutritional needs, were considered in deciding when to initiate renal replacement therapy and the modality of therapy.[108]

Table 17-2 COMPARISON OF RENAL REPLACEMENT THERAPIES

	PD	HD	CVVH or CVVHD
Solute removal	Good	Excellent	Fair (excellent)
Fluid removal	Good	Excellent	Excellent (excellent)
Toxin removal	Fair	Excellent	Fair (good)
Removal of potassium	Fair	Excellent	Fair (good)
Removal of ammonia	Fair	Excellent	Fair (good)
Need for hemodynamic stability	No	Yes	No (no)
Need for anticoagulation	No	Yes	Variable (variable)
Ease of access	Easy	Variable	Variable (variable)
Continuous	Yes	No	Yes (yes)
Respiratory compromise	Occasional	No	No (no)
Risk for peritonitis	Yes	No	No (no)
Risk for hypotension	Low	High	High (high)
Disequilibrium	No	Yes	No (no)
Reverse osmosis water	No	Yes	No (no)

CVVH, continuous venovenous; CVVHD, continuous venovenous hemodiafiltration; HD, hemodialysis; PD, peritoneal dialysis.

The indications to initiate renal replacement therapy are not absolute and take into consideration a number of factors, including the cause of kidney injury, the rapidity of the onset of kidney injury, the severity of fluid and electrolyte abnormalities, and the nutritional needs of the neonate. Because neonates and infants have less muscle mass than older children, they require initiation of renal replacement therapy at lower serum levels of serum creatinine and BUN compared with older children. The presence of fluid overload unresponsive to diuretic therapy and the need for enteral feedings or hyperalimentation to support nutritional needs is an important factor in considering the initiation of renal replacement therapy.

Peritoneal Dialysis

Peritoneal dialysis has been a major modality of therapy for AKI and CKD in neonates because vascular access is difficult to maintain in neonates. Advantages of peritoneal dialysis are that it is relatively easy to perform and does not require heparinization, and the newborn does not need to be hemodynamically stable to undergo peritoneal dialysis. The disadvantages include a slower correction of metabolic parameters and the potential for peritonitis. To increase the efficiency of peritoneal dialysis, frequent exchanges as often as every hour, and the use of dialysate with higher glucose concentrations, will remove more solute and water, respectively. Relative contraindications include recent abdominal surgery and massive organomegaly or intraabdominal masses as well as ostomies, which may increase the risk of peritonitis.

Access to the peritoneal cavity is usually through a Tenckhoff catheter. Alternately, several VLBW neonates were successfully dialyzed by using a 14-gauge vascular catheter to access the peritoneal fluid.[109] Commercially available 1.5%, 2.5%, and 4.25% glucose solutions are available for use in peritoneal dialysis. In older children, peritoneal dialysis is usually initiated with volumes of 15 to 20 mL/kg body weight; in neonates, it is usually initiated with slightly lower volumes of 5 to 10 mL/kg body weight. Low-volume peritoneal dialysis has a milder effect on the hemodynamic status of neonates and has been shown to effectively control uremia and promote ultrafiltration in neonates and older children.[110-113] The dialysate volume can be increased depending on the need for additional solute and fluid removal and the cardiovascular and respiratory status. If the neonate has lactate acidosis, dialysis with the standard solutions will increase the lactate load and aggravate the acidosis. Peritoneal dialysis with a bicarbonate-buffered dialysate solution should be used in neonates with lactate acidosis.

Substantial fluid and electrolyte imbalances can occur during peritoneal dialysis, especially when using frequent exchanges, and prolonged use of hypertonic glucose solutions can result in hyperglycemia, hypernatremia, and hypovolemia. Peritonitis (dialysate white blood cell count >100/mm^3) is another complication of acute peritoneal dialysis and can be treated with intraperitoneal antibiotics. If the neonate develops hypokalemia or hypophosphatemia during the course of dialysis, then 3 to 5 mEq/L of KCl or 2 to 3 mEq/L of potassium phosphate can be added to the dialysate. To avoid hypothermia in neonates, the dialysate should be warmed to body temperature before infusion into the peritoneal cavity.

Although technically challenging, long-term peritoneal dialysis has been carried out in VLBW infants with a weight as low as 930 g,[114] and short-term peritoneal dialysis has been used in smaller premature newborns.[110-113] Peritoneal dialysis has been shown to provide adequate clearance in neonates with AKI after cardiopulmonary bypass.[111] The majority of infants who have undergone long-term peritoneal dialysis were found to have normal developmental milestones or attended regular school and had good growth and development.[112] Neonates and infants with oliguria and with extrarenal abnormalities and a higher mortality rate compared with infants with isolated kidney disease and nonoliguric kidney injury.[113]

Hemodialysis

Hemodialysis has also been used for several years in the treatment of AKI and CKD during childhood.[115,116] Hemodialysis has the advantage that metabolic abnormalities can be corrected rather quickly and hypervolemia can be corrected by rapid ultrafiltration as well. The disadvantages of hemodialysis include the requirement for heparinization, the need for maximally purified water by a reverse osmosis system, and the need for skilled nursing personnel. Hemodialysis is commonly used for treatment of metabolic disorders associated with hyperammonemia from urea cycle defects.[116] Relative contraindications include hemodynamic instability and severe hemorrhage.

During hemodialysis, rapid ultrafiltration may also result in hypotension, which has also been shown to result in additional renal ischemia and potentially prolong the episode of AKI. Rapid removal of BUN and other uremic products can result in dialysis disequilibrium, particularly if the child begins hemodialysis with a high BUN (>120–150 mg/dL [42.8–53.5 mmol/L]). The pathogenesis of this syndrome is complex and multifactorial, but may be related to removal of urea from the blood while brain levels decline slower such that disequilibrium occurs; symptoms include restlessness, fatigue, headache, nausea, vomiting leading to confusion, seizures, and coma.[117] This severe complication of hemodialysis can be prevented by slowly lowering the BUN during hemodialysis and by the prophylactic infusion of mannitol (0.5–1 g/kg body weight) during hemodialysis to counteract the decline in the serum osmolality that occurs during hemodialysis.

Whereas vascular access in newborns can be provided by umbilical vessels, older infants and children require catheterization of a large vessel to obtain blood flows adequate for hemodialysis. Catheters can be placed in the internal or external jugular veins or in the femoral vein. To avoid hypotension, the total volume of the dialysate circuit, including the dialyzer and tubing, should not exceed 10% of the child blood volume. Blood flow rates to achieve clearances of 1.5 to 3.0 mL/kg/min are used depending on the indications for dialysis, the initial BUN level and degree of azotemia, and the clinical status of the child. Again, depending on the clinical status of the child and the degree of azotemia, clearances can be increased to 3 to 5 mL/kg/min in subsequent dialysis sessions. To maintain adequate control of azotemia and to allow for adequate nutrition during AKI, frequent hemodialysis (as often as daily) may be needed in neonates.

Hemofiltration

Over the past several years, renal replacement therapy with hemofiltration, including continuous venovenous hemofiltration (CVVH) or with the addition of a dialysis circuit to the hemofilter and continuous venovenous hemodiafiltration (CVVHD), has become increasingly popular in the treatment of AKI during childhood.[118-121] Whereas hemofiltration without dialysis (CVVH) follows the principle of removal of large quantities of ultrafiltrate from plasma with replacement of an isosmotic electrolyte solution, hemofiltration with dialysis (CVVHD) also results in solute removal via the added dialysis circuit. The advantages of hemofiltration (with or without a dialysis circuit) include that it can result in rapid fluid removal; does not require the patient to be hemodynamically stable; and is continuous, avoiding rapid solute and fluid shifts that occur in hemodialysis. The disadvantages include that hemofiltration may require constant heparinization, and there is a potential for severe fluid and electrolyte abnormalities because of the large volume of fluid removed and subsequently replaced. In neonates at risk of bleeding, regional anticoagulation with citrate can be performed to minimize the risk of bleeding. Hemofiltration and hemodiafiltration were found to allow good control of fluid, electrolyte, and acid–base balance and have been used in newborns with inborn errors of metabolism.[120] The survival rate in children weighing up to 10 kg undergoing CVVH is similar to that of older children and adolescents.[121] As in hemodialysis, catheterization of a large vessel is necessary to obtain blood flows adequate for hemofiltration. Catheters can be placed in the internal or external jugular veins or in the femoral vein. CVVH can also be performed in neonates and children on extracorporeal membrane oxygenation (ECMO) by adding a filter in the ECMO circuit or by inserting a continuous renal replacement therapy machine.[122]

Prognosis

In neonates, the prognosis and recovery from AKI is highly dependent on the underlying etiology of the AKI.[9-14] Factors that are associated with mortality include multiorgan failure, hypotension, a need for pressors, hemodynamic instability, and a need for mechanical ventilation and dialysis.[9-14] Overall, mortality in newborns with AKI ranges from 10% to 61% and is highest in infants with multiorgan failure.[9-14] In infants maintained by peritoneal dialysis for AKI, mortality was 64% in oligo/anuric infants compared with 20% in infants with adequate urine output.[12] Other recent studies have shown that AKI in VLBW infants was independently associated with mortality.[123] Long-term follow-up of children with AKI has shown that death and kidney sequelae are common 3 to 5 years after AKI in pediatric patients, suggesting that the detrimental effects of AKI are long lasting.[124]

It is well known that neonates with congenital disease such as dysplasia with or without obstructive uropathy, cortical necrosis, or cystic kidney diseases are at risk for later development of CKD. In contrast, it has been thought that ischemic and nephrotoxic kidney injury is reversible with kidney function returning to normal. However, recent studies have shown that hypoxic ischemic and nephrotoxic insults can result in alterations that can lead to kidney disease at a later time.[1-3,69-72] Thus, AKI from any cause is a risk factor for subsequent kidney disease. AKI in full-term neonates is associated with kidney disease later in life.[69] In one study of six older children with a history of AKI not requiring dialysis in the neonatal period, only two were normal, three had CKD, and one was on dialysis.[43] Although the number of children studied was small, this study raises concern about the long-term kidney outcome for such children. An inverse relationship between the development of hypertension and proteinuria during adulthood and birth weight has been reported.[70,73]

The long-term effect of AKI in neonates is potentially compounded when the insult occurs before the full complement of nephrons has developed in utero.

Because nephrogenesis proceeds until 34-35 weeks weeks of gestation, AKI before this time may result in a reduced nephron number. Indeed, it has been shown that preterm neonates with AKI have a high incidence of a low GFR and increasing proteinuria several years later,[71] and morphologic studies have shown decreased nephron number and glomerulomegaly.[72] Several studies in animal models and some human studies have documented that hyperfiltration of the remnant nephron may eventually lead to progressive glomerulosclerosis of the remaining nephrons. Typically, the late development of CKD first becomes apparent with the development of hypertension, proteinuria, and eventually an elevated BUN and creatinine.

When premature neonates were investigated during childhood (ages 6.1–12.4 years), defects in tubular reabsorption of phosphorus (TRP) were evident, the TRP was significantly lower and the urinary excretion of phosphorus significantly higher compared with control children.[125] Urinary calcium excretion was also higher in children born prematurely compared with control children. Others have found nearly identical findings, and the investigators attributed these alterations to aminoglycoside nephrotoxicity.[126,127] Recent studies have also shown that low birth weight is a risk factor for focal segmental glomerulosclerosis.[128] In addition, extrauterine as well as intrauterine growth retardation was associated with impaired renal function in children who were born very preterm.[129] In view of these alterations in kidney function, increasing proteinuria, and tubular dysfunction, neonates with AKI and nephrotoxic insults need lifelong monitoring of their kidney function, blood pressure, and urinalysis.[1-3,130]

17

References

1. Goldstein SL, Devarajan P. Acute kidney injury in childhood: should we be worried about progression to CKD? *Pediatr Nephrol.* 2011;26:509-522.
2. Basile D. Rarefaction of peritubular capillaries following ischemic acute renal failure: a potential factor predisposing progressive nephropathy. *Curr Opin Nephrol and Hypertens.* 2004;13:1-13.
3. Andreoli SP. Acute kidney injury in children. *Pediatr Nephrol.* 2009;24:253-263.
4. Lip GYH, Churchill D, Beevers M, et al. Angiotensin converting enzyme inhibitors in early pregnancy. *Lancet.* 1997;350:1446.
5. Martinovic J, Benachi A, Laurent N, et al. Fetal toxic effects and angiotensin-II-receptor antagonists. *Lancet.* 2001;358:241.
6. Cooper WO, Hernandez-Diaz S, Arbogast PG, et al. Major congenital malformations after first-trimester exposure to ACE inhibitors. *N Eng J Med.* 2006;354:2443.
7. Benini D, Fanos V, Cuzzolin L, et al. In utero exposure to nonsteroidal anti-inflammatory drugs: Neonatal acute renal failure. *Pediatr Nephrol.* 2004;19:232-234.
8. Hui-Stickle S, Brewer ED, Goldstein SL. Pediatric ARF Epidemiology at a Tertiary Care Center from 1999 to 2001. *Am J Kidney Dis.* 2005;45:96-101.
9. Mathews DE, West KW, Rescorla FJ, et al. Peritoneal dialysis in the first 60 days of life. *J Pediatr Surg.* 1990;25:110-116, 1990.
10. Andreoli SP. Acute renal failure. *Curr Opin Pediatr.* 2002;17:713-717.
11. Mogal NE, Brocklebank JT, Meadow SR. A review of acute renal failure in children: incidence, etiology and outcome. *Clin Nephrol.* 1998;49:91-95.
12. Karlowivz MG, Adelman RD. Nonoliguric and oliguric acute renal failure. *Pediatr Nephrol.* 1995;9:718-722.
13. Andreoli SP. Renal Failure in the Newborn Unit. In: Polin RA, Yoder MC, Berg FD, eds. *Workbook in Practical Neonatology.* Philadelphia, PA: W.B. Saunders Company; 2007:329-344.
14. Gouyon JB, Guignard JP. Management of acute renal failure in newborns. *Pediatr Nephrol.* 2000;14:1037-1044.
15. Vanpee M, Blennow M, Linne T, et al. Renal function in very low birth weight infants: normal maturity reached during childhood. *J Pediatr.* 1992;121:784-788.
16. Drukker A, Guignard JP. Renal aspects of the term and preterm infant: a selective update. *Curr Opinin Pediatr.* 2002;14:175-182.
17. Devarajan P. Emerging biomarkers of AKI. *Contr Nephrol.* 2007;156:203-312.
18. Al-Ismaili Z, Palijan A, Zappitelli M. Bisomarkers of acute kidney injury in children: discovery, evaluation, and clinical application. *Pediatr Nephrol.* 2011;26:29-40.
19. Lavery AP, Meinzen-Derr JK, Anderson E, et al. Urinary NGAL in Premature Infants. *Pediatric Res.* 2008;64:423-428.
20. Parravicini E. The clinical utility of urinary neutrophil gelatinase-associated lipocalin in the neonatal ICU. *Curr Opin Pediatr.* 2010;22:146-150.
21. Zaffanello M, Antonucci R, Cuzzolin L. Early diagnosis of acute kidney injury with urinary biomarkers in the newborn. *J Mat-Fet Med.* 2009;22(Suppl 3):62-66.
22. Bellomo R, Ronco C, Kellum JA, et al. Acute renal failure – definition, outcomes measures, animal models, fluid therapy and information technology needs. *Crit Care.* 2004;8:R204-212.

23. Akcan-Arikan A, Zappitelli M, Loftis LL, et al. Modified RIFLE criteria in critically ill children with acute kidney injury. *Kid Int*. 2007;71:1028-1035.
24. Duzova A, Bakkaloglu A, Dalyoncu M, et al. Etiology and outcome of acute kidney injury in children. *Pediatr Nephrol*. 2010;25:1453-1461.
25. Askenazi DJ, Ambalavannan N, Goldstein SL. Acute kidney injury in critically ill newborns: What do we know? What do we need to learn? *Pediatr Nephrol*. 2009;24:265-274.
26. Goldstein SL. Pediatric acute kidney injury: it's time for real progress. *Pediatr Nephrol*. 2006;21:891-895.
27. Martin-Ancel A, Garcia-Alix A, Gaya F, et al. Multiple organ involvement in perinatal asphyxia. *J Pediatr*. 1995;127:786-793.
28. Cataldi L, Leone R, Moretti U, et al. Potential risk factors for the development of acute renal failure in preterm newborn infants: a case controlled study. *Arch Dis Child Fetal Neonatal Ed*. 2005;90:514-519.
29. Aggarwal A, Kumar P, Chowkhary G, et al. Evaluation of renal function in asphyxiated newborns. *J Trop Pediatr*. 2005;51:295-299, 2005.
30. Cuzzolin L, Fanos V, Pinna B, et al. Postnatal renal function in preterm newborns: a role of diseases, drugs and therapeutic interventions. *Pediatr Nephrol*. 2006;21:931-938.
31. Durkan AM, Alexander RT. Acute kidney injury post neonatal asphyxia. *J Pediatr*. 2011;158:e29-33.
32. Airede A, Bello M, Werasingher HD. Acute renal failure in the newborn: incidence and outcome. *J Paediatr Child Health*. 1997;33:246-249.
33. Nobilis A, Kocsis I, Toth-Heyn P, et al. Variance of ACE and AT1 receptor genotype does not influence the risk of neonatal acute renal failure. *Pediatr Nephrol*. 2001;16:1063-1066.
34. Vasarhelyi B, Toth-Heyn P, Treszl A, et al. Genetic polymorphism and risk for acute renal failure in preterm infants. *Pediatri Nephrol*. 2005;20:132-135.
35. Treszl A, Toth-Heyn P, Koscic I. Interleukin genetic variants and the risk of renal failure in infants with infection. *Pediatr Nephrol*. 2002;17:713-717.
36. Fekkete A, Treszl A, Toht-Heyn P, et al. Association between heat shock protein 72 gene polymorphism and acute renal failure in neonates. *Pediatric Research*. 2003;54:452-455.
37. Kelly KJ, Baird NR, Greene AL. Induction of stress response proteins and experimental renal ischemia/reperfusion. *Kidney Int*. 2001;59:1798-1802.
38. Toth-Heyhn P, Dukker A, Guignard JP. The stressed neonatal kidney: from pathophysiology to clinical management of neonatal vasomotor nephropathy. *Pediatr Nephrol*. 2000;14:227-239.
39. Andreoli SP. Acute renal failure in the newborn. *Sem Perinat*. 2004;28:112-123.
40. Badr KF, Ichikawa I. Prerenal failure: a deleterious shift from renal compensation to decompensation. *N Engl J Med*. 1998;319:623-628.
41. van Bel F, Guit GL, Schipper J, et al. Indomethacin-induced changes in renal blood flow velocity waveform in premature infants investigated with color Doppler imaging. *J Pediatr*. 1991;118:621-626.
42. Cifuentes RF, Olley PR, Balfe JW, et al. Indomethacin and renal function in premature infants with persistent patent ductus arteriosus. *J Pediatr*. 1979;95:583-587.
43. Allegaert K, Vanhole C, de Hoon J, et al. Nonselective cyclo-oxygenase inhibitors and glomerular filtration rate in preterm infants. *Pediatr Nephrol*. 2005;20:1557-1561.
44. Zanardo V, Vedovato S, Lago P, et al. Urinary ET-1, AVP and sodium in premature infants treated with indomethacin and ibuprofen for patent ductus arteriosus. *Pediatr Nephrol*. 2005;20:1552-1556.
45. Gersony WM, Peckham GJ, Ellison RC, et al. Effects of indomethacin in premature infants with paten ductus arteriosus: results of a national collaborative stud. *J Pediatr*. 1983;102:895-906.
46. Itabashi K, Ohno T, Nishda H. Indomethacin responsiveness of patent ductus arteriosus and renal abnormalities in preterm infants treated with indomethacin. *J Pediatr*. 2003;143:203-207.
47. Guignard JP. The adverse effects of prostaglandin-synthesis inhibitors in the newborn rabbit. *Sem Perinat*. 2002;26:398-405.
48. Perazella MA, Eras J. Are selective COX–2 inhibitors nephrotoxic? *Am J Kidney*. 2000;35:937-940.
49. Tack ED, Perlman JM. Renal failure in sick hypertensive premature infants receiving captopril therapy. *J Pediatr*. 1988;112:805-810.
50. Wood EG, Bunchman TE, Lynch RE. Captopril-induced reversible acute renal failure in an infant with coarctation of the aorta. *Pediatrics*. 1991;88:816-818.
51. Basile DP. The endothelial cell in ischemic acute kidney injury: implications for acute and chronic function. *Kidney Int*. 2007;72:151-156.
52. Sutton TA, Fisher CJ, Molitoris BA. Microvascular endothelial injury and dysfunction during ischemic acute renal failure. *Kidney Int*. 2002;62:1539-1549.
53. Molitoris BA. Putting the actin cytoskeleton into perspective: pathophysiology of ischemic alterations. *Am J Physiol*. 1997;272:F430-F433.
54. Andreoli SP. Reactive oxygen molecules, oxidant injury and renal disease. *Pediatr Nephrol*. 1991;5:733-742.
55. Andreoli SP, McAteer JA. Reactive oxygen molecule mediated injury in endothelial cells and renal tubular epithelial cells in vitro. *Kidney Int*. 1990;38:785-794.
56. Kelly KJ, Williams WW, Colvin RB, Bonventre JV. Antibody to intercellular adhesion molecule-1 protects the kidney against ischemic injury. *Proc Natl Acad Sci USA*. 1994;91:812-817.

57. Goligorsky MS, Brodsky SV, Noiri E. Nitric oxide in acute renal failure: NOS versus NOS. *Kidney Int.* 2002;61:855-861.

58. Gorligosky MS, Noiri E. Duality of nitric oxide in acute renal failure. *Semin Nephrol.* 1999;19:263-271.

59. Radi R, Pueluffo G, Noel MA, et al. Unraveling peroxynitrite fomranion in biological systems. *Free Radic Biol Med.* 2001;30:463-488.

60. Wilhelm SM, Simonson MS, Robinson AV, et al. Endothelin up regulation and localization following renal ischemia and reperfusion. *Kidney Int.* 1999;55:1011-1018.

61. Ruschitzka F, Shaw S, Gygi D, et al. Endothelial dysfunction in acute renal failure: role of circulating and tissue endothelin-1. *J Am Soc Nephrol.* 1999;10:953-962.

62. Forbes JH, Hewitson TD, Becker GJ, et al. Simultaneous blockage of endothelin A and B receptors in ischemic acute renal failure is detrimental to long term kidney function. *Kidney Int.* 2001;59: 1333-1341.

63. Zuk A, Bonventre JV, Brown D, et al. Polarity, integrin and extracellular matrix dynamics in the post ischemic rat kidney. *Am J Physiol.* 1998;275:C711-C731.

64. Kwon O, Corrigan G, Meyers BD, et al. Sodium reabsorption and distribution of Na+K+ATPase during post-ischemic injury to the renal allograft. *Kidney Int.* 1999;55:963-975.

65. Van Why SK, Mann AS, Radio T, et al. Hsp27 associates with actin and limits injury in energy depleted renal epithelial. *J Am Soc Nephrol.* 2002;13:2667-2680.

66. Luster AD. Chemokines: chemotactic cytokines that mediate inflammation. *New Engl J Med.* 1998;338:436-445.

67. Heinzelmann M, Mercer-Jones MA, Passsmore JC. Neutrophils and renal failure. *Am J Kid Dis.* 1999; 34:384-399.

68. Himmelfarb J, McMonagle E, Freedjman S, et al. The PICARD Group. Oxidative stress is increased in critically ill patients with acute renal failure. *J Am Soc Nephrol.* 2004;15:2449-2456.

69. Polito C, Papale MR, LaManna AL. Long-term prognosis of acute renal failure in the full term newborn. *Clin Pediatr.* 1998;37:381-386.

70. Tulassay T, Vasarheleyi B. Birth Weight and renal function. *Curr Opin Nephrol Hypertension.* 2002;11:347-352.

71. Abitbol CL, Bauer CR, Montane B, et al. Long term follow-up of extremely low birth weight infants with neonatal renal failure. *Pediatr Nephrol.* 2003;18:887-893.

72. Rodriguez MM, Gomez A, Abitbol C, et al. Comparative renal histomorphometry: a case study of oliogonephropathy of prematurity. *Pediatr Nephrol.* 2005;20:945-949.

73. Keijzer-Veen MG, Schrevel M, Finken MJ, et al. Dutch POPS-19 Collaborative Study Group. Micro-albuminuria and lower glomerular filtration rate at young adult age in subjects born very prematurely and after intrauterine growth retardation. *J Am Soc Nephrol.* 2005;16:2762-2765.

74. Payne RM, Martin TC, Bower RJ, et al. Management and follow-up of arterial thrombosis in the neonatal period. *J Pediatr.* 1989;114:853-858.

75. Ellis D, Kaye RD, Bontempo FA. Aortic and renal artery thrombosis in a neonate: recovery with thrombolytic therapy. *Pediatr Nephrol.* 1997;11:641-644.

76. Christensen AM, Daouk GH, Norling LL, et al. Postnatal transient renal insufficiency in the feto-fetal transfusion syndrome. *Pediatr Nephrol.* 1999;13:117-120.

77. Cincotta RB, Gray PH, Phythian G, et al. Long term outcome of twin-twin transfusion syndrome. *Arch Dis Child Fetal Med.* 2000;83:F171-F176.

78. Beck M, Graf C, Ellenrieder B, et al. Long-term outcome of kidney function after twin-twin transfusion syndrome treated by intrauterine laser coagulation. *Pediatr Nephrol* 2005; 20:1657-1659.

79. Ogunlesi TA, Akdkanmbi F. Evaluating and managing neonatal acute kidney injury in a resource-poor setting. *Indian J Pediatrics.* 2009;76:293-296.

80. Jenik AG, Ceriani Cernadas JM, Gorenstein A, et al. A randomized, double-blind, placebo-controlled trail of the effects of prophylactic theophylline on renal function in term neonates with perinatal asphyxia. *Pediatrics.* 2000;105:E45-E48.

81. Bhat M, Shah ZA, Makidoomi MS, et al. Theophylline for renal function in term neonates with perinatal asphyxia: a randomized, placebo controlled trial. *J Pediatr.* 2006;149:180-184.

82. Bakr AF. Prophylactic theophylline to prevent renal dysfunction in newborns exposed to perinatal asphyxia – a study in a developing country. *Pediatr Nephrol.* 2005;20:1249-1252.

83. Gouyon JB, Guignard JP. Theophylline prevents the hypoxemia-induced renal hemodynamic changes in rabbits. *Kidney Int.* 1988;33:1078-1083.

84. Kellum JA. Use of diuretics in the acute care setting. *Kidney Int.* 1998;53:67-70.

85. Denton MD, Chertow GM, Brady HR. "Renal-dose" dopamine for the treatment of acute renal failure: Scientific rationale, experimental studies and clinical trials. *Kidney Int.* 1996;49:4-14.

86. Chertow GM, Sayegh MH, Allgren RL, et al. Is the administration of dopamine associated with adverse or favorable outcomes in acute renal failure? *Am J Med.* 1996;101:49-53.

87. Bellomo R, Chapman M, Finfers S, et al. Clinical Trials Group: low dose dopamine in patients with early renal dysfunction: a placebo controlled trial. *Lancet.* 2000;356:2139-2143.

88. Kellum JA, Decker JM. Use of dopamine in acute renal failure: a meta-analysis. *Crit Care Med.* 2001;29:1526-1531.

89. Galley HF. Renal dose dopamine: will the message get through? *Lancet.* 2000;356:2112-2113.

90. Lauschke A, Teichgraber UKM, Frei U, et al. "Low-dose" dopamine worsens renal perfusion in patients with acute renal failure. *Kidney Int.* 2006;69:1669-1674.

17

91. Marthur VS, Swan SK, Lambrecht LJ, et al. The effects of fenoldopam, a selective dopamine receptor agonist, on systemic and renal hemodynamics in normotensive subjects. *Crit Care Med*. 1999;27: 1832-1837.

92. Landoni G, Biondi-Zoccai GGL, Tumlin JA. Beneficial impact of fenoldopam in critically ill patients with or at risk for acute renal failure: a meta-analysis of randomized clinical trials. *Am J Kidney Dis*. 2007;49:56-68.

93. Knoderer CA, Leiser JD, Nailescu C, et al. Fenoldopam for acute kidney injury in children. *Pediatr Nephrol*. 2008;23:495-498.

94. Rodriguez-Soriano J. Potassium homeostasis and its disturbances in children. *Pediatr Nephrol*. 1995;9:364-374.

95. Malone TA. Glucose and insulin versus cation-exchange resin for the treatment of hyperkalemia in very low birth weight infants. *J Pediatr*. 1991;118:121-123.

96. Singh BS, Sadiq HF, Noguchi A, et al. Efficacy of albuterol inhalation in treatment of hyperkalemia in premature neonates. *J Pediatr*. 2002;121:16-20.

97. Bunchman TE, Wood EG, Schenck MH, et al. Pretreatment of formula with sodium polystyrene sulfonate to reduce dietary potassium intake. *Pediatr Nephrol*. 1991;5:29-32.

98. Gerstman BB, Kirkman R, Platt R. Intestinal necrosis associated with postoperative orally administered sodium polystyrene sulfonate in sorbitol. *Am J Kid Dis*. 1992;20:159-161.

99. Andreoli SP, Dunson JW, Bergstein JM. Calcium carbonate is an effective phosphorus binder in children with chronic renal failure. *Am J Kidney Dis*. 1987;9:206-210.

100. Kohda Y, Chiao H, Starr RA. A melanocyte stimulating hormone protects against renal injury after ischemia in mice and rats. *Curr Opin Nephrol Hypertens*. 1998;99:1165-1172.

101. Weston CE, Feibelman MB, Kouting W, et al. Effect of oxidant stress on growth factor stimulation of proliferation in cultured human proximal tubular cells. *Kidney Int*. 1999;56:1274-1276.

102. Chatterjee PK, Cuzzocreas S, Brown P, et al. Tempol, a membrane permeable radical scavenger reduces oxidant stress mediated renal dysfunction and injury in the rat. *Kidney Int*. 2000;58: 568-673.

103. Lange C, Togel F, Ittrich H, et al. Administered mesenchymal stem cells enhance recovery from ischemic/reperfusion-induced acute renal failure in rats. *Kidney Int*. 2005;68:1613-1617.

104. Allgren RL, Marbury TC, Rahman SN, et al. Anaritide in acute tubular necrosis. *N Engl J Med*. 1997;336:828-834.

105. Hirschberg R, Kopple J, Lipsett P, et al. Multicenter clinical trial of recombinant human insulin like growth factor in patients with acute renal failure. *Kidney Int*. 1999;55:2423-2432.

106. Molitoris BA. Transitioning to therapy in ischemic acute renal failure. *J Am Soc Nephrol*. 2003; 14:165-267.

107. Jo SK, Rosner MH, Okusa MD. Pharmacologic treatment of acute kidney injury: why drugs haven't worked and what is on the horizon. *Clin J Am Soc Nephrol*. 2007;2:356-365.

108. Belsha CW, Kohaut EC, Warady BA. Dialytic management of childhood acute renal failure: a survey of North American pediatric nephrologists. *Pediatr Nephrol*. 1995;9:361-363.

109. Yu JE, Park MS, Pai KS. Acute peritoneal dialysis in very low birth weight neonates using a vascular catheter. *Pediatr Nephrol*. 2010;25:367-371.

110. Golej J, Kitzmueller E, Herman M, et al. Low-volume peritoneal dialysis in 116 neonatal and paediatic critical care patients. *Eur J Pediatr*. 2002;161;385-389.

111. McNiece KL, Ellis EE, Drummond-Webb JJ, et al. Adequacy of peritoneal dialysis in children following cardiopulmonary bypass surgery. *Pediatric Nephrol*. 2005;20:972-976.

112. Ledermann SE, Scanes ME, Fernando ON, et al. Long-term outcome of peritoneal dialysis in infants. *J Pediatric*. 2000;136:24-29.

113. Ellis EN, Pearson D, Champion B, et al. Outcome of infants on chronic peritoneal dialysis. *Adv Perit Dial*. 1995;11:266-269.

114. Rainey KE, DiGeronimo R, Pascaul-Baralt J. Successful long term peritoneal dialysis in a very low birth weight infant with renal failure secondary to feto-fetal transfusion syndrome. *Pediatrics*. 2000;106:849-852.

115. Sadowski RH, Harmon WE, Jabs K. Acute hemodialysis of infants weighing less than five kilograms. *Kidney Int*. 1994;45:903-906.

116. Wigand C, Thompson T, Bock GH, et al. The management of life-threatening hyperammonemia. *J Pediatr*. 1980;116:125-128.

117. Silver SM, Sterns RH, Halperin ML. Brain swelling after dialysis: old urea or new osmoles? *Am J Kidney Dis*. 1996;28:113.

118. Ronco C, Brendolan A, Bragantini L, et al. Treatment of acute renal failure in newborns by continuous arterio-venous hemofiltration. *Kidney Int*. 1986;29:908-915.

119. Zobel G, Rod S, Urlesberger B, et al. Continuous renal replacement therapy in critically ill neonates. *Kidney Int*. 1998;53:S169-S173.

120. Falk MC, Knight JF, Roy LP, et al. Continuous venovenous hemofiltration in the acute treatment of inborn errors of metabolism. *Pediatr Nephrol*. 1994;8:330-333.

121. Symons JM, Brophy PD, Gregory MJ, et al. Continuous renal replacement therapy in children up to 10 kg. *Am J Kid Dis*. 2003;41:984-989.

122. Santigo MJ, Sanchez A, Lopez-Herce J. The use of continuous renal replacement therapy in series with extracorporeal membrane oxygenation. *Kidney Int*. 2009;76:1289-1299.

123. Askenazi DJ, Griffin R, McGwin G, et al. Acute kidney injury is independently associated with mortality in very low birth weight infants: a matched case-control study. *Pediatr Nephrol*. 2009; 24:991-997.

124. Askenazi DJ, Feig DI, Graham NM, et al. 3-5 year longitudinal follow up of pediatric patients with acute renal failure. *Kidney Int.* 2006;69:184-189.
125. Rodriguez-Soriano J, Aguirre M, Oliveros R, et al. Long-term follow-up of extremely low birth weight infants. *Pediatr Nephrol.* 2005;20:579-584.
126. Jones CA, Bowden LS, Watling R, et al. Hypercalciuria in ex-preterm children aged 7-8 years. *Pediatr Nephrol.* 2001;16:665-671.
127. Jones C, Judd B. Long term follow-up of extremely low birth weight infants. *Pediatr Nephrol.* 2006;21:299-303.
128. Hodgin JB, Rasoulpour M, Markowitz GS, D'Agati VD. Very low birth weight is a risk factor for focal segmental glomerulosclerosis. *Clin J Am Soc Nephrol.* 2009;4:71-76.
129. Bacchetta J, Harambat J, Dubourg L, et al. Both extrauterine and intrauterine restriction impair renal function in children born very preterm. *Kidney Int.* 2009;76:445-452.
130. Hsu CW, Symoms JM. Acute kidney injury: can we improve prognosis? *Pediatr Nephrol.* 2010;25:2401-2412.

17

CHAPTER 18

Hereditary Tubulopathies

Israel Zelikovic, MD

Hereditary tubular transport disorders comprise a group of diseases that lead to profound derangements in the homeostasis of electrolytes, minerals, or organic solutes in the body and can be associated with significant morbidity.[1-4]

For decades, the study of inherited tubular transport disorders has focused on the physiologic and metabolic alterations leading to impaired solute handling by the tubular epithelial cell. Over the past decade, the breakthrough in molecular biology and molecular genetics has provided the tools to investigate hereditary tubulopathies at the molecular level. As a result, exciting discoveries have been made, and the underlying molecular defects in many of these disorders have been defined.[1-4] The molecular study of hereditary tubulopathies has been important not only in clarifying the genetic basis of these disorders but also in providing new and important insight into the function of specific transport proteins and into the physiology of renal tubular reclamation of solutes.

Generally, tubular transport disorders are subdivided into two large groups: (1) *primary isolated tubulopathies*, which are mostly hereditary and involve an impairment in a single tubular function, and (2) *generalized tubulopathies*, which are hereditary or acquired and are caused by complex tubular derangements involving more than one transport system. A variety of primary inherited tubulopathies alter specific renal epithelial transport functions.[1,2] In most instances, the change in transport function leads to the loss of an essential substance in the urine and either impaired homeostasis of this substance in the body (as in renal tubular acidosis [RTA] or Bartter syndrome) or precipitation of the substance in the kidney (as in cystinuria or hypercalciuria). In some of these disorders, however, the defect in tubular function leads to accumulation of a substance in the body (as in Liddle syndrome).

Hereditary tubulopathies can affect children at all ages, but usually, children with these disorders present in the neonatal period or in the first year of life. Clinical manifestations of hereditary tubulopathies are commonly nonspecific and may include failure to thrive, stunted growth, poor feeding, recurrent vomiting, diarrhea, constipation, polyuria, polydipsia, or recurrent febrile episodes.[1] In some instances, however, more specific manifestations such as rickets, urolithiasis, or hypertension aid in the diagnosis of a specific tubulopathy. In most of these disorders, the principle of therapy is replacement of the substance lost in the urine or prevention of precipitation of the substance in the kidney. Some of the tubulopathies (e.g., isolated glycosuria) are benign and require no therapy. In addition to a detailed history and careful examination of the child, simultaneous and accurate assessment of the serum and urine concentration of the substance involved in the tubulopathy hold the key to the correct diagnosis.[1] Renal ultrasonography and bone radiography are helpful studies in most tubulopathies.

This chapter summarizes the general characteristics of hereditary tubular transport disorders, reviews the molecular pathophysiology and genetic aspects of the diseases, describes the clinical feature of the tubulopathies, and briefly summarizes their therapy. The focus of this chapter is on disorders resulting from primary gene defects in transporters or channels operating along the renal tubule. Some tubular transport disorders secondary to defects in receptors (e.g., as Ca^{2+}-sensing receptor or antidiuretic hormone [ADH] receptor) or enzymes (e.g., with no K [lysine] serine-threonine protein kinases, WNKs) resulting in isolated tubulopathies are also discussed. Generalized tubulopathies involving several transport systems (e.g., Fanconi syndrome) are not discussed or only briefly mentioned. In Tables 18-1 through 18-4, the disorders reviewed are summarized and grouped by the nephron segment affected.

Proximal Tubule

Proximal Renal Tubular Acidosis

General Characteristics

Proximal renal tubular acidosis (pRTA) (RTA type 2) is characterized by normal anion gap, hyperchloremic metabolic acidosis caused by impaired capacity of the proximal tubule to reabsorb HCO_3^- (Fig. 18-1).[4-6] Thus, at normal plasma HCO_3^- concentration, large amounts of HCO_3^- (>15% of the filtered load) escape proximal reabsorption and reach the distal tubule. This load overwhelms the limited capacity of the distal tubule to reabsorb HCO_3^-, substantial bicarbonaturia occurs, urine pH increases, net acid secretion ceases, and metabolic acidosis develops.[6,7] This HCO_3^- wasting is a transient phenomenon, and when the serum HCO_3^- level stabilizes in the acidemia range, the smaller amounts of HCO_3^- lost in the proximal tubule are completely reabsorbed by the distal tubule, and urine pH decreases to less than 5.5.[5,6] In pRTA, serum K^+ level is usually diminished. Hypokalemia develops because increased delivery of Na^+ to the distal nephron results in enhanced secretion of K^+

Text continued on page 313.

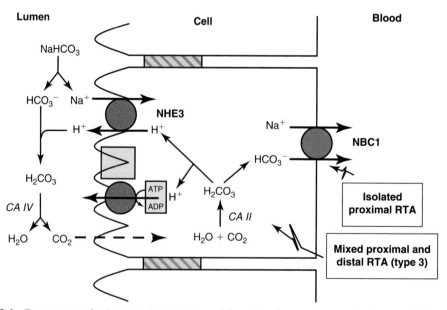

Figure 18-1 Transport mechanisms participating in acid–base handling in a proximal tubular cell. H^+ and HCO_3^- are formed in the cell as a result of carbonic anhydrase II (CAII) action. H^+ exits the cell via the apical Na^+/H^+ exchanger (NHE3) and H^+-ATPase pump. HCO_3^- exit occurs via the basolateral Na^+/HCO_3^- cotransporter (NBC1). Hereditary renal tubular acidosis syndromes caused by defects in NBC1 and CAII, respectively, are depicted.

Table 18-1 HEREDITARY TUBULOPATHIES CAUSED BY TRANSPORT DEFECTS IN THE PROXIMAL TUBULE

Disorder	Defective Gene	Locus	Defective Protein	Mode of Inheritance	Localization of Defect	Clinical Features	OMIM No.*
Isolated proximal RTA (type 2)	SLC4A4	4q21	Na$^+$-HCO$_3^-$ cotransporter, NBC1	AR	Basolateral	Normal anion gap metabolic acidosis, failure to thrive, hypokalemia, polyuria, polydipsia, dehydration, muscle weakness, ocular abnormalities	604278
Classic cystinuria Type I Non type I	SLC3A1 SLC7A9	2p163 19q13.1	rBAT b$^{0,+}$AT	AR Incomplete AR	Luminal Luminal	Urinary stones, obstruction, infection	220100 600918
Lysinuric protein intolerance	SLC7A7	14q11	y$^+$LAT-1	AR	Basolateral	Failure to thrive, protein intolerance, vomiting, hypotonia, hyperammonemia, seizures, coma	222700
Hartnup disease	SLC6A19	5p15.33	AA transport system B^0	AR	Luminal	Skin rash, cerebellar ataxia, psychiatric illnesses	234500
Isolated hereditary glycosuria	SLC5A2	16p11.2	SGLT2	AR	Luminal	None	233100
Fanconi-Bickel syndrome	SLC2A2	3q26.1	GLUT2	AR	Basolateral	Failure to thrive, proximal tubulopathy, hepatomegaly, fasting hypoglycemia, postprandial hyperglycemia	227810

*Online Mendelian Inheritance in Man (database at http://www.ncbi.nlm.nih.gov/Omim).
  AA, amino acid; AD, autosomal dominant; AR autosomal recessive; b$^{0,+}$AT, light subunit of AA transport system b$^{0,+}$; GLUT2, facilitative glucose transporter; rBAT, heavy subunit of AA transport system b$^{0,+}$; SGLT2, Na$^+$-glucose cotransporter; y$^+$LAT-1, light subunit of AA transport system y$^+$L.

18

D

Table 18-2 TUBULOPATHIES CAUSED BY TRANSPORT DEFECTS IN THE LOOP OF HENLE

Disorder	Defective Gene	Locus	Defective Protein	Localization of Defect	Mode of Inheritance	Clinical Features	OMIM No.*
Antenatal Bartter syndrome (type I)	SLC12A1	15q21	Na⁺, K⁺, 2Cl⁻ cotransporter, NKCC2	Luminal	AR	Renal salt wasting, hypokalemia, hypochloremic metabolic alkalosis, failure to thrive, polyuria, dehydration, muscle weakness, hypercalciuria	241200
Antenatal Bartter syndrome (type II)	KCNJ1	11q24	K⁺ channel, ROMK	Luminal	AR	Renal salt wasting, hypokalemia, hypochloremic metabolic alkalosis, failure to thrive, polyuria, dehydration, muscle weakness, hypercalciuria	601678
Classic Bartter syndrome (type III)	CLCNKB	1p36	Cl⁻ channel, ClC-Kb	Basolateral	AR	Renal salt wasting, hypokalemia, hypochloremic metabolic alkalosis, failure to thrive, polyuria, dehydration, muscle weakness, ± hypercalciuria	602023
Bartter syndrome with deafness (type IV)	BSND	1p31	Barttin (β subunit of ClC-Ka/ClC-Kb)	Basolateral	AR	Renal salt wasting, hypokalemia, hypochloremic metabolic alkalosis, failure to thrive, polyuria, dehydration, muscle weakness, ± hypercalciuria, chronic renal failure, sensorineural deafness	602522
AD hypocalcemia with Bartter Syndrome (type V)	CASR	3q21	CaSR	Basolateral	AD	Renal salt wasting, hypokalemia, hypochloremic metabolic alkalosis, failure to thrive, polyuria, dehydration, muscle weakness, hypercalciuria	601198
Familial benign hypercalcemia/neonatal severe primary hyperparathyroidism	CASR	3q21	CaSR	Basolateral	AD/AR	Mild or severe hypercalcemia, hypermagnesemia, hypocalciuria, hypomagnesiuria	145980 /259200
Familial hypomagnesemia–hypercalciuria–nephrocalcinosis syndrome	CLDN16 CLDN19	3q28 1p34	Claudin-16 (paracellin1), claudin-19	Tight junction	AR	Muscle weakness, tetany, urinary stones, ocular abnormalities (in particular in CLDN19 defect)	603959 610036

*Online Mendelian Inheritance in Man (database at http://www.ncbi.nlm.hih.gov/Omim).

AD, autosomal dominant; AR, autosomal recessive; CaSR, Ca²⁺/Mg²⁺ sensing receptor; ClC-Ka, basolateral Cl⁻ channel; ClC-Kb, basolateral Cl⁻ channel; NKCC2, Na⁺, K⁺, 2Cl⁻ co-transporter; ROMK, renal outer medullary potassium channel.

Table 18-3 HEREDITARY TUBULOPATHIES CAUSED BY TRANSPORT DEFECTS IN THE DISTAL CONVOLUTED TUBULE

Disorder	Defective Gene	Locus	Defective Protein	Localization of Defect	Mode of Inheritance	Clinical Features	OMIM No.*
Gitelman syndrome	SLC12A3 CLCNKB	16q13 1p36	Na+-Cl- cotransporter, TSC (NCCT) Cl- channel, ClC-Kb	Luminal Basolateral	AR	Mild renal salt wasting, hypokalemia, hypochloremic metabolic alkalosis, muscle weakness, tetany, hypomagnesemia, hypocalciuria	263800
Hypomagnesemia with secondary hypocalcemia	TRPM6	9q22	Mg^{2+} channel, TRPM6	Luminal	AR	Severe hypomagnesemia, hypocalcemia, mental retardation, epilepsy	602014
AD hypomagnesemia	KCNA1	12p13	K+ channel, Kv1.1	Luminal	AD	Severe hypomagnesemia, episodic ataxia	160120
Isolated AR hypomagnesemia	EGF	4q25	Pro-EGF	Basolateral	AR	Severe hypomagnesemia, mental retardation, epilepsy	611718
Isolated dominant hypomagnesemia	FXYD2	11q23	γ subunit of Na+, K+-ATPase	Basolateral	AD	Severe hypomagnesemia, hypocalciuria	154020
Maturity onset diabetes of the young, type 5	HNF1B	17q12	HNF1B	Nuclear/ basolateral	AD	Hypomagnesemia, cystic kidneys, diabetes mellitus	137920
EAST, SESAME syndrome	KCNJ10	1q23	K+ channel, Kir4.1	Basolateral	AR	Hypomagnesemia, hypocalciuria, epilepsy, ataxia, sensorineural deafness	612780
Pseudohypoaldosteronism type 2 (Gordon syndrome)	WNK4 WNK1	17q21 12p13	WNK4 WNK1	Cytoplasmic/ luminal	AD	Thiazide-sensitive hypertension, hyperkalemia, hyperchloremic metabolic acidosis	601844 605232

*Online Mendelian Inheritance in Man (database at http://www.ncbi.nlm.nih.gov/Omim)

AR, autosomal recessive; AD, autosomal dominant; ClC-kb, basolateral Cl- channel; EAST, epilepsy, ataxia, sensorineural deafness and tubulopathy; EGF, epidermal growth factor; HNF1B, hepatocyte nuclear factor 1B; NKCC2, Na+, K+, 2Cl- co-transporter; SESAME, seizures, sensorineural deafness, ataxia, mental retardation, and electrolyte imbalance; WNK, with no K [lysine] serine-threonine protein kinase.

18

TABLE 18-4 HEREDITARY TUBULOPATHIES CAUSED BY TRANSPORT DEFECTS IN THE CORTICAL COLLECTING DUCT

Disorder	Defective Gene	Locus	Defective Protein	Cell Type Involved	Localization of Defect	Clinical Features	OMIM No.*
Distal RTA (Type 1)							
AD distal RTA	SLC4A1	17q21-22	AE1	α-Intercalated	Basolateral	Mild metabolic acidosis, hypokalemia, hypercalciuria, hypocitraturia, nephrolithiasis, nephrocalcinosis, rickets or osteomalacia	179800
AR distal RTA	SLC4A1	17q21-22	AE1	α-Intercalated	Basolateral	Metabolic acidosis, hemolytic anemia (Southeast Asia only)	602722
AR distal RTA with deafness	ATP6V1B1	2p13	B_1 subunit of H^+-ATPase	α-Intercalated	Luminal	Early metabolic acidosis, nephrocalcinosis, vomiting, dehydration, growth retardation, rickets, bilateral sensorineural hearing loss	267300
AR distal RTA without or with late-onset deafness	ATP6VOI4	7q33	a4 subunit of H^+-ATPase	α-Intercalated	Luminal	Early metabolic acidosis, nephrocalcinosis, vomiting, dehydration, growth retardation, rickets, late-onset sensorineural hearing loss or normal hearing	267300
Mixed proximal and distal RTA (type 3)	CA2	8q22	CAII	Proximal tubule and α-intercalated	Cytoplasm	Metabolic acidosis, hypokalemia, osteopetrosis, blindness, deafness, early nephrocalcinosis	259730
Hyperkalemic RTA Type 4							
AD pseudohypoaldosteronism type 1	MR	4q31	Mineralocorticoid receptor	Principal	Cytoplasm	Mild hyponatremia, hyperkalemia, metabolic acidosis	600983
AR pseudohypoaldosteronism type 1	SCNN1A SCNN1B SCNN1C	12p13,1 16p13 16p12	Na^+ channel ENaC (α, β, γ subunits)	Principal	Luminal	Neonatal salt wasting, severe dehydration, hyperkalemic metabolic acidosis, hyponatremia, respiratory disease	264350
Nephrogenic Diabetes Insipidus							
X-linked NDI	AVPR2	Xq28	V2R	Principal	Basolateral	Polydipsia, polyuria, hyposthenuria, hypernatremic dehydration, failure to thrive, neurologic deficit	304800
AR or ADNDI	AQP2	12q13	H_2O channel, AQP2	Principal	Luminal	Polydipsia, polyuria, hyposthenuria, hypernatremic dehydration, failure to thrive, neurologic deficit	125800
NSIAD	AVPR2	Xq28	V2R	Principal	Basolateral	Hyponatremia, seizures, hypertonic urine	300539

*Online Mendelian Inheritance in Man (database at http://www.ncbi.nlm.nih.gov/Omim).
AD, autosomal dominant; AE1, anion exchanger 1; AQP2, aquaporin 2; AR, autosomal recessive; CAII, carbonic anhydrase II; ENaC, epithelial Na^+ channel; NDI, nephrogenic diabetes insipidus; NSIAD, nephrogenic syndrome of inappropriate diuresis; RTA, renal tubular acidosis; V2R, vasopressin type 2 receptor.

in the principal cell of the cortical collecting duct (CCD), and mild volume depletion secondary to Na^+ loss results in secondary hyperaldosteronism that increases K^+ secretion.[6,7]

pRTA occurs either as a manifestation of a generalized proximal tubular dysfunction (Fanconi syndrome) or as an isolated entity. Inheritance of isolated pRTA is autosomal recessive and occurs consistently in association with ocular abnormalities, including glaucoma, band keratopathy, and cataracts (Table 18-1 and Fig. 18-1).[8-10] Additional manifestations include short stature, calcification of the basal ganglia, and mental retardation (see later discussion).[4,9]

Molecular Pathophysiology

Normally, most (80%–90%) of the filtered load of HCO_3^- is reabsorbed in the proximal tubule. Several membrane transport proteins participate in acid–base handling in the proximal tubule (Fig. 18-1).[5-7] H^+ and HCO_3^- are formed in the proximal tubular cell as a result of the action of intracellular carbonic anhydrase II (CAII). H^+ efflux from cell to lumen occurs via the epical Na^+/H^+ exchanger (NHE3) and to a small extent via the apical H^+-ATPase pump. HCO_3^- exit to blood is mediated by the basolateral membrane Na^+- HCO_3^- cotransporter (NBC1).

The Na^+/HCO_3^- cotransporter NBC1 (Fig. 18-1), encoded by the *SLC4A4* gene located on chromosome 4q21, has been implicated in autosomal recessive proximal RTA.[8,9] NBC1 belongs to the HCO_3^- transporter superfamily, to which the Cl^-/HCO_3^- exchanger also belongs.[5,11] Igarashi et al[8] identified two homozygous missense mutations in kidney NBC1 in two individuals with autosomal recessive pRTA and ocular abnormalities (Table 18-1). Both patients had cataracts, glaucoma, and band keratopathy. A number of other mutations have subsequently been described.[12] In addition to reduced functional activity, defects of intracellular trafficking have been demonstrated for some of these mutations.[12,13] It is possible that defective corneal NBC1 function in these patients results in impaired HCO_3^- transport, which in turn leads to abnormal calcium carbonate deposition in the cornea and band keratopathy.[9,10]

Clinical Features

The most prominent clinical feature of pRTA is failure to thrive. Other manifestations, which are related to untreated hypokalemia, include polyuria, polydipsia, dehydration, vomiting, anorexia, constipation, and muscle weakness (Table 18-1).[5,6] Hypercalciuria, nephrocalcinosis, and nephrolithiasis typically are not observed. Metabolic bone disease usually occurs in patients with Fanconi syndrome and is attributed to hypophosphatemia and impaired vitamin D metabolism, but may also be induced by the bone Ca^{2+}-depleting effect of chronic acidosis in isolated pRTA.[4,9]

The diagnosis of pRTA is usually straightforward and can be based on several simple laboratory data. These include (1) normal anion gap, hyperchloremic metabolic acidosis; (2) hypokalemia; (3) low urine pH during acidemia; and (4) a negative urinary anion gap (calculated as $[Na^+]+[K^+]-[Cl^-]$) indicating substantial urinary ammonium concentration, in the absence of extrarenal losses of HCO_3^- such as gastroenteritis[14] (as opposed to the positive urinary anion gap in distal RTA; see later discussion). Although usually not necessary, demonstration of increased (>15%) fractional excretion of HCO_3^- by the HCO_3^- titration curve can support the diagnosis. Children with pRTA require large doses of alkali (up to 20 mEq/kg/day). Hypokalemia should be treated by correcting hypovolemia and by using KCl supplements.[14]

Hereditary Aminoacidurias

Only negligible amounts of amino acids are normally present in the final urine, reflecting very efficient reabsorption mechanisms for these organic solutes in the proximal tubule. Aminoacidurias are a group of disorders in which a single amino acid or a group of amino acids are excreted in excess amounts in the urine.[15] The defective tubular reabsorption is assumed to result from a genetic defect in a specific transport system that directs the reabsorption of these amino acids under normal conditions. Some of these disorders also involve a similar transport abnormality in the intestine. As opposed to inborn errors of amino acid metabolism, in which plasma levels of amino acids are elevated, resulting in overflow aminoaciduria, plasma levels of amino acids in hereditary aminoacidurias are largely normal. The aminoacidurias are generally categorized into five major groups according to the group-specific transport pathway presumed to be affected.[15] Discussed in this chapter are the cationic aminoacidurias, classic cystinuria and lysinuric protein intolerance (LPI), as well as the neutral aminoaciduria, Hartnup disease (Table 18-1 and Fig. 18-1). The genetic defects in these three membrane transport disorders, which are associated with significant morbidity, have been identified.

Classic Cystinuria
General Characteristics
Cystinuria is a disorder of amino acid transport characterized by excessive urinary excretion of cystine and the dibasic amino acids lysine, arginine, and ornithine.[15] The pathogenic mechanism of cystinuria is defective transepithelial transport of these amino acids in the proximal tubule and the small intestine.[15-17] The high-affinity, low-capacity amino acid transport system shared by cystine and the dibasic amino acids (i.e., $b^{0,+}$) (Fig. 18-2) is defective in classic cystinuria.[15,18]

The very low solubility of cystine in the urine results in cystine stone formation in homozygous patients. Urinary cystine calculi may produce considerable morbidity, including urinary obstruction; colic; infection; and in severe cases, loss of kidney function. Cystinuria accounts for 1% to 2% of all urolithiasis and 6% to 8% of urolithiasis in children.[18]

Classic cystinuria is inherited in an autosomal recessive fashion. It is a common disorder with an overall prevalence of one in 7000 to one in 15,000 and an estimated gene frequency of 0.01.[16] A very high prevalence, one in 2500, is observed in Israeli Jews of Libyan origin.[15,18]

Cystinuria has been classified into three phenotypes based on the degree of intestinal uptake of cystine by homozygotes and the level of urinary dibasic amino acids in heterozygotes.[18,19] Type I cystinuria is inherited as an autosomal recessive trait, and obligate heterozygotes have normal urinary amino acid profiles. In

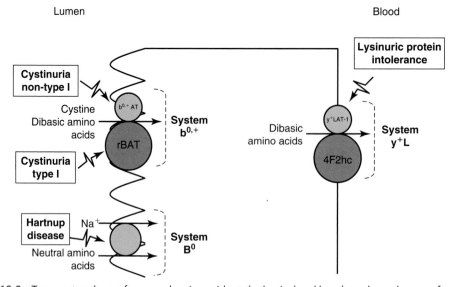

Figure 18-2 Transport pathways for several amino acids at the luminal and basolateral membranes of a proximal tubular cell. *Large circles* represent the heavy subunits and *small circles* the light subunits of the heteromeric dibasic amino acid transporters $b^{0,+}$ and y^{+}L. Depicted are hereditary aminoacidurias cause by defects in these transporters.

contrast, obligate heterozygotes for type II and type III cystinuria show various degrees of hyperexcretion of cystine and dibasic amino acids in the urine. In addition, genetic compounds of cystinuria, such as types I/III, can occur.[19]

Molecular Pathophysiology

Type I cystinuria is caused by mutations in the gene *SLCA3A1* localized to chromosome 2p21. The gene encodes a protein termed rBAT, which constitutes the heavy subunit of the proximal tubular, brush-border membrane-bound, heteromeric dibasic amino acid transporter $b^{0,+}$ (Fig. 18-2).[15,20] To date, more than 130 different rBAT mutations have been reported in patients with type I cystinuria.[18] These mutations include nonsense, missense, splice site, frameshift mutations and large deletions.[18,21] Cystinuria types II and III are caused by mutations in the gene *SLC7A9*, which is localized to chromosome 19q13.1 and encodes the $b^{0,+}$ AT protein that constitutes the light subunit of the heteromeric amino acid transporter $b^{0,+}$ (Fig. 18-2).[5,22] To date, more than 90 different mutations have been identified in non–type I cystinuria patients.[18]

Clinical Features

The simplest diagnostic test in cystinuria is the microscopic examination of the urinary sediment of a freshly voided morning urine.[16] The presence of typical flat hexagonal cystine crystals is diagnostic. The best screening procedure is the cyanide–nitroprusside test.[16] The definite test is a measurement of cystine and the dibasic amino acids concentrations by ion exchange chromatography.

Cystine stones are radiopaque because of the density of the sulfur molecule, and on radiography, they appear smooth. Cystine also may act as nidus for calcium oxalate, so mixed stones may be found.[15]

The disease usually presents with renal colic. Occasionally, infection, hypertension, or renal failure may be the first manifestation (Table 18-1).[16,17] Most patients have recurrent stone formation. Cystinuric patients who receive a kidney transplant have normal urinary cystine and dibasic amino acid excretion after transplantation.[15]

Treatment

Cystine crystalluria occurs when the cystine content of the urine exceeds 300 mg/L at a pH of 4.5 to 7.0. Cystine solubility increases sharply at a urine pH above 7.0.[16] The major therapeutic approaches to cystinuria are designed to increase the solubility of cystine, reduce excretion cystine, and convert cystine to more soluble compounds.[16,18] Therapies used in the management of cystinuria include the following:

1. Increased oral fluid intake to increase urine volume and cystine solubility. Because patients with cystinuria excrete 0.5 to 1.0 g/day of cystine, intake of at least twice normal maintenance fluid volume for age could be required to keep the urinary cystine concentration below 300 mg/L.[15,16]
2. Oral alkali in addition to high fluid intake to further increase cystine solubility in the urine.[15] A urine pH of 7.5 to 8.0 can be maintained by the provision of 1 to 2 mEq/kg/day of bicarbonate or citrate in divided doses. Because high sodium intake increases cystine excretion, potassium citrate is preferred.[16] Because urine alkalinization may result in formation of mixed Ca^{2+}-containing stones, adherence to high fluid intake is crucial.
3. Na^{+} restriction to reduce cystine excretion. Dietary Na^{+} restriction is recommended in patients with cystinuria because urinary excretion of cystine and dibasic amino acids correlates with urinary Na^{+} excretion.[23]
4. Pharmacologic therapy to increase cystine solubility and decrease cystine excretion. The sulfhydryl-binding compound d-penicillamine (β-dimethylcysteine) leads to the formation of the mixed disulfide penicillamine–cysteine after a disulfide exchange reaction. This mixed disulfide is far more water soluble than cystine. Unfortunately, penicillamine produces serious side effects, including rashes, fever, arthralgia, nephrotic

syndrome, pancytopenia, and loss of taste.[16,24] Mercaptopropionyl glycine (MPG), another agent undergoing a disulfide exchange reaction, is as effective as d-penicillamine in the treatment of patients with cystinuria. Because of the lower toxicity of MPG, this compound is the pharmacologic agent of choice in the therapy of cystinuria.[18,25] It has been proposed that meso-1,3 dimercaptosuccinic acid (DMSA), an additional compound forming disulfide linkage with cysteine, might also be a useful therapeutic agent in those with cystinuria.[15]

5. Urologic procedures that have been used to treat cysteine stones include chemolysis of stones by irrigation through a percutaneous nephrostomy, extracorporal shockwave lithotripsy, and lithotomy.[18]

Lysinuric Protein Intolerance

General Characteristics

Lysinuric protein intolerance (LPI) is a rare autosomal recessive disorder characterized by excessive urinary excretion of dibasic amino acids (especially lysine), normal cystine excretion, and poor intestinal absorption of dibasic amino acids.[15] Plasma values of dibasic amino acids are subnormal. The disease is relatively common in Finland, where the prevalence of the disease is one 60,000, and in Italy. Homozygous patients show massive dibasic aminoaciduria, as well as hyperammonemia after a protein overload. The clinical manifestations in homozygotes for LPI are protein malnutrition and postprandial hyperammonemia. They include failure to thrive, marked protein intolerance, vomiting, diarrhea, hepatosplenomegaly, muscle hypotonia, interstitial lung disease, osteoporosis, seizures, and coma (Table 18-1).[15,26]

Molecular Pathophysiology

The pathogenic mechanism of LPI appears to be defective, high-affinity, dibasic amino acid transport system y⁺L (Fig. 18-2) at the basolateral membrane of renal and intestinal epithelial cells, resulting in impaired efflux of these amino acids from cell to interstitium.[15,26] Non-epithelial cells such as hepatocytes, granulocytes, and cultures akin fibroblasts from patients with LPI also show impaired transport of dibasic amino acids. The defective hepatic transport of dibasic amino acids is associated with disturbances in the urea cycle and consequent hyperammonemia.[26]

LPI is caused by mutations in the gene *SLC7A7* encoding y⁺LAT-1, a member of the family of light subunits that combine with 4F2hc (a heavy subunit) to form heteromeric amino acid transporters.[5] The 4F2hc / y⁺LAT-1 transporter has been shown to have the activity of amino acid transport system y⁺L that is responsible for the efflux of basic amino acids at the basolateral plasma membrane of epithelial cells (Fig. 18-2).[27] The *SLC7A7* gene is localized to chromosome 14q11-13. To date, more than 40 *SLC7A7* mutations, spread along the entire gene, have been found in LPI patients from different ethnic groups.[28,29]

Treatment

Therapy of patients with LPI consists of protein restriction to prevent hyperammonemia, as well as oral supplements of arginine, ornithine, and (most important) citrulline.[30] Administration of the latter amino acid, which corrects the hepatic deficiency in ornithine and arginine, results in clinical improvement and catch-up growth.

Hartnup Disease

General Characteristics

Hartnup disease, which may have afflicted Julius Caesar and his family,[31] was first recognized in two siblings in England in 1956.[32] This disease is characterized by intestinal malabsorption and massive aminoaciduria of the neutral monoamino monocarboxylic amino acids alanine, serine, threonine, valine, leucine, isoleucine, phenylalanine, tyrosine, tryptophan, histidine, glutamine, and asparagine (see Table 18-1).[33] Most patients also have increased excretion of indolic compounds that originate in the gut from bacterial degradation of tryptophan.[33] Transport of other neutral amino acids, including cystine, imino acids, glycine, and β-amino acids, is unaffected. The disease is inherited as an autosomal recessive trait and has an estimated incidence of one in 20,000 live births. Heterozygotes have normal urinary acid excretion under physiologic conditions. Clinical features in homozygotes may include photosensitive rash, cerebellar ataxia, and a variety of psychiatric manifestations resembling the features of pellagra (Table 18-1).[23] These pellagra-like manifestations are primarily caused by intestinal malabsorption and urinary loss of tryptophan, an amino acid that is required for niacin synthesis. The diagnosis should be suspected in any patient with pellagra who has no history of niacin or nicotinamide deficiency and should be made by chromatographic analysis of the urine.[33]

Molecular Pathophysiology

A defect in the broad-specificity neutral, α-amino acid transport mechanism in the renal and intestinal brush-border membrane was presumed to be the pathogenic mechanism underlying this disorder.[15] The transport characteristics and the epithelial distribution of the Na^+-dependent neutral amino acid transport B^o (see Fig. 18-2) have led to the conclusion that this transporter is the defective one in Hartnup disorder. In 2001, the gene responsible for Hartnup disease was localized to chromosome 5p15.[34] Subsequently, Bröer's group[35] cloned from the syntenic region in the mouse the B^oAT1 (*SLC6A19*) gene. This *SLC6* gene encodes a Na^+-dependent neutral amino acid transporter, which is expressed in the brush-border membrane of the early proximal tubule and the intestine and corresponds to the B^o transport system.[36]

In 2004, two groups[37,38] cloned the human *SLCA19* gene from chromosome 5p15 and have found several mutations in this gene in British, Japanese, and Australian patients with Hartnup disease, thereby identifying *SLCA19* as the disease-causing gene. To date, a total of 17 mutations have been identified that cause Hartnup disorder.[15] Interestingly, it has been demonstrated[15] that most of the probands with Hartnup disease analyzed so far display allelic heterogeneity in that they are compound heterozygotes for the *SLC6A19* mutation.

Treatment

Patients with Hartnup disease respond well to oral therapy with 40 to 100 mg/day of nicotinamide.[15] Oral administration of tryptophan ethylester, a lipid-soluble form of tryptophan, has been shown to increase serum tryptophan and reverse clinical symptoms in patients with Hartnup disease.[39]

Hereditary Glycosurias

Glycosurias are a group of disorders in which specific defects in glucose transporters in the renal tubule result in excretion of significant quantities of glucose in the urine.[15] This group includes hereditary isolated glycosuria and Fanconi-Bickel syndrome (Table 18-1 and Fig. 18-3).

Hereditary Isolated Glycosuria
General Characteristics

Hereditary isolated glycosuria is an abnormality in which variable amounts of glucose are excreted in the urine at normal concentrations of blood glucose.[15,40] The renal defect is specific for glucose, and there is no increase in the urinary excretion of other sugars. Renal glycosuria is a benign condition without symptoms or physical consequences except during pregnancy or prolonged starvation—when dehydration and ketosis may develop.[40] The metabolism, storage, and use of carbohydrates, as well as insulin secretion are normal. The condition exists from infancy throughout adult life, and diagnosis usually is done on routine urine analysis. The distinction between renal glycosuria and diabetes mellitus is made with a fasting blood glucose level and a glucose tolerance test. The genetic pattern in renal glycosuria is autosomal recessive.[15,40]

PROXIMAL CONVOLUTED TUBULE

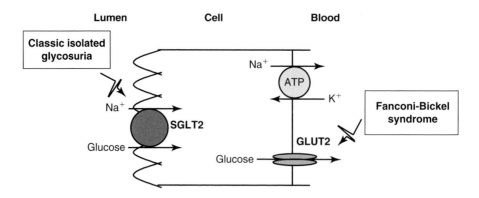

PROXIMAL STRAIGHT TUBULE

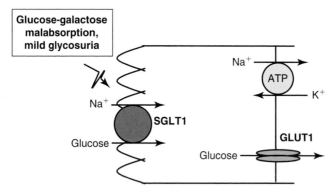

Figure 18-3 Schematic model for the distribution of glucose transporters in renal tubular epithelium. Glucose transport from lumen to cell in the proximal convoluted tubule and the proximal straight tubule is mediated by the luminal Na⁺-dependent glucose transporters SGLT2 and SGLT1, respectively. Glucose exit from cells in these two nephron segments occurs via the basolateral, facilitative Na⁺-independent glucose transporters GLUT2 and GLUT1, respectively. Depicted are hereditary glycosurias caused by defects in these transporters. (Adapted with permission from Zelikovic I. Aminoaciduria and glycosuria. In: Avner ED, Harmon N, Niaudet P, Yoshikawa N, eds. *Pediatric Nephrology*, 6th ed. Heidelberg: Springer-Verlag, 2009, pp. 889-927.)

Molecular Pathophysiology

Transport of glucose at the brush-border membrane of the convoluted segment of the proximal tubule occurs by a low-affinity, high-capacity Na⁺-glucose cotransporter, SGLT2 (Fig. 18-3), which reabsorbs the bulk (90%) of the filtered glucose.[15,41] The residual glucose reabsorption occurs in the straight segment of the proximal tubule by the high-affinity, low-capacity Na⁺-glucose cotransporter SGLT1.[41] Both SGLT2 and SGLT1 are members of the SLC5 Na⁺/glucose cotransport family.[41] Glucose exit from proximal tubular cells is mediated by the facilitative, Na⁺-independent glucose transporters GLUT2 and GLUT1, which belong to the SLC2 family of facilitative haxose transporters and are located in the basolateral membrane of the proximal convoluted and the proximal straight segments, respectively (Fig. 18-3).[15,42]

Hereditary isolated glycosuria is caused by mutations in the gene *SLC5A2*, which is located on chromosome 16p11.2 and encodes SGLT2 (Table 18-1 and Fig. 18-3). To date, more than 30 different *SLC5A2* mutations have been identified in patients with isolated glycosuria.[15,43,44] In some cases, the glycosuria in patients with *SLC5A2* mutations is accompanied by aminoaciduria, the pathophysiology of which is unknown.[44]

It is important to consider the relationships between renal glycosuria, a benign condition, and intestinal glucose–galactose malabsorption, a potentially lethal disease. Glucose–galactose malabsorption, an autosomal recessive disease, is characterized in homozygotes by a neonatal onset of severe watery diarrhea that results in death unless glucose and galactose are removed from the diet.[40] Glucose–galactose malabsorption is caused by mutations in the intestinal brush-border SGLT1 Na$^+$-glucose cotransporter.[45] Patients with glucose–galactose malabsorption who have been studied show a mild defect in renal tubular reabsorption of glucose.[15,40] In contrast, patients with isolated renal glycosuria show no defect in intestinal D-glucose absorption. This has indicated that the SGLT1 Na$^+$-glucose cotransporter affected in glucose–galactose malabsorption is shared between the intestine and the kidney (Fig. 18-3).

Fanconi-Bickel Syndrome

Mutations in the gene for GLUT2 (*SLC2A2*), the facilitative glucose transporter operating in all membranes of various tissues, including the hepatocyte and proximal convoluted tubule, are associated with glycosuria in the Fanconi-Bickel syndrome (Table 18-1 and Fig. 18-3).[15,46] This autosomal recessive disorder is characterized by hepatorenal glycogen accumulation, Fanconi syndrome including proximal RTA, fasting hypoglycemia, postprandial hyperglycemia, impaired utilization of glucose and galactose, rickets, and markedly stunted growth.[46,47] The renal loss of glucose is attributable to the transport defect for monosaccharides across the renal basolateral membrane, which also leads to accumulation of glucose and secondarily glycogen within proximal tubular cells, resulting in toxic effects on these cells. To date, more than 30 different mutations in *SLC2A2* have been detected in patients with Fanconi-Bickel syndrome.[47] Therapy of patients with Fanconi-Bickel syndrome is symptomatic and includes stabilization of glucose homeostasis and replacement of renal solute losses.

Loop of Henle

Bartter Syndrome

General Characteristics

Bartter syndrome is a group of closely related hereditary tubulopathies. All variants of the syndrome share several clinical characteristics, including renal salt wasting, hypokalemic metabolic alkalosis, hyperreninemic hyperaldosteronism with normal blood pressure, and hyperplasia of the juxtaglomerular apparatus.[48-50] All forms of the syndrome are transmitted as autosomal recessive traits.

Molecular Pathophysiology

Generally, Bartter syndrome results from defective transepithelial transport of Cl$^-$ in the thick ascending limb of the loop of Henle (TAL) or the distal convoluted tubule (DCT).[48,50] Transepithelial Cl$^-$ transport in the TAL is a complex process that involves coordinated interplay among the luminal, bumetanide-sensitive Na$^+$, K$^+$, 2Cl$^-$ co-transporter (NKCC2); the luminal, K$^+$ channel (renal outer medullary potassium channel [ROMK]); the basolateral Cl$^-$ channel (ClC-Kb); as well as other cotransporters and channels (Fig. 18-4).[48,51-53] Chloride is reabsorbed across the luminal membrane of the TAL cell by the activity of NKCC2. This cotransporter is driven by the low intracellular Na$^+$ and Cl$^-$ concentration generated by Na$^+$, K$^+$-ATPase and ClC-Kb, respectively. In addition, ROMK enables functioning of NKCC2 by recycling K$^+$ back to the renal tubular lumen. Normally, the lumen-to-cell flux of Cl$^-$ via the NKCC2 cotransporter in the TAL and the exit of K$^+$ from cell to lumen generate lumen-positive electrical potential, which in turn drives paracellular Ca^{2+} and Mg^{2+} transport from the lumen to the blood (Fig. 18-4). The Ca^{2+}/Mg^{2+}-sensing receptor (CaSR), a G protein–coupled receptor expressed in the basolateral membrane of the TAL,[54-56] also appears to participate in electrolyte and mineral handling in this nephron segment. Activation of the CaSR by hypercalcemia or

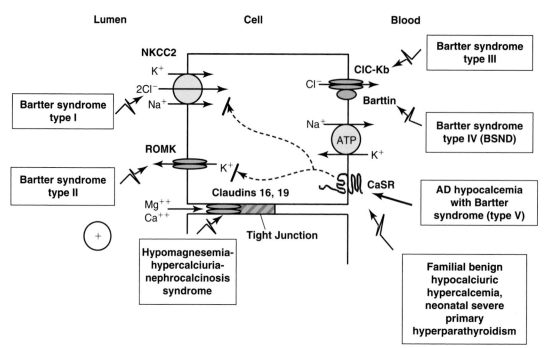

Figure 18-4   Transcellular and paracellular transport pathways in the TAL. Cl⁻ reabsorption across the luminal membrane occurs via the Na⁺, K⁺, 2Cl⁻ cotransporter (NKCC2). This cotransporter is driven by the low intracellular Na⁺ and Cl⁻ concentrations generated by the basolateral Na⁺, K⁺-ATPase and ClC-Kb, respectively. In addition, renal outer medullary potassium channel (ROMK) enables function of NKCC2 by recycling K⁺ back to the lumen. The lumen-positive electrical potential, which is generated by Cl entry into the cell and K⁺ exit from the cell, drives paracellular, claudin-16–, and claudin-19–mediated Ca^{2+} and Mg^{2+} transport from lumen to blood. Activation of the basolateral calcium sensing receptor (CaSR) by high concentrations of extracellular Ca^{2+} or Mg^{2+} triggers a series of intracellular signaling events, resulting in an inhibition of the luminal ROMK channel and the luminal NKCC2 channel. This in turn results in decreased NaCl reabsorption and (secondary to the reduction in the intra-luminal positive potential) increased urinary Ca^{2+} and Mg^{2+} excretion. Hereditary tubulopathies caused by defects in these transport mechanisms are depicted. AD, autosomal dominant; BSND, Bartter syndrome with deafness.

hypermagnesemia triggers a series of intracellular signaling events. This action inhibits NKCC2 and ROMK activity, decreases Cl⁻ reabsorption, reduces lumen positive voltage, and hence inhibits Mg^{2+} and Ca^{2+} reabsorption in the TAL, which results in urinary loss of these divalent cations (see later discussion) (Fig. 18-4).[54,55] Chloride transport in the DCT occurs primarily via the luminal, thiazide-sensitive NaCl cotransporter (TSC) (Fig. 18-5).[51,52] Cl⁻ exit to blood in the DCT is mediated via basolateral Cl⁻ channels.

The genetic variants of Bartter syndrome that have been identified include (Table 18-2 and Figs. 18-4 and 18-5):[48,49,57-60]

1. Bartter syndrome type I is caused by mutations in the NKCC2 gene, *SLC12A1*. This gene belongs to the family of electroneutral chloride-coupled cotransporter genes[61] and resides on chromosome 15q15-21. This genetic variant leads to antenatal Bartter syndrome, which is the most severe form of the disease. It is characterized by polyhydramnios, premature birth, life-threatening episodes of salt and water loss in the neonatal period, hypokalemic alkalosis and failure to thrive, as well as osteopenia, hypercalciuria, and early-onset nephrocalcinosis.[48,57,62]

2. Bartter syndrome type II is caused by mutations in the ROMK gene (*KCNJ1*), which is located on chromosome 11q24-25.[48] ROMK mutations lead to the clinical phenotype of antenatal Bartter syndrome.[58]

3. Bartter syndrome type III is caused by mutations in the ClC-Kb gene, *CLCNKB*.[59] This gene, which is located on chromosome 1p36, belongs to the family of genes encoding voltage-gated Cl⁻ channels.[48,50] Patients with

Lumen   Cell   Blood

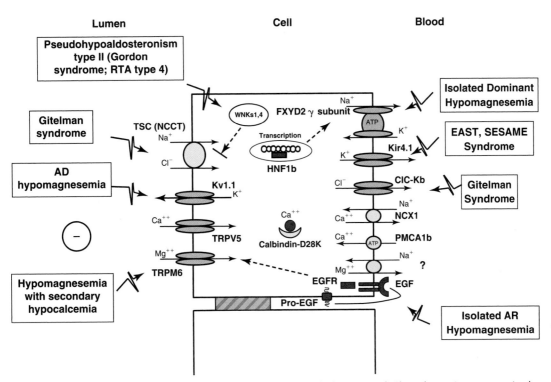

Figure 18-5 Transport mechanisms in the distal convoluted tubule. Na$^+$ and Cl$^-$ reabsorption occurs via the luminal, thiazide-sensitive NaCl cotransporter (TSC; NCCT), the activity of which is modulated, among other factors, by the action of the intracellular serine/threonine protein kinases WNK4 and WNK1. Na$^+$ exits the cell via the basolateral Na$^+$, K$^+$-ATPase and Cl$^-$ exit to blood is mediated by the basolateral Cl$^-$ channel ClC-Kb. Ca^{2+} enters the cell via the luminal Ca^{2+} channel TRPV5, is transported transcellularly by vitamin D–dependant calbindin-D28K and exits the cell via the Ca^{2+}-ATPase, PMCA1B, and the Na$^+$/Ca^{2+} exchange, NCX1. Mg^{2+} enters the cell via the luminal Mg^{2+} channel, TRPM6, and exits the cell via a putative basolateral Na$^+$/Mg^{2+} exchanger. TRPM6-mediated Mg^{2+} entry into the cell is promoted by the negative intracellular membrane potential, which is maintained by the activity of the Na$^+$, K$^+$-ATPase as well as by the action of the luminal K$^+$ channel Kv1.1 and the basolateral K$^+$ channel Kir 4.1. The latter channel recycles K$^+$ entering the cell via the Na$^+$, K$^+$-ATPase back into the interstitium. The γ subunit of Na$^+$, K$^+$-ATPase, FXYD2, which is transcriptionally regulated by the hepatocyte nuclear factor 1b (HNF1b), modulates the activity of Na$^+$, K$^+$-ATPase by affecting its affinity to K$^+$ and Na$^+$. The basolateral EGF receptor (EGFR) activates TRPM6 by shuttling it from intracellular compartments to the apical membrane. Hereditary tubulopathies caused by defects in these transport mechanisms are depicted. AD, autosomal dominant; AR, autosomal recessive.

CLCNKB mutation usually have classic Bartter syndrome, which occurs in infancy or early childhood. It is characterized by marked salt wasting and hypokalemia, leading to polyuria, polydipsia, volume contraction, muscle weakness, and growth retardation. Hypercalciuria and nephrocalcinosis may occur.[48,50]

4. Bartter syndrome type IV is caused by mutations in the barttin gene, *BSND*. Barttin serves as a β subunit for ClC-Ka and ClC-Kb chloride channels (see Fig. 18-4).[63,64] A hereditary defect in barttin leads to antenatal Bartter syndrome associated with sensorineural deafness and renal failure. Barttin colocalizes with the subunit of the Cl$^-$ channel in basolateral membranes of the renal tubule and inner ear epithelium.[64]

5. Bartter syndrome type V is caused by gain-of-function mutations in the gene *CASR*, encoding CaSR (Fig. 18-4). This genetic defect leads to autosomal dominant hypocalcemia with Bartter syndrome.[65,66] As indicated earlier, activation of the basolateral CaSR inhibits the luminal NKCC2 cotransporter and the ROMK channel, resulting in decreased NaCl reabsorption and increased urinary Ca^{2+} and Mg^{2+} excretion.

6. Gitelman syndrome is caused by mutations in the gene *SLC12A3* encoding the thiazide-sensitive NaCl cotransporter (NCCT) operating in the DCT (see later discussion).

Recent data, however, have suggested that the genotype–phenotype correlation is not so clear cut and that phenotypic overlap may occur. It has been shown that mutations in *CLCNKB* can also cause phenotypes that overlap with either antenatal or Gitelman syndrome.[67,68]

The loss-of-function mutations in the genes of TAL cell transporters in Bartter syndrome lead to derangements in tubular handling of minerals observed in this syndrome.[48,51-53] Normally, the NKCC2-mediated entry of Cl^- from lumen to the TAL cell and the ROMK-mediated K^+ exit from cell to lumen generate lumen-positive electrical potential, which in turn drives paracellular Ca^{2+} and Mg^{2+} transport from lumen to blood (see earlier) (Fig. 18-4). Impaired function of MKCC2 or ROMK in antenatal Bartter syndrome results in reduction of intra-luminal positive charge, which leads to hypercalciuria and nephrocalcinosis. However, normal serum Ca^{2+} levels are maintained. Possible mechanisms responsible for the maintenance of normocalcemia include a 1.25(OH) vitamin tD –induced increase in intestinal Ca^{2+} absorption and parathyroid hormone (PTH)– induced retrieval of Ca^{2+} from bone.[51,52] The transport defect in the TAL should have resulted in inhibition of Mg^{2+} reabsorption and hypomagnesemia. The absence of hypomagnesemia in patients with antenatal Bartter syndrome has been explained by compensatory stimulation of Mg^{2+} reabsorption in the distal convoluted tubule induced by the high level of aldosterone, which is a characteristic of the syndrome.[48]

Therapy

Treatment of patients with all variants of Bartter syndrome involves correction of hypovolemia as well as supplementation of lost electrolytes. This therapy includes increased oral fluid and salt intake and KCl supplements. Occasionally, Aldactone or amiloride (or both) can be added to correct the hypokalemia. Indomethacin therapy should be used only in neonatal Bartter syndrome or severe cases of Bartter syndrome unresponsive to other therapies. However, attention should be paid to potential gastrointestinal or renal toxicity of this drug. Patients with Gitelman syndrome should also receive $MgSO_4$ or $MgCl_2$ supplementation.

Familial Hypomagnesemia with Hypercalciuria and Nephrocalcinosis

General Characteristics

Familial hypomagnesemia with hypercalciuria and nephrocalcinosis syndrome (FHHNC, Michellis-Castrillo syndrome) is a rare autosomal recessive disorder.[69,70] The disease is characterized by marked renal Mg^{2+} wasting, which leads to severe hypomagnesemia.[53,70] Patients also have hypercalciuria, resulting in nephrocalcinosis and renal failure. In addition, ocular abnormalities, such as myopia and horizontal nystagmus, may occur.[53]

Molecular Pathophysiology

In 1999, Simon et al[71] first reported that FHHNC was caused by mutations in the gene *CLDN16* (also known as *PCLN-1*). The gene encodes a protein, claudin-16 (paracellin-1), that is located in the paracellular tight junctions of the TAL (Fig. 18-4) and is a member of the claudin family of tight junction proteins.[72] Claudin-16, which appears to regulate the paracellular transport of Mg^{2+} in the TAL, is the first reported tight junction protein involved in ion resorption. Mutations in the gene *CLDN16* render the claudin-16 protein either nonfunctional[71,73] or, when occurring in the PDZ domain, cause mislocalization of the protein to lysosomes.[74] The disease mutations found in claudin-16 result in an increase in the permeability of the tight junction to anions, thereby dissipating the transepithelial voltage gradient and selectively impeding Mg^{2+} (and Ca^{2+}) resorption.[75] Despite the concomitant impairment in Ca^{2+} reabsorption, these patients maintain normal serum Ca^{2+}, most likely by using alternative routes of renal and intestinal Ca^{2+} reclamation.

More recently, FHHNC associated with severe ocular abnormalities has been shown to be caused also by mutations in *CLDN19*, the gene encoding the tight junction protein claudin-19 (Fig. 18-4).[76] Claudin-19 colocalizes with claudin-16 in the TAL, the two proteins interact in conferring a tight junction with cation selectivity and hence control divalent ion reabsorption.[77,78]

Autosomal Dominant Hypocalcemic Hypercalciuria

Normally, extracellular Ca^{2+} regulates PTH activity by interacting with the CaSR located on the surface of parathyroid cells.[79] Autosomal dominant hypocalcemic hypercalciuria (ADHH) is caused by heterozygous activating mutations of the CaSR gene, which cause the receptor to be hyperresponsive to extracellular calcium, thereby decreasing PTH production.[79,80] Patients with ADHH have mild hypocalcemia, low PTH levels, and occasionally hypomagnesemia.[65,66] In addition, the activation of renal CaSR inhibits Ca^{2+} and Mg^{2+} reabsorption in the TAL, leading to hypercalciuria and hypermagnesiuria (Fig. 18-4). In some cases, because of the effect of CaSR on TAL transporters, ADHH is associated with Bartter-like syndrome (Bartter syndrome type V; see earlier discussion).

Familial Benign Hypocalciuric Hypercalcemia and Neonatal Severe Primary Hyperparathyroidism

Patients with familial benign hypocalciuric hypercalcemia (FHH) or severe neonatal primary hyperparathyroidism (NSHPT) have inactivating mutations in the CaSR gene that are heterozygous and homozygous, respectively.[79,81] These mutations shift the setpoint of Ca^{2+} in this condition, blunting the normal ability to reduce PTH secretion in response to elevated Ca^{2+} and Mg^{2+} levels and directly increasing renal Ca^{2+} and Mg^{2+} reabsorption (Table 18-2 and Fig. 18-4).[79,82] Whereas FHH is a mild disease inherited in an autosomal dominant fashion, NSHPT is a severe, life threatening condition caused by homozygous CaSR mutations.[81] The genetic defect in both diseases "leads" to elevated or "inappropriately normal" PTH levels, hypercalcemia, hypermagnesemia, and an inappropriate reduction in urinary Ca^{2+} and Mg^{2+} excretion. Renal hyperabsorption of divalent cations is partly caused by increased circulating PTH levels and partly by reduced functionality of the CaSR in the TAL.[83] The persistence of hypocalciuria even after parathyroidectomy in FHH patients confirms the role of CaSR in regulating renal calcium handling.[84]

Distal Convoluted Tubule

Gitelman Syndrome

General Characteristics

Gitelman syndrome, which is a variant of Bartter syndrome, is characterized by a mild clinical presentation in older children and adults.[48,49] Patients may be asymptomatic and present with transient muscle weakness, abdominal pain, symptoms of neuromuscular irritability, or unexplained hypokalemia. Hypocalciuria and hypomagnesemia are typical (Table 18-3).[48,49]

Molecular Pathophysiology

Gitelman syndrome is usually caused by mutations in the gene *SLC12A3* encoding the DCT apical membrane thiazide-sensitive NCCT (Fig. 18-5).[60] Hence, the Gitelman phenotype is mimicked by prolonged treatment with thiazide, a potent NCC blocker. However, mutations in the gene *CLCNKB* encoding the basolateral membrane Cl^- channel ClC-Kb have also been reported to result in Gitelman syndrome phenotype.[67,68]

The exact mechanism underlying the hypocalciuria and hypomagnesemia in Gitelman syndrome remain to be elucidated. It has been hypothesized that the loss-of-function mutation in NCCT causes hypocalciuria by the same mechanism as thiazides (Fig. 18-5).[5,85] According to this hypothesis, impaired Na^+ reabsorption across the luminal membrane of the DCT cell, coupled with continued exit of intracellular Cl^- through basolateral ClC-Kb channels, causes the cell to hyperpolarize. This in turn stimulates entry of Ca^{2+} into the cell via the luminal voltage-activated Ca^{2+} channels, TRPV5.[85,86] In addition, the lowering of intracellular Na^+ concentration facilitates Ca^{2+} exit via the basolateral Na^+/Ca^{2+} exchanger, NCX1, and the Ca^{2+}-ATPase, PMCA1b.[86] Other studies have suggested that the hypocalciuria in Gitelman syndrome or in chronic thiazide administration is secondary to volume contraction, which increases proximal tubular Na^{2+} reabsorption and hence facilitates hyperabsorption of Ca^{2+} in the proximal tubule.[52,87] The reasons for renal Mg^{2+} wasting and hypomagnesemia typical of Gitelman syndrome are unknown.

Pseudohypoaldosteronism Type II
General Characteristics

Pseudohypoaldosteronism type II (PHAII), or Gordon syndrome, is an autosomal dominant disorder characterized by hypertension, hyperkalemia, hyperchloremic metabolic acidosis (RTA type 4; see later), and low plasma aldosterone levels.[88-90] The underlying pathogenic mechanism is chloride-dependent Na^+ retention, and the disease is highly responsive to low-dose thiazide treatment.[89,90]

Molecular Pathophysiology

Pseudohypoaldosteronism type II is caused by mutations in the genes encoding the WNKI and WNK4 serine-threonine protein kinases, which are particular subtypes of these kinases "lacking" a lysine residue at the active site (WNK means with no K [lysine]) (Table 18-3 and Fig. 18-5).[91,92] WNK1 and WNK4 serve as both intracellular [Cl^-] sensors and ion transport regulators[92,93] with an inhibitory activity on the thiazide-sensitive NCCT of the DCT (Fig. 18-5). Both genetic types of PHAII increase surface expression and activity of the NCCT in the DCT.[89,94] Consequent decreased Na^+ delivery to the CCD results in reduced Na^+ reabsorption, which in turn results in decreased electrogenic secretion of H^+ and K^+.

Hypomagnesemia with Secondary Hypocalcemia

Hypomagnesemia with secondary hypocalcemia (HSH) is a rare autosomal recessive disorder that is characterized by very low serum Mg^{2+} and Ca^{2+} levels and manifests in early infancy with seizures, tetany, and muscle spasms (Table 18-3).[53,95,96] Affected patients have evidence of both defective intestinal absorption and impaired renal reabsorption of Mg^{2+}.[95,96] The hypocalcemia, which is secondary to Mg^{2+} deficiency–induced parathyroid failure, is resistant to Ca^{2+} or vitamin D therapy.[52] The hypomagnesemia and the hypocalcemia respond to large doses of oral or parenteral Mg^{2+}.[96] The disorder is caused by a mutation in the gene *TRPM6*, which is localized on chromosome 9q22, and encodes the transient receptor potential Mg^{2+} channel, TRPM6, that is exclusively expressed in the apical membrane of the DCT (Fig. 18-5) and the small intestine.[95,96] TRPM6 appears to constitute the apical Mg^{2+} entry channel in transcellular Mg^{2+} reabsorption in the DCT.[53,97] Although the hypomagnesemia of HSH appears to be primarily the result of deficient TRPM6-mediated intestinal Mg^{2+} absorption, there is also evidence for renal Mg^{2+} leak.[95,96]

Isolated Dominant Hypomagnesemia

Isolated dominant hypomagnesemia (IDH) is a rare disorder characterized by renal Mg^{2+} wasting, mild hypomagnesemic symptoms, and as hypocalciuria (Table 18-3).[53,98] Linkage analysis has mapped the syndrome to chromosome 11q23.[53] Subsequent molecular analysis[97] has identified the gene *FXYD2* encoding the Na^+, K^+-ATPase γ subunit, also termed *FXYD2*, as the mutated gene in this disorder (Fig. 18-5). The FXYD2 protein is localized on the basolateral membrane of the DCT (Fig. 18-5).[99] Isolated renal Mg^{2+} wasting is the first human disease in which a mutation in a gene encoding a Na^+, K^+-ATPase subunit has been implicated. FXYD2 proteins are a family of single transmembrane proteins known to modulate Na^+, K^+-ATPase function.[100] The FXYD2 protein changes the Na^+, K^+-ATPase kinetics by reducing the affinity for Na^+ while increasing that for K^+. In IDH, the dominant negative mutant FXYD2 protein binds to wild-type FXYD2 proteins and retains them inside the cell.[101] It has been hypothesized that this retention results in reduced outward basolateral Na^+ transport in the polarized DCT cell, which in turn reduces intracellular voltage, thereby reducing inward electric driving force for Mg^{2+} entry via TRPM6.[52]

Recently, mutations in the gene encoding the hepatocyte nuclear factor 1B (*HNF1B*) implicated in maturity-onset diabetes of the young (MODY) type 5 have been shown to result in hypomagnesemia and renal Mg^{2+} wasting as well as hypocalciuria (Table 18-3).[53,102] The *HNF1B* gene encodes a transcription factor that regulates the *FXYD2* gene (Fig. 18-5).[53] Defective transcription of *FYXD2* appears to promote renal Mg^{2+} wasting.

Isolated Autosomal Recessive Hypomagnesemia

Isolated autosomal recessive hypomagnesemia (IRH) was first reported in two siblings who showed renal Mg^{2+} wasting, normal urinary Ca^{2+} excretion, and epileptic seizures and psychomotor deficit (Table 18-3).[103] The molecular defect in these patients was identified as a mutation in the epidermal growth factor (EGF) gene causing a defect in the routing of pro-EGF to the basolateral membrane of the DCT cell (Fig. 18-5).[104,105] Normally, the binding of EGF protein to the EGF receptor located in the basolateral membrane is essential for the function of the apical membrane–bound Mg^{2+} channel, TRPM6.[105,106] The EGF mutation results in disruption of this pathway, dysfunction of TRPM6 and renal Mg^{2+} wasting. EGF is the first reported autocrine and paracrine magnesiotropic hormone.[52]

Autosomal Dominant Hypomagnesemia

Autosomal dominant hypomagnesemia is a rare disease that was recently reported in a large Brazilian family.[107] The patients displayed recurrent muscle cramps, tetany, tremor, muscle weakness, cerebellar atrophy, and hypomagnesemia (Table 18-3). A mutation was found in the gene *KCNA1* encoding the voltage-gated K^+ channel (Kv1.1).[107] This channel colocalizes with TRPM6 in the apical membrane of DCT cells (Fig. 18-5), drives apical K^+ efflux from cells, and generates the inside negative voltage essential for TRPM6-meidated Mg^{2+} entry into cells. A heterozygous Kv1.1 N255D mutation results in a nonfunctional channel with a dominant negative effect on the wild-type Kv1.1 channel, an effect that is in line with the dominant negative inheritance pattern of this disorder.[53]

EAST or SESAME Syndrome

Recently, two groups reported a new syndrome of hereditary hypomagnesemia. EAST (epilepsy, ataxia, sensorineural deafness and tubulopathy) or SESAME (seizures, sensorineural deafness, ataxia, mental retardation, and electrolyte imbalance) syndrome includes the indicated central nervous system and inner ear manifestations and a Gitelman syndrome–like tubulopathy with normotensive hypokalemic metabolic alkalosis and hypomagnesemia (Table 18-3).[108,109] The syndrome is caused by a defect in the gene *KCNJ10* encoding the basolateral K^+ channel Kir4.1 (Fig. 18-5). Kir4.1 malfunction leads to reduced basolateral K^+ cycling, which in turn impedes electrogenic Na^+, K^+-ATPase transport.[53] This results in depolarization of the DCT apical membrane and inhibition of NCCT-driven NaCl reabsorption and TRPM6-driven Mg^{2+} reabsorption explaining the Gitelman syndrome–like phenotype.

Mitochondrial Hypomagnesemia

In 2004, a large white family was identified with hypomagnesemia, hypercholesterolemia, and hypertension.[110] A pattern of maternal transmission suggested a mitochondrial disease, and indeed, mutation analysis discovered a thymine-to-cytidine conversion near the anticodan of the isoleucine tRNA.[110] Family members with hypomagnesemia had evidence of renal Mg^{2+} wasting. The authors have speculated on impaired energy metabolism of DCT cells as the consequence of the mitochondrial defect, which could impede transcellular Mg^{2+} transport.[111]

Collecting Duct

Distal Renal Tubular Acidosis

General Characteristics

Distal renal tubular acidosis (dRTA) (RTA type 1) is characterized by normal anion gap, hyperchloremic metabolic acidosis caused by failure of hydrogen ion secretion in the distal nephron (Fig. 18-6).[4,7,12] Patients fail to appropriately lower pH even in the presence of systemic acidosis.[4,7] Urine pH usually remains above 6. The defective H^+ secretion results in persistent bicarbonaturia (5%–15% of filtered load in infants and children), reduced net acid secretion (see later discussion), and metabolic acidosis.[7,12] Untreated dRTA is characterized by renal wasting of Na^+ and K^+. As in proximal RTA, the urinary K^+ loss in dRTA is caused by extracellular fluid volume contraction and secondary hyperaldosteronism.[6,7]

Distal RTA in children is most commonly a primary entity. Primary dRTA is inherited as either an autosomal dominant or autosomal recessive trait (see Table 18-4).[5,12] Whereas patients with the autosomal dominant form usually have a mild

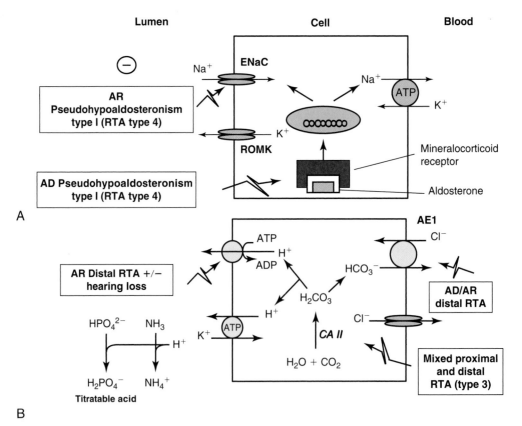

Figure 18-6 Transport mechanisms involved in electrolyte and acid–base handling in principal cell (**A**) and α-intercalated cell (**B**) of the cortical collecting duct. **A.** Aldosterone-mineralocorticoid receptor complex interacts with hormone-responsive elements of DNA in the nucleus of the principal cell. This results in production of specific proteins, which stimulate epithelial Na^+ channel (ENaC)–mediated Na^+ entry (and renal outer medullary potassium channel [ROMK]–mediated K^+ exit) at the luminal membrane and Na^+, K^+-ATPase at the basolateral membrane. **B.** H^+ and HCO_3^- are formed in the α-intercalated cell as a result of intracellular carbonic anhydrase (CAII) action. H^+ is secreted into the lumen via H^+-ATPase and H^+-K^+-ATPase and binds to the major urinary buffers, HPO_4^{2-} and NH_3 to form titratable acid and ammonium ion, respectively. Depicted are hereditary renal tubular acidosis syndromes caused by defects in these transport mechanisms. AD, autosomal dominant; AR, autosomal recessive.

disease, those with autosomal recessive dRTA may be severely affected in infancy with growth retardation and early nephrocalcinosis, leading to renal failure.[5,12] Autosomal recessive dRTA is subdivided into two variants with or without sensorineural hearing loss (see later discussion) (Table 18-4).[4,12,112,113]

Molecular Pathophysiology

Acid–base handling in the distal tubule occurs primarily in the CCD. There are two classes of cells in the CCD, which can be distinguished by morphologic and functional criteria: the principal cell and the intercalated cell (Fig. 18-6).[112] The principal cells are involved in sodium, potassium, and water transport, and the intercalated cells, which make up one-third of the cells in the CCD, are responsible for acid–base transport (i.e., proton and bicarbonate secretion and reabsorption) in this nephron segment.[114,115]

H$^+$ and HCO$_3^-$ are formed in the CCD cell as a result of the action of intracellular carbonic anhydrase (Fig. 18-6). The CCD is capable of secreting H$^+$ or HCO$_3^-$ depending on the acid–base status of the body.[115,116] Two functionally distinct subtypes of intercalated cells have been identified in the CCD: α (or type A) and β (or type B). α (or type A) intercalated cells secrete protons to the lumen and reabsorb HCO$_3^-$ to the blood (Fig. 18-6).[117] These cells harbor the H$^+$-ATPase (proton pump) and the H$^+$/K$^+$- ATPase in the luminal membrane and the kidney splice variant of anion exchanger 1 (AE1), a Cl$^-$/ HCO$_3^-$ exchanger, in the basolateral membrane. β (or type B) intercalated cells (not depicted) operate in the reverse orientation: they reabsorb protons to the blood and secrete HCO$_3^-$ (in exchange for Cl$^-$) across the apical membrane into the lumen.[115,117]

Secretion of H$^+$ in the α intercalated cells results in (1) reabsorption of 10% to 20% of the filtered HCO$_3^-$ that escaped absorption in the proximal tubule, and (2) titration of the major urinary buffers HPO$_4^{2-}$ and NH$_3$ to form H$_2$PO$_4^-$ (titratable acid) and ammonium ion (NH$_4$), respectively (Fig. 18-6). NH$_3$ is synthesized primarily in the proximal tubule and reaches the distal tubular lumen by a series of specialized transport processes.[6,116]

H$^+$ secretion into the tubular lumen is mediated by two mechanisms: (1) H$^+$-ATPase located at the luminal membrane of the α intercalated cells and (2) the lumen negative electrical potential difference created by electrogenic, epithelial Na$^+$ channel (ENaC)–mediated Na$^+$ reabsorption in the principal cells[6,116] (Fig. 18-6). These cells are also responsible for K$^+$ secretion.

Autosomal Dominant Distal Renal Tubular Acidosis

The AE1 gene, SLC4A1, located on chromosome 17q21-22 and a member of the anion exchanger SLC4 gene family, has been implicated in autosomal dominant dRTA (Table 18-4).[4,12,118] The AE1 gene product, also termed band 3, consists of 12 to 14 transmembrane domains and functions as an anion exchanger in erythroid cells and in the basolateral membrane of α-intercalated cells (Fig. 18-6). Erythrocyte AE1 (eAE1) is 65 amino acids longer at its NH$_2$ terminus than the kidney isoform (kAE1).[118] Several mutations in this N-terminal region of band 3 have been identified as the cause of hereditary spherocytosis and Southeast Asian ovalocytosis and normal acid–base handling.[4,119] However, various missense and deletion mutations of AE1 have been found in the COOH terminus and other regions of AE1 in several families with autosomal dominant dRTA (Fig. 18-6).[120,121] It has been demonstrated that AE1 mutations associated with autosomal dominant dRTA have normal function, but cause abnormalities in trafficking and targeting of AE1 to the renal basolateral membrane.[4,121] It is noteworthy that AE1 mutations causing autosomal recessive dRTA in association with hemolytic anemia have been demonstrated in Southeast Asian kindreds.[4,12]

Autosomal Recessive Distal Renal Tubular Acidosis

The ATP6V1B1 gene, localized on chromosome 12q13 and encoding the B$_1$-subunit of the apical proton pump expressed in α-intercalated cells, has been implicated in autosomal recessive dRTA with early-onset sensorineural deafness (Table 18-4 and Fig. 18-6).[122-124] The B$_1$-containing H$^+$-ATPase is a member of the vacuolar

(V)-ATPase family that has a complex structure of at least 10 subunits.[124,125] An intracellular domain of H+-ATPase, which, among other subunits, contains three B subunits, catalyzes ATP hydrolysis, providing energy for active H+ transport across the membrane-spanning Vo domain.[4,125] Various mutations causing autosomal recessive dRTA with sensorineural deafness have been identified within the *ATP6V1B1* gene.[4,12,123] Consistent with the finding of hearing loss, expression of *ATP6V1B1* in the cochlea and endolymphatic sac has been demonstrated.[4,122] This suggests that mutations in inner ear H+-ATPase likely affect auditory function by altering the normally acidic endolymphatic pH.[4,122]

Several homozygous mutations in the *ATP6V0A4* gene, located on chromosome 7q33-34 and encoding the a4 accessory subunit of H+-ATPase, were found to cause dRTA without or with later onset deafness (Table 18-4).[126,127]

Clinical Features

Prominent clinical manifestations of dRTA include failure to thrive, polyuria, polydipsia, constipation, vomiting, dehydration, muscle weakness, nephrocalcinosis, and nephrolithiasis.[6,14] The factors promoting the nephrocalcinosis and stone formation in dRTA are hypercalciuria, hypocitraturia, and alkaline urine. The hypercalciuria is probably related to chronic accumulation of acid that is buffered by Ca^{2+} release from bone as well as inhibition of distal tubular Ca^{2+} reabsorption by chronic metabolic acidosis.[4] The hypocitraturia is secondary to intracellular acidosis that promotes citrate uptake from the tubular lumen.[128]

The diagnosis of primary, classical dRTA can be based on (1) normal anion gap, hyperchloremic metabolic acidosis; (2) hypokalemia (as opposed to the hyperkalemia observed in voltage-dependent defect); (3) urine pH greater than 5.5 during spontaneous acidosis; and (4) a positive urinary anion gap (see proximal RTA) indicating low urinary ammonium concentration.[6,14] Although usually not necessary, the diagnosis of dRTA can be substantiated by the demonstration of an inability to maximally acidify the urine after NH_4Cl loading or by the finding of urine–blood PCO_2 (U-BPCO_2 <20 mm Hg after alkali loading).[14] The evaluation of dRTA should include examination of urinary Ca^{2+} and citrate levels as well as renal ultrasonography to investigate for the presence of nephrocalcinosis.

Treatment

The goals of dRTA therapy are to improve growth, prevent nephrocalcinosis and nephrolithiasis, and prevent progressive renal insufficiency. Infants and young children with dRTA may require up to 5 mEq/kg/day of alkali to correct acidemia, depending on the magnitude of renal HCO_3^- wasting.[6] As renal HCO_3^- wasting decreases with age, alkali requirements decrease. Hypokalemia, which can be significant, should be corrected. Provision of HCO_3^- by using citrate salts provides the additional advantage of exogenous citrate to prevent nephrocalcinosis and nephrolithiasis.[14]

Mixed Proximal and Distal Renal Tubular Acidosis (Type 3)

This variant of RTA shares the features of both proximal (reduced HCO_3^- reabsorption) and distal (impaired urine acidification) RTA (Table 18-4) (Figs. 18-1 and 18-6). It is caused by autosomal recessive mutations of the *CAII* gene located on chromosome 8q22 and expressed in kidney, bone, and brain.[6,129,130] Because CAII is present in the cytosol of both proximal and distal tubules, these mutations lead to this mixed syndrome. Because the expression of *CAII* is affected also in bone and brain, additional manifestations include osteopetrosis, cerebral calcifications, and mental retardation.[129,130] The osteopetrosis, which is secondary to osteoclast dysfunction, is a condition of increased bone density but also increased bone fragility leading to increased fracture risk.[4] Excess bone growth leads to conductive deafness and can also cause blindness through compression of the optic nerve.

Hyperkalemic Renal Tubular Acidosis (Type 4)

Hyperkalemic RTA is characterized by a normal ability to acidify the urine during acidosis, but reduced urinary concentration of ammonium and hence of net acid.[4,6,7]

The primary pathogenic mechanism in type 4 RTA is aldosterone deficiency or resistance that results in impairment of H^+ and K^+ secretion in the principal cells of the collecting tubule (Fig. 18-6). The ensuing hyperkalemia leads to an impairment of ammonium production. Decreased ENaC-mediated Na^+ reabsorption by principal cells also contributes to impaired electrogenic secretion of H^+ by intercalated cells.

Two hereditary aldosterone resistance states, PHAI and PHAII (discussed earlier; see Distal Convoluted Tubule) lead to type 4 RTA (Table 18-4).

Pseudohypoaldosteronism Type I

General Characteristics and Clinical Features

Pseudohypoaldosteronism type I (PHAI) is a rare inherited disorder characterized by renal salt wasting and end-organ unresponsiveness to mineralocorticoids.[5,6,131] The manifestations of the disease include hyponatremia, hyperkalemia, hyperchloremic metabolic acidosis, and elevated plasma aldosterone and plasma renin activity. The disorder is divided into two forms of inheritance with distinct pathophysiologic and clinical features. The autosomal dominant form is a relatively mild disease that remits with age, is restricted to the kidney, and is caused by heterozygous loss-of-function mutations in the mineralocorticoid receptor gene (Fig. 18-6).[132] The autosomal recessive form presents with severe Na^+ transport defects in all aldosterone target tissues, including the kidney, colon, and salivary and sweat glands, as well as in the lungs.[5,133,134] Autosomal recessive PHAI is characterized by neonatal salt wasting with dehydration, hypotension, life-threatening hyperkalemia, type 4 RTA, and failure to thrive.[131,133,134] The sweat test result is usually positive. The manifestations of the disease do not respond to mineralocorticoids, but do improve with salt supplementation. Neonatal respiratory distress syndrome and respiratory tract infections in affected children are common.[135]

Molecular Pathophysiology

The amiloride-sensitive ENaC, located at the apical membrane of Na^+ transporting epithelia such as the kidney, colon, lung, and ducts of the exocrine glands, plays an essential role in Na^+ and fluid reabsorption. In the kidneys, ENaC, which is composed of a combination of three similar subunits, α, β, and γ, is found primarily in the principal cells of the collecting duct, where it mediates the entry of Na^+ across the luminal membrane, a process driven by the basolateral Na^+, K^+-ATPase (Fig. 18-6).[133,134] Hence, ENaC has a central role in controlling extracellular fluid homeostasis and blood pressure. The activity of ENaC is under the tight control of hormones, such as aldosterone (Fig. 18-6) and vasopressin. Autosomal recessive PHAI is caused by homozygous or compound heterozygous loss-of-function mutations, which have been described in each of the three subunits α, β, and γ of ENaC (Fig. 18-6).[5,133,136,137]

Nephrogenic Diabetes Insipidus

General Characteristics and Clinical Features

Congenital nephrogenic diabetes insipidus (NDI) is characterized by an inability of the kidney to concentrate urine in response to the ADH arginine vasopressin (AVP).[138,139] Polydipsia and polyuria, hyposthenuria, dehydration, constipation, and hypernatremia are the hallmarks of NDI in infants and children.[139,140] Failure to thrive is common, and recurrent episodes of dehydration may cause severe neurologic sequelae. Older children can present with poor growth, nocturia and enuresis, and learning and behavior difficulties.[139,140]

Clinical diagnosis of NDI can be established by a water deprivation test demonstrating inappropriate urinary concentration unresponsive to DDAVP (desmopressin) administration. The evaluation of an infant or a child with NDI should include renal ultrasonography to evaluate for NDI secondary to disorders that result in impaired ability to concentrate the urine. These include conditions such as dysplastic and polycystic kidneys, renal scars, and nephrocalcinosis.[140]

Molecular Pathophysiology

The movement of water across the renal tubular epithelial membrane is of central importance in maintaining water and electrolyte balance. Reabsorption of water in the renal tubule occurs mainly through aquaporin (AQP) water channels, the activity of which is controlled by the vasopressin type 2 receptor (V2R) (see below). AQPs are members of a large family of pore-forming intrinsic membrane proteins.[141] There are now 13 well-characterized mammalian AQPs, AQP 0-12, of which eight (AQPs 1, 2, 3, 4, 6, 7, 8, and 11) are expressed in the kidney.[138,141] Ultrastructural studies have shown that AQPs have a barrel-like structure and are assembled in tetramers.[141,142]

Aquaporin 2 is the vasopressin-responsive AQP in the principal cells of the renal collecting duct, where 10% of the filtered volume is reabsorbed (Fig. 18-7). AQP2 is localized to the apical side of the principal cell (whereas AQP3 and AQP4 are expressed at the basolateral membrane).[139] Binding of the antidiuretic hormone AVP to the vasopressin type 2 receptor (V2R) at the basolateral side of the principal cell activates G protein (G_s) and increases intracellular cyclic adenosine monophosphate (cAMP) levels, resulting in phosphorylation of AQP2 by cAMP-dependent protein kinase (Fig. 18-7). This in turn triggers intracellular vesicles containing AQP2 to fuse with the apical membrane, rendering the cell water permeable. Upon dissociation of AVP from its receptor, AQP2 is internalized by endocytosis, and the cell returns to its water-impermeable state.[141]

X-Linked Nephrogenic Diabetes Insipidus

X-linked ND1 is caused by mutations in the V2 receptor gene, AVPR2, which resides on the long arm of chromosome X (Xq28).[143,144] Most (>90%) of the patients with congenital NDI have mutations in the AVPR2 gene. To date, more than 190 different putative disease causing mutations in the AVPR2 gene have been reported.[139,144] When studied in vitro, most AVPR2 mutations lead to receptors that are trapped in the endoplasmic reticulum and are unable to reach the plasma membrane.[144]

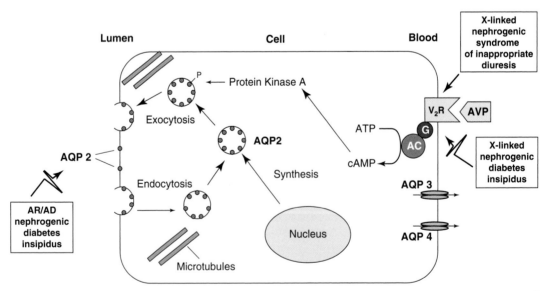

Figure 18-7   Regulation of aquaporin 2 (AQP2) recycling in a principal cell of the collecting duct. Binding of arginine vasopressin (AVP) to vasopressin type 2 receptor (V_2R) at the basolateral membrane triggers a signaling cascade, which results in protein kinase A-induced phosphorylation of AQP2 in intracellular vesicles. After phosphorylation, AQP2-containing vesicles translocate to the apical membrane (a process that involves the microtubular machinery), thereby increasing the water permeability of the membrane. Upon dissociation of AVP from its receptor, AQP2 is retrieved endocytically from the apical membrane, and the cell returns to its water-impermeable state. Hereditary tubulopathies caused by defects in these pathways are depicted. (Modified with permission from Zelikovic I. Renal tubular disorders. In: Hogg RJ, ed. *Kidney Disorders in Children and Adolescents*. 1st ed. London: Taylor & Francis, 2006: 165-180.)

Autosomal Recessive and Autosomal Dominant Nephrogenic Diabetes Insipidus

Nephrogenic diabetes insipidus can be transmitted as an autosomal recessive or autosomal dominant trait. In these cases, the disease is caused by mutations in the *AQP2* gene, located on chromosome 12q13.[145,146] To date, 40 different putative disease-causing mutations in the *AQP2* gene have been reported in autosomal recessive NDI.[139,141] Most of these are missense mutations. Similar to AVPR2 mutants, mutations in the *AQP2* gene lead to an impaired routing of channel proteins to the plasma membrane caused by misfolding and retention in the endoplasmic reticulum.

At present, eight NDI families with autosomal dominant inheritance have been identified.[141] This form of NDI is caused by various mutations in the *AQP2* gene that change the transport signal of the AQP2 protein with consequent misrouting to the Golgi compartment or to late endosomes.[139,141]

Therapy

The hallmarks of therapy of NDI include[139,140] (1) replacement of urinary water losses by adequate supply of fluid (if necessary, via nasogastric or gastric tube); (2) reduction of dietary solute load by restricting Na$^+$ intake and by providing protein intake not higher than the recommended daily allowance; and (3) pharmacologic therapy, including thiazide, amiloride, and (if indicated) indomethacin. Finally, of great interest are recent studies investigating the yield of pharmacologic chaperones in rescuing misfolded V2R and AQP2 proteins trapped in the endoplasmic reticulum.[147,148] The findings of these studies may provide a basis for future design of therapeutic strategies for some forms of NDI.

Nephrogenic Syndrome of Inappropriate Diuresis

General Characteristics

The nephrogenic syndrome of inappropriate diuresis (NSIAD) is a rare, recently described genetic disorder of water balance affecting male infants.[149,150] The clinical and laboratory features of NSIAD resemble those of the syndrome of inappropriate secretion of antidiuretic hormone (SIADH) and include hyponatremia, seizures, and inappropriately hypertonic urine.[151,152] However, in contrast to the markedly elevated plasma AVP levels in SIADH, NSIAD is characterized by undetectable or very low AVP levels in plasma.[149,152]

Molecular Pathophysiology

The NSIAD is caused by a gain of function mutation in the V2R receptor gene, *AVPR2*, located on chromosome xq28, which leads to constitutive activation of the receptor (see Table 18-4 and Fig. 18-7).[149] The two unrelated male infants included in the first report on this syndrome,[149] as well as the few cases subsequently reported,[152] display missense mutations, resulting in the substitution of arginine to cysteine or leucine in codon 137. The mechanism whereby these mutations cause constitutive activation of the receptor is unclear. Interestingly, the manifestations of the disease mostly occur after the age of a few months. It has been suggested that limited concentrating capacity of the renal tubule in neonates combined with high insensible water loss might have a protective role and postpone the appearance of the disease.[152]

Therapy

The simplest therapy of NSIAD is fluid restriction that, however, is not feasible during early life because of its consequence of caloric deficiency.[150,152] Administration of urea to induce osmotic diuresis or furosemide with salt supplementation, both therapies used in SIAPH,[151 153] are potential therapies in NSIAD that have not been tested in this syndrome and can lead to serious side effects. Of a great interest is a recent functional study in renal cells demonstrating AVP-induced internalization of the mutant V2R.[153] The findings of the study raise the possibility that administration

18

of vasopressin could have a therapeutic value for NSIAD by reducing steady-state surface receptor levels, thus lowering basal cAMP production and accumulation that most likely underlies NSIAD.

Conclusion

In the past decade, remarkable progress has been made in our understanding of the molecular pathogenesis of hereditary tubulopathies. Molecular genetics and molecular biology studies have led to the identification of numerous tubular disease-causing mutations, have provided important insight into the defective molecular mechanisms underlying various tubulopathies, and have greatly increased our understanding of the physiology of renal tubular transport. Nevertheless, numerous issues remain unsettled and warrant additional research. Future studies will shed more light on the molecular mechanisms and functional defects underlying the impaired transport in various tubulopathies. These studies may significantly improve our understanding of the mechanisms underlying renal salt homeostasis, urinary mineral excretion, and blood pressure regulation in health and disease. The identification of the molecular defects in inherited tubulopathies may provide a basis for future design of targeted therapeutic interventions and, possibly, strategies for gene therapy of these complex disorders.

Acknowledgment

I am indebted to Mrs. Ora Bider for her expert secretarial assistance.

References

1. Devuyst O, Konrad M, Jeunemaitre X, et al. Tubular disorders of electrolyte regulation. In: Avner ED, Harmon WE, Niaudet P, et al, eds. *Pediatric Nephrology*. 6th ed. Heidelberg: Springer Verlag; 2009:929-977.
2. Hildebrandt F. Genetic kidney diseases. *Lancet*. 2010;375:1287-1295.
3. Bonnardeaux A, Bichet DG. Inherited disorders of the renal tubule. In: *Brenner & Rector's The kidney*. 8th ed. Philadelphia: W.B. Saunders Company; 2008:1390-1427.
4. Fry AC, Karet FE. Inherited renal acidoses. *Physiology*. 2007;22:202-211.
5. Zelikovic I. Molecular pathophysiology of tubular transport disorders. *Pediatr Nephrol*. 2001; 16:919-935.
6. Soriano JR. Renal tubular acidosis: the clinical entity. *J Am Soc Nephrol*. 2002;13:2160-2170.
7. Krapf R, Seldin DW, Alpern RJ. Clinical syndromes of metabolic acidosis. In: Alpern RJ, Hebert SC, eds. *Seldin and Giebisch's The Kidney, Physiology and Pathophysiology*. 4th ed. Philadelphia: Saunders Elsevier; 2008:1667-1720.
8. Igarashi T, Inatomi J, Sekine T, et al. Mutations in SLC4A4 cause permanent isolated proximal renal tubular acidosis with ocular abnormalities. *Nat Genet*. 1999;23:264-266.
9. Igarashi T, Sekine T, Inatomi J, et al. Unraveling the molecular pathogenesis of isolated proximal renal tubular acidosis. *J Am Soc Nephrol*. 2002;13:2171-2177.
10. Usui T, Hara M, Satoh H, et al. Molecular basis of ocular abnormalities associated with proximal renal tubular acidosis. *J Clin Invest*. 2001;108:107-115.
11. Soleimani M, Burnham CE. Physiologic and molecular aspects of the Na+/ HCO3- cotransporter in health and disease processes. *Kidney Int*. 2000;57:371-384.
12. Alper SL. Familial renal tubular acidosis. *J Nephrol*. 2010;23:S57-S76.
13. Toye AM, Parker MD, Daly CM, et al. The human NBCe1-A mutant R881C, associated with proximal renal tubular acidosis, retains function but is mistargeted in polarized renal epithelia. *Am J Physiol Cell Physiol*. 2006;291:C788-C801.
14. Zelikovic I. Renal tubular acidosis. *Pediatr Ann*. 1995;24:48-54.
15. Zelikovic I. Aminoaciduria and glycosuria. In: Avner ED, Harmon N, Niaudet P, Yoshikawa N, eds. *Pediatric Nephrology*. 6th ed. Heidelberg: Springer-Verlag; 2009:889-927.
16. Palacin M, Goodyer P, Nunes V, et al. Cystinuria. In: Scriver CR, Beaudet AL, Sly WS, et al, eds. *The metabolic and molecular bases of inherited disease*. New York: McGraw-Hill; 2001:4909-4932.
17. Mattoo A, Goldfarb DS. Cystinuria. *Semin Nephrol*. 2008;28:181-191.
18. Chillaron J, Font-Llitjos M, Fort J, et al. Pathophysiology and treatment of cystinuria. *Nat Rev Nephrol*. 2010;6:424-434.
19. Goodyer P, Saadi I, Ong P, et al. Cystinuria subtype and the risk of nephrolithiasis. *Kidney Int*. 1998; 54:56-61.
20. Chillaron J, Roca R, Valencia A, et al. Heteromeric amino acid transporters: biochemistry, genetics, and physiology. *Am J Physiol*. 2001;281:F995-F1018.
21. Palacin M, Borsani G, Sebastio G. The molecular bases of cystinuria and lysinuric protein intolerance. *Curr Opin Genet Dev*. 2001;11:328-335.
22. Wagner CA, Lang F, Bröer S. Function and structure of heterodimeric amino acid transporters. *Am J Physiol*. 2001;281:C1077-C1093.

23. Jaeger P, Portmann L, Saunders A, et al. Anticystinuric effects of glutamine and of dietary sodium restriction. *N Engl J Med*. 1986;315:1120-1123.
24. Jaffe IA. Adverse effects profile of sulfhydryl compounds in man. *Am J Med*. 1986;80:471-476.
25. Pak CYC, Fuller C, Sakhaee K, et al. Management of cystine nephrolithiasis with alpha-mercaptopropionylglycine. *J Urol*. 1986;136:1003-1008.
26. Simell O. Lysinuric protein intolerance and other cationic aminoacidurias. In: Scriver CR, Beaudet AL, Sly WS, et al. eds. *The Metabolic and Molecular Bases of Inherited Disease*. New York: McGraw-Hill; 2001:4933-4956.
27. Palacin M, Bertran J, Zorzano A. Heteromeric amino acid transporters explain aminoacidurias, *Curr Opin Nephrol Hypertens*. 2000;9:547-553.
28. Palacin M, Nunes V, Font-Llitjos M, et al. The genetics of heteromeric amino acid transporters. *Physiology (Bethesda)*. 2005;20:112-124.
29. Sperandeo MP, Andria G, Sebastio G. Lysinuric protein intolerance: update and extended mutation analysis of the SLC7A7 gene. *Hum Mutat*. 2008;29:14-21.
30. Rajantie J, Simell O, Rapola J, et al. Lysinuric protein intolerance: a two year trial of dietary supplementation therapy with citrulline and lysine, *J Pediatr*. 1980;97:927-932.
31. Dirckx JH. Julius Caesar and the Julian emperors: a family cluster with Hartnup disease? *Am J Dermatopathol*. 1986;8:351-357.
32. Baron DN, Dent CE, Harris H, et al. Hereditary pellegra-like skin rash with temporary cerebellar ataxia, constant renal aminoaciduria and other bizarre biochemical features. *Lancet*. 1956;1:421-428.
33. Levy HL. Hartnup disorder. In: Scriver CR, Beaudet Al, Sly WS, et al, eds. *The Metabolic and Molecular Bases of Inherited Disease*. New York: McGraw-Hill; 2001:4957-4969.
34. Nozaki J, Dakeishi M, Ohura T, et al. Homozygosity mapping to chromosome 5p15 of a gene responsible for Hartnup disorder. *Biochem Biophys Res Comm*. 2001;284:255-260.
35. Bröer A, Klingel K, Kowalczuk S, et al. Molecular cloning of mouse amino acid transport system B^0, a neutral amino acid transporter related to Hartnup disorder. *J Biol Chem*. 2004;279:24467-24476.
36. Bröer S. Amino acid transport across mammalian intestinal and renal epithelia. *Physiol Rev*. 2008;88:249-280.
37. Kleta R, Romeo E, Ristic Z, et al. Mutations in SLC6A19, encoding B0AT1, cause Hartnup disorder. *Nature Genet*. 2004;36:999-1002.
38. Seow HF, Bröer S, Bröer A, et al. Hartnup disorder is caused by mutations in the gene encoding the neutral amino acid transporter SLC6A19. *Nature Genet*. 2004;36:1003-1007.
39. Jonas AJ, Butler IJ. Circumvention of defective neutral amino acid transport in Hartnup disease using tryptophan ethyl ester. *J Clin Invest*. 1989;84:200-204.
40. Wright E, Martin MG, Turk E. Familial glucose-galactose malabsorption and hereditary glycosuria. In: Scriver CR, Beaudet AL, Sly WS, et al, eds. *The Metabolic and Molecular Bases of Inherited Disease*. New York: McGraw-Hill; 2001:4891-4908.
41. Wright EM, Turk E. The sodium/glucose cotransport family SLC5. *Pflugers Arch*. 2004;447:510-518.
42. Uldry M, Thorens B. The SLC2 family of facilitated hexose and polyol transporters. *Pflugers Arch*. 2004;447:480-489.
43. Santer R, Kinner M, Lassen CL, et al. Molecular analysis of the SGLT2 gene in patients with renal glucosuria. *J Am Soc Nephrol*. 2003;14:2873-2882.
44. Magen D, Sprecher E, Zelikovic I, et al. A novel missense mutation in SLC5A2 encoding SGLT2 underlies autosomal recessive renal glucosuria and aminoaciduria. *Kidney Int*. 2005;67:34-41.
45. Turk E, Zabel B, Mundlos S, et al. Glucose/galactose malabsorption caused by a defect in the Na$^+$/glucose cotransporter. *Nature*. 1991;350:354-356.
46. Santer R, Schneppenheim R, Dombrowski A, et al. Mutations in GLUT2, the gene for the liver-type glucose transporter, in patients with Fanconi-Bickel syndrome, *Nat Genet*. 1997;17:324-326.
47. Santer R, Groth S, Kinner M, et al. The mutation spectrum of the facilitative glucose transporter gene SLC2A2 (GLUT2) in patients with Fanconi-Bickel syndrome. *Hum Genet*. 2002;110:21-29.
48. Zelikovic I. Hypokalemic salt-losing tubulopathies: an evolving story. *Nephrol Dial Transpl*. 2003;18:1696-1700.
49. Knoers NVAM. Gitelman syndrome. *Adv Chronic Kidney Dis*. 2006;13:148-154.
50. Seyberth HW. An improved terminology and classification of Bartter-like syndromes. *Nat Clin Pract Nephrol*. 2008;4:560-567.
51. Mount DB, Yu ASL. Transport of inorganic solutes: sodium, chloride, potassium, magnesium, calcium, and phosphate. In: Brenner BM, ed. *The Kidney*. 8th ed. Philadelphia: Saunders Elsevier; 2008:156-213.
52. Dimke H, Hoenderop JG, Bindels RJ. Hereditary tubular transport disorders: implications for renal handling of Ca2+ and Mg2+. *Clin Sci (Lond)*. 2009;118:1-18.
53. Cristobal PS, Dimke H, Hoenderop JGJ, et al. Novel molecular pathways in renal Mg2+ transport: a guided tour along the nephron. *Curr Opin Nephrol Hypertens*. 2010;19:456-462.
54. Brown EM, MacLeod RJ. Extracellular calcium sensing and extracellular calcium signaling. *Physiol Rev*. 2001;81:237-239.
55. Riccardi D, Brown EM. Physiology and pathophysiology of the calcium-sensing receptor in the kidney. *Am J Physiol Renal Physiol*. 2010;298:F485-F499.
56. Huang H, Miller RT. Novel Ca receptor signaling pathways for control of renal ion transport. *Curr Opin Nephrol Hypertens*. 2010;19:106-112.

18

57. Simon DB, Karet FE, Hamdan JM, et al. Bartter's syndrome, hypokalemic alkalosis with hypercalciuria, is caused by mutations in the Na-K-2Cl contransporter NKCC2. *Nat Genet*. 1996;13:183-188.

58. Simon DB, Karet FE, Rodriguez-Soriano J, et al. Genetic heterogeneity of Bartter's syndrome revealed by mutations in the K+ channel, ROMK. *Nat Genet*. 1996;14:152-156.

59. Simon DB, Bindra RS, Mansfield TA, et al. Mutations in the chloride channel gene, CLCNKB, cause Bartter's syndrome type III. *Nat Genet*. 1997;17:171-178.

60. Simon DB, Nelson-Williams C, Bia MJ, et al. Gitelman's variant of Bartter's syndrome, inherited hypokalemic alkalosis, is caused by mutations in the thiazide-sensitive Na-Cl contransporter. *Nat Genet*. 1996;12:24-30.

61. Gamba G. Electroneutral chloride coupled cotransporters. *Curr Opin Nephrol Hypertens*. 2000;9:535-540.

62. Seyberth HW, Rascher W, Schweer H, et al. Congenital hypokalemia with hypercalciuria in pre-term infants: a hyperprostaglandinuric tubular syndrome different from Bartter syndrome. *J Pediatr*. 1985;107:694-701.

63. Birkenhager R, Otto E, Schurmann MJ, et al. Mutation of BSND causes Bartter syndrome with sensorineural deafness and kidney failure. *Nat Genet*. 2001;29:310-314.

64. Estevez R, Boettger T, Stein V, et al. Barttin is a Cl$^-$ channel beta-subunit crucial for renal Cl$^-$ reabsorption and inner ear K+ secretion. *Nature*. 2001;414:558-561.

65. Vargas-Poussou R, Huang C, Hulin P, et al. Functional characterization of a calcium-sensing receptor mutation in severe autosomal dominant hypocalcemia with a Bartter-like syndrome. *J Am Soc Nephron*. 2002;13:2259-2266.

66. Watanabe S, Fukumoto S, Chang H, et al. Association between activation mutations of calcium-sensing receptor and Bartter's syndrome. *Lancet*. 2002;360:692-694.

67. Jeck N, Konrad M, Peters M, et al. Mutations in the chloride channel gene, CLCNKB, leading to a mixed Bartter-Gitelman phenotype. *Pediatr Res*. 2000;48:754-758.

68. Zelikovic I, Szargel R, Hawash A, et al. A novel mutation in the chloride channel gene, CLCNKB, as a cause of Gitelman and Bartter syndromes. *Kidney Int*. 2003;63:24-32.

69. Michelis MF, Drash AL, Linarelli LG, et al. Decreased bicarbonate threshold and renal magnesium wasting in a sibship with distal renal tubular acidosis. Evaluation of the pathophysiological role of parathyroid hormone. *Metab Clin Exp*. 1972;21:905-920.

70. Praga M, Vara J, Gonzalez-Parra E, et al. Familial hypomagnesemia with hypercalciuria and nephrocalcinosis. *Kidney Int*. 1995;47:1419-1425.

71. Simon DB, Lu Y, Chaote KA, et al. Paracellin-1, a renal tight junction protein required for paracellular Mg2+ resorption. *Science*. 1999;285:103-106. http://sanfrancisco.cbslocal.com/2011/08/29/stockton-mom-accused-of-beating-up-principal-over-dress-code/.

72. Anderson JM. Molecular structure of tight junctions and their role in epithelial transport. *News Physiol Sci*. 2001;16:126-130.

73. Weber S, Schneider L, Peters M, et al. Novel paracellin-1 mutations in 25 families with familial hypomagnesemia with hypercalciuria and nephrocalcinosis. *J Am Soc Nephrol*. 2001;12:1872-1881.

74. Muller D, Kausalya PJ, Claverie-Martin F, et al. A novel claudin16 mutation associated with childhood hypercalciuria abolishes binding to ZO-1 and results in lysosomal mistargeting. *Am J Hum Genet*. 2003;73:1293-1301.

75. Hou J, Paul DL, Goodenough DA. Paracellin-1 and the modulation of ion selectivity of tight junctions. *J Cell Sci*. 2005;118:5109-5118.

76. Konrad M, Schaller A, Seelow DJ, et al. Mutations in the tight-junction gene claudin-19 (CLDN19) are associated with renal magnesium wasting, renal failure and severe ocular involvement. *Am J Hum Genet*. 2006;79:949-957.

77. Hou J, Renigunta A, Konrad M, et al. Claudin-16 and claudin-19 interact and form a cation-selective tight junction complex. *J Clin Invest*. 2008;118:619-628.

78. Hou J, Renigunta A, Gomes AS, et al. Claudin-16 and claudin-19 interaction is required for their assembly into tight junctions and for renal reabsorption of magnesium. Proc Natl Acad Sci USA. 2009;106:15350-15355.

79. Brown EM, Hebert SC. Inherited diseases of the calcium-sensing receptor: impact on parathyroid and renal function. In: Lifton RP, Somlo S, Giebisch GH, et al, eds. *Genetic Diseases of the Kidney*. Philadelphia: Saunders Elsevier; 2009:263-278.

80. Pollak MR, Brown EM, Estep HL, et al. Autosomal dominant hypocalcaemia caused by a Ca (2+)-sensing receptor gene mutation. *Nat Genet*. 1994;8:303-307.

81. Egbuna OI, Brown EM. Hypercalcaemic and hypocalcaemic conditions due to calcium-sensing receptor mutations. *Best Pract Res Clin Rheumatol*. 2008;22:129-148.

82. Auwerx J, Demedts M, Bouillon R. Altered parathyroid set point to calcium in familial hypocalciuric hypercalcaemia. *Acta Endocrinol*. 1984;106:215-218.

83. Hebert SC. Extracellular calcium-sensing receptor: implications for calcium and magnesium handling in the kidney. *Kidney*. 1996;50:2129-2139.

84. Pollak MR, Seldman CE, Brown EM. Three inherited disorders of calcium sensing. *Medicine (Baltimore)*. 1996;75:115-123.

85. Friedman PA. Codependence of renal calcium and sodium transport. *Annu Rev Physiol*. 1998;60:179-197.

86. Van de Graaf SFJ, Bindels RJM, Hoenderop JGJ. Physiology of epithelial Ca^{2+} and Mg^{2+} transport. *Rev Physiol Biochem Pharmacol*. 2007;158:77-160.

87. Nijenhuis T, Vallon V, Van der Kemp AW, et al. enhanced passive Ca^{2+} reabsorption and reduced Mg^{2+} channel abundance explains thiazide-induced hypocalciuria and hypomagnesemia. *J Clin Invest*. 2005;115:1651-1658.

88. Bonny O, Rossier BC. Disturbances of Na/K balance: pseudohypoaldosteronism revisited. *J Am Soc Nephrol*. 2002;13:2399-2414.

89. Kahle KT, Wilson FH, Lifton RP. The syndrome of hypertension and hyperkalemia (pseudohypoaldosteronism type II): WNK kinases regulate the balance between renal salt reabsorption and potassium secretion. In: Lifton RP, Somlo S, Giebisch GH, et al, eds. *Genetic diseases of the kidney*. Philadelphia: Saunders Elsevier; 2009:313-329.

90. Proctor G, Linas S. Type 2 pseudohypoaldosteronism: new insights into renal potassium, sodium, and chloride handling. *Am J of Kidney Dis*. 2006;48:674-693.

91. Wilson FH, Disse-Nicodeme S, Choate KA, et al. Human hypertension caused by mutations in WNK kinases. *Science*. 2001;293:1107-1112.

92. Peng JB, Warnock DG. WNK4-mediated regulation of renal ion transport proteins. *Am J Physiol Renal Physiol*. 2007;293:F961-F973.

93. Kahle KT, Ring AM, Lifton RP. Molecular physiology of the WNK kinases. *Annu Rev Physiol*. 2008;70:11.1-11.27.

94. Cai H, Cebotaru V, Wang YH, et al. WNK4 kinase regulates surface expression of the human sodium chloride cotransporter in mammalian cells. *Kidney Int*. 2006;69:2162-2170.

95. Schlingmann KP, Weber S, Peters M, et al. Hypomagnesemia with secondary hypocalcemia is caused by mutations in TRPM6, a new member of the TRPM gene family. *Nature Genetics*. 2002;31:166-170.

96. Walder RY, Landau D, Meyer P, et al. Mutation of TRPM6 causes familial hypomagnesemia with secondary hypocalcemia. *Nat Genet*. 2002;31:171-174.

97. Voets T, Nilius B, Hoefs S, et al. TRPM6 forms the Mg^{2+} influx channel involved in intestinal and renal Mg^{2+} absorption. *J Biol Chem*. 2004;279:19-25.

98. Meij IC, Koendering JB, van Bokhoven H, et al. Dominant isolated renal magnesium loss is caused by misrouting of the Na^+-K^+-ATPase gamma-subunit. *Nat Genet*. 2000;26:265-266.

99. Sweadner KJ, Rael E. The FXYD gene family of small ion transport regulators or channels: cDNA sequence, protein signature sequence, and expression. *Genomics*. 2000;68:41-56.

100. Beguin P, Wang X, Firsov D, et al. The gamma subunit is a specific component of the Na^+-K^+-ATPase and modulates its transport function. *EMBO J*. 1997;16:4250-4260.

101. Cairo ER, Friedrich T, Swarts HG, et al. Impaired routing of wild type FXYD2 after oligomerisation with FXYD2-G41R might explain the dominant nature of renal hypomagnesemia. *Biochim Biophys Acta*. 2008;1778:398-404.

102. Adalat S, Woolf AS, Johnstone KA, et al. HNF1B mutations associate with hypomagnesemia and renal magnesium wasting. *J Am Soc Nephrol*. 2009;20:1123-1131.

103. Geven WB, Monnens LA, Willems JL, et al. Isolated autosomal recessive renal magnesium loss in two sisters. *Clin Genet*. 1987;32:398-402.

104. Muallem S, Moe OW. When EGF is offside, magnesium is wasted. *J Clin Invest*. 2007;117:2086-2089.

105. Thebault S, Alexander RT, Tiel Groenestege WM, et al. EGF increases TRPM6 activity and surface expression. *J Am Soc Nephrol*. 2009;20:78-85.

106. Groenestege WM, Thebault S, van der Wijst J, et al. Impaired basolateral sorting of pro-EGF causes isolated recessive renal hypomagnesemia. *J Clin Invest*. 2007;117:2260-2267.

107. Glaudemans B, van der Wijst J, Scola RH, et al. A missense mutation in the Kv1.1 voltage-gated potassium channel-encoding gene KCNA1 is linked to human autosomal dominant hypomagnesemia. *J Clin Invest*. 2009;119:936-942.

108. Bockenhauer D, Feather S, Stanescu HC, et al. Epilepsy, ataxia, sensorineural deafness, tubulopathy, and KCNJ10 mutations. *N Engl J Med*. 2009;360:1960-1970.

109. Scholl UI, Choi M, Liu T, et al. Seizures, sensorineural deafness, ataxia, mental retardation, and electrolyte imbalance (SeSAME syndrome) caused by mutations in KCNJ10. *Proc Natl Acad Sci USA*. 2009;106:5842-5847.

110. Wilson FH, Hariri A, Farhi A, et al. A cluster of metabolic defects caused by mutation in a mitochondrial tRNA. *Science*. 2004;306:1190-1194.

111. Reilly RF, Ellison DH. Mammalian distal tubule: physiology, pathophysiology, and molecular anatomy. *Physiol Rev*. 2000;80:277-313.

112. Donckerwolcke RA, van Biervliet JP, Koorevaar G, et al. The syndrome of renal tubular acidosis with nerve deafness. *Acta Paediatr Scand*. 1976;65:100-104.

113. Brown MT, Cunningham MJ, Ingelfinger JR, et al. Progressive sensorineural hearing loss in association with distal renal tubular acidosis. *Arch Otolaryngol Head Neck Surg*. 1993;119:458-460.

114. Madsen KM, Nielsen S, Tisher CC. Anatomy of the kidney. In: Brenner BM, ed. *The Kidney*. 8th ed. Philadelphia: Saunders Elsevier; 2008:25-90.

115. Schwartz GJ. Plasticity of intercalated cell polarity: effect of metabolic acidosis. *Nephron*. 2001;87:304-313.

116. Hamm LL, Alpern RJ, Preisig PA. Cellular mechanisms of renal tubular acidification. In: Alpern RJ, Hebert SC, eds. *Seldin and Giebisch's The Kidney, Physiology and Pathophysiology*. 4th ed. Philadelphia: Saunders Elsevier; 2008:1539-1585.

117. Wagner CA. Renal acid-base transport: old and new players. *Nephron Physiol*. 2006;103:1-6.

118. Alper SL. Molecular physiology of SLC4 anion exchangers. *Exp Physiol*. 2006;91:153-161.

119. Gallagher PG. Red cell membrane disorders. *Hematology Am Soc Hematol Educ Program*. 2005;13-18.

120. Bruce LJ, Cope DL, Jones GK, et al. Familial distal renal tubular acidosis is associated with mutations in the red cell anion exchanger (Band 3 AE1) gene. *J Clin Invest.* 1997;100:1693-1707.
121. Shayakul C, Alper SL. Inherited renal tubular acidosis. *Curr Opin Nephrol Hypertens.* 2000;9:541-546.
122. Karet FE, Finberg KE, Nelson RD, et al. Mutations in the gene encoding B1 subunit of H⁺-ATPase cause renal tubular acidosis with sensorineural deafness. *Nat Genet.* 1999;21:84-90.
123. Blake-Palmer KG, Karet FE. Cellular physiology of the renal H⁺ ATPase. *Curr Opin Nephrol Hypertens.* 2009;433-438.
124. Wagner CA, Finberg KE, Breton S, et al. Renal vacuolar-ATPase. *Physiol Rev.* 2004;84:1263-1314.
125. Jefferies KC, Cipriano DJ, Forgac M. Function, structure and regulation of the vacuolar (H⁺)-ATPases. *Arch Biochem Biophys.* 2008;476:33-42.
126. Smith AN, Skaug J, Choat KA, et al. Mutation in ATP6N1B, encoding a new kidney vacuolar proton pump 116-kD subunit, cause recessive distal renal tubular acidosis with preserved hearing. *Nat Genet.* 2000;26:71-75.
127. Stover EH, Borthwick KJ, Bavalia C, et al. Novel ATP6V1B1 and ATP6V0A4 mutations in autosomal recessive distal renal tubular acidosis with new evidence for hearing loss. *J Med Genet.* 2002;39:796-803.
128. Rothstein M, Obialo C, Hruska KA. Renal tubular acidosis. *Endocrinol Metab Clin North Am.* 1990;19:869-887.
129. Sly WS, Hewett-Emmett D, Whyte MP, et al. Carbonic anhydrase II deficiency identified as the primary defect in the autosomal recessive syndrome of osteopetrosis with renal tubular acidosis and cerebral calcification. *Proc Natl Acad Sci USA.* 1983;80:2752-2756.
130. Roth DE, Venta PJ, Tashian RE, et al. Molecular basis of human carbonic anhydrase H deficiency. *Proc Natl Acad Sci USA.* 1992;89:1804-1808.
131. Scheinman SJ, Guay-Woodford LM, Thakker RV, et al. Genetic disorders of renal electrolyte transport. *N Engl J Med.* 1999;340:1177-1187.
132. Geller DS, Rodriguez-Soriano J, Vallo A, et al. Mutations in the mineralocorticoid receptor gene cause autosomal dominant pseudohypoaldosteronism Type I. *Nat Genet.* 1998;19:279-281.
133. Rossier BC. Cum grano salis: the epithelial sodium channel and the control of blood pressure. *J Am Soc Nephrol.* 1997;8:980-992.
134. Bonny O, Hummler E. Dysfunction of epithelial sodium transport: from human to mouse. *Kidney Int.* 2000;57:1313-1318.
135. Kerem E, Bistritzer T, Hanukoglu A, et al. Pulmonary epithelial sodium channel dysfunction and excess airway liquid in pseudohypoaldosteronism. *New Eng J Med.* 1999;341:156-162.
136. Bonny O, Rossier BC. Disturbances of Na/K balance: pseudohypoaldosteronism revisited. *J Am Soc Nephrol.* 2002;13:2399-2414.
137. Chang SS, Grunder S, Hanukoglu A, et al. Mutations in subunits of the epithelial sodium channel cause salt wasting with hyperkalaemic acidosis, pseudohypoaldosteronism type 1. *Nat Genet.* 1996;12:248-253.
138. Fujiwara TM, Bichet DG. Molecular biology of hereditary diabetes insipidus. *J Am Soc Nephrol.* 2005;16:2836-2846.
139. Knoers NVAM, Levtchenko EN. Nephrogenic diabetes insipidus. In: Avner ED, Harmon WE, Niaudet P, et al, eds. *Pediatric Nephrology.* 6th ed. Heidelberg: Springer Verlaag; 2009:1005-1018.
140. Linshaw MA. Congenital nephrogenic diabetes insipidus. *Pediatr in Rev.* 2007;28:372-380.
141. Loonen AJM, Knoers NVAM, Van Os CH, et al. Aquaporin 2 mutations in nephrogenic diabetes insipidus. *Semin Nephrol.* 2008;28:252-265.
142. Kozono D, Yasui M, King LS, et al. Aquaporin water channels: Atomic structure molecular dynamics meet clinical medicine. *J Clin Invest.* 2002;109:1395-1399.
143. Rosenthal W, Seibold A, Antaramian A, et al. Molecular identification of the gene responsible for congenital nephrogenic diabetes insipidus. *Nature.* 1992;359:233-235.
144. Bichet DG. Vasopressin receptor mutations in nephrogenic diabetes insipidus. *Semin in Nephrol.* 2008;28:245-251.
145. Deen PMT, Verdijk MA, Knoers NVAM, et al. Requirement of human renal water channel aquaporin-2 for vasopressin-dependent concentration of urine. *Science.* 1994;264:92-95.
146. Mulders SM, Knoers AVAM, van Leiburg AF, et al. New mutations in the AQP2 gene in nephrogenic diabetes insipidus resulting in functional but misrouted water channels. *J Am Soc Nephrol.* 1997;8:242-248.
147. Cohen FE, Kelly JW. Therapeutic approaches to protein-misfolding diseases. *Nature.* 2003;426:905-909.
148. Bernier V, Morello J, Zarruk A, et al. Pharmacologic chaperones as a potential treatment for x-linked nephrogenic diabetes insipidus. *J Am Soc Nephrol.* 2006;17:232-243.
149. Feldman BJ, Rosenthal SM, Vargas GA, et al. Nephrogenic syndrome of inappropriate antidiuresis. *N Engl J Med.* 2005;352:1884-1890.
150. Gitelman SE, Feldman BJ, Rosenthal SM. Nephrogenic syndrome of inappropriate antidiuresis: a novel disorder in water balance in pediatric patients. *Am J Med.* 2006;119:S54-S58.
151. Ellison DH, Berl T. The syndrome of inappropriate antidiuresis. *N Engl J Med.* 2007;356:2064-2072.
152. Levtchenko EN, Monnens LAH. Nephrogenic syndrome of inappropriate antidiuresis. *Nephrol Dial Transplant.* 2010;25:2839-2843.
153. Rochdi MD, Vargas GA, Carpentier E, et al. Functional characterization of vasopressin type 2 receptor substitutions (R137H/C/L) leading to nephrogenic diabetes insipidus and nephrogenic syndrome of inappropriate antidiuresis: implications for treatments. *Mol Pharmacol.* 2010;77:836-845.

CHAPTER 19

Obstructive Uropathy: Assessment of Renal Function in the Fetus

Robert L. Chevalier, MD

19

- **Pathogenesis of Congenital Obstructive Uropathy**
- **Differential Diagnosis of Fetal Hydronephrosis: Introduction to the Controversies**
- **Fetal Renal Development and Physiology**
- **Evaluation of the Fetal Urinary Tract**
- **Evaluation of Fetal Renal Function**
- **Fetal Surgical Intervention for Obstructive Uropathy**
- **Histology of the Fetal Kidney in Obstructive Uropathy**
- **Postnatal Follow-up**
- **Long-term Implications of Congenital Obstructive Uropathy**
- **The Future**
- **Summary and Conclusions**

Obstructive uropathy comprises the greatest identifiable cause of renal insufficiency and renal failure in infants and children.[1] This group of disorders creates significant diagnostic and therapeutic challenges for obstetricians, perinatologists, neonatologists, pediatric nephrologists, and pediatric urologists. The hallmark of obstructive uropathy is hydronephrosis, which is most often first detected by fetal ultrasonography. The etiology of the lesions responsible for congenital urinary tract obstruction remains undetermined in most cases, although mutations in certain genes have been implicated in a variety of urinary tract malformations[2,3] and malformation syndromes.[4] The natural history of obstructive uropathy remains poorly defined, and an improved understanding of pathophysiology will be necessary to advance diagnosis and management.

Although the focus of this review is the assessment of renal function in fetuses, the rationale for measuring fetal renal function is as important as the evaluation itself. Moreover, renal function is inextricably linked to renal growth, development, and adaptation to injury (e.g. obstruction of the urinary tract). A physician caring for a fetus with obstructive uropathy must be aware of not only the fetal and neonatal outcome but also the potential function of the kidneys and urinary tract throughout life (Fig. 19-1). The consequences of urinary tract maldevelopment include not only the challenges of dialysis and transplantation, but also those of recurrent urinary tract infections (UTIs) and urinary incontinence. Any fetal intervention must, therefore, take into account its potential impact on the patient's expected quality of life through adulthood. For these reasons, the determination of renal function in fetuses is considered in the broad context of congenital obstructive uropathy.

Pathogenesis of Congenital Obstructive Uropathy

The relative contribution of primary renal maldevelopment and altered renal development secondary to obstruction of urine flow remains unclear. Studies in animals

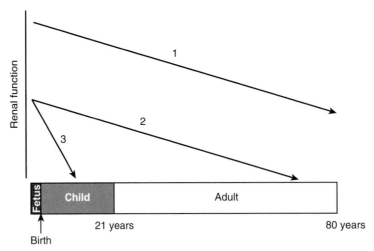

Figure 19-1 Schematic showing the long-term impact of congenital obstructive uropathy. The urinary tract abnormality develops in embryonic and fetal life, but if mild (1), the consequences of the condition may become apparent only later in adulthood, if at all. If moderate (2), progression of renal insufficiency may develop earlier in adulthood. If severe (3), renal failure develops in infancy or childhood. Fetal intervention should take into account not only the health and welfare of fetus and mother, but also the long-term implications of perinatal management.

have shown that experimentally-induced fetal ureteral or urethral obstruction can result in dysplastic renal changes (generally after obstruction early in gestation) or hydronephrosis with varying degrees of impairment of renal growth and function (after obstruction later in gestation).[5,6] The consequences of obstruction to urine flow during renal development are highly complex, involving tubular dilatation and altered epithelial–mesenchymal interaction, apoptosis, and cyst formation.[7] If initiated early in fetal life, urinary tract obstruction alters branching morphogenesis, leading to altered induction of glomeruli, podocyte apoptosis, and glomerular cysts (Fig. 19-2). The result of these events is a decrease in nephron number. The severity of obstructive uropathy depends on the severity and timing of obstruction, as well as the site and duration of obstruction.[8]

Differential Diagnosis of Fetal Hydronephrosis: Introduction to the Controversies

Even the definition of *clinically significant urinary tract obstruction* is subject to debate. Peters has offered the following: "Obstruction is a condition of impaired urinary drainage, which, if uncorrected, will limit the ultimate functional potential of a developing kidney."[9] Although this definition accounts for the relationship between renal function and renal development, it does not provide a useful clinical guide to determine a critical degree of urinary tract obstruction in a fetus or infant. In a fetus or infant with hydronephrosis, urinary tract obstruction must be distinguished from vesicoureteral reflux (VUR) and from physiologic renal pelvic dilatation.[8] Additional nonobstructive causes of hydronephrosis include congenital extrarenal pelvis and nonrefluxing nonobstructed megaureter (Table 19-1).[10]

Ureteropelvic junction obstruction (UPJO) is the most common lesion resulting in congenital obstructive uropathy. Although it is most often unilateral, the contralateral kidney may be subject to other abnormalities, such as VUR.[11] The major controversy surrounding the evaluation of UPJO is the selection of patients for surgical pyeloplasty (as well as the timing of the procedure), with the objective of maximizing long-term renal function. Ureterovesical obstruction and ureterocele with ectopic ureter are additional sites for a congenital obstructive lesion and must also be distinguished from uncomplicated VUR. Less commonly encountered, retrocaval ureter, primary obstructive megaureter, or midureteral stricture can also result in

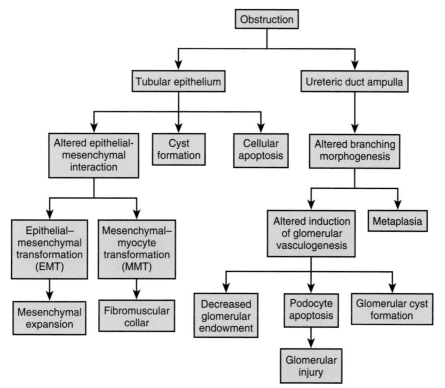

Figure 19-2 Pathogenesis of obstructive renal dysplasia based on experimental fetal sheep and monkey studies. The effects of obstruction involve a combination of renal maldevelopment and injury: first, there is abnormal branching morphogenesis leading directly to a reduction in glomerular development. Second, there are podocyte apoptosis, tubular apoptosis and epithelial–mesenchymal transformation, and interstitial cell transformation to myofibroblasts, which contribute to ongoing nephron loss. (From Woolf AS, Thiruchelvam N. Congenital obstructive uropathy: its origin and contribution to end-stage renal disease in children [review]. *Adv Ren Replace Ther* 8:157, 2001, with permission.)

Table 19-1 CAUSES OF ANTENATAL HYDRONEPHROSIS

Anomalous UPJ or UPJO
Multicystic kidney
Retrocaval ureter
Primary obstructive megaureter
Nonrefluxing nonobstructed megaureter
Vesicoureteral reflux
Midureteral stricture
Ectopic ureterocele
Ectopic ureter
Posterior urethral valves
Prune belly syndrome
Urethral atresia
MMIHS
Hydrocolpos
Pelvic tumor
Cloacal abnormality

MMIHS, megacystis–microcolon–intestinal hypoperistalsis syndrome; UPJ, ureteropelvic junction; UPJO, ureteropelvic junction obstruction
Adapted from Elder JS. Antenatal hydronephrosis: fetal and neonatal management. *Pediatr Clin North Am.* 44:1299, 1997.

fetal hydronephrosis (Table 19-1). Multicystic dysplastic kidney can be confused sonographically with UPJO and is thought to result from ureteral atresia and severe obstructive uropathy in early fetal development.[12] These kidneys are nonfunctional, generally involute either before or after parturition, and can be followed by serial ultrasonography. Other cystic kidney disorders, such as solitary cysts and polycystic kidney disease, are generally easier to differentiate from obstructive uropathy.

Although less common, bladder outlet obstruction constitutes a more serious cause of obstructive uropathy because both kidneys are compromised. The differential diagnosis of obstructive lesions in this site includes posterior urethral valves (PUVs), prune belly syndrome, and urethral atresia (Table 19-1). Dilatation of the fetal bladder and renal pelves but with normal amniotic fluid volume suggests megacystis–microcolon-–intestinal hypoperistalsis syndrome, a rare and lethal condition that, unlike most obstructive nephropathy, is far more common in girls.[13] The major controversy in the management of these lower tract lesions also relates to patient selection and the timing of surgical intervention, including fetal urinary diversion (discussed later).[14] Finally, hydrocolpos, neoplasms (e.g., sacrococcygeal tumors), or cloacal abnormalities may rarely account for congenital urinary tract obstruction (Table 19-1).

Fetal Renal Development and Physiology

To understand the assessment of renal function in a fetus with potential obstructive uropathy, it is first necessary to review normal fetal renal physiology. Because function follows morphology, it is useful to examine human fetal renal development (Fig. 19-3).[15] After the initial appearance and disappearance of the pronephros and mesonephros in early embryonic life, the metanephros begins development at the end of the first trimester (Fig. 19-3). Nephrogenesis undergoes most rapid growth

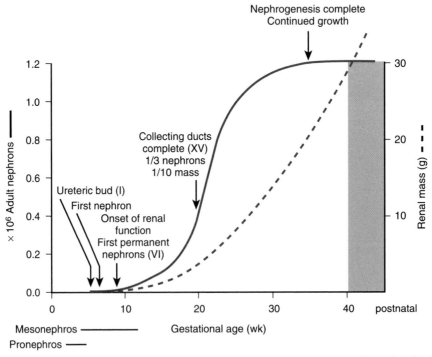

Figure 19-3 Human fetal renal development. The pronephros and mesonephros are formed in the first weeks of embryonic life and are replaced by the metanephros, which begins to produce urine at about the 10th week of gestation. The most rapid period of nephrogenesis is in the midtrimester, with nephrogenesis being complete by the 34th week. Renal mass follows an exponential increase throughout the second and third trimesters. (From Harrison MR, Golbus MS, Filly RA, et al. Management of the fetus with congenital hydronephrosis. *J Pediatr Surg* 17:728, 1982, with permission.)

during the second trimester, with completion by 34 weeks' gestation; renal mass increases exponentially throughout the second and third trimesters (Fig. 19-3). Fetal urine production normally increases dramatically in the third trimester, reaching rates of approximately 50 mL/hr at term (Fig. 19-4).[16] For a 2.5-kg infant, this amounts to a urine flow rate of 20 mL/kg/hr that would translate to a high rate of diuresis in the neonate. As described later, the high fetal urine flow rate contributes significantly to amniotic fluid volume (Fig. 19-5),[17] which becomes compromised in severe bilateral fetal obstructive uropathy.

Fetal renal blood flow increases linearly throughout the second half of pregnancy, from less than 20 mL/min at 20 weeks to 40 to 100 mL/min at 40 weeks (Fig. 19-6).[18] Fetal glomerular filtration rate (GFR) also increases progressively during the second half of gestation and has been calculated from data obtained from a clinical fetal research center.[19,20] Estimated fetal creatinine clearance increases from less than 1 mL/min below 25 weeks to greater than 4 mL/min at term (Fig. 19-7A).[21] Urine concentrating capacity is reduced in fetuses because of anatomic immaturity of the renal medulla, decreased medullary concentration of sodium chloride and urea, and diminished responsiveness of collecting ducts to vasopressin.[22] Recent studies show that this is partly attributable to reduced density of aquaporins (AQPs) in fetuses.[23,24] Fractional excretion of sodium (FENa) decreases progressively throughout the second half of gestation, but remains at 5% to 20% of the filtered load (Fig. 19-7B).[21] This is partly attributable to progressive maturation of sodium channels in the collecting duct.[25] These changes lead to a progressive decrease in fetal urine sodium concentration from 16 to 36 weeks' gestation (Fig. 19-8).[26] Renal

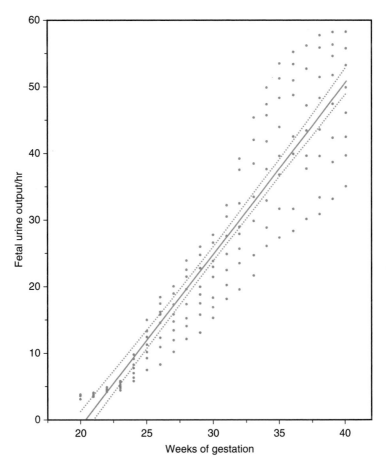

Figure 19-4   Values of hourly urine production (mL) by normal fetuses plotted with mean and 95% confidence limits of the slope. (From Mitra SC. Effect of cocaine on fetal kidney and bladder function. *J Maternal-Fetal Med.* 8:262, 1999, with permission.)

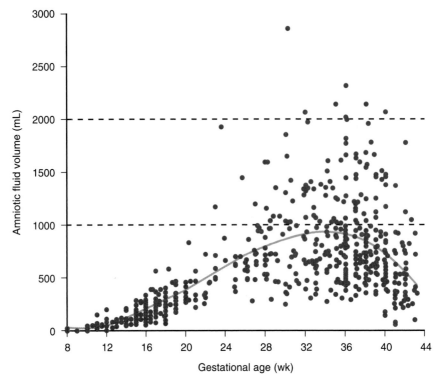

Figure 19-5 Amniotic fluid volume in human pregnancies in the second and third trimesters (individual data points [n = 705 pregnancies]). *Solid line* is polynomial regression. (From Brace RA, Wolf EJ. Normal amniotic fluid volume changes throughout pregnancy. *Am J Obstet Gynecol.* 161:382, 1989, with permission.)

adaptation to parturition is revealed by a marked reduction in FENa in neonates compared with fetuses of similar gestational age (Fig. 19-7B).[27]

Because postnatal bladder dysfunction is a major cause of morbidity in infants with bladder outlet obstruction, increasing attention is being paid to fetal bladder physiology. Ultrasound studies have revealed a progressive increase in duration of fetal bladder cycles from approximately 25 minutes at 20 weeks gestation to 60 minutes at 40 weeks.[16]

Evaluation of the Fetal Urinary Tract

The assessment of a fetus with hydronephrosis should first involve a detailed evaluation of the sonogram of the kidneys and urinary tract. The severity of fetal renal

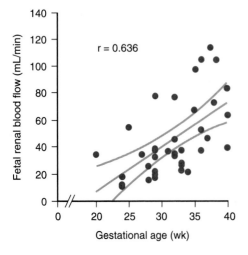

Figure 19-6   Renal blood flow in human fetuses in the second half of gestation measured by color-pulsed Doppler evaluation of the renal artery (individual data points [n = 22 fetuses, each studied three times], with lines showing mean and 95% confidence intervals). (From Veille JC, Hanson RA, Tatum K, et al. Quantitative assessment of human fetal renal blood flow. *Am J Obstet Gynecol.* 169:1399, 1993, with permission.)

Figure 19-7 Renal function in human fetuses (*pink circles*) and neonates (*red circles*) in the second half of gestation. **A.** Estimated creatinine clearance. **B.** Calculated fractional sodium excretion. Fetal values were calculated from several groups of data from a single human fetal research center,[19,20,123] and postnatal values were previously reported by Al-Dahhan et al.[27] (From Haycock GB. Development of glomerular filtration and tubular sodium reabsorption in the human fetus and newborn. *Br J Urol.* 81(suppl 2):33, 1998, with permission.)

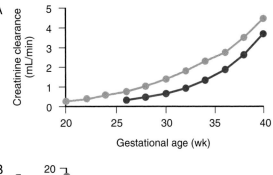

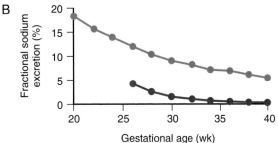

pelvic dilatation does not always correlate well with renal functional outcome,[28] but an anteroposterior renal pelvic diameter exceeding 7 mm in the third trimester appears to be predictive of obstructive uropathy, with a 69% to 92% positive predictive value.[29,30] Of note, variability in the measurement of fetal renal pelvic diameter averages 4 mm, such that 70% of fetuses had both "normal" and "abnormal" values during a 2-hour study period.[31] A meta-analysis of antenatal renal ultrasound results revealed that oligohydramnios and renal cortical appearance provide the best predictive value for postnatal renal function (sensitivity, 0.6; specificity. 0.8) (Table 19-2).[32] Comparison of renal pelvic diameters measured by antenatal ultrasonography grouped by ultimate outcome shows a broad range for each gestational age, but discrimination clearly improves with gestational and postnatal age.[33] Increased renal echogenicity or effacement of the corticomedullary junction on the fetal ultrasound have been associated with dysplastic changes in the kidney and, therefore, an unfavorable prognosis.[34] Although a correlation between gross renal anatomy (revealed by ultrasonography) and renal function (measured by postnatal diuretic renography) would be expected, this is often not the case. In fact, studies have shown that the relationship between renal histology and renal function in children with UPJO is

Figure 19-8 Fetal urinary sodium concentration based on data from 26 human fetuses 16 to 36 weeks' gestation with normal urinary tracts (mean and 95% confidence intervals). (From Nicolini U, Fisk NM, Rodeck CH, et al. Fetal urine biochemistry: an index of renal maturation and dysfunction. *Br J Obstet Gynaecol.* 99:46, 1992, with permission.)

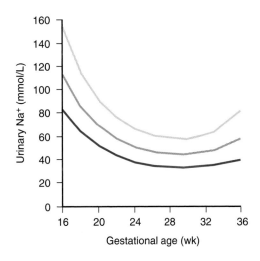

Table 19-2 SUBGROUP META-ANALYSIS (RANDOM EFFECTS MODEL) OF ANTENATAL ULTRASOUND DIAGNOSTIC MEASURES TO PREDICT POOR POSTNATAL RENAL FUNCTION IN SURVIVORS WITH CONGENITAL LOWER URINARY TRACT OBSTRUCTION

Diagnostic Measure	Sensitivity (95% CI)	Specificity (95% CI)	P	AUC
Oligohydramnios	0.63 (0.51–0.74)	0.76 (0.65–0.85)	19.67, (0.02)	0.74
Renal cortical appearance	0.57 (0.37–0.76)	0.84 (0.71–0.94)	10.29, (0.04)	0.78
Gestation at diagnosis <24 weeks	0.48 (0.26–0.70)	0.82 (0.66–0.92)	3.88, (0.14)	0.68

AUC, area under receiver operating characteristic curve; CI, confidence intervals.

With permission from Morris RK, Malin GL, Khan KS, et al. Antenatal ultrasound to predict postnatal renal function in congenital lower urinary tract obstruction: systematic review of test accuracy [review]. BJOG 116:1290, 2009.

very poor.[35] There is evidence that fetal renal artery Doppler examination can distinguish nonfunctioning cystic kidneys from normal,[36] but studies documenting a reliable estimate of renal blood flow in fetal obstructive uropathy are lacking. Even postnatal measurement of the intrarenal resistive index has not proved reliable for the evaluation of obstructive uropathy.[37]

Fetal ultrasonography also permits the examination of the lower urinary tract, paying particular attention to dilatation and thickening of the bladder, both of which are increased with significant bladder outlet obstruction, which occurs with PUV. Ultrasound measurement of fetal bladder sagittal diameter is also helpful in predicting postnatal outcome. The fetal bladder can be measured in the first trimester; a diameter exceeding 15 mm is associated with a poor prognosis.[38] There is a tight relationship between bladder diameter and gestational age, with measurements exceeding the 95% confidence interval defined as "dilated" and those larger than 10 mm defined as "megacystis" (Fig. 19-9). When coupled with renal pelvic changes (pyelectasis vs. hydronephrosis), the combination of megacystis and hydronephrosis carries the worst prognosis.[39] Whereas the association of bladder diameter greater than 40 mm with hydronephrosis before 28 weeks is predictive of PUV, the absence of hydronephrosis and bladder diameter less than 40 mm is predictive of urethral atresia or stenosis.[40] The prognosis is more dependent on the obstructive

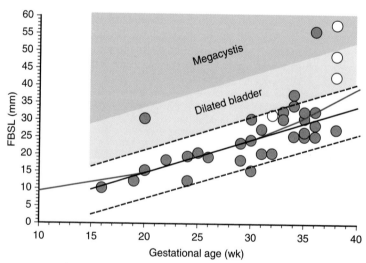

Figure 19-9 Exact exponential and approximate linear regression models of normal fetal bladder sagittal length (FBSL) reveal that the exact exponential regression (*curved line*) relationship of FBSL and gestational age can be approximated by a linear regression model (*solid line*). Outliers (*open circles*) often showed megaureter in newborns. Regions defining enlarged bladder as dilated bladder or megacystis are shown above 95% confidence intervals. *Filled circles* indicate normal values. (From Maizels M, Alpert SA, Houston JTB, et al. Fetal bladder sagittal length: a simple monitor to assess normal and enlarged fetal bladder size, and forecast clinical outcome. J Urol. 172:1995, 2004, with permission.)

lesion than on renal ultrasound or biochemical profiles; urethral atresia is less favorable than PUV.[40] Examination of the bladder after emptying by vesicocentesis is also helpful. Fetuses with urethral atresia or completely obstructed PUV demonstrate symmetrically round and thick-walled bladders.[41] In addition, ultrasonography provides an estimation of amniotic fluid volume, which is decreased in the second and third trimester in any condition associated with decreased fetal urine production. This includes bilateral renal agenesis, renal hypoplasia, dysplasia, polycystic kidney disease, or obstructive uropathy. Severe oligohydramnios is associated with pulmonary hypoplasia, which becomes a major cause of neonatal mortality in fetal obstructive uropathy.[42] This is important because the prevention of pulmonary hypoplasia (rather than the prevention of renal insufficiency, as described later) constitutes the major justification for the clinical measurement of renal function in human fetuses.

Fetal urinary tract ultrasonography may be limited by severe oligohydramnios, fetal complex malformation syndromes, or maternal obesity. In such cases, measurement of the water apparent diffusion coefficient by magnetic resonance imaging (MRI) can be helpful, but must be factored for gestational age.[43] This technique can be used to complement sonography and to clarify the diagnosis, sometimes modifying the decision to continue or terminate the pregnancy.[44]

After the condition has been detected by maternal ultrasonography, the mother of a fetus with urinary tract anomalies and oligohydramnios should receive consultation by appropriate specialists, including a perinatologist, genetic counselor, pediatric urologist, and pediatric nephrologist. Delivery of these infants should optimally be planned for a tertiary care center with the necessary experience and multidisciplinary team.

Evaluation of Fetal Renal Function

The clinical evaluation of fetal renal function is challenging and must be measured indirectly. As described above, fetal urine flow can be determined from timing fetal bladder filling and emptying,[16] and amniotic fluid volume provides an estimate of fetal urine production in the second and third trimester.[17] Fetal urine sampling provides information regarding fetal renal function (Table 19-3). As stated previously, however, the rationale for measuring fetal renal function is to confirm which fetuses with severe oligohydramnios have salvageable renal function and, therefore, require intervention to permit pulmonary maturation.[45]

Table 19-3 CONCENTRATIONS OF BIOMARKERS OF FETAL RENAL FUNCTION ASSOCIATED WITH A FAVORABLE RENAL PROGNOSIS

Fetal serum markers	
β_2-microglobulin (mg/L)[46-48]	<5.6
Fetal urine markers	
Sodium (mmol/L)[46]	<100
Chloride (mmol/L)[51]	<90
Calcium (mmol/L)[26]	<1.2
Osmolality (mOsm/L)[51]	<200
β_2-microglobulin (mg/L)[49]	<2
Total protein (mg/dL)[51]	<20
N-acetyl-β-D-glucosaminidase (nmol/mL/hr)[50]	<100
Cystatin-C (mg/L)[55]	<1
Amniotic fluid markers	
Cystatin-C (mg/L)[56]	<1

Fetal serum β_2-microglobulin, normally less than 5.6 mg/l (Table 19-3), serves as a measure of glomerular function and does not change with gestational age.[46,47] This parameter can also be a useful predictor of renal injury in fetuses with obstructive uropathy (Fig. 19-10).[47] Although sampling of fetal serum β_2-microglobulin is more difficult than urine, sensitivity and specificity are 80% and 99%, respectively,[48] and it allows serial tracking of fetal renal function before and after surgical intervention. In contrast, fetal urinary β_2-microglobulin is increased as a consequence of tubular dysfunction, with values exceeding 2 mg/L suggesting a poor renal outcome (Table 19-3).[49] Similarly, fetal urinary N-acetyl-β-D-glucosaminidase (NAG) concentration is elevated in severe obstructive uropathy (>100 nmol/mL/hr) (Table 19-3), although neither β_2-microglobulin nor NAG can be used independently to discriminate between fetuses with renal damage and those with normal function.[50]

Urinary calcium concentration exceeding 1.2 mmol/L has also been reported to correlate with poor renal outcome (Table 19-3).[26] After the beginning of metanephric function at the end of the first trimester (Fig. 19-3), tubular function matures throughout gestation, and urine becomes progressively hypotonic, with decreasing urinary sodium concentration from 16 to 30 weeks' gestation (Fig. 19-8).[26] It should be noted that in the early second trimester, fetal urine sodium concentration is normally similar to plasma, so the effects of obstructive uropathy would not be detectable at 16 weeks (Fig. 19-8). However, because urine sodium concentration decreases throughout the second and third trimesters, values above 100 mEq/L beyond 20 weeks' gestation should be considered abnormal (Table 19-3).[46] In addition to urine sodium, urine chloride concentration has also been shown to be a useful marker of fetal renal dysfunction, with values above 90 mEq/L being abnormal (Table 19-3).[51] Similarly, urine osmolality exceeding 200 mOsm/L and total protein exceeding 20 mg/dL were found to be associated with significant fetal renal dysfunction (Table 19-3), with superior sensitivity and specificity to urine β_2-microglobulin or sodium concentration.[51]

Although fetal urine sodium and calcium concentration can discriminate severe renal dysfunction secondary to obstructive uropathy, these markers are less helpful in predicting moderate renal dysfunction.[52] Although requiring sophisticated analytical equipment, proton nuclear magnetic resonance spectroscopy can provide superior resolution of potential biomarkers in 0.5 mL of fetal urine from patients subsequently followed for at least 1 year with either normal GFR, decreased GFR,

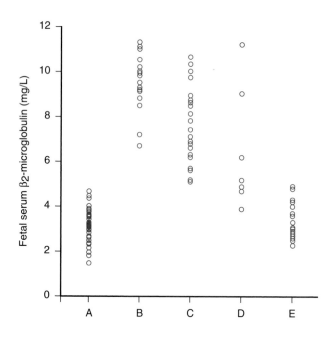

Figure 19-10 Fetal serum β_2-microglobulin concentration. **A.** Control participants ($n = 67$). **B.** Bilateral renal agenesis ($n = 18$). **C.** Termination of pregnancy because of bilateral renal dysplasia ($n = 26$). **D.** Infants with postnatal serum creatinine greater than 50 μmol/L ($n = 6$). **E.** Infants with postnatal serum creatinine less than 50 μmol/L ($n = 28$). (From Dommergues M, Muller F, Ngo S, et al. Fetal serum B2-microglobulin predicts postnatal renal function in bilateral uropathies. *Kidney Int.* 58:312, 2000, with permission.)

Figure 19-11 Urine samples from human fetuses with bilateral urinary tract obstruction examined by proton nuclear magnetic resonance. Group 1 (*n* = 21, *squares*) consisted of survivors for longer than 1 year with serum creatinine below 50 µmol/L. Group 2 (*n* = 17, *triangles*) consisted of survivors with serum creatinine above 50 µmol/L. Group 3 (*n* = 18, *crosses*) consisted of those with histologic dysplasia associated with fetal (termination of pregnancy) or neonatal death. **A.** Relationship between fetal urinary concentration of β_2-microglobulin and sodium concentration. **B.** Relationship between fetal urinary valine and threonine concentration. (From Eugene M, Muller F, Dommergues M, et al. Evaluation of postnatal renal function in fetuses with bilateral obstructive uropathies by proton nuclear magnetic resonance spectroscopy. *Am J Obstet Gynecol.* 170:595, 1994, with permission.)

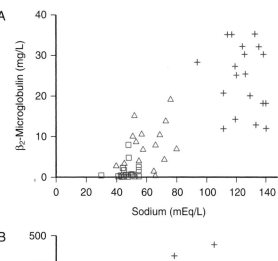

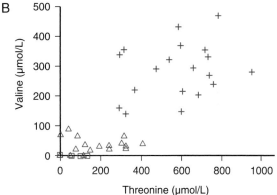

or severe renal dysplasia associated with fetal or neonatal death.[53] High-resolution magnetic resonance spectroscopy has also been used to measure amino acids, glucose, and creatinine in second- and third-trimester amniotic fluid.[54] Although amino acids and glucose decrease with gestational age, creatinine increases: combinations of these may prove useful as biomarkers of fetal renal maturation.[54] Two-dimensional representation of fetal urine β_2-microglobulin and sodium concentration discriminates between those with normal and decreased GFR (but survival) with 76% sensitivity, 81% specificity, and 81% negative predictive value (Fig. 19-11A).[53] Fetal urine valine-threonine concentration discriminates with 88% sensitivity, 86% specificity, and 90% negative predictive value (Fig. 19-11B).[53]

Recently, cystatin C has been investigated as a promising marker of fetal renal function. Cystatin C is a low-molecular-weight protein (13.3 kDa) that is produced by all nucleated human cells, does not cross the placenta and is filtered by the glomerulus and completely reabsorbed by the tubule.[55] Fetal *urine* cystatin C has a similar sensitivity and specificity to urinary sodium and β_2-microglobulin in distinguishing severe renal dysfunction, but has the advantage of not varying with gestational age (Fig. 19-12A).[55] In contrast, studies have shown that *amniotic fluid* cystatin C concentration normally decreases with gestational age from 22 to 36 weeks (Fig. 19-12B), but that concentrations of cystatin C in amniotic fluid from pregnancies with fetal uropathies are significantly higher (1.1–1.8 mg/L) than normal (0.5–0.8 mg/L) (Table 19-3).[56] Similar conclusions were reached in a recent report comparing fetal urine and amniotic fluid cystatin C concentrations.[57]

An enhancement of sensitivity in discrimination by urinary biomarkers has been achieved by sequential sampling of three fetal bladder aspirations, each 48 hours apart.[58] The rationale for this is as follows: the first urine sample represents "bladder" urine, the second represents urine that was flushed into the bladder from the dilated upper urinary tracts, and the third represents newly produced urine that

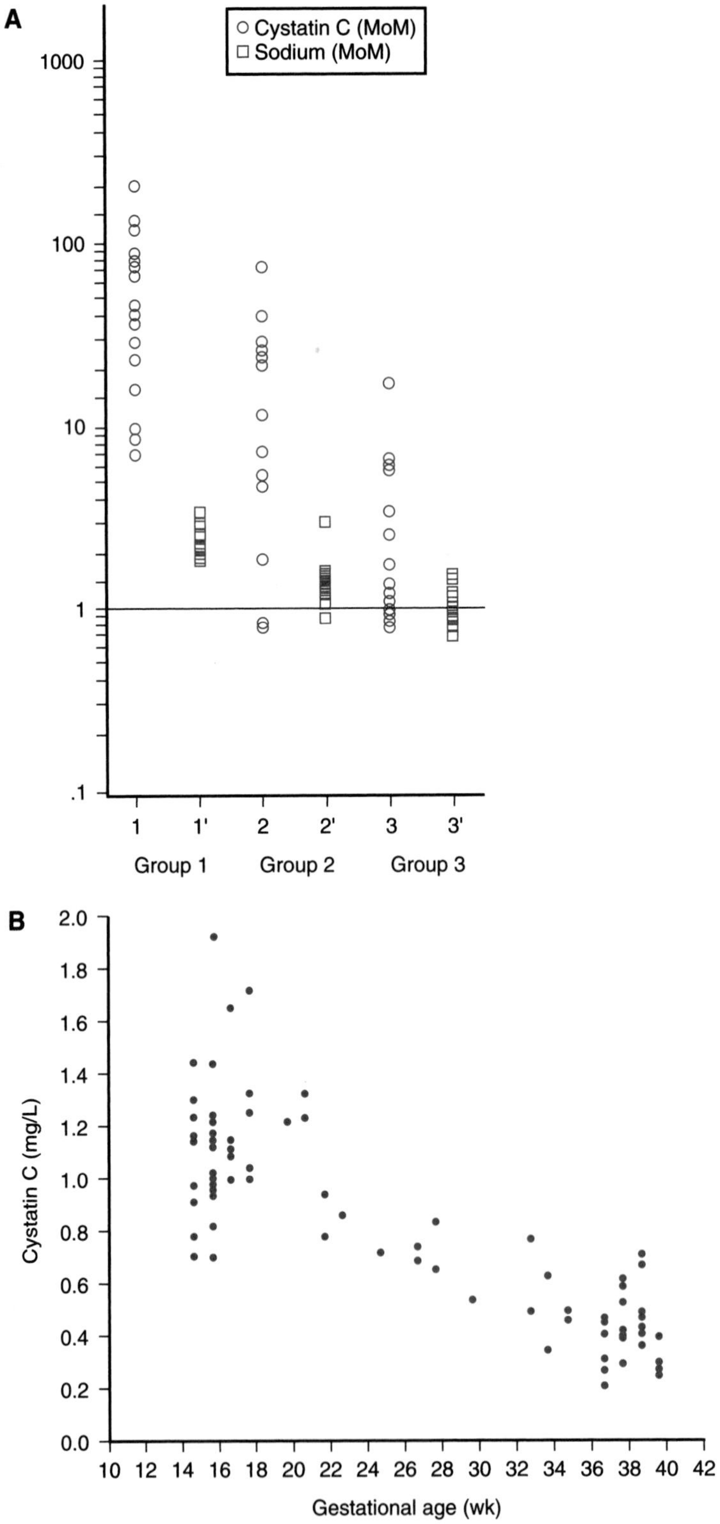

Figure 19-12 Fetal urine and amniotic fluid cystatin C concentration. **A.** Fetal urine cystatin C and sodium concentration expressed as multiples of the median (MoM) on a logarithmic scale. Group 1 (*n* = 19) consisted of termination of pregnancy or neonatal death because of bilateral renal dysplasia. Group 2 (*n* = 19) consisted of infants with postnatal serum creatinine above 50 μmol/L. Group 3 (*n* = 33) consisted of infants with postnatal creatinine below 50 μmol/L. **B.** Amniotic fluid cystatin C in the second and third trimesters for normal fetuses (*n* = 96). Values for 22- to 36-week fetuses with obstructive uropathy ranged from 1.08 to 1.75 mg/L. (From Muller F., Bernard MA, Benkirane A, et al. Fetal urine cystatin C as a predictor of postnatal renal function in bilateral uropathies. *Clin Chem.* 45:2292, 1999; and Mussap M, Fanos V, Pizzini C, et al. Predictive value of amniotic fluid cystatin C levels for the early identification of fetuses with obstructive uropathies. *Intl J Obstet Gynaecol.* 109:778, 2002, with permission.)

drained into the bladder after temporary relief of obstruction by the bladder aspirations.[51,58] It should be recalled that with bladder outlet obstruction, renal function is often impaired asymmetrically. Thus, bladder urine indices reflect function of the more severely affected kidney and may underestimate the recoverability of the less damaged kidney. For this reason, if there is a marked difference in hydronephrosis between kidneys, aspiration of the renal pelves can be performed.[45]

Fetal renal maturation can also be inferred from biochemical profiles of amniotic fluid, which is more easily obtained than fetal urine or blood. Amniotic fluid α1-microglobulin, β_2-microglobulin, glucose, and uric acid concentration provided good correlation with fetal renal maturation, but their utility in distinguishing postnatal prognosis has not been confirmed.[59,60]

Three variables have been identified as independent predictors of adverse outcome in fetal hydronephrosis: oligohydramnios, postnatal GFR below 20 mL/min, and prematurity.[61] The nadir plasma creatinine concentration is a useful marker of prognosis: whereas fetuses with a nadir of greater than 1.0 mg/dL all progressed to renal failure, 75% of those with a nadir serum creatinine of less than 0.8 mg/dL maintained normal GFR for more than 4 years.[45] Although oligohydramnios and reduced GFR are directly linked to functioning renal mass, the role of prematurity is less obvious. Fetuses with significant bladder outlet obstruction are more likely to be born before term.[62] Of greater concern is the recent discovery that nephrogenesis may not progress postnatally in very low birth weight infants, such that the ultimate number of nephrons may remain permanently decreased.[63,64] Because severe congenital bladder outlet obstruction can itself significantly reduce the number of nephrons in the human fetus,[65] the added complication of prematurity becomes an important variable.

A recent meta-analysis of fetal urine analytes to predict renal outcome included 23 articles (total of 572 women) that met selection criteria.[66] The two most accurate tests were urine calcium and sodium concentration, with β_2-microglobulin being less accurate (Fig. 19-13).[66] It is important to use gestation-specific thresholds.

Fetal Surgical Intervention for Obstructive Uropathy

In the setting of oligohydramnios with bladder distension and bilateral hydronephrosis, after other serious anomalies have been ruled out by fetal ultrasonography (with amnioinfusion if necessary), fetal karyotype should be obtained from chorionic villus sampling or amniotic fluid (Fig. 19-14).[67] A minimum of three serial fetal urine samples may then be obtained at 48- to 72-hour intervals as described previously, and fetuses are characterized as having a good prognosis (Table 19-3), borderline prognosis (maximum of 2 abnormal values), or poor prognosis (maximum of 3 abnormal values). Parents are then offered the option of prenatal intervention if the karyotype is normal male with isolated lower urinary tract obstruction and good or borderline urine markers.[67] Vesicoamniotic shunting is a temporary percutaneous intervention that provides diversion of fetal urine to the amniotic space and has been described in detail.[14] As discussed later, the ultimate outcome of patients undergoing fetal intervention for obstructive uropathy is variable, with survival largely depending on the specific underlying diagnosis and the criteria for patient selection.[67-69] Meta-analysis of the benefits of prenatal bladder drainage on the outcome of fetal lower urinary tract obstruction suggests improved survival of those with poor predicted prognosis (Fig. 19-15), although when considering the effect on long-term survival with normal postnatal renal function, the results suggest a trend favoring no treatment.[70] A sobering conclusion was reached by a European group reviewing the outcome of feto-amniotic shunting in a 9-year study (1993–2001) compared with a prior 4-year study (1988–1992): "The indications, complications and management of feto-amniotic shunting did not change profoundly."[71] Systematic reviews of fetal medicine have suffered from methodologic flaws such as assessing validity of included studies.[72] In the absence of a large prospective study, the impact of vesicoamniotic shunting on even pulmonary maturation remains to be established conclusively. Recruitment for the Percutaneous shunting in Lower

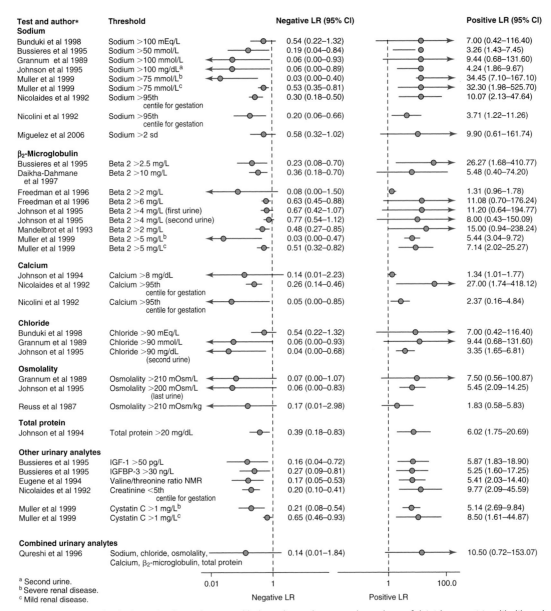

Test and author*	Threshold	Negative LR (95% CI)	Positive LR (95% CI)
Sodium			
Bunduki et al 1998	Sodium >100 mEq/L	0.54 (0.22–1.32)	7.00 (0.42–116.40)
Bussieres et al 1995	Sodium >50 mmol/L	0.19 (0.04–0.84)	3.26 (1.43–7.45)
Grannum et al 1989	Sodium >100 mmol/L	0.06 (0.00–0.93)	9.44 (0.68–131.60)
Johnson et al 1995	Sodium >100 mg/dL[a]	0.06 (0.00–0.89)	4.24 (1.86–9.67)
Muller et al 1999	Sodium >75 mmol/L[b]	0.03 (0.00–0.40)	34.45 (7.10–167.10)
Muller et al 1999	Sodium >75 mmol/L[c]	0.53 (0.35–0.81)	32.30 (1.98–525.70)
Nicolaides et al 1992	Sodium >95th centile for gestation	0.30 (0.18–0.50)	10.07 (2.13–47.64)
Nicolini et al 1992	Sodium >95th centile for gestation	0.20 (0.06–0.66)	3.71 (1.22–11.26)
Miguelez et al 2006	Sodium >2 sd	0.58 (0.32–1.02)	9.90 (0.61–161.74)
β₂-Microglobulin			
Bussieres et al 1995	Beta 2 >2.5 mg/L	0.23 (0.08–0.70)	26.27 (1.68–410.77)
Daikha-Dahmane et al 1997	Beta 2 >10 mg/L	0.36 (0.18–0.70)	5.48 (0.40–74.20)
Freedman et al 1996	Beta 2 >2 mg/L	0.08 (0.00–1.50)	1.31 (0.96–1.78)
Freedman et al 1996	Beta 2 >6 mg/L	0.63 (0.45–0.88)	11.08 (0.70–176.24)
Johnson et al 1995	Beta 2 >4 mg/L (first urine)	0.67 (0.42–1.07)	11.20 (0.64–194.77)
Johnson et al 1995	Beta 2 >4 mg/L (second urine)	0.77 (0.54–1.12)	8.00 (0.43–150.09)
Mandelbrot et al 1993	Beta 2 >2 mg/L	0.48 (0.27–0.85)	15.00 (0.94–238.24)
Muller et al 1999	Beta 2 >5 mg/L[b]	0.03 (0.00–0.47)	5.44 (3.04–9.72)
Muller et al 1999	Beta 2 >5 mg/L[c]	0.51 (0.32–0.82)	7.14 (2.02–25.27)
Calcium			
Johnson et al 1994	Calcium >8 mg/dL	0.14 (0.01–2.23)	1.34 (1.01–1.77)
Nicolaides et al 1992	Calcium >95th centile for gestation	0.26 (0.14–0.46)	27.00 (1.74–418.12)
Nicolini et al 1992	Calcium >95th centile for gestation	0.05 (0.00–0.85)	2.37 (0.16–4.84)
Chloride			
Bunduki et al 1998	Chloride >90 mEq/L	0.54 (0.22–1.32)	7.00 (0.42–116.40)
Grannum et al 1989	Chloride >90 mmol/L	0.06 (0.00–0.93)	9.44 (0.68–131.60)
Johnson et al 1995	Chloride >90 mg/dL (second urine)	0.04 (0.00–0.68)	3.35 (1.65–6.81)
Osmolality			
Grannum et al 1989	Osmolality >210 mOsm/L	0.07 (0.00–1.07)	7.50 (0.56–100.87)
Johnson et al 1995	Osmolality >200 mOsm/L (last urine)	0.06 (0.00–0.83)	5.45 (2.09–14.25)
Reuss et al 1987	Osmolality >210 mOsm/kg	0.17 (0.01–2.98)	1.83 (0.58–5.83)
Total protein			
Johnson et al 1994	Total protein >20 mg/dL	0.39 (0.18–0.83)	6.02 (1.75–20.69)
Other urinary analytes			
Bussieres et al 1995	IGF-1 >50 pg/L	0.16 (0.04–0.72)	5.87 (1.83–18.90)
Bussieres et al 1995	IGFBP-3 >30 ng/L	0.27 (0.09–0.81)	5.25 (1.60–17.25)
Eugene et al 1994	Valine/threonine ratio NMR	0.17 (0.05–0.53)	5.41 (2.03–14.40)
Nicolaides et al 1992	Creatinine <5th centile for gestation	0.20 (0.10–0.41)	9.77 (2.09–45.59)
Muller et al 1999	Cystatin C >1 mg/L[b]	0.21 (0.08–0.54)	5.14 (2.69–9.84)
Muller et al 1999	Cystatin C >1 mg/L[c]	0.65 (0.46–0.93)	8.50 (1.61–44.87)
Combined urinary analytes			
Qureshi et al 1996	Sodium, chloride, osmolality, Calcium, β₂-microglobulin, total protein	0.14 (0.01–1.84)	10.50 (0.72–153.07)

[a] Second urine.
[b] Severe renal disease.
[c] Mild renal disease.

Figure 19-13 Individual results for index tests likely to be at least moderately useful (either positive likelihood ratio >5 or negative likelihood ratio <0.2) in prediction of poor postnatal renal function in fetuses with obstructive uropathy. CI, confidence interval; IGF, insulin-like growth factor; LR, likelihood ratio; NMR, nuclear magnetic resonance. (From Morris RK, Quinlan-Jones E, Kilby MD, et al. Systematic review of accuracy of fetal urine analysis to predict poor postnatal renal function in cases of congenital urinary tract obstruction. [Review]. *Prenat Diagn*. 27:900, 2007, with permission.) *References in table refer to those in original paper.

Urinary Tract Obstruction (PLUTO) study will continue until 2013 and may provide answers regarding 5-year impact of intervention.[73]

Histology of the Fetal Kidney in Obstructive Uropathy

Kidneys from human fetuses with severe bladder outlet obstruction showed both dysplastic and cystic changes, with increased apoptosis of mesenchymal and tubular cells (Fig. 19-2).[74] Examination of kidneys from human fetuses with severe bladder outlet obstruction or multicystic dysplasia with ureteral atresia showed expansion

Figure 19-14 Algorithm for the prenatal evaluation and management of fetuses with suspected lower urinary tract obstruction. (From Biard JM, Johnson MP, Carr MC, et al. Long-term outcomes in children treated by prenatal vesicoamniotic shunting for lower urinary tract obstruction. *Obstet Gynecol.* 106:503, 2005, with permission.)

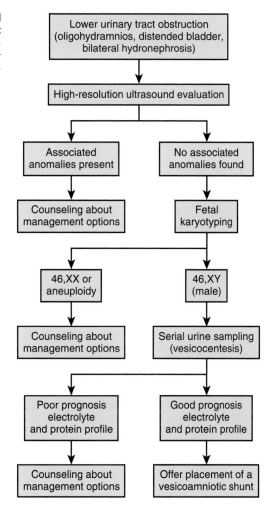

19

of glomerular and tubular cysts with retention of the macula densa and primitive loop structure, suggesting that the abnormalities developed after initial nephron differentiation.[75] In another study of human fetuses of 14 to 37 weeks' gestation with severe bilateral hydronephrosis, histologic findings revealed a range of dysplastic changes, including cessation of nephrogenesis, disappearance or myofibroblastic differentiation of metanephric blastema, and increased expression of α-smooth muscle actin by mesenchymal cells.[76] These changes are clearly irreversible and correlate with oligohydramnios, ultrasound evidence of renal dysplasia (loss of corticomedullary differentiation, renal hyperechogenicity, and presence of renal cortical cysts), and abnormal fetal urine sodium or β_2-microglobulin concentration.[76]

Attempts to perform renal biopsies in fetuses with obstructive uropathy have been of marginal usefulness. In the largest series reported to date, a successful renal specimen was obtained by percutaneous needle aspiration in five of 10 biopsies performed in fetuses with bilateral obstructive uropathy.[77] Normal fetal renal histology was found in four of these cases, with renal dysplasia being found in the remaining patient, who went on to develop renal failure despite a fetal urine sodium concentration of 60 mEq/L.[77] The authors conclude that although the technique is feasible and safe, it is limited by the difficulties in obtaining an adequate sample and the concern that needle biopsy does not provide representative samples of the entire kidney.[77]

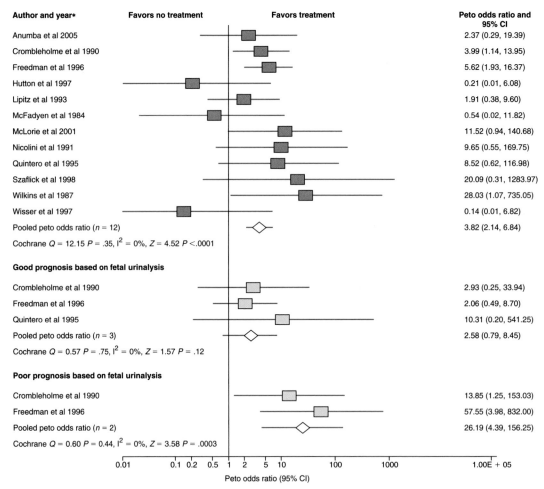

Figure 19-15 Effect of antenatal intervention on perinatal survival compared with no treatment (including voluntary termination of pregnancies) stratified by predicted prognosis. CI, confidence interval. (From Morris RK, Malin GL, Khan KS, et al. Systematic Review of the effectiveness of antenatal intervention for the treatment of congenital lower urinary tract obstruction. [Review]. *BJOG*. 117:382, 2010, with permission.*References in table refer to those in original paper.)

Postnatal Follow-up

Bilateral Hydronephrosis

Infants with antenatal diagnosis of bilateral hydronephrosis should have prompt postnatal abdominal ultrasonography, voiding cystourethrography (VCUG), and nuclide renography to determine whether there is evidence for bilateral upper tract obstruction or VUR or bladder outlet obstruction. In such patients, continuous bladder drainage through an indwelling catheter is necessary to determine the renal functional potential before deciding on definitive surgical intervention.[11] During the transition from fetal to extrauterine life, infants with severe obstructive uropathy (especially after relief of obstruction) may manifest an exaggeration of the normal postnatal diuresis and natriuresis.[78] This is caused by the altered expression of renal sodium transporters and AQPs in bilateral obstructive uropathy[79,80] and mediated by upregulation of cyclooxygenase-2 in the renal medulla.[81]

Unilateral Hydronephrosis

Ultrasonography of the kidneys and urinary tract should be performed after birth in all infants with suspected antenatal hydronephrosis (Fig. 19-16). In the immediate postnatal period, infants with renal pelvic diameters less than 15 mm were found

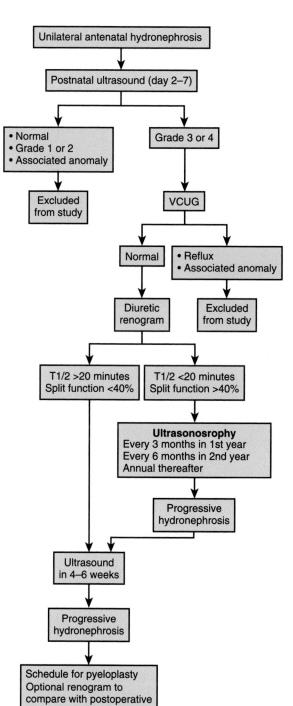

Figure 19-16   Algorithm for the postnatal evaluation and management of infants with unilateral hydronephrosis determined by antenatal ultrasonography. Ultrasound grading of hydronephrosis is that of the Society for Fetal Urology.[85] T1/2, nuclide clearance half-time; VCUG, voiding cystourethrogram. (From Hafez AT, Mclorie G, Bägli D, et al. Analysis of trends on serial ultrasound for high grade neonatal hydronephrosis. J Urol. 168:1518, 2002, with permission.)

not to have significant renal abnormalities, but of those with greater pelvic dilatation, 79% had urinary tract obstruction or VUR.[82] Although there is concern that physiologic volume contraction in the early postnatal period could underestimate hydronephrosis if neonatal ultrasonography is performed within the first 2 days of life, there is no significant difference in ultimate outcome gained by waiting until 7 to 10 days of life.[83] However, to enhance the reliability of the neonatal study, most practitioners suggest a delay.[83] Follow-up of fetuses with persistent postnatal hydronephrosis should include VCUG to rule out VUR, and diuretic renography to determine the severity of functional obstruction (Fig. 19-16).[84] A progressive increase in the severity of hydronephrosis by ultrasonography may be a more reliable index of severity of obstruction than the pattern of diuretic renography.[84,85] Calyceal dilatation on ultrasound examination may be a better index of progression than the measured pelvic diameter, although all infants with pelvic diameter exceeding 50 mm should have pyeloplasty regardless of calyceal dilatation.[86]

A significant controversy has developed regarding the indications for pyeloplasty in infants with a diagnosed UPJO. Koff and his associates argue that close monitoring by renal ultrasonography and diuretic renography[87] can avert surgical intervention in all but approximately 25% of patients with unilateral UPJO[88] and 35% of bilateral UPJO.[87-89] There are several concerns with this "conservative" approach, which has been termed *aggressive observation* by DiSandro and Kogan.[90] Substantial experimental and clinical evidence indicate that the severity of renal injury from UPJO can be related to the duration of obstruction.[11,90] Retrospective studies of patients with UPJO detected prenatally had better outcomes than those diagnosed postnatally,[91-93] and in one study, pyeloplasty resulted in improved function only in the group diagnosed prenatally.[93] Therefore, waiting for measurable functional deterioration may lead to irreversible nephron loss. Of particular concern is the failure of patients' families to adhere to a schedule of follow-up studies, which may contribute to an even greater incidence of renal deterioration in patients for whom pyeloplasty is deferred.[94]

Long-term Implications of Congenital Obstructive Uropathy

The management of obstructive uropathy in fetuses and neonates should be governed by the expected long-term outcomes for these patients. Although patients with unilateral disease and a normal contralateral kidney should enjoy normal long-term renal function, there may be an increased prevalence of abnormalities of the contralateral kidney that may not be detected initially.[11] Children with antenatally diagnosed hydronephrosis have smaller maximum bladder volume, larger residual volume, and larger bladder wall thickness than normal, suggesting that immaturity of the ureteropelvic junction may be associated with bladder dysfunction in these infants.[95] Even after pyeloplasty, patients with either unilateral or bilateral hydronephrosis may manifest ongoing tubular dysfunction, such as renal tubular acidosis or a renal concentrating defect.[96] In patients with PUV and normal renal function, distal renal tubular acidosis can persist long after ablation of the valves.[97]

Although ongoing postnatal renal maturation of children with bilateral severe obstructive uropathy can permit a period of years of life with conservative medical management, the needs of continued growth often lead to renal failure and the need for renal replacement therapy.[98] Thus, relentless progression of renal insufficiency characterizes many cases of PUV, with the onset of renal failure by the second decade of life.[98] In a recent report, the long-term outcome among patients with antenatal diagnosis of PUV was not different from those detected postnatally.[99] Although prenatal surgical intervention for fetal obstructive uropathy was developed in San Francisco 25 years ago to avoid this outcome, the experience has been variable. In a retrospective review of the San Francisco program from 1981 to 1999, 14 fetuses with PUV and "favorable" urinary electrolytes underwent surgery; of these, six died, with five of the survivors developing chronic renal insufficiency.[68] The investigators concluded that favorable urinary electrolytes and surgical intervention may not change the outcome.[68] The experience for prenatal intervention for lower urinary tract obstruction at Detroit, another major center, was similar: 38% died, and 50% lived beyond 2 years of age, with 57% of these developing chronic renal insufficiency or renal failure.[69] Disturbingly, height was below the fifth percentile in 50%, although "acceptable continence" was achieved in 50%.[69] A long-term additional complication of survivors includes chronic respiratory disorders.[45] In the most recent report from Children's Hospital of Philadelphia (a third major center for fetal intervention in obstructive uropathy), the 1-year survival rate was 91%, with 18 surviving candidates yielding fetal urinary prognostic indices that were good in 13 cases and borderline or poor in five cases.[67] Six of the 18 children developed renal failure, eight had persistent respiratory problems, nine had musculoskeletal problems, and nine had frequent UTIs.[67] There is increasing awareness of the importance of managing bladder function: patients with increased nadir creatinine or severe bladder dysfunction have significantly greater probability of developing renal failure.[100,101] For this reason, fetoscopic transuterine release of PUV may allow for fetal bladder cycling and better long-term bladder function. Neurologic development was normal in all but three patients, and the patients and their families reported that their lives were worthwhile, with "quality of life" scores not different from those of the healthy population.[67] This last outcome measure is perhaps more meaningful than any of the other statistical analysis that we can apply to our patients.

The Future

The current state of the art allows us to visualize the fetal urinary tract as well as to evaluate renal function in fetuses throughout the second half of gestation. Unfortunately, for severe forms of obstructive uropathy, much of the damage sustained by the kidneys as a result of obstruction occurs between 8 and 16 weeks of gestation. Analysis of amniotic fluid creatinine, γ-glutamyltransferase, and β_2-microglobulin concentration during this interval shows an abrupt increase after 10 weeks' gestation[102] that likely reflects the onset of glomerular filtration by the newly formed metanephros (Fig. 19-3). Unfortunately, fetal kidneys are difficult to visualize during the first trimester, and because of nephron immaturity, fetal urine or amniotic fluid indices cannot reflect significant renal maldevelopment at this point (Figs. 19-3, 19-5, and 19-8).

Many factors converge to impact the delicate process of renal morphogenesis in fetuses. In addition to the genome of fetuses, which may contain mutations in genes expressed by the developing metanephros, maternal and uterine environmental factors can alter gene activity (Fig. 19-17).[103] Considerable experimental data support a major role for fetal urinary flow impairment as another factor that significantly alters gene activity (Fig. 19-17).

Advances in imaging and the discovery of new biomarkers of fetal renal function and injury should lead to new diagnostic and therapeutic approaches to

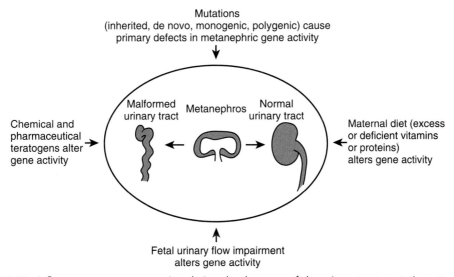

Figure 19-17 Influences on gene expression during development of the urinary tract: mutations, teratogens, alterations in the maternal diet, and obstruction to urine flow in fetuses. (From Woolf AS. A Molecular and genetic view of human renal and urinary tract malformations. *Kidney Int.* 58:500, 2000, with permission.)

congenital urinary tract obstruction. Three-dimensional ultrasonography can provide improved resolution of fetal gross anatomy[104] and may enhance prenatal evaluation of obstructive uropathy. There is also increasing appreciation of the complex alterations in renal gene expression and cellular responses to congenital urinary tract obstruction.[11] Microarray analysis of renal gene expression in mice or rats with experimental or spontaneous ureteral obstruction has revealed significant upregulation or downregulation of many molecules.[105-107] Preliminary microarray analysis of human fetal and infant kidneys with congenital urinary tract obstruction is consistent with patterns found in the animal models.[108] Further study of such changes can lead to the development of new biomarkers of obstructive uropathy.[109]

Candidate markers that are upregulated in the kidneys of experimental animals with ureteral obstruction include transforming growth factor-β1, tumor necrosis factor-α, and monocyte chemoattractant protein-1; epidermal growth factor is downregulated.[110,111] The urinary excretion of these molecules is altered in children with unilateral UPJO and may, therefore, prove useful also in fetal urine assays.[112-114] Using combined capillary electrophoresis and mass spectrometry, a matrix of polypeptides was identified in urine that enabled prediction (with 94% precision) of renal deterioration in infants with UPJO.[115] Another European group using this approach reported similar success in predicting renal deterioration in urine of infants with UPJO younger than 1 year of age (sensitivity, 83%; specificity, 92%), but in older patients, sensitivity decreased to 20% and specificity to 66%.[116] These results suggest that the normal pattern of urinary biomarkers changes with renal development and maturation, and standards will need to be established for changing fetal and postnatal ages. Over the past 5 years, the renal expression of dozens of molecules has been shown to be altered by urinary tract obstruction[105-107] and experimental manipulation of some pathways can attenuate the renal lesions.[117] Some of the salutary effects in experimental models have been achieved by gene therapy.[117] Because much of the renal injury resulting from congenital obstructive uropathy takes place in the prenatal or early perinatal period, fetal gene therapy is theoretically an attractive option.[118] Moreover, fetuses have larger populations of less differentiated cells (e.g., stem cells) that may be more responsive to such an approach and are immunologically naïve and, therefore, susceptible to induction of tolerance.[118]

Finally, certain human gene polymorphisms of the renin–angiotensin system predict the development and progression of congenital uropathies. Mutations in the angiotensin type 2 receptor gene are associated with an increased incidence of congenital anomalies of the kidney and urinary tract in several populations.[119,120] Italian children with congenital uropathies and renal parenchymal lesions have a higher prevalence of the D/D genotype of angiotensin-converting enzyme than patients without parenchymal lesions.[120] European children with chronic renal failure caused by renal malformations and the D/D genotype have a more rapid rate of loss of GFR than those with I/D or I/I genotype (Fig. 19-18).[121] Similarly, Indian children with

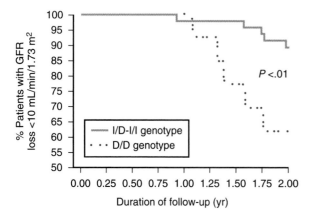

Figure 19-18 Renal "survival" analysis in children with chronic renal failure caused by renal malformations (n = 59). During 2 years of follow-up, loss of glomerular filtration rate above 10 mL/min/1.73 m² was observed in 39% of patients with angiotensin-converting enzyme D/D genotype compared with only 11% in those with I/D or I/I genotypes. (From Hohenfellner K, Wingen A-M, Nauroth O, et al. Impact Of ACE I/D gene polymorphism on congenital renal malformations. *Pediatr Nephrol.* 16:356, 2001, with permission.)

congenital uropathies (including PUV) and D allele also have an adverse prognosis.[122] Fetal testing for such polymorphisms may lead to improved long-term management of patients with congenital obstructive uropathy.

Summary and Conclusions

Assessment of renal function in fetuses with obstructive uropathy is a complex and multidisciplinary process that requires an understanding of fetal renal development and physiology, as well as of the causes and consequences of maldevelopment of the urinary tract. This review addresses a number of major questions relating to the evaluation and management of congenital obstructive uropathy and provides arguments for the following conclusions:

1. **What is the natural history of obstructive uropathy?** Based on animal models as well as the follow-up of infants born with urinary tract obstruction, the evolution of this group of disorders is extremely heterogeneous and dependent on many variables. These include the timing and location of the obstructive lesion, the severity of obstruction, and the gestational age at birth.

2. **What is the relative contribution of primary renal maldevelopment versus altered renal development secondary to obstructive injury?** The patient's genome as well as the fetal–maternal environment are shared determinants of the renal functional outcome. A better understanding of mutations accounting for altered renal morphogenesis as well as polymorphisms modulating the progression of secondary renal injury will lead to better preventive measures. Advances in understanding the cellular and molecular mechanisms responsible for both abnormal renal development and the secondary adaptive responses will lead to improved therapies.

3. **What constitutes a definition of *significant urinary tract obstruction*?** Significant obstruction "is a condition of impaired urinary drainage, which, if uncorrected, will limit the ultimate functional potential of a developing kidney."[9] This definition emphasizes the importance of long-term outcome in any evaluation or intervention of affected fetuses.

4. **What is the correlation of fetal renal pelvic dilatation with functional outcome?** Unfortunately, with the exception of extreme hydronephrosis, the lack of precision in the measurement of fetal renal pelvic dilatation results in a poor correlation between this parameter and renal functional outcome. Improved imaging techniques (e.g., MRI) and standardization of procedures are needed.

5. **What is the correlation of fetal renal histologic changes with functional outcome?** Attempts to correlate fetal histologic changes with renal prognosis have been disappointing. Even postnatal renal histology in children with unilateral UPJO shows poor correlation with relative renal function. Refined approaches, such as immunohistochemistry or laser capture microscopy, are needed.

6. **Which patients should undergo pyeloplasty for UPJO, and what should be the criteria?** Fetuses with unilateral hydronephrosis and normal amniotic fluid volume should not undergo measurement of renal function or intervention before birth. Infants with high-grade progressive hydronephrosis should undergo early postnatal pyeloplasty regardless of relative renal function.

7. **Which patients should undergo fetal intervention for obstructive nephropathy, and what should be the criteria?** Selected fetuses with bilateral hydronephrosis, distended bladder, and oligohydramnios may undergo karyotyping, serial ultrasonography, and urine sampling. Those with favorable sonographic and urine biomarker profiles should be considered for placement of a vesicoamniotic shunt by an experienced team of specialists in an established center. At the present time, fetal intervention cannot be mandated in any individual patient, and a rigorous prospective controlled study (i.e., PLUTO) is currently underway.[73]

8. **What is the impact of fetal intervention on the long-term prognosis?** In properly selected patients, the prevention of pulmonary hypoplasia is the most important outcome of successful fetal intervention for severe obstructive uropathy, and survival can be 90% at 1 year. Optimization of renal function is difficult to document, and 30% to 60% of survivors develop chronic renal insufficiency or renal failure.

9. **What will the future bring?** Advances in imaging and the discovery of new biomarkers of renal development and injury (proteomics) will allow evaluation in the first trimester. Progress in genomics should permit the identification of mutations or polymorphisms predictive of renal malformations or risk of progression of the renal lesions of obstructive uropathy. Gene therapy is also theoretically more likely to be effective in fetuses than postnatally.

References

1. Seikaly MG, Ho PL, Emmett L, et al. Chronic renal insufficiency in children: the 2001 annual report of the NAPRTCS. *Pediatr Nephrol.* 2003;18:796.
2. Woolf AS, Winyard PJ. Molecular mechanisms of human embryogenesis: developmental pathogenesis of renal tract malformations. [Review] [235 Refs]. *Pediatr Dev Pathol.* 2002;5:108.
3. Woolf AS, Thiruchelvam N. Congenital obstructive uropathy: its origin and contribution to end-stage renal disease in children. [Review] [75 Refs]. *Adv Ren Replace Ther.* 2001;8:157.
4. Woolf AS. Emerging roles of obstruction and mutations in renal malformations. [Review] [61 Refs]. *Pediatr Nephrol.* 1998;12:690.
5. Peters CA. Obstruction of the fetal urinary tract. *J Am Soc Nephrol.* 1997;8:653.
6. Peters CA. Animal models of fetal renal disease. *Prenat Diagn.* 2001;21:917.
7. Matsell DG, Tarantal AF. Experimental models of fetal obstructive nephropathy. *Pediatr Nephrol.* 2002;17:470.
8. Chevalier RL, Peters CA. Obstructive uropathy, Chap. 56. In: Avner ED, Harmon WE, Niaudet P, Yoshikawa N, eds. *Pediatr Nephrol.* 6th ed. Berlin: Springer; 2009:1337-1377.
9. Peters CA. Urinary tract obstruction in children. *J Urol.* 1995;154:1874.
10. Elder JS. Antenatal hydronephrosis—fetal and neonatal management. *Pediatr Clin North Am.* 1997;44:1299.
11. Chevalier RL, Roth JA. Obstructive uropathy, Chap. 55. In: Avner ED, Harmon WE, Niaudet P, eds. *Pediatric Nephrology.* 5th ed. Philadelphia: Lippincott Williams And Wilkins; 2004:1049-1076.
12. Woolf AS. Unilateral multicystic dysplastic kidney. *Kidney Int.* 2006;69:190.
13. Bornstein E, Atkins K, Fishman S, et al. Severe uropathy and normal amniotic fluid volume in a male fetus. *J Ultrasound Med.* 2008;27:1099.
14. Johnson MP. Fetal Obstructive uropathy, Chap. 18. In: Harrison MR, Evans MI, Adzick NS, Holzgreve W, eds. *The unborn patient.* 3rd ed. Philadelphia: W.B. Saunders Co.; 2001:259-286.
15. Harrison MR, Golbus MS, Filly RA, et al. Management of the fetus with congenital hydronephrosis. *J Pediatr Surg.* 1982;17:728.
16. Mitra SC. Effect of cocaine on fetal kidney and bladder function. *J Maternal-Fetal Med.* 1999;8:262.
17. Brace RA, Wolf EJ. Normal amniotic fluid volume changes throughout pregnancy. *Am J Obstet Gynecol.* 1989;161:382.
18. Veille JC, Hanson RA, Tatum K, et al. Quantitative assessment of human fetal renal blood flow. *Am J Obstet Gynecol.* 1993;169:1399.
19. Nicolaides KH, Cheng HH, Snijders RJM, et al. Fetal urine biochemistry in the assessment of obstructive uropathy. *Am J Obstet Gynecol.* 1992;166:932.
20. Moniz CF, Nicolaides KH, Bamforth FJ, et al. Normal reference ranges for biochemical substances relating to renal, hepatic, and bone function in fetal and maternal plasma during pregnancy. *J Clin Pathol.* 1985;38:468.
21. Haycock GB. Development of glomerular filtration and tubular sodium reabsorption in the human fetus and newborn. *Br J Urol.* 1998;81(Suppl. 2):33.
22. Stanier MW. Development of intra-renal solute gradients in foetal and postnatal life. *Pfluegers Arch.* 1972;336:263.
23. Devuyst O, Burrow CR, Smith BL, et al. Expression of aquaporins-1 and -2 during nephrogenesis and in autosomal dominant polycystic kidney disease. *Am J Physiol.* 1996;271:F169-F183.
24. Wintour EM, Earnest L, Alcorn D, et al. Ovine AQP1: cDNA cloning, ontogeny, and control of renal gene expression. *Pediatr Nephrol.* 1998;12:545.
25. Watanabe S, Matsushita K, Mccray PBJ, et al. Developmental expression of the epithelial Na+ channel in kidney and uroepithelia. *Am J Physiol Renal Physiol.* 1999;276:F304-F314.
26. Nicolini U, Fisk NM, Rodeck CH, et al. Fetal urine biochemistry: an index of renal maturation and dysfunction. *Br J Obstet Gynaecol.* 1992;99:46.
27. Al-Dahhan J, Haycock GB, Chantler C. Sodium homeostasis in term and preterm neonates. *Arch Dis Child.* 1983;58:335.
28. Hanna MK. Antenatal hydronephrosis and ureteropelvic junction obstruction: the case for early intervention. *Urology.* 2000;55:612.
29. Ismaili K, Hall M, Donner C, et al. Results of systematic screening for minor degrees of fetal renal pelvis dilatation in an unselected population. *Am J Obstet Gynecol.* 2003;188:242.

30. Kent A, Cox D, Downey P, et al. A study of mild fetal pyelectasia—outcome and proposed strategy of management. *Prenat Diagn*. 2000;20:206.
31. Persutte WH, Hussey M, Chyu J, et al. Striking findings concerning the variability in the measurement of the fetal renal collecting system. *Ultrasound Obst Gynecol*. 2000;15:186.
32. Morris RK, Malin GL, Khan KS, et al. Antenatal ultrasound to predict postnatal renal function in congenital lower urinary tract obstruction: systematic review of test accuracy. [Review] [46 Refs]. *BJOG*. 2009;116:1290.
33. Clautice-Engle T, Anderson NG, Allan RB, et al. Diagnosis of obstructive hydronephrosis in infants: comparison sonograms performed 6 days and 6 weeks after birth. *Am J Roentgenol*. 1995;164:963.
34. Mouriquand PDE, Troisfontaines E, Wilcox DT. Antenatal and perinatal uro-nephrology: current questions and dilemmas. *Pediatr Nephrol*. 1999;13:938.
35. Zhang PL, Peters CA, Rosen S. Ureteropelvic junction obstruction: morphological and clinical studies. *Pediatr Nephrol*. 2000;14:820.
36. Gill B, Bennett RT, Barnhard Y, et al. Can fetal renal artery doppler studies predict postnatal renal function in morphologically abnormal kidneys? A preliminary report. *J Urol*. 1996;156:190.
37. Rawashdeh YF, Djurhuus JC, Mortensen J, et al. The intrarenal resistive index as a pathophysiological marker of obstructive uropathy. *J Urol*. 2001;165:1397.
38. Yiee J, Wilcox D. Abnormalities of the fetal bladder. [Review] [46 Refs]. *Semin Fetal Neonat Med*. 2008;13:164.
39. Maizels M, Alpert SA, Houston JTB, et al. Fetal bladder sagittal length: a simple monitor to assess normal and enlarged fetal bladder size, and forecast clinical outcome. *J Urol*. 2004;172:1995.
40. Robyr R, Benachi A, Daikha-Dahmane F, et al. Correlation between ultrasound and anatomical findings in fetuses with lower urinary tract obstruction in the first half of pregnancy. *Ultrasound Obstet Gynecol*. 2005;25:478.
41. Wu S, Johnson MP. Fetal lower urinary tract obstruction. [Review] [38 Refs]. *Clin Perinatol*. 2009;36:377.
42. Nakayama DK, Harrison MR, De Lorimier AA. Prognosis of posterior urethral valves presenting at birth. *J Pediatr Surg*. 1986;21:43.
43. Savelli S, Di MM, Perrone A, et al. MRI with diffusion-weighted imaging (DWI) and apparent diffusion coefficient (ADC) assessment in the evaluation of normal and abnormal fetal kidneys: preliminary experience. *Prenat Diagn*. 2007;27:1104.
44. Cassart M, Massez A, Metens T, et al. Complementary role of MRI after sonography in assessing bilateral urinary tract anomalies in the fetus. *AJR*. 2004;182:689.
45. Freedman AL, Johnson MP, Gonzalez R. Fetal therapy for obstructive uropathy: past, present … future? *Pediatr Nephrol*. 2000;14:167.
46. Nicolini U, Spelzini F. Invasive assessment of fetal renal abnormalities: urinalysis, fetal blood sampling and biopsy. *Prenat Diagn*. 2001;21:964.
47. Dommergues M, Muller F, Ngo S, et al. Fetal serum B2-microglobulin predicts postnatal renal function in bilateral uropathies. *Kidney Int*. 2000;58:312.
48. Berry SM, Lecolier B, Smith RS, et al. Predictive value of fetal serum beta 2-microglobulin for neonatal renal function. Lancet. 1995;345:1277.
49. Muller F, Dommergues M, Mandelbrot L, et al. Fetal urinary biochemistry predicts postnatal renal function in children with bilateral Obstructive uropathies. *Obstet Gynecol*. 1993;82:813.
50. Tassis BMG, Trespidi L, Tirelli AS, et al. In Fetuses with isolated hydronephrosis, urinary beta2-microglobulin and N-acetyl-beta-D-glucosaminidase (NAG) have a limited role in the prediction of postnatal renal function. *Prenat Diagn*. 1996;16:1087.
51. Johnson MP, Bukowski TP, Reitleman C, et al. In utero surgical treatment of fetal obstructive uropathy: a new comprehensive approach to identify appropriate candidates for vesicoamniotic shunt therapy. *Am J Obstet Gynecol*. 1994;170:1770.
52. Guez S, Assael BM, Melzi ML, et al. Shortcomings in predicting postnatal renal function using prenatal urine biochemistry in fetuses with congenital hydronephrosis. *J Pediatr Surg*. 1996;31:1401.
53. Eugene M, Muller F, Dommergues M, et al. Evaluation of postnatal renal function in fetuses with bilateral obstructive uropathies by proton nuclear magnetic resonance spectroscopy. *Am J Obstet Gynecol*. 1994;170:595.
54. Cohn BR, Joe BN, Zhao S, et al. Quantitative metabolic profiles of 2nd and 3rd trimester human amniotic fluid using HR-MAS spectroscopy. *Magn Reson Mater Phy*. 2009;22:343.
55. Muller F, Bernard MA, Benkirane A, et al. Fetal urine cystatin C as a predictor of postnatal renal function in bilateral uropathies. *Clin Chem*. 1999;45:2292.
56. Mussap M, Fanos V, Pizzini C, et al. Predictive value of amniotic fluid cystatin C levels for the early identification of fetuses with obstructive uropathies. *Intl J Obstet Gynaec*. 2002;109:778.
57. Acar O, Uluocak N, Ziylan O, et al. Is cystatin C a promising parameter to determine postnatal outcome of prenatally diagnosed infravesical obstruction? *J Urol*. 2009;182:1542.
58. Johnson MP, Corsi P, Bradfield W, et al. Sequential urinalysis improves evaluation of fetal renal function in obstructive uropathy. *Am J Obstet Gynecol*. 1995;173:59.
59. Oliveira FR, Barros EG, Magalhaes JA. Biochemical profile of amniotic fluid for the assessment of fetal and renal development. *Braz J Med Biol Res*. 2002;35:215.
60. Cagdas A, Aydinli K, Irez T, et al. Evaluation of the fetal kidney maturation by assessment of amniotic fluid alpha-1 microglobulin levels. *Eur J Obstet Gynecol Reprod Biol*. 2000;90:55.
61. Oliveira EA, Diniz JSS, Cabral ACV, et al. Prognostic factors in fetal hydronephrosis: a multivariate analysis. *Pediatr Nephrol*. 1999;13:859.

62. Hedrick HL, Flake AW, Crombleholme TM, et al. History of fetal diagnosis and therapy: Children's Hospital of Philadelphia experience. *Fetal Diagn Ther.* 2003;18:65.

63. Rodriguez MM, Gomez A, Abitbol C, et al. Comparative renal histomorphometry: a case study of oligonephropathy of prematurity. *Pediatr Nephrol.* 2005;20:945.

64. Rodriguez MM, Gomez AH, Abitbol CL, et al. Histomorphometric analysis of postnatal glomerulogenesis in extremely preterm infants. *Pediatr Devel Pathol.* 2004;7:17.

65. Gasser B, Mauss Y, Ghnassia JP, et al. A quantitative study of normal nephrogenesis in the human fetus: its implication in the natural history of kidney changes due to low obstructive uropathies. *Fetal Diagn Ther.* 1993;8:371.

66. Morris RK, Quinlan-Jones E, Kilby MD, et al. Systematic review of accuracy of fetal urine analysis to predict poor postnatal renal function in cases of congenital urinary tract obstruction. [Review] [65 Refs]. *Prenat Diagn.* 2007;27:900.

67. Biard JM, Johnson MP, Carr MC, et al. Long-Term outcomes in children treated by prenatal vesicoamniotic shunting for lower urinary tract obstruction. *Obstet Gynecol.* 2005;106:503.

68. Holmes N, Harrison MR, Baskin LS. Fetal surgery for posterior urethral valves: long-term postnatal outcomes. *Pediatrics.* 2001;108:36.

69. Freedman AL, Johnson MP, Smith CA, et al. Long-term outcome in children after antenatal intervention for obstructive uropathies. *Lancet.* 1999;354:374.

70. Morris RK, Malin GL, Khan KS, et al. Systematic review of the effectiveness of antenatal intervention for the treatment of congenital lower urinary tract obstruction. [Review] [43 Refs]. *BJOG.* 2010; 117:382.

71. Blaicher W, Hausler M, Gembruch U, et al. Feto-amniotic shunting – experience of six centres. *Ultraschall In Der Medizin.* 2005;26:134.

72. Knox EM, Thangaratinam S, Kilby MD, et al. A review of the methodological features of systematic reviews in fetal medicine. [Review] [94 Refs]. *Eur J Obstet Gynecol Reprod Biol.* 2009;156:121.

73. Morris RK, Kilby MD. An overview of the literature on congenital lower urinary tract obstruction and introduction to the PLUTO trial: percutaneous shunting in lower urinary tract obstruction. [Review] [27 Refs]. *Aust N Z J Obstet Gynaecol.* 2009;49:6.

74. Poucell-Hatton S, Huang M, Bannykh S, et al. Fetal obstructive uropathy: patterns of renal pathology. *Pediatr Devel Pathol.* 2000;3:223.

75. Shibata S, Shigeta M, Shu Y, et al. Initial pathological events in renal dysplasia with urinary tract obstruction in utero. *Virchows Arch Int J Pathol.* 2001;439:560.

76. Daiekha-Dahmane F, Dommergues M, Muller F, et al. Development of human fetal kidney in obstructive uropathy: correlations with ultrasonography and urine biochemistry. *Kidney Int.* 1997;52:21.

77. Bunduki V, Saldanha LB, Sadek L, et al. Fetal renal biopsies in obstructive uropathy: feasibility and clinical correlations—preliminary results. *Prenat Diagn.* 1998;18:101.

78. Terzi F, Assael BM, Claris Appiani A, et al. Increased sodium requirement following early postnatal surgical correction of congenital uropathies in infants. *Pediatr Nephrol.* 1990;4:581.

79. Li CL, Wang WD, Kwon TH, et al. Altered expression of major renal Na transporters in rats with bilateral ureteral obstruction and release of obstruction. *Am J Physiol Renal Physiol.* 2003;285: F889-F901.

80. Li C, Wang W, Kwon TH, et al. Downregulation of AQP1, -2, and -3 after ureteral obstruction is associated with a long-term urine-concentrating defect. *Am J Physiol.* 2001;281:F163-F171.

81. Norregard R, Jensen BL, Li C, et al. COX-2 inhibition prevents downregulation of key renal water and sodium transport proteins in response to bilateral ureteral obstruction. *Am J Physiol.* 2005;289: F322-F333.

82. Johnson CE, Elder JS, Judge NE, et al. The accuracy of antenatal ultrasonography in identifying renal abnormalities. *Am J Dis Child.* 1992;146:1181.

83. Wiener JS, O'Hara SM. Optimal timing of initial postnatal ultrasonography in newborns with prenatal hydronephrosis. *J Urol.* 2002;168:1826.

84. Hafez AT, Mclorie G, Bägli D, et al. Analysis of trends on serial ultrasound for high grade neonatal hydronephrosis. *J Urol.* 2002;168:1518.

85. Fernbach SK, Maizels M, Conway JJ. Ultrasound grading of hydronephrosis: introduction to the system used by the society for fetal urology. *Pediatr Radiol.* 1993;23:478.

86. Dhillon HK. Prenatally diagnosed hydronephrosis: the great ormond street experience. *Br J Urol.* 1998;81:39.

87. Conway JJ, Maizels M. The "well tempered" diuretic renogram: a standard method to examine the asymptomatic neonate with hydronephrosis or hydroureteronephrosis. *J Nucl Med.* 1992; 33:2047.

88. Ulman I, Jayanthi VR, Koff SA. The long-term followup of newborns with severe unilateral hydronephrosis initially treated nonoperatively. *J Urol.* 2000;164:1101.

89. Onen A, Jayanthi VR, Koff SA. Long-term followup of prenatally detected severe bilateral newborn hydronephrosis initially managed nonoperatively. *J Urol.* 2002;168:1118.

90. Disandro MJ, Kogan BA. Ureteropelvic junction obstruction. *Urol Clin Noth Am.* 1998;25:187.

91. Mcaleer IM, Kaplan GW. Renal function before and after pyeloplasty: Does it improve? *J Urol.* 1999;162:1041.

92. Capolicchio G, Leonard MP, Wong C, et al. Prenatal diagnosis of hydronephrosis: impact on renal function and its recovery after pyeloplasty. *J Urol.* 1999;162:1029.

93. Chertin B, Fridmans A, Knizhnik M, et al. Does early detection of ureteropelvic junction obstruction improve surgical outcome in terms of renal function? *J Urol.* 1999;162:1037.

94. Eskild-Jensen A, Jorgensen TM, Olsen LH, et al. Renal function may not be restored when using decreasing differential function as the criterion for surgery in unilateral hydronephrosis. *BJU Int.* 2003;92:779.
95. Leung VYF, Rasalkar DD, Liu JX, et al. Dynamic ultrasound study on urinary bladder in infants with antenatally detected fetal hydronephrosis. *Pediatr Res.* 2010;67:440.
96. Chandar J, Abitbol C, Zilleruelo G, et al. Renal tubular abnormalities in infants with hydronephrosis. *J Urol.* 1996;155:660.
97. Sharma RK, Sharma AP, Kapoor R, et al. Prognostic factors for persistent distal renal tubular acidosis after surgery for posterior urethral valve. *Am J Kid Dis.* 2001;38:488.
98. Roth KS, Carter WH Jr, Chan JCM. Obstructive nephropathy in children: long-term progression after relief of posterior urethral valve. *Pediatrics.* 2001;107:1004.
99. Ylinen E, Ala-Houhala M, Wikstrom S. Prognostic factors of posterior urethral valves and the role of antenatal detection. *Pediatr Nephrol.* 2004;19:874.
100. Ansari MS, Gulia A, Srivastava A, et al. Risk factors for progression to end-stage renal disease in children with posterior urethral valves. *J Pediatr Urol.* 2010;6:261.
101. Defoor W, Clark C, Jackson E, et al. Risk factors for end stage renal disease in children with posterior urethral valves. *J Urol.* 2008;180:1705.
102. Gulbis B, Jauniaux E, Jurkovic D, et al. Biochemical investigation of fetal renal maturation in early pregnancy. *Pediatr Res.* 1996;39:731.
103. Woolf AS. A molecular and genetic view of human renal and urinary tract malformations. *Kidney Int.* 2000;58:500.
104. Hsieh YY, Chang CC, Lee CC, et al. Fetal renal volume assessment by three-dimensional ultrasonography. *Am J Obstet Gynecol.* 2000;182:377.
105. Higgins DF, Lappin DWP, Kieran NE, et al. DNA oligonucleotide microarray technology identifies fisp-12 among other potential fibrogenic genes following murine unilateral ureteral obstruction (UUO): modulation during epithelial-mesenchymal transition. *Kidney Int.* 2003;64:2079.
106. Silverstein DM, Travis BR, Thornhill BA, et al. Altered expression of immune modulator and structural genes in neonatal unilateral ureteral obstruction. *Kidney Int.* 2003;64:25.
107. Seseke F, Thelen P, Ringert RH. Characterization of an animal model of spontaneous congenital unilateral obstructive uropathy by cDNA microarray analysis. *Eur Urol.* 2004;45:374.
108. Liapis H. Biology of congenital obstructive nephropathy. *Exp Nephrol.* 2003;93:87.
109. Chevalier RL. Biomarkers of congenital obstructive nephropathy: past, present and future. *J Urol.* 2004;172:852.
110. Misseri R, Meldrum DR, Dinarello CA, et al. TNF-alpha mediates obstruction-induced renal tubular cell apoptosis and proapoptotic signaling. *Am J Physiol.* 2004;288:F406-F411.
111. Stephan M, Conrad S, Eggert T, et al. Urinary concentration and tissue messenger rna expression of monocyte chemoattractant protein-1 as an indicator of the degree of hydronephrotic atrophy in partial ureteral obstruction. *J Urol.* 2002;167:1497.
112. El Sherbiny MT, Mousa M, Shokeir AA, et al. Role of urinary transforming growth factor-b1 concentration in the diagnosis of upper urinary tract obstruction in children. *J Urol.* 2002;168:1798.
113. Valles P, Pascual L, Manucha W, et al. Role of endogenous nitric oxide in unilateral ureteropelvic junction obstruction in children. *Kidney Int.* 2003;63:1104.
114. Grandaliano G, Gesualdo L, Bartoli F, et al. MCP-1 and EGF renal expression and urine excretion in human congenital obstructive nephropathy. *Kidney Int.* 2000;58:182.
115. Decramer S, Wittke S, Mischak H, et al. Predicting the clinical outcome of congenital unilateral ureteropelvic junction obstruction in newborn by urinary proteome analysis. *Nature Med.* 2006;12:398.
116. Drube J, Zurbig P, Schiffer E, et al. Urinary proteome analysis identifies infants but not older children requiring pyeloplasty. *Pediatr Nephrol.* 2010;25:1673.
117. Chevalier RL. Obstructive nephropathy: towards biomarker discovery and gene therapy. *Nat Clin Prac Nephrol.* 2006;2:157.
118. Yang EY, Flake AW, Adzick NS. Prospects for fetal gene therapy. *Sem Perinatol.* 1999;23:524.
119. Pope JC, Brock JW III, Adams MC, et al. Congenital anomalies of the kidney and urinary tract —role of the loss of function mutation in the pluripotent angiotensin type 2 receptor gene. *J Urol.* 2001;165:196.
120. Rigoli L, Chimenz R, Di Bella C, et al. Angiotensin-converting enzyme and angiotensin type 2 receptor gene genotype distributions in italian children with congenital uropathies. *Pediatr Res.* 2004;56:988.
121. Hohenfellner K, Wingen A-M, Nauroth O, et al. Impact of ACE I/D gene polymorphism on congenital renal malformations. *Pediatr Nephrol.* 2001;16:356.
122. Bajpai M, Pratap A, Somitesh C, et al. Angiotensin converting enzyme gene polymorphism in asian indian children with congenital uropathies. *J Urol.* 2004;171:838.
123. Rabinowitz R, Peters MT, Vyas S, et al. Measurement of fetal urine production in normal pregnancy by real-time ultrasonography. *Am J Obstet Gynecol.* 1989;161:1264.

Index

Page numbers followed by *f* indicate figures; *t*, tables.